P9-DNR-514

Teaching Today's Health

Teaching Today's Health

SEVENTH EDITION

David J. Anspaugh, Pe.D, EdD, CHES, AAHE fellow

PROFESSOR EMERITUS, UNIVERSITY OF MEMPHIS

**PROFESSOR AND CHAIR,
TRI STATE UNIVERSITY, ANGOLA, INDIANA**

Gene Ezell, EdD, CHES, AAHE fellow

**PROFESSOR, UNIVERSITY OF TENNESSEE
AT CHATTANOOGA**

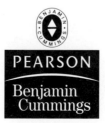

PEARSON

Benjamin
Cummings

San Francisco Boston New York
Cape Town Hong Kong London Madrid Mexico City
Montreal Munich Paris Singapore Sydney Tokyo Toronto

Publisher: Daryl Fox
Acquisitions Editor: Deirdre McGill
Project Editor: Cheryl Cechvala
Associate Editor: Michelle Cadden
Marketing Manager: Sandra Lindelof
Development Manager: Claire Brassert
Production Editor: Steven Anderson
Project Coordination and Composition: The Left Coast Group
Copy Editor: Carla Breidenbach
Proofreader: Deborah Kopka
Text Designer: Kaelin Chappell
Photo Research: Brian Donnelly, Cypress Integrated Systems
Cover Designer: Yvo Riezebos
Manufacturing Buyer: Stacey Weinberger
Cover Printer: Coral Graphics
Printer: R. R. Donnelley

Cover Photo: Yellow Dog Productions/Getty Images

Photo credits can be found on page 809.

ISBN 0-8053-5495-6

Copyright © 2004 by Pearson Education, Inc., publishing as Pearson Benjamin Cummings, San Francisco, CA 94111. All rights reserved. Printed in the United States of America. This publication is protected by Copyright and permission should be obtained from the publisher prior to any prohibited reproduction, storage in a retrieval system, or transmission in any form or by any means, electronic, mechanical, photocopying, recording, or likewise. For information regarding permission(s), write to: Pearson Education, Inc., Rights and Permissions Department.

Library of Congress Cataloging-in-Publication Data
Anspaugh, David J.
 Teaching today's health/David Anspaugh, Gene Ezell.—7th ed.
  p. cm.
Includes bibliographical references and index.
 ISBN 0-8053-5495-6 (hardcover)
1. Health education (Elementary) — United States. I. Ezell, Gene. II.
Title.
 LB1588.U6A83 2004
372.3'7—dc21   2003004326

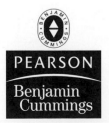

PEARSON
Benjamin
Cummings

www.aw.com/bc   2 3 4 5 6 7—DOH—07 06 05 04

This book is dedicated to my wife Susan, for her love and support, and for making my life special.

—DJA

A special dedication to Megan Ezell, for your excellent contribution in writing the Environmental Health chapter for this edition.

—GE

Brief Contents

Contents

CHAPTER FIVE

Measurement and Evaluation of Health Education 103

CHAPTER SIX

Mental Health and Stress Reduction 122

CHAPTER SEVEN

Strategies for Teaching Mental Health and Stress Reduction 153

Preface

With each new edition of *Teaching Today's Health,* we strive to offer a better product to our students. Each attempt at rewriting is really an effort to better explain our philosophy of teaching health education and what we as teachers must do to ensure that elementary and middle school students are better served, provided correct information, and ensured personalizing opportunities to assess their value system. Ultimately, we want students to develop positive lifestyles. If students do not understand the value of health information, they will have no incentive to adopt a healthy lifestyle. To assure this outcome, teachers must give students opportunities for critical thinking and provide an environment that fosters positive self-esteem, a sense of self-efficacy, and an internal locus of control. Finally, teachers should provide a model for making effective decisions.

Like previous editions, the seventh edition of *Teaching Today's Health* presents the background, content, and strategies necessary for optimal teaching of health education in elementary and middle schools. Health education must originate from a solid knowledge base. From this cognitive base, teachers can provide multiple opportunities for students to personalize information. It is through the personalizing of basic information that children begin to make value-related decisions that will ultimately result in positive health habits. Ingrained in these concepts is the continuing development of critical thinking skills.

Drug abuse, teenage pregnancies, and sexually transmitted infections such as HIV/AIDS are threats to our nation and to this generation of youth. Conditions that were unknown only a few years ago are currently classified as epidemic. Teachers continually deal with controversy and are bombarded by new information in many areas. Clearly, it is difficult to remain on the cutting edge of the health field. Recognizing this need, we have attempted to include the material needed for a solid foundation in teaching elementary and middle school health.

ORGANIZATION

As with previous editions, the seventh edition of *Teaching Today's Health* is organized to present a strong foundation of health education theory along with an abundance of strategies to help teachers develop the skills required to become competent health teachers. Chapters 1 through 5 discuss the necessity for health education, the role of the teacher, planning effective health education, strategies for teaching, and implementing effective evaluation. All these topics are covered within the framework of the contemporary theory of wellness and optimal well-being.

Chapters 6 through 26 consist of specific content areas followed by strategies for making the content come alive for students. The strategies include values clarification activities, dramatizations, decision stories, experiments and demonstrations, puzzles, games, and bulletin board suggestions. With this new edition, suggested grade levels have been added to all activities in the strategies chapters, and many activities that require worksheets, puzzles, or game boards are accompanied by Teaching in Action boxes to illustrate how a sample teaching tool could be used.

Finally, we have retained the critical thinking questions, recommended Web sites, videos and other additional resources that can make teaching health education more effective, and have consolidated all references in a section in the back of the text for ease of use. Within this framework, the main theme of the value of establishing lifelong knowledge and positive practices pervades the text.

We wish to give special acknowledgement to Megan Ezell, who wrote the chapter on environmental health in this edition. Her knowledge and expertise in writing this chapter are most appreciated. Also, a note of gratitude to Kelly McClanahan for her administrative help with this edition.

It is our sincere desire that a great many elementary and middle school children will benefit from the information gathered in this text.

Finally, we appreciate the worthwhile comments and suggestions of our reviewers: Darwin Dennison, UNC Wilmington; Anita Ellowitz, University of Utah; Bonnie Luft, Baylor University; Vic Sbarbaro, CSU Chico; and Steve Sedbrook, Fort Hays State University.

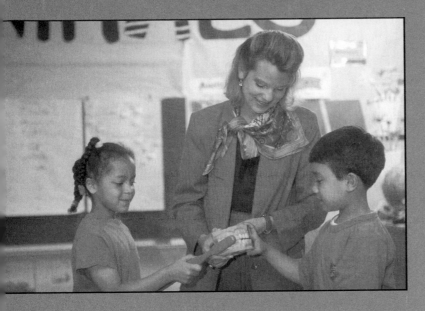

CHAPTER ONE

The Need for Health Education

School health programs offer the opportunity to provide the services and knowledge necessary to enable children to be productive learners and to develop skills to make healthy decisions for the rest of their lives.

—National School Boards Association et al. (1995)

VALUED OUTCOMES

After reading this chapter, you should be able to:

- define health, health education, and health promotion
- list and describe the components that make up wellness
- identify why health education is a necessary component in the nation's schools
- discuss the significance of the Youth Risk Behavior Surveillance System
- identify the components of a comprehensive school education
- discuss the components of a coordinated school health education program

The raising of a child requires much love, care, and concern from many different sources, including the home, community, community agencies, and school. As you read this chapter, think of how and in what manner these components of our society can provide positive support and guidance for children and their families. How can the family become part of the coordinated school program? How can other agencies provide input and services? What is the role of the school health team?

The Evolution of Health Education

Formal health education first took the form of instruction in anatomy and physiology. Health was taught purely as a science, and emphasis was placed on retention of facts. As health education evolved, health teachers became more concerned with the attitudinal and behavioral aspects of students' health. Today, the emphasis is on a preventive approach, as opposed to the crisis-oriented approach of just a few years ago. It is interesting to note that, since the 1970s, early-age death rates have declined at a significant rate. This decline reflects a decrease in deaths due to cardiovascular disease and coincides with the declining use of tobacco, the reduction in dietary intake of fats and cholesterol, and increased exercise among adults. Society is in a period where lifestyle, more than medicine, can lead to decreases in death rates.

Americans are currently in the middle of a health promotion movement. It is virtually impossible to read a magazine, listen to radio, or view television without being bombarded with information on some health-related topic or activity.

As teachers, the charge today is to motivate students to improve their own health status through positive self-direction. Health education offers students an opportunity for personal growth and enhancement that is not duplicated anywhere else in the school curriculum.

WHAT IS HEALTH?

Health topics are everywhere. On television, radio, the Internet, and in popular magazines, Americans are continually bombarded with health-related information. For years, the World Health Organization's (WHO) 1947 definition of health—"a state of complete physical, mental and social well-being and not merely the absence of disease or infirmity" (WHO 2002)—was the accepted definition. A newer definition formulated by the Joint Committee on Health Education Terminology (1991) points to the essence of the concept. The committee stated that **health** "is an integrated method of functioning which is oriented toward maximizing the potential of which the individual is capable. It requires that the individual maintain a continuum of balance and purposeful direction with the environment where he (sic) is functioning." This concept goes beyond

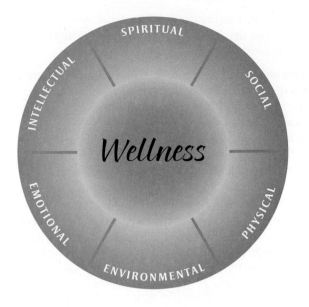

Figure 1.1
The Components of Wellness

simply not being ill or sick. It implies, as Hoyman suggested in 1975, that health has several dimensions, each having its own continuum.

Obviously, the definition of health has evolved over the years. H. L. Dunn (1991), a physician, provides a definition that is almost identical to one developed by the Joint Committee on Health Education Terminology (1991). Dunn refers to this conceptualization as **wellness,** implying that individuals engage in attitudes and behaviors that enhance quality of life and maximize personal potential. Figure 1.1 shows a conceptualization of these components.

1. **Spiritual**—the belief in some force that unites human beings. This force can include nature, science, religion, or a higher power. It includes morals, values, and ethics. Optimal spirituality is the ability to discover, articulate, and act on a (your) basic purpose in life (Chapman 1987).

2. **Social**—the ability to interact successfully with people and one's personal environment. It is the ability to develop and maintain intimacy with others and to have respect/tolerance for those with different opinions and beliefs.

3. **Physical**—the ability to carry out daily tasks, develop cardiovascular fitness, muscular fitness, maintain adequate nutrition and proper weight, avoid abusing drugs/alcohol, and not use tobacco products.

4. **Environmental**—maintaining safe water, food, and air. It involves having a safe emotional and physical environment in which we can live and carry out our daily activities.

5. **Emotional**—the ability to control stress and to express emotions appropriately and comfortably. It is the ability to recognize and accept feeling and to not be defeated by setbacks and failures.

6. **Intellectual**—the ability to learn and use information effectively for personal, family, and career development. It means striving for continued growth and learning to deal with new challenges effectively.

The first assumption of the wellness approach to living is that good health is achieved by balancing each of these dimensions. A second assumption is that each individual is ultimately responsible for her or his well-being. That is, we—not the government, physicians, nurses, or some other institution—must accept personal responsibility. Each person must foster attitudes that will improve the quality of life and expand the human potential. To accomplish this, teachers must empower their students to see themselves as being *in control* of improving their quality of life. Such students have an internal **locus of control.** (This trait contrasts with external locus of control, in which an individual believes that he or she cannot control many of the factors that contribute to a higher level of wellness.)

Another vital concept in a wellness lifestyle is **self-efficacy.** Self-efficacy is the belief in one's ability to accomplish a specific task or behavior. Self-efficacy is something each student can give him- or herself, if the teacher can provide the support and encouragement necessary to acquire a personal sense of competence.

The sooner children begin the lifelong process of becoming healthy, the greater the possibility they will be successful. Teachers must recognize that children bring to schools many values and behaviors. These values represent both the beneficial and negative aspects of a child's living practices. At the same time, teachers should be aware of the powerful influence they exert on the lives of their students. Nowhere in the entire educational spectrum can a teacher make such an impression as at the elementary level. Consequently, the teacher who exemplifies a lifestyle conducive to high-level wellness, who exhibits a style of living that is physically, socially, and psychologically healthy, enhances the probability that his or her students will attempt to incorporate those beneficial aspects in their own lives.

What Is Health Education and Health Promotion?

As with the term **health, health education** has taken on new meanings over the years. Although there are many ways of defining health education, the Joint Committee on Health Education Terminology stated that the health education process is the "continuum of learning which enables people, as individual members of social structures, to voluntarily make decisions, modify, and change social conditions in ways which are health enhancing" (1991, 103). Green and Kreuter (1999) provide yet another definition. They define health education as "any combination of learning experiences designed to facilitate voluntary actions conducive to health."

The term **health promotion** is sometimes used incorrectly in reference to health education. Health promotion is defined by the Joint Committee on Health Education Terminology as "the aggregate of all purposeful activities designed to improve personal and public health through a combination of strategies, including the competent implementation of behavioral change strategies, health education, health protection measures, risk factor detection, health enhancement and health maintenance" (1991, 102). Health promotion is therefore broader in scope than health education, and health education is an intricate part of health promotion. Health education is one of several different formats that can be used to influence health and quality of life for people.

From the elementary teacher's perspective, health education is the process of developing and providing planned learning experiences in such a way as to supply information, change attitudes, and influence behavior. In other words, health education is helping children develop the concept of wellness (discussed in the previous section). This process should result in children developing a sense of individual responsibility for their health, leading to health enhancement or high-level wellness. As part of this process, a child should develop self-esteem, self-confidence, and a sense that he or she can achieve success not only in health-related matters, but also in life in general.

All this is accomplished through the teacher creating and facilitating learning experiences that develop the child's decision-making ability. With good decision-making skills, the child will make better choices about the personal, family, peer, and societal factors that influence the quality of life. An effective school health program must have a direct influence on children's lives and behavior.

Health education is a lifelong process. As people develop awareness of the many components of health and incorporate them into their own lives, they

- assume responsibility for their own health and health care and actively participate with a medical professional in the decision-making process
- respect the benefits of medical technology but are not in awe of medical equipment and tests to the point that they do not question medical professionals on their use of the technology
- try new behaviors and modify others
- are skeptical of health fads and trends
- ask questions, seek evidence, and evaluate information regarding health matters
- strive for self-reliance in personal health matters
- voluntarily adopt practices consistent with a healthy lifestyle

Accomplishing Health Education

With the school day already crowded, many elementary teachers wonder how to find time to teach health education. But time must be found. Our nation's children are an invaluable resource. Health education can help ensure that this generation is fit physically, psychologically, and socially to assume the difficult tasks of adulthood. Still, the problem remains: When and how should health education be taught in the classroom? How can it be accomplished?

Health education that is relevant and motivating for the student requires careful planning. The quality of health instruction is reflected in the amount of planning and organization done by the teacher. There are many approaches to teaching health, several of which will be discussed in Chapter 4. However, the responsibility rests with each teacher to create and facilitate direct instruction in health and to infuse other health-related topics whenever the opportunity arises.

As previously stated, time must be allotted for direct health instruction during the school day. There is no substitute for this. However, if the time that can be allotted is minimal, health instruction can be incorporated into other parts of the curriculum, such as reading, mathematics, science, geography, art, social studies, and physical education. There are some advantages to integrating a part of health instruction into other subject areas, including opportunities for a significant amount of creativity in learning and teaching. However, the greatest need is for health to receive its just place in the elementary school day.

To accomplish health education, the topic selected must be appropriate to the developmental level of the child. Health must be taught every semester at every grade level from kindergarten through grade six. The planned curriculum must be sequential and address the physical, emotional, mental, and social dimensions of the child's health at a particular grade level. Only in this way can it become a meaningful part of each child's learning experience. Meaningful health education is education that influences a child's decision-making skills. To do this, health instruction must blend information giving with attitudinal experiences. G. I. Brown describes this balance of information and attitude assessment as confluent education, which he defines as "the integration of cognitive learning with affective learning" (1990, 4). In short, a child will be better able to make personal decisions concerning health behavior if the teacher has provided cognitive and affective opportunities for growth. Part of this process is providing children with a decision-making model with ample opportunities to practice decision making.

Presenting factual information alone—the cognitive aspect of health education—is not enough. Knowledge of facts *alone* does not lead to changes in behavior. The failure of many cognitive drug education programs in the past is evidence of this. Knowledge must become personalized if it is to have an effect. This personalization is the affective aspect of health education. Strategies for accomplishing this personalization component will be presented throughout this text.

To accomplish its objectives, health education must be:

Sequential—instruction should be provided throughout the educational experience, grades K through 12. The curriculum at each level should be based on what has been learned in previous years and serve as the basis for curricula in future years.

Planned—instruction should be based on goals, outcome-related objectives, and evaluation criteria. It should be taught within the total curriculum framework, not substituted for by teaching within other subjects such as science.

Comprehensive—instruction should include all the identified health content areas. More important than the individual subjects, however, is an understanding of how all subjects interrelate with the components of high-level wellness and quality of life.

Taught by qualified health teachers—individuals who have a concern for the total wellness of their students and who have been trained in the content as well as the strategies of health education. Effective health teaching requires more than the accumulation of knowledge. It requires that students have opportunities to personalize and incorporate positive health habits into their daily lives.

The need for health education continues to grow each year. It is important to remember that in the last twenty years, topics such as drug abuse, smoking, heart disease prevention, teenage pregnancy, adolescent suicide, stress control, incest, child abuse, human immunodeficiency virus (HIV), and cardiopulmonary resuscitation (CPR) have been added to an already long list of topics that includes nutrition, disease, mental health, sexuality, personal health, environmental health, first aid, and quackery.

It would seem that the task of creating health education programs is overwhelming. How does the school help children acquire knowledge, develop awareness and skills, provide personalizing experiences, and reinforce healthful behaviors? Equally important, how does the school interact with the community and the family to maximize the potential for assuming healthful behaviors?

Conceptually, the family, community, and school all play important roles in children's learning, and each segment must seek to cooperate with the others to provide opportunities to learn, practice, and reinforce healthful lifestyles. It is imperative that schools recognize the importance of working within the community and with the family in attaining the healthy development of each child. This process is discussed more completely in the section dealing with the coordinated school health program on pages 14–17.

Why Health Education?

Perhaps the best argument for teaching health education is that health behaviors are the most important determinant of health status. Since health-related behaviors are both learned and changeable, there is no better time to start formal health education than in the elementary school years, when the child is more flexible and more apt to accept positive health behaviors. In addition, many of the negative aspects of a lifetime of abuse could be avoided. This avoidance becomes increasingly important with mounting evidence that most health problems are due to smoking, poor nutrition, being overweight, lack of exercise, stress, abuse of drugs and alcohol, and unsafe personal behavior.

The Centers for Disease Control and Prevention (CDC) has indicated that during chldhood and adolescence, behaviors are established that later contribute significantly to heart disease, cancer, and injuries. The behaviors identified included the use of tobacco products, unhealthy eating habits, inactivity, use of alcohol and drugs, and unprotected sex. The unprotected sex is manifesting in HIV infections, sexually transmitted infections (STI), and unintended pregnancies (CDC 2002a).

For the five- to twenty-four-year-old age group, almost three-quarters of all mortality and much of the morbidity and social problems can be attributed to four causes. Motor vehicle crashes account for 29 percent of all deaths among this age group with 40 percent of these deaths being alcohol related. Homicide accounts for 20 percent, suicide accounts for 12 percent, and other injuries such as fires, drownings, and falls account for 11 percent. Not listed in these statistics is the fact that nearly 25 percent of new HIV infections and 25 percent of all new STIs are within this age group and that nearly one million teenagers become pregnant each year. Further, the CDC reports that among adults (ages twenty-five and older) two-thirds of all mortality and a substantial portion of morbidity result from only three causes: heart disease causes 34 percent of all deaths, cancer causes 25 percent, and stroke is responsible for 7 percent. The three categories of behaviors that contribute to these are tobacco use, dietary patterns, and physical inactivity (CDC 2002b).

Unfortunately, health education still suffers from a lack of importance in the school curriculum and a lack of adequately trained teachers. If we wish to help prevent many of the conditions that are now the leading causes of death (accidents, cardiovascular disease, cancer, and so on), then we must emphasize prevention in our educational efforts. Table 1.1 shows the leading causes of death by ages.

Not every area of concern in a comprehensive health education program has been covered here, but it is hoped that the pressing need for health education has been established. The scope of health education is a broad one. Personal, family, and community problems must be effectively addressed if we are to live personally and socially satisfying lives. The time to begin effective health education is in the elementary school.

Today parents, administrators, and students no longer perceive health education as a peripheral or secondary activity. More than 90 percent of administrators believe that it is at least as useful as other subjects in the curriculum. Parents and students alike believe that the same amount, or even more time, should be devoted to teaching health education relative to other subjects taught in the curriculum (Seffrin 1994). The window of opportunity is there for providing comprehensive health education. As teachers, parents, and as a society, we must begin to effectively deal with the challenges facing children and youth today. The Health Highlight boxes found on pages 14 and 18–19 illustrate some facts and statistics that help emphasize the continuing need for health education.

More tragic is the loss in human potential. Today, the diseases that are killing Americans are the chronic diseases such as cancer, heart disease, and AIDS. Many of these deaths could be prevented by helping people alter their lifestyles through improved eating habits, regular exercise, eliminating smoking, and practicing safer sex. Decreasing the incidence of these diseases will be achieved

Table 1.1   *Leading Causes of Death by Ages, 1998*

Rank	Ages 1–4	Ages 5–9	Ages 10–14	Ages 15–24
1	Unintentional injuries (1,935)	Unintentional injuries (1,544)	Unintentional injuries (1,710)	Unintentional injuries (13,349)
2	Congenital anomalies (564)	Malignant neoplasms (487)	Malignant neoplasms (526)	Homicide (5,506)
3	Homicide (399)	Congenital anomalies (198)	Suicide (317)	Suicide (4,135)
4	Malignant neoplasms (365)	Homicide (170)	Homicide (290)	Malignant neoplasms (1,699)
5	Heart disease (214)	Heart disease (156)	Congenital anomalies (173)	Heart disease (1,057)
6	Pneumonia and influenza (146)	Pneumonia and influenza (70)	Heart disease (170)	Congenital anomalies (450)
7	Septicemia (89)	Chronic lower respiratory disease (54)	Chronic lower respiratory disease (98)	Chronic lower respiratory disease (239)
8	Perinatal period (75)	Benign neoplasms (52)	Pneumonia and influenza (51)	Pneumonia and influenza (215)
9	Cerebrovascular (57)	Cerebrovascular (35)	Cerebrovascular (47)	HIV (194)
10	Benign neoplasms (53)	HIV (29)	Benign neoplasms (32)	Cerebrovascular (178)

SOURCE: National Center for Injury Prevention & Control 2002

not through additional medical care or greater medical expenditures, but through educating people to live healthful lives and, thereby, prevent disease. As a nation, our resources must be invested in helping people take control of their lives.

National Initiatives for Comprehensive School Health

Several national initiatives have created support for a comprehensive school health education program. A most important document was *Healthy People 2010: National Health Promotion and Disease Prevention Objectives* (Office of Disease Prevention and Health Promotion 2002). This document focused on improving the quality of life for all citizens of the United States. Many of the objectives either relate directly to, or have implications for, coordinated school health education. The focus areas for Healthy People Framework 2010 are found in Table 1.2.

Other initiatives that have followed help to emphasize the importance of coordinated school health programs. They include The National Education

Table 1.2　　*Focus Areas of the Healthy People Framework—2010*

1. Access to quality health services	15. Injury and violence prevention
2. Arthritis, osteoporosis and chronic back conditions	16. Maternal, infant, and child health
3. Cancer	17. Medical product safety
4. Chronic kidney disease	18. Mental health and mental disorders
5. Diabetes	19. Nutrition
6. Disability and secondary conditions	20. Occupational safety and health
7. Educational and community-based programs	21. Oral health
8. Environmental health	22. Physical activity and fitness
9. Family planning and sexual health	23. Public health infrastructure
10. Food safety	24. Respiratory diseases
11. Health communication	25. Sexually transmitted diseases
12. Heart disease and stroke	26. Substance abuse
13. HIV	27. Tobacco use
14. Immunizations and infectious diseases	28. Vision and hearing

SOURCE: Office of Disease Prevention and Health Promotion 2002

Goals for 2000 and the federally enacted Safe and Drug-Free Schools and Communities Act (SDFSCA) of 1994. Two of the eight goals set forth by the National Education Goals for the Year 2000 emphasize health education (National Education Goals Panel 2002). Goal 1 states that "All children [in America] will start school ready to learn." A component of this goal states that every child would receive nutrition, physical activity experiences, and health care to enable them to arrive at school with healthy minds and bodies. Goal 7 states that "Every school in the United States will be free of drugs, violence, and the unauthorized presence of firearms and alcohol and will offer a disciplined environment conducive to learning." The objectives for this goal include implementing a firm and fair policy on possession, use, and distribution of drugs and alcohol; having parent, business, government, and community organizations work together to provide a learning environment free of violence, drugs, crime, and the presence of weapons; schools should provide a healthy environment and safe haven for all; all local educational agencies should develop a sequential comprehensive kindergarten through twelfth grade (K through 12) drug and alcohol program; community-based teams should be organized to provide support for students and teachers; and every school should work to eliminate sexual harassment (Joint Committee on Health Education Standards 1995).

To help achieve the health-related goals mentioned above, the SDFSCA was signed in 1994 to provide grants to local school districts to help carry out projects for up to two years to ensure the fulfillment of the goals. The Act allows for a variety of activities, from identifying school violence, addressing discipline problems, developing comprehensive violence-prevention programs, and training personnel, to hiring security guards.

Health Highlight

WHAT IS COMPREHENSIVE SCHOOL HEALTH EDUCATION CURRICULUM?

This is the Division of Adolescent and School Health's definition of the key elements of a comprehensive school health education (CSHE). These guidelines should serve as measures as to whether states, school districts, and individual schools provide a CSHE program. They are:

1. A documented, planned, and sequential program of health instruction for students in grades K through 12.

2. A curriculum that addresses and integrates education about a range of categorical health problems and issues at developmentally appropriate ages.

3. Activities that help young people develop the skills they need to avoid: tobacco use and dietary patterns that contribute to disease; sedentary lifestyle; sexual behaviors that result in unintentional and intentional injuries.

4. Instruction provided for a prescribed amount of time at each grade level.

5. Management and coordination by an educational professional trained to implement the program.

6. Instruction from teachers who are trained to teach the subject.

7. Involvement of parents, health professionals, and other concerned community members. *(Part of a coordinated school health program)

8. Periodic evaluation, updating, and improvement.

*Author added
SOURCE: CDC 1993

The Youth Risk Behavior Surveillance System

The Youth Risk Behavior Surveillance System (YRBSS) provides information on the health behaviors practiced by young people. It is another source of information that helps educators determine the health practices and status of American youth. The YRBSS also serves to illustrate the necessity for a coordinated school health program. This system was developed by the CDC along with cooperation and collaboration with federal, state, and private-sector partners. It includes a national survey as well as surveys conducted by state and local education agencies. The CDC conducts national surveys every two years to produce data representative of students in grades 9 through 12 in both public and private schools in the fifty states and the District of Columbia. In 1999 more than 15,000 students in forty-one states and four territories took the survey. Summary results certainly indicate the need for beginning a coordinated school health education in the elementary school. Tables 1.3, 1.4, and 1.5 on pages 12 and 13. provide information on risk behaviors that improved, worsened, or either did not change or demonstrated inconsistent patterns of change. The data represent the years in which the YRBSS was given; the 2001 survey had not been analyzed at the time of this publication.

Table 1.3   *Youth Risk Behavior Trends: Risk Behaviors That Improved,[1] 1991–1999*

	1991	1993	1995	1997	1999
Injury-related behaviors					
Never or rarely wore a seat belt	25.9	19.1	21.7	19.3	16.4
Never or rarely wore a bicycle helmet[2]	96.2	92.8	92.8	88.4	85.3
Rode with a drunk driver[3]	39.9	35.3	38.8	36.6	33.1
Carried a gun[4]	NA	7.9	7.6	5.9	4.9
Carried a weapon on school property[4]	NA	11.8	9.8	8.5	6.9
Involved in a physical fight[5]	42.5	41.8	38.7	36.6	35.7
Involved in a physical fight on school property[5]	NA	16.2	15.5	14.8	14.2
Seriously considered suicide[6]	29.0	24.1	24.1	20.5	19.3
Tobacco Use					
Current smokeless tobacco use[4]	NA	NA	11.4	9.3	7.8
Sexual behaviors					
Ever had sexual intercourse	54.1	53.0	53.1	48.4	49.9
Had four or more sexual partners	18.7	18.7	17.8	16.0	16.2
Used a condom at last sexual intercourse[7]	46.2	52.8	54.4	56.8	58.0
Had been taught about HIV/AIDS in school	83.3	86.1	86.3	91.5	90.6
Physical Activity					
Participated in strengthening exercise[8]	47.8	51.9	50.3	51.4	53.6

1. Significant linear change, $p < .05$.
2. Among students who rode bicycles during the 12 months preceding the survey.
3. ≥ 1 times during the 30 days preceding the survey.
4. On ≥ 1 of the 30 days preceding the survey.
5. ≥ 1 time during the 12 months preceding the survey.
6. During the 12 months preceding the survey.
7. Among currently sexually active students.
8. On ≥ 3 of the 7 days preceding the survey.
NA: data not collected.

SOURCE: CDC 2002

Table 1.4   *Youth Risk Behavior Trends: Risk Behaviors That Worsened,[1] 1991–1999*

	1991	1993	1995	1997	1999
Tobacco use					
Frequent cigarette use[3]	12.7	13.8	16.1	16.7	16.8
Alcohol and other drug use					
Episodic heavy drinking[4]	31.3	30.0	32.6	33.4	31.5
Lifetime marijuana use	31.3	32.8	42.4	47.1	47.2
Current cocaine use[5]	1.7	1.9	3.1	3.3	4.0
Lifetime illegal steroid use	2.7	2.2	3.7	3.1	3.7

continued

Table 1.4   *continued*

	1991	1993	1995	1997	1999
Sexual behaviors					
Used birth control pills at last sexual intercourse[7]	20.8	18.4	17.4	16.6	16.2
Physical activity					
Attended physical education class daily	41.6	34.3	25.4	27.4	29.1

1. Significant linear change, $p < .05$.
2. On ≥ 1 of the 30 days preceding the survey.
3. On ≥ 20 of the 30 days preceding the survey.
4. Drank ≥ 5 drinks of alcohol on at least one occasion on $\geq$ 1 of the 30 days preceding the survey.
5. ≥ 1 times during the 30 days preceding the survey.
6. During the 12 months preceding the survey.
7. Among currently sexually active students.

NA: data not collected.

SOURCE: CDC 2002

Table 1.5   *Youth Risk Behavior Trends: Risk Behaviors That Did Not Change or Demonstrated Inconsistent Patterns of Change, 1991–1999*

	1991	1993	1995	1997	1999
Injury-related behaviors					
Felt too unsafe to go to school[1]	NA	4.4	4.5	4.0	5.2
Threatened or injured with a weapon on school property[2]	NA	7.3	8.4	7.4	7.7
Attempted suicide[2]	7.3	8.6	8.7	7.7	8.3
Tobacco use					
Lifetime cigarette use[3]	70.1	69.5	71.3	70.2	70.4
Alcohol and other drug use					
Current alcohol use[1]	50.8	48.0	51.6	50.8	50.0
Alcohol use on school property[1]	NA	5.2	6.3	5.6	4.9
Marijuana use on school property[4]	NA	5.6	8.8	7.0	7.2
Sexual behaviors					
Currently sexually active[5]	37.5	37.5	37.9	34.8	36.3
Physical activity					
Participated in vigorous physical activity[6]	NA	65.8	63.7	63.8	64.7
Enrolled in physical education class	48.9	52.1	59.6	48.8	56.1

1. On ≥ 1 of the 30 days preceding the survey.
2. ≥ 1 times during the 12 months preceding the survey.
3. Ever tried cigarette somoking, even 1 or 2 puffs.
4. ≥ 1 times during the 30 days preceding the survey.
5. Sexual intercourse during the 3 months preceding the survey.
4. For at least 20 minutes on ≥ 3 of the 7 days preceding the survey.

NA: data not collected.

SOURCE: CDC 2002

Health Highlight

KEY FACTS ABOUT AMERICAN CHILDREN (2001)

1	Young person under 25 dies from HIV infection	825	Babies are born at low birthweight (less than 5 pounds, 8 ounces)
5	Children or youth under 20 commit suicide	1,310	Babies are born without health insurance
9	Children or youth under 20 are homicide victims	1,329	Babies are born to teen mothers
9	Children or youth under 20 die from firearms	2,019	Babies are born into poverty
34	Children or youth under 20 die from accidents	2,319	Babies are born to mothers who are not high school graduates
77	Babies die	2,861	High school students drop out of school*
157	Babies are born at very low birthweight (less than 3 pounds, 4 ounces)	3,585	Babies born to unmarried mothers
		4,248	Children are arrested
180	Children are arrested for violent crimes	7,883	Children are reported abused or neglected
367	Children are arrested for drug abuse	17,297	Public school students are suspended*
401	Babies are born to mothers who had late or no prenatal care		

*Based on calculations per school day (180 days of 7 hours each).
SOURCE: Children's Defense Fund ©2002

The Coordinated School Health Program

A total school health program is needed if the school is to function as an effective institution for promoting high-level wellness. As shown in Figure 1.2, a coordinated school health program includes eight components: (1) a healthful school environment, (2) school health instruction, (3) school health services, (4) physical education, (5) nutrition and food services, (6) school-based counseling (psychological and social services), (7) schoolsite health promotion for staff, and (8) school, family, and community health promotion partnerships (Marx, Wooley, and Northrop 1998). Each component involves planning, administration, and evaluation. Adequate planning for all eight components ensures their comprehensiveness. Effective leadership coordinates the components and ensures proper staffing, budgeting, policy fulfillment, and evaluation.

A HEALTHFUL SCHOOL ENVIRONMENT

This aspect of the school health program includes the physical and psychological environment in which students and faculty exist. Issues addressed include the emotional and social environment of the classroom, the development of

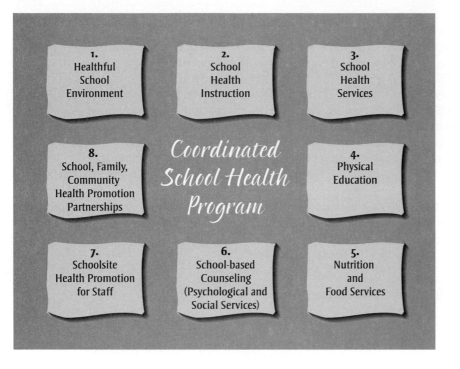

Figure 1.2
The Coordinated School Health Program

1. Healthful School Environment
2. School Health Instruction
3. School Health Services
8. School, Family, Community Health Promotion Partnerships
Coordinated School Health Program
4. Physical Education
7. Schoolsite Health Promotion for Staff
6. School-based Counseling (Psychological and Social Services)
5. Nutrition and Food Services

self-worth and self-esteem, and the fostering of positive relationships for students and school personnel. In addition, safety hazards on the school grounds and within the buildings are of concern. This includes chemical agents, temperature, humidity, noise, lighting, and radiation found within the building and classroom environment.

Few teachers are fortunate enough to be able to work in ideal situations. However, it is desirable to do all that is possible to enhance the teaching environment. The classroom should be physically adequate, pleasant, attractive, and comfortable for the children. When the classroom setting is bright, lively, and dynamic, morale is improved.

Teachers should require a quality environment in which to work. This is important not only for the teaching/learning process, but also for teacher and student morale. Whenever possible, teachers should volunteer as consultants in planning and maintaining the school site and surroundings. Fostering a cooperative relationship with the custodial staff, lunchroom staff, and administrators in charge of the various aspects of the environment is beneficial. Working with the custodians by keeping the classroom sanitary and by diplomatically suggesting improvements can enhance the environment significantly.

The psychological setting is just as important as the physical one, and the teacher is responsible for establishing the emotional tone within the classroom. The overall atmosphere should be one of acceptance, one in which the teacher knows the children well and is sensitive to their individual needs. The classroom should be nonthreatening. Stress is reduced when there is a relaxed approach to instruction, one in which there is less emphasis on competition that pits child against child. Students should feel free to express their feelings honestly without fear of ridicule or rebuke. They should also feel free to fail occasionally without punishment. A teacher can promote the children's well-being by being kind but fair in promoting teacher–pupil relationships, setting reasonable goals for each student, praising positive behavior, challenging children within their capabilities, and tolerating occasional frustration. Allowing the students to assist in planning health learning opportunities is also very important. If they are involved in planning, they will become more interested in the subject matter. When children are interested, discipline is less likely to become a problem.

Although emphasis in this section has been on the classroom environment, there are other considerations that are part of the healthy school environment. An issue of particular importance is the safety of students when transported on school buses. Guidelines are needed for daily bus rides, as well as for special occasions, such as field trips or extracurricular events. Safety in the classroom, the cafeteria, the gymnasium, and within the general school physical plant is an important aspect of a healthful school environment.

SCHOOL HEALTH INSTRUCTION

The second area of the school health program is health instruction, in which information is presented to students in a way that fosters desirable health knowledge, attitudes, and practices. Strategies, information, and methods concerning this aspect of a coordinated school health program are described later in the text.

SCHOOL HEALTH SERVICES

These programs seek to promote the children's health through screening, intervention, and remediation of various health conditions. The school nurse most often coordinates and provides the services of this component. Screenings for visual or auditory problems and scoliosis, as well as first-aid procedures, illness protocol, and services for the handicapped are part of health services. Professionals who make up the school health services team include the school physician, dentist, social worker, speech pathologist, and the nurse.

PHYSICAL EDUCATION

A comprehensive physical education program is one that offers a daily program of activities. These programs should be based on developing cardiovascular fitness, strength, flexibility, and agility. A sound program can help reduce stress and promote social development.

NUTRITION AND FOOD SERVICES

This component involves training the food preparation personnel and developing nutritionally sound food programs for the school. Part of this component is helping children to select nutritionally balanced meals and ensuring that food served in the school cafeteria is nutritious, attractive, and palatable.

SCHOOL-BASED COUNSELING

This aspect of the comprehensive health program seeks to meet the needs of children by providing psychological and social services such as assertiveness, problem solving, and self-esteem training. Services also are provided by school psychologists for children who experience learning difficulties and behavioral problems.

SCHOOLSITE HEALTH PROMOTION

Programs for faculty and staff can provide benefits by reducing health care costs, improving morale, and increasing productivity of the faculty and staff. Health promotion programs are a natural for the school, because facilities and personnel for conducting programs are already in place. Health educators, physical educators, nurses, counselors, and nutritionists are available to aid in program development.

SCHOOL, FAMILY, AND COMMUNITY HEALTH PROMOTION PARTNERSHIPS

An effective strategy for promoting the health of school-age students is the development of collaborative efforts between the community agencies and the school. These coalitions can coordinate and advocate for improving the various aspects of the comprehensive school health program.

Teachers should consider themselves as part of a team whose main mission is to provide optimal conditions to enhance the wellness of each student. Each member of the health team has a particular role to play. Like a chain, the health team is only as strong as its weakest link. Everyone involved with the health of students, including the students themselves, must take that personal responsibility seriously. Each member must work cooperatively with other members in order to reach the ultimate goal of total high-level health.

School-Based Health Centers— The School Nurse

School-based health centers (SBHCs) are a fairly recent innovation in the health care of children. The concept is for students to receive primary and preventive care in the school setting and thus to increase quality care. Currently there are more than 600 SBHCs nationally, with some of these facilities serving as primary care providers while others are preventive in function (Making the Grade 1995). A U.S. General Accounting Office report in 1994 indicated that SBHCs do improve students' access to quality care by helping overcome financial barriers, lack of health insurance, and transportation difficulties associated with students receiving appropriate health care. Many problems are associated with establishing SBHCs in the school setting. Most current facilities have links with health maintenance organizations (HMOs). Problems with reimbursement,

Health Highlight

INDICATORS OF AMERICAN CHILDREN'S WELL-BEING

America's Children: Key National Indicators of Well-Being, 2000 is the fourth annual report to the nation on the condition of our most precious resource, our children. Included are eight contextual measures that describe the changing population, family characteristics, and context in which children are living and 23 indicators of well-being in the areas of economic security, health, behavior and social environment, and education. This year, two special features are presented on kindergartners' knowledge and skills and youth participation in volunteer activities.

Part I: Population and Family Characteristics

- In 1999, there were 70.2 million children under age 18 in the United States, or 26 percent of the population, down from a peak of 36 percent at the end of the baby boom (1964). Children are expected to remain a stable percentage of the total population as they are projected to compose 24 percent of the population in 2020.

- The racial and ethnic diversity of America's children continues to increase. In 1999, 65 percent of U.S. children were white, non-Hispanic; 15 percent were black, non-Hispanic; 4 percent were Asian or Pacific Islander; and 1 percent were American Indian or Alaska Native. The number of Hispanic children has increased faster than that of any other racial or ethnic group, growing from 9 percent of the child population in 1980 to 16 percent in 1999.

- The family structures of children have become more varied. The percentage of children living with one parent increased from 20 percent in 1980 to 27 percent in 1999. Most children living with single parents live with a single mother. However, the proportion of children living with single fathers doubled over this time period, from 2 percent in 1980 to 4 percent in 1999. Some children live with a single parent who has a cohabiting partner: 16 percent of children living with single fathers and 9 percent of children living with single mothers also lived with their parents' partners.

- In 1999, 54 percent of children from birth through third grade received some form of child care on a regular basis from persons other than their parents, up from 51 percent in 1995.

Part II: Indicators of Children's Well-Being
Economic Security Indicators

- The poverty rate for related children dropped from 19 percent in 1997 to 18 percent in 1998. The poverty rate for children has fluctuated since the early 1980s: It reached a high of 22 percent in 1993 and has since decreased to 18 percent, a rate comparable to that seen in 1980.

- The percentage of children living with their parents where at least one parent was working full time all year increased slightly in 1998 to 77 percent, from 76 percent in 1997.

- Many children live in households that have housing problems, such as physically inadequate housing, crowded housing, or a high cost burden. The percentage of households with children that have these problems has been increasing since 1978; 36 percent had one or more housing problems in 1997, up from 30 percent in 1978.

- The percentage of children experiencing food insecurity decreased in 1999. However, nearly one-third of children in poverty experienced food insecurity.

permission to treat, nature of services, and financing are just some of the obstacles to establishing effective SBHCs (Hacker 1996). Yet despite the many problems, the school-based health center approach to student health care may gain much greater acceptance in the future.

Even if such facilities are not available on a broad scale, schools should have access to a school nurse. Unfortunately, many school districts have been

- While the percentage of children without health insurance remained steady at 15 percent, the percentage with private insurance increased to 68 percent in 1998.

Health Indicators

- The percentage of children born with low birthweight (less than about 5.5 pounds) or very low birthweight (less than about 3.3 pounds) has steadily increased since 1984. About 7.6 percent of infants were low birthweight and 1.4 percent were very low birthweight in 1998. The increase in the proportion of low-birthweight infants is partly due to the rising number of twins and other multiple births.

- Death rates for children continued to drop in 1998. For children ages 1 to 4 and 5 to 14, the death rates were 34 and 20 per 100,000 children in each age group, respectively. The leading cause of death in these age groups was unintentional injuries, with most of these fatal injuries resulting from car crashes. Birth defects, cancer, and homicide were also leading causes of death for children ages 1 to 14.

- Deaths among adolescents ages 15 to 19 also continued to decline. In 1997, the adolescent mortality rate was 75 per 100,000 youth ages 15 to 19. Declines in deaths from firearm injuries between 1994 and 1997 contributed to the overall drop in mortality for adolescents.

- The birth rate for adolescents dropped by more than one-fifth between 1991 and 1998. In 1998, the birth rate for 15- to 17-year-olds was 30 per 1,000 females ages 15 to 17, the lowest it has been in at least 40 years.

Behavior and Social Environment Indicators

- The prevalence of heavy drinking among adolescents has been stable over the past few years. In 1999, 31 percent of 12th-graders, 26 percent of 10th-graders, and 15 percent of 8th-graders reported having five or more drinks in a row at least once during the past 2 weeks.

- Violent crimes committed by young people have dropped sharply. In 1998, the serious violent crime offending rate for youth was 27 crimes per 1,000 adolescents ages 12 to 17, totaling 616,000 such crimes involving juveniles—a drop by more than half from the 1993 high, and the lowest level since data were first collected in 1973.

Education Indicators

- In 1999, 53 percent of children ages 3 to 5 were read to daily by a family member, the same as in 1993 after increasing to 57 percent in 1996.

- Between 1996 and 1999, the percentage of children ages 3 to 5 not yet in kindergarten who were enrolled in early childhood centers rose from 55 to 59 percent. The largest increases were among children living in poverty, children with mothers who were not in the labor force, and black, non-Hispanic children.

- The overall high school completion rate for young adults ages 18 to 24 declined from 86 percent in 1997 to 85 percent in 1998. This decline was most pronounced among Hispanics.

Special Features

- Upon entering kindergarten in 1998, 66 percent of children were able to recognize letters and 29 percent knew the sounds made by letters that begin words—important skills in developing the ability to read.

- Fifty-five percent of high school students participated in volunteer activities in 1999, up from 50 percent in 1996. In 1999, 16 percent of these teens performed 35 or more hours of service throughout the school year.

SOURCE: Federal Interagency Forum on Child and Family Statistics 2000

forced to cut back or underdevelop the role of the school nurse by assigning one nurse responsibility for several schools. This does not allow nurses sufficient time in a given school to completely develop the school health service. Even worse, in some communities school health services are performed by parents, school secretaries, or some other untrained person.

The services provided by school nurses are extremely important to the children's welfare. Most frequently, they provide direct care to sick or injured children. Important functions are information gathering through assessment of the children, recordkeeping, and routine assessments. These assessments should help provide for appropriate follow-up care and some type of interpretation to the parent.

Nurses are excellent resources. They should be included on any health education curriculum planning committee and should be involved in planning the education of special populations. Nurses have become increasingly involved in planning the educational programs of handicapped children. Nurses can assist these children in becoming self-sufficient in the classroom and help alleviate the fears and concerns of the teachers. Finally, the nurse should see that emergency procedures for injuries, accidents, and sickness are developed because of legal concerns when undertaking aid in any of these situations. The nurse can help ensure proper care by helping to develop guidelines and workshops for teachers, aids, and office personnel in emergency procedures.

Summary

- Health is defined as an integrated method of functioning that is oriented toward maximizing personal potential.

- Wellness implies that individuals engage in attitudes and behaviors that enhance quality of life and maximize personal potential.

- Wellness consists of six components: spiritual, social, emotional, intellectual, physical, and environmental.

- To achieve wellness, students must feel they can control their lives (locus of control) and believe in their ability to accomplish a specific task or behavior (self-efficacy).

- Self-esteem, self-confidence, and a sense that students can achieve success are key to optimal learning.

- Health promotion is the aggregate of all purposeful activities designed to improve personal and public health through a combination of strategies, including health education, health-protection measures, health enhancement, and health maintenance.

- Health education is the process of developing and providing planned experiences to supply information, change attitudes, and influence behavior.

- To accomplish its goals, health education must be sequential, planned, comprehensive, and taught by qualified teachers.

- Quality health education includes providing a decision-making model that helps students make informed, appropriate decisions concerning their health.

- Factual information does not ensure behavioral change.

- Opportunities must be provided for personalizing the information learned so that attitudes can be formulated as precursors to behavior.

- The CDC has identified six categories of risk behaviors: behaviors that may result in unintentional and intentional injuries; tobacco use; alcohol and other drug use; sexual behaviors that result in HIV infections, other STIs, and unintended pregnancy; unhealthy dietary behaviors; and inadequate physical activity.

- A comprehensive school health education program has a planned, sequential K through 12 program; addresses a range of categorical health problems and issues; helps students develop skills to avoid negative behaviors; provides for a prescribed amount of time at each grade level; is managed/coordinated by a trained professional to implement the program; contains instruction from teachers who are trained to teach health; involves parents and health professionals; and includes periodic evaluation, updating, and improvement.

- Several national initiatives have created support for a coordinated school health program.

- The YRBSS is an excellent source of information that helps identify the need for a comprehensive school health education curriculum and coordinated health program.

- Problems that indicate the need for comprehensive health education include child and adolescent accident rates, transmission of HIV and other STIs, smoking, lack of activity, poor nutrition, alcohol and drug use, problem pregnancies, suicides, and chronic diseases.

- An effective coordinated school health program has eight components: healthful school environment; school health instruction; school health services; physical education; nutrition and food services; school-based counseling (psychological and social services); schoolsite health promotion; and school, family and community health promotion partnerships.

- A school-based health center can be an important component of an effective school health program.

DISCUSSION QUESTIONS

1. Discuss the various definitions of health and the implications of the definitions.
2. Define the term *wellness*; discuss the implications of the different components.
3. What is the difference between health promotion and health education?
4. How would you justify the need for health education in the elementary school?
5. What are some of the initiatives that support the need for health education?
6. Why is prevention the best approach to affecting the quality of life?
7. Why is self-responsibility so important to develop when teaching health?
8. Discuss why the YRBSS is an important tool for all classroom teachers as well as health educators.
9. What are the various components of a coordinated school health program, and why are they important?
10. How can the classroom teacher aid in the development of a healthy school environment?

WEB SITE ACTIVITY

Select one of the Web sites listed below and search for position papers on various health education concerns. Review one of the position papers to determine if it reflects the way health is currently taught.

WEB SITES OF INTEREST

American Association for Health Education
   www.aahperd.org

American Medical Association
   www.ama-assn.org

American School Health Association
   www.ashaweb.org

CDC's Comprehensive School Activities
   www.cdc.gov/needphd/comprehe.htm

Children's Defense Fund
   www.childrensdefense.org

Youth Risk Behavior Surveillance System (YRBSS)
   www.cdc.gov/needphp/dash/yrbs

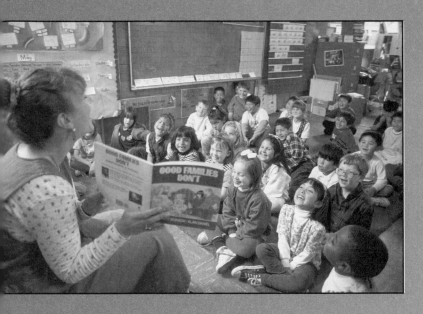

CHAPTER TWO

The Role of the Teacher in Coordinated School Health Programs

Comprehensive health education, offered early and reinforced throughout a student's school career, is fundamental to promoting healthy behaviors.

—Marx and Northrop (1995)

VALUED OUTCOMES

After reading this chapter, you should be able to:

- discuss the academic and personal qualifications of an effective health educator
- describe how a teacher of health has an opportunity to be a significant model in students' lives
- explain the unique challenges health educators face
- explain the barriers that make health instruction more difficult to teach than other subjects
- discuss the minimum competencies needed by a health educator
- describe the legal liability associated with teaching
- discuss how the educator can work with other members of the school staff to enhance the wellness of each student

Because of their important status as role models for children, and their responsibilities *in loco parentis* (in the place of parents), teachers are expected to live up to higher social standards and expectations than people in other occupations. As you read through this chapter, reflect on your personal qualities relative to the material being discussed. Are there areas in which you could improve? Is it fair to ask teachers to "measure up" to some of the expected qualities? Are the legal and ethical responsibilities fair?

The Challenge of Health Education

Health education professionals and professional organizations have been working for more than twenty years to improve the preparation and competency of health educators. This work has led to the use of voluntary certification as the method of national credentialing to designate that individuals have met or exceeded established standards (Sciacca et al. 1999, 42). Health education has become a focal point during the last few years as our nation has worked toward reaching specific health goals (such as the Healthy People 2010 objectives for the nation, discussed in Chapter 1) for the citizens of our country. The emphasis on health education has, in turn, led to an increased awareness of the need for effective health educators.

To be effective, an educator must concentrate not only on academic preparation, but also on personal qualifications. Personal qualifications of an educator are important because of the significance of and emphasis on the teacher's behavior and attitudes.

Teaching health is unlike teaching any other topic in the curriculum. For example, in other classes the teacher may get immediate feedback from the students regarding the learning of a concept. However, in health education the teacher may never know if a student actually applies a health concept in his or her life, because the opportunity to apply that concept may not surface until several years later. Furthermore, the methodology used in health education is unlike other subject areas in that it demands an open, accepting environment in the classroom during instruction.

A philosophy that should govern every teacher is the following: "Every teacher is a health teacher"; that is, every teacher in the school is a health teacher, regardless of what discipline he or she is actually teaching. This implies that, regardless of the subject matter you happen to be teaching, you are making an impact on your students through your behavior. Health education may be the only subject matter in which the teacher must embody the content. You can teach as much by what you do as what you say in the classroom. In other words, you as a teacher are on display before your students, and you have the opportunity to portray a positive health image through your behavior. For example, if the students observe you eating a good diet in the lunchroom, they will see that health, at least that aspect, is important to you; therefore, they are more likely to adopt the same value.

Elementary school children are very impressionable, and you can teach skills and influence behavior positively through your own behavior and attitudes. You have an excellent opportunity to become a good health role model by practicing safe and healthy habits.

You must emphasize to students that they cannot become healthy passively. Involving them in active learning opportunities, in which they are allowed to clarify their values and taught how to make wise decisions, will personalize their health education. Your students will then be better able to make their own responsible choices for healthful behavior.

BARRIERS TO SUCCESSFUL HEALTH TEACHING

Planning and implementing school health education that is comprehensive often demands perseverance, commitment by an individual, and sometimes a fair amount of good luck. Health educators face shrinking budgets and competing priorities and must be aware of and responsive to cultural diversity and value differences. Almost every school that decides to implement a new health education program will face challenges (Marx and Northrop 1995).

For example, elementary education majors in most colleges receive very little instruction in health content and in methodology that specifically relates to health instruction. Because the elementary teacher must teach many subjects, most college programs emphasize methods and materials instead of specific subject areas. This puts the elementary teacher at a distinct disadvantage because teaching health requires a different methodology from other subjects. Teaching content alone is not sufficient in health education.

Students may be able to pass a paper-and-pencil test on health knowledge, but this does not ensure that they will put that knowledge into practice. This phenomenon, known as cognitive dissonance, concerns the discrepancy between personal health knowledge and general health behavior. For example, there is a common knowledge regarding protective factors related to wearing safety belts in cars, yet a significant number of Americans do not wear them regularly.

Therefore, health instruction requires an active involvement of the student in the learning process; that is, you must give the student opportunities to experience situations (even though they may be simulated) in which they focus their values and make decisions regarding health behavior. Again, this teaching process is no guarantee that every student will make a healthy decision in each case, but it will more effectively help the student learn the concept being taught as well as apply the concept to his or her lifestyle.

Health instruction further demands the inclusion of teaching methodologies that enable the student to consider a healthy behavior valuable enough to incorporate into his or her lifestyle. To overcome these specific barriers, take as many courses as you can that emphasize health content and health instruction. For a more detailed discussion of value-based instruction, see Chapter 4.

Effective health instruction is hindered by the tremendous wealth of health information currently available. Health education is by its nature interdisciplinary in that it borrows not only from educational theory but also from many social sciences, such as psychology and sociology, as well as from physical science, biology, and even religion. It is difficult enough for a health education specialist to stay current in health, much less the elementary teacher, who must master several other subject areas.

This previous barrier is compounded by the fact that health information is changing constantly—the results of new studies related to health information appear virtually every day. The teacher has an obligation to follow these new developments. One way to do so is to attend educational seminars and workshops.

Further, some health information is conflicting; two studies on the same health topic might reach different conclusions. Some physicians consider megadoses of vitamin C to be the answer to preventing colds; other physicians disagree. Such disagreements between authorities cause a dilemma for the conscientious teacher who wishes to present *all* the information. Also, the conflicting information can be confusing for the student who is trying to make a wise, informed decision.

Another problem surfaces when teachers must deal with information that is inconclusive. For example, much information about AIDS appears contradictory. Normally, teachers think it is imperative to know everything in order to command the respect of students; but this is impossible in situations where even the authorities have not discovered all the answers.

Another barrier to effective health instruction is that so many issues in health education are controversial. Teachers who handle controversial issues risk offending students and/or parents. Even in some subjects that would not appear controversial, such as nutrition, you might offend some groups, say vegetarians, if you teach that servings of meat are recommended for a balanced diet. Further, controversial topics tend to polarize students. The more controversial the topic, the more emotional the students become about the issue. When this occurs, there is a greater likelihood of dissension and ill feeling among the students. Such dissension can disrupt the optimal teaching/learning environment that is necessary in health instruction.

Many times, as an instructor, you will be battling against students' negative image of health and health education. Health educators are sometimes viewed as "warriors against pleasure," which means that students think of health educators as those who tell them to quit doing what they like to do, such as eating desserts, and to do what they don't like to do, such as exercising. This may translate into negative feelings that the teacher must overcome, especially when the student perceives that the teacher's ideas conflict with those of parents or the peer group. Also, some students come into the health education classroom with preconceived notions, habits, and misconceptions about health information. This misinformation might have come from the home, media, older siblings, or peers. Teachers should be very knowledgeable of their students' backgrounds and subcultural perspectives. This understanding is critical in understanding a student's behavior and knowing what will motivate a student.

This makes the job of the educator doubly difficult because not only must she or he provide the correct information, but she or he also may be spending much of the time in the classroom dispelling many myths that the students bring with them.

Health Highlight

FUTURE LICENSING—INDIANA DEPARTMENT OF EDUCATION
QUALIFICATIONS FOR TEACHERS OF HEALTH EDUCATION

The State of Indiana is one of the few states in the process of requiring specific qualifications for health educators. Each qualification includes "knowledges," "performances," and "dispositions." More information can be found at *www.in.gov/psb/standards/HealthPhysEdContStds.html*. Some of these qualifications are listed below.

Standard 1A: Content Knowledge for Health Education

The teacher understands the content areas of health education and the tools of inquiry and skills related to the development of a health-literate person.

Standard 1B: Content Knowledge for Physical Education

The teacher understands the concept and content of physical education and the tools of inquiry related to the development of a physically educated person.

Standard 2: Growth and Development

The teacher understands how individuals learn and develop and provides opportunities that support mental, physiological, social, emotional, and moral development.

Standard 3: Instructional Strategies

The teacher plans and implements a variety of developmentally appropriate instructional strategies based upon the curriculum goals in order to develop learners' critical thinking, problem-solving, and performance skills.

Standard 4: Communication

The teacher uses knowledge of effective verbal, nonverbal, and multimedia communication techniques to foster inquiry, collaboration, and engagement in the learning process.

Standard 5: Management and Motivation

The teacher uses an understanding of individual and group motivation and behavior to create a learning environment that encourages positive social interaction, active engagement in learning, and self-motivation.

Standard 6: Diverse Learners

The teacher understands how individuals differ in their approaches to learning and creates appropriate instruction adapted for diverse learners.

Standard 7: Assessment

The teacher understands and uses formal, informal, and authentic assessment strategies to evaluate and ensure the learner's physical, mental, social, and emotional development.

Standard 8: Reflection

The teacher is a reflective practitioner who seeks opportunities for professional growth and evaluates the effects of his or her actions on learners, parents/guardians, and other professionals.

Standard 9: Collaboration

The teacher fosters relationships with colleagues, parents/guardians, and community agencies to support the learners' growth and well-being.

SOURCE: Indiana Professional Standards Board 2002

Finally, some administrators place a low priority on health education by allowing other activities to substitute for health instruction or by not placing health education in the curriculum at all. One way to overcome this problem is to help other teachers integrate health education with the other main subjects in the curriculum. There are many ways to integrate health into content and activities at the elementary level. For example, figuring one's heart rate can be integrated into mathematics. For language arts, the students can read a story about a health topic. The students can do many experiments in health class that are related to science.

Professional Preparation

In an effort to strengthen the professional preparation of health educators, health education was formally joined with the National Council for Accreditation of Teacher Education (NCATE) in 1986. The purpose for this alliance was to establish an accreditation process for teacher training programs. It involved (1) assessment of the competencies for health educators, (2) the inclusion of the recognized ten content areas of comprehensive school health instruction (see Chapter 1), and (3) key professional issues relative to health education in a school setting. These three components are included in the criteria for accreditation standards for health education. These standards provide university health education teacher training programs with guidance in planning, implementing, and evaluating their professional preparation programs (Smith et al. 1999).

Although standards for professional training of health educators have been set in the past, school health education has been criticized as being ineffective. This is largely the result of poorly prepared teachers.

Ideally, a preschool or elementary school health teacher should be a specialist, but this is not feasible when so many subjects must be taught. Therefore, the elementary teacher is forced to teach subjects such as health with less professional preparation than his or her secondary colleagues. Many states still allow teachers with dual certification in health and physical education to teach health at the secondary level and those with a general elementary certification to teach health at the elementary level.

There are several reasons for recommending that a teacher of health be a certified specialist. Health is different from other subjects in that the content comes from a variety of sources and is not limited to one distinct discipline. Also, the behavioral outcomes desired of the student in a health class differ remarkably from other subjects. Because these outcomes are not easily measured, a health teacher should have specific training in making empirical observations that indicate whether the desired outcomes are being acquired.

Even when a teacher is dually prepared—say, in health and physical education—the health portion is typically slighted in favor of the physical education portion. The reduced number of courses in this dual major hinders effective teacher preparation.

A course dealing with the personal health of the individual is also desirable. In this course, prospective teachers learn more about their own personal behavior. Further, a basic course in first aid and emergency skills is very helpful.

The National Task Force on the Preparation and Practice of Health Educators, composed of professionals from several national organizations with an interest in health education, has been working since 1978 to develop a framework of minimum competencies that should be required of health educators. These competencies are included in the document *A Framework for the Development of Competency-based Curricula for Entry-Level Health Educators* (later revised and retitled *A Competency-Based Curriculum Framework for the Professional Preparation of Entry-Level Health Educators*—National Task Force 1988) and are intended to guide certifying institutions in the professional preparation of students intending to teach health. This curriculum was developed with a generic health educator in mind, that is, an individual who might be teaching health in a variety of settings, including the school classroom. Eventually, NCATE accreditation of teacher credential programs in health will require the use of the guidelines specified in this framework.

As an outgrowth of the work of this task force, the National Commission for Health Education Credentialing (NCHEC) was formed to oversee the professional credentialing process for health educators. Certification is granted through a process of both meeting basic academic eligibility requirements and receiving a passing score on the certified health education specialist national examination. The certification exam itself consists of questions developed around responsibilities of health educators.

As discussed earlier, a teacher's preparation does not end upon receipt of a diploma and teaching certificate. You can continue to educate yourself by taking graduate courses, either in specific content areas or in advanced teaching methods; joining local, state, regional, and national health education professional organizations; and attending professional health conferences. Staying current also requires reading up-to-date textbooks, journals, and other health education publications. Finally, in-service workshops that deal with health-related topics are extremely valuable. To continue professional development beyond undergraduate training, many school health educators join one of the following professional associations:

- American Association for Health Education (AAHE), 1900 Association Drive, Reston, VA 22091-1599. This organization is housed currently under the umbrella of the American Alliance for Health, Physical Education, Recreation and Dance. This organization began as a professional organization for the health and physical education teacher. Its current emphasis includes the health professional in several types of work environments, such as K through 12 school, university, hospital, business and industry, and community.

- American School Health Association (ASHA), 7263 State Route 43, P.O. Box 708, Kent, OH 44240. This professional organization emphasizes all areas of school health, including services and environment as well as education. Therefore, its membership includes health educators as well as school nurses, physicians, dentists, and dental hygienists.

Becoming a Quality Health Teacher

There are many influences on a child, such as the media and peer pressure, that may be detrimental. Teachers should be positive role models, because educators are an important factor in students' health behavior development. Students desire positive role models who are honest, sincere, energetic, knowledgeable, and caring. The following discussion lists actions that will help you become a quality health educator.

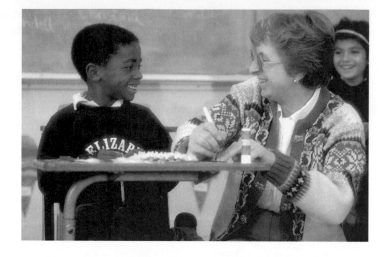

A teacher's task is to motivate students to want to learn.

Stay Motivated. Examples start with the teacher. If you hope to motivate your students to work hard, your own efforts should reflect your commitment to hard work. Motivation for teachers includes finding ways to get students to do things they might not want to do on their own. This means finding ways to get students to do more than "know" health—to get them to put into action what they know. It is necessary to consider motivating techniques to discover new ways to persuade youngsters to act in healthy ways. If the students are motivated about the subject, we can teach them the skills they'll need to make healthy decisions and to act in healthy ways. No small part of our task as teachers has become to motivate them beyond apathy. The problem lies in fostering the kind of attitude that includes sacrifice and discipline—among the students and yourselves.

There is probably no phase of teaching health that is more grossly misunderstood by teachers than the area of motivation. Teachers tend to be highly motivated individuals, and they sometimes have trouble understanding or dealing with students who do not share equally their enthusiasm and love for education or health behaviors.

Realize that you can motivate dedicated students and students who believe in you and your program. You cannot motivate students who feel no sense of responsibility or commitment to you or your program. Your task, then, is obvious—to motivate your students to want to learn and to want to be healthy. Students will more likely be motivated when they know you care enough about them to work as hard as you can to try to improve their skills.

In too many cases, we as health educators accept as truth the contention that students don't care about acting in healthy ways. Many young people are simply waiting for someone to guide them and care about them, and those are the students we have to find and motivate. If we accept as true that none of them will accept the challenge of excelling in an age of mediocrity, we're doing them a grave disservice—we're prejudging them toward the same mediocrity we want them to avoid. Not all young people are selfish and apathetic; many have not had the opportunity to challenge themselves to a higher purpose beyond mediocrity.

The best teachers are, always have been, and always will be, those teachers who work hardest to motivate their students. Motivation is as important a part of any teacher's teaching as any part of his or her lesson plan. One cannot overstate or overestimate the effect of motivation (or lack of motivation) on the level of intensity of a student's performance.

Be Organized. Students, especially young students, want and need the kind of guidance, leadership, and professionalism that is evidenced in teachers' efforts to organize their classes. Practice organization and attention to detail. Convey your concern for your program to your students in terms more vivid than you could ever express in words.

Good organization is a habit. Anyone can become more organized by making lists of tasks to accomplish and assigning priorities to those that are most important. Then, approximate the amount of time needed for each task, and try to work through the list in order of priority.

Be Consistent in Your Relations with Your Students. This doesn't mean that you have to treat all students alike. Students are not alike, and you should not treat them as if they are. Their motivations as well as their personalities vary widely. Some students thrive on praise and compliments, while others react as if a compliment were a signal that it's all right to quit working in class. Be aware of the differences in your students, and learn what motivates them best.

Students have the right to fair and equitable treatment, attention, and discipline. Treat all of them with dignity and respect.

Avoid Forming Hasty (or Permanent) Negative Opinions of Students. This sometimes happens when we pay attention to the teacher's lounge gossip about students who we are going to have in class. When we prejudge, the student never has a chance. Once we label a student, he or she tends to live up (or down) to that level of expectation.

Never Be Too Busy to Listen to Your Students. Communication is a two-way street. Students are expecting—or demanding through various forms of behavior—that teachers be concerned about them as human beings as well as students. When a student has a problem, the teacher should be willing to talk with him or her about it and to give the student a chance to talk it out. Sometimes all a youngster needs is an adult to give him a loving pat on the back that says, "I care," and to listen when the youngster needs to talk. Genuine communication does not always require words; it grows out of a mutual sense of concern for others.

Show Love, Care, and Concern to Your Students. Teachers may view their teaching as just a job, but students need guidance and a sense of belonging that grows out of a teacher's personal and professional behavior toward his or her students. Many teachers prefer not to become involved in the personal lives of their students. Increasingly, however, teachers are being required to deal with problems in students' personal lives that affect their in-class performances.

Be a Success Yourself. Success, like inventions, is 1 percent inspiration and 99 percent perspiration. Successful people invest in themselves. They go to seminars, read a lot, and consult with others. They are natural and eager learners. This doesn't mean they must go back to school, but they believe there's something to be learned from every encounter they have with other people and their ideas. Successful people believe they're in control of their own lives (internal locus of control) and their fates. They know that effort means more than luck ("Luck is the loser's way of explaining the winner's victory"). Good luck comes from hard work. A surprising number of opportunities seem to open up for those people who work hardest at putting themselves on a successful path.

Successful people have self-confidence. They believe they can overcome obstacles.

Be Positive. A key ingredient of success is the ability to eliminate from your own environment things that tend to put you in a negative or unresourceful state, while installing positive ones in yourself and in others. Positive thinking and unswerving dedication to making a dream a reality will provide the incentive to carry through whatever hard times and negativism on the part of others that lies in your path. Change your vocabulary. Instead of "Why don't they do something about it?" make it "I know what I'm going to do." Expect, anticipate, and welcome change. Change is normal and inevitable. With every change there is the unfamiliar and the unexpected. Risk it!

Use positive self-talk on a daily basis. Think uplifting thoughts. This is especially true regarding your students.

Seek Role Models. Benefit from others—if you think about why you are the way you are, chances are it has a lot to do with trying to be like someone you admired. Teachers usually have a teacher in their past who inspired them to become teachers.

We never stop needing role models. Even superstars study them, copy them, compete with them, and try to surpass them. Goad yourself to meet new challenges, set new goals, then top your previous behavior.

Set Goals. Another key to success is knowing what you want. People's abilities to fully tap their resources are directly affected by their goals. Before you can operate efficiently, you must develop specific goals. Outline your goals clearly. Concrete goals are easily understood by you and by students. Goals don't have to be elaborate. Set goals and develop a plan to achieve those goals.

Work Hard. The road to success is never easy. To be a success, you have to work. This is not popular advice. Work and achievement are irrevocably linked.

Stay Mentally Fresh. No matter how well you are doing what you are doing, you can do it better by exposing yourself to interests and ideas outside your immediate, day-to-day activities. These ideas will spark your imagination and give you ideas you can use in your own work. One excellent way to stay mentally fresh and get physically healthy at the same time is to exercise.

Health Highlight

THE 34TH ANNUAL PHI DELTA KAPPA/GALLUP POLL OF THE PUBLIC'S ATTITUDES TOWARD THE PUBLIC SCHOOLS

- For the first time in the thirty-three-year history of these polls, a majority of respondents assign either an A or a B (strongly agree and agree) to the schools in their communities.

- As has been the case in all past polls, the closer people are to the public schools, the better they like them.

- Seventy-two percent of Americans want to reform the existing system.

- Poll findings confirm the decline in support for using public money to fund attendance at private or parochial schools.

- The public is relatively uninformed about charter schools. Last year's poll found that only about half of the respondents had heard or read about such schools.

- Sixty-seven percent of respondents disapprove of allowing students to earn high school credits over the Internet without attending a regular school.

- Topping the list of perceived problems facing the public schools are lack of school funding and lack of discipline. Fighting/violence/gangs and overcrowded schools tied for third.

- Sixty-five percent favor awarding more state and federal dollars to schools that show progress toward state standards, while only 32 percent favor withholding funds to those schools.

SOURCE: Rose and Gallup 2002

The Teacher as Part of the Health Team

LEGAL RESPONSIBILITIES OF THE TEACHER

One major concern of today's teacher is liability because we live in a litigious society. Negligence can be charged when children are under your care and supervision, such as in the classroom, on the playground, and entering or departing buses. You are considered *in loco parentis* when a child is under your supervision. Your primary responsibility is to act responsibly to prevent injury to students. You should be well aware of first-aid and emergency procedures in order to care for a student in your charge so as not to aggravate an existing injury or illness.

You should follow your school system's procedure for filing a report for each accident. Each school should provide in-service preparation of faculty for preventing and handling accidents and should have an active safety program. (Safety procedures and accident reports are discussed further in Chapter 19.)

WORKING WITH STUDENTS

One of the teacher's responsibilities is counseling students in health-related matters. Counseling should be straightforward and free of moral judgment, preaching, or scare tactics. In the role of counselor, you must develop good listening skills and communication skills. Sometimes it is difficult to get to the heart of the problem; these skills will help you offer sound advice. Also, you need to show genuine sympathy toward a student's problem.

No matter how concerned you are about a student's problem, you must recognize the limitations of your ability to help. Do not try to diagnose or assign blame for a health problem. Either of these actions can lead to legal problems. If you perceive that a student is having problems, it is best to record your observations, without personal opinions, and discuss them with an administrator. The student may require additional guidance beyond the initial crisis counseling you can supply. Make sure you are familiar with available services in the school or community so you can refer the student to the most appropriate one. Most teachers are not professionally trained in counseling, nor are they expected to replace those who are.

WORKING WITH PARENTS

Always notify a student's parents when an illness or serious deviation from normal health occurs. School policy should be followed when parents are notified. Some schools require teachers to contact parents through the administrative offices. A good policy is to ensure that a member of the school administration is present at any parent–teacher conference. The third party can clear up any confusion in communication and can serve as an arbitrator in case of misunderstanding. The teacher should share his or her observations without including personal opinions or diagnoses. He or she should explain to the parents the significance of the child's health condition and encourage them to obtain needed care for the child. If a parent asks for guidance in seeking care, refer the person to the proper agency or individual. Be sure to take an active role in following up on any case reported to parents.

Health educators can involve parents in the health education of their children by sending information home in a newsletter and designing activities in which the parents help the children.

WORKING WITH OTHER TEACHERS AND THE SCHOOL ADMINISTRATION

A major responsibility of the health teacher is to keep the other teachers and the administrators informed of health matters related to the community and students. This information will help the other faculty members and the administration to understand the students and to recognize the need for health education in the school.

The educator can represent the school on health-related committees of teacher–parent and community organizations. You can help other faculty and administrators be aware of the environmental conditions in the school that

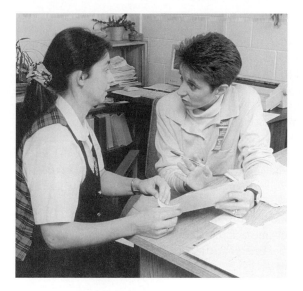

Health educators can keep other professionals informed of health matters.

might be unhealthy to the students, staff, and faculty. You should also attempt to become involved in textbook selection committees. Look for sound, up-to-date content, but beware of textbooks that propagate stereotypes.

A primary duty of the health educator is to plan the health education curriculum and make recommendations to the administration regarding the health education program within the school. You can help interpret and implement any state requirement for the health curriculum. Also make suggestions concerning the health service program and health environment.

The teacher must also work closely with the school administration when notifying parents about a child's health, referring parents to appropriate health resources, and following up on student cases. Principals often request that the teacher be included in health-related referrals. The teacher should keep the administration informed about a child's progress in school after the child returns from an illness.

WORKING WITH THE SCHOOL OR CLINIC NURSE

Because you daily observe each child in your class, you can help the school nurse understand the health behavior of students. You can also assist the nurse in various aspects of the screening program—by preliminary screening in the classroom, by preparing students for screening tests to reduce their anxiety, and by referring students who are in particular need of screening. Teacher and nurse can participate in in-service workshops for the other faculty members. Finally, teachers who are properly trained can complement the school's emergency care program by offering their services when needed.

WORKING WITH OUTSIDE AGENCIES

One of your objectives should be to promote health education and awareness in the community. You can help volunteer organizations educate the community in health matters. Many of these agencies, such as the American Heart Association and American Dental Association, have health curricula and need help to implement their programs in the schools. Through this cooperation, you can learn about other health professionals in your community and can acquaint yourself with the services offered to students by these agencies. Determine which agencies will provide services for paying students and which will provide services for students for a reduced or waived fee. You should also become involved with the local public health department and cooperate with department staff members in providing services to the students and community.

Finally, in this time of budget cuts and termination of health programs, you are strongly urged to become active in lobbying for health services and programs. Work with local teacher groups to educate legislators about health matters.

Summary

- Health education has evolved from a diverse background over the past 170 years.
- The nation's emphasis on health education has, in turn, led to a need for effective educators.
- An effective educator must concentrate on academic preparation and personal qualifications.
- Teaching health is different from teaching other disciplines in the curriculum.
- Teachers must be aware that they are modeling health behavior to students through their own lifestyles.
- There are several barriers to successfully implementing health education.
- There are several unique challenges to teaching health education.
- Teachers can overcome these hindrances by keeping their knowledge of health current, learning how to present controversial information in the classroom, and helping administrators see how health education can be integrated with other required subjects.
- Educators who model good health behavior have a positive impact on their students.
- Several specific characteristics and actions will help a teacher become a quality educator.
- Teamwork with parents, the school nurse, the school physician, administrators, community organizations, and students is the key to a successful school health program.

- As part of the team, the teacher
    - is aware of his or her legal responsibilities
    - observes each student for any deviation from normal health
    - reports to the proper authority within the school
    - is available to refer the student and parent to the appropriate community resource or to counsel the student and/or parent concerning the child's health.

DISCUSSION QUESTIONS

1. Describe the challenges in the role of the health teacher.
2. How does health education differ from other subject area instruction?
3. Discuss the interdisciplinary nature of health as a barrier to implementing good health instruction.
4. Describe the role of the NCHEC in promoting the health education profession.
5. How can a teacher be a positive role model in health behavior to the students?
6. List the characteristics and actions that will help you become a quality educator.
7. Discuss the ways in which a teacher can work with other teachers to improve the coordinated school health program.
8. Why should an administrator be present at any parent–teacher conference?
9. Describe the teacher qualities needed to work effectively with handicapped students.
10. Discuss how a teacher can involve parents in their child's health education.

CRITICAL THINKING QUESTIONS

1. What do you consider to be the greatest challenge for today's health educator?
2. How would you propose to overcome the barriers to successful health teaching as described in this chapter?
3. What do you consider to be the primary benefits of becoming a certified health educator? What are the drawbacks?
4. Considering the list of personal qualities detailed in this chapter, can these be developed within a teacher?
5. Describe the process you would use in scheduling and implementing a teacher–parent–administrator meeting.

WEB SITE ACTIVITY

Use the Web site: *www.aahperd.org/aahe/pdf_files/standards.pdf.* Determine what to teach in a fifth grade health education class regarding Health Education Standard 7: "Students will demonstrate the ability to advocate for personal, family and community health."

WEB SITES OF INTEREST

American Association for Health Education (AAHE): *www.aahperd.org/aahe*
AAHE is dedicated to providing opportunities for networking and to providing you the best health-education resources.

American College Health Association (ACHA): *www.acha.org*
ACHA offers several programs and services designed to help student health services maintain the highest standards of quality. If you are preparing for accreditation, considering staff or budget changes, or would simply like to know how your health center compares to others, the Consultation Services Program offers a detailed, professional, and objective analytical report.

American Public Health Association (APHE): *www.apha.org*
Throughout its history APHA has been in the forefront of numerous efforts to prevent disease and promote health. APHA brings together researchers, health service providers, administrators, teachers, and other health workers in a unique, multidisciplinary environment of professional exchange, study, and action.

American School Health Association (ASHA): *www.ashaweb.org*
ASHA unites the many professionals working in schools who are committed to safeguarding the health of school-age children. The Association, a multidisciplinary organization of administrators, counselors, dentists, health educators, physical educators, school nurses, and school physicians, advocates high-quality school health instruction, health services, and a healthful school environment.

Society for Public Health Education (SOPHE): *www.sophe.org*
SOPHE is a 501(c)(3) professional organization founded in 1950 to provide leadership to the profession and to promote the health of all people by: stimulating research on the theory and practice of health education; supporting high-quality performance standards for the practice of health education and health promotion; advocating policy and legislation affecting health education and health promotion; and developing and promoting standards for professional preparation of health education professionals.

The National Commission for Health Education Credentialing (NCHEC):
   www.nchec.org
The mission of NCHEC is to improve the quality of health education practice through the establishment, implementation, and maintenance of a certification process for health education specialists, and through the promotion of scientific, ethical, and state-of-the-art programs of professional preparation and continuing education.

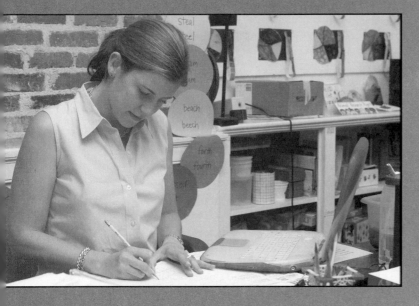

CHAPTER THREE

Planning for Health Instruction

When it comes to the
education of our children . . .
failure is not an option.

—President George W. Bush
(2001)

VALUED OUTCOMES

After reading this chapter, you should be able to:

- list the content areas of health education
- describe the scope and sequence of health education
- identify the National Health Standards and understand why they are important
- identify the curricular approaches approved by National Diffusion Network
- discuss why outcome-based education and performance indicators are important to health education
- write instructional objectives
- develop an effective lesson plan

As you read this chapter, reflect on why it is necessary to begin to utilize the concepts of outcome-based education (OBE) and performance indicators in planning and teaching the health education curriculum. What are the advantages and disadvantages of this approach? What might be the concerns of teachers in implementing such an approach? Can the National Health Education Standards really enhance the teaching of health?

Content Areas in the Elementary School

Teaching health education, like teaching any subject, requires careful planning. Teachers must know what to teach, when to teach it, and how to teach it so that the content is internalized, or personalized, by the students. First-graders are vastly different from eighth-graders. Health instruction at each grade level must be tailored to the maturational, intellectual, and interest levels of the students.

Virtually every state department of education has a health education curriculum that can be used as a guide for planning. It should be read carefully, for in it can be found a recommended list of topics to be presented at each grade level. Teachers must recognize the complexity of life and attempt to incorporate the dimensions of wellness (physical, social, intellectual, emotional, environmental, and spiritual) into health instruction.

The general public often visualizes elementary health instruction merely in terms of rules for brushing teeth and riding bicycles safely. It is, of course, far more than that. Various health education authorities cite from ten to twenty different content areas, depending on how the areas are grouped or separated. Most health educators agree on these content areas for elementary health instruction:

- mental/emotional health
- personal health
- nutrition
- family health
- prevention of substance use and abuse
- injury prevention and safety
- growth and development
- consumer and community health
- prevention and control of disease
- environmental health

The ultimate reason for all health education is to increase each student's **health literacy,** or "the capacity of the individual to obtain, interpret, and understand basic health information and services and the competence to use such information and services in ways which are health enhancing" (AAHE 1995, 75). Content areas and topics also change in emphasis to reflect current knowledge and health concerns.

Grade Placement for Health Education Topics

Once basic content areas have been charted, it must be determined how much emphasis will be placed on each area at each grade level. Emphasis within each content area should be based on the developmental level, health needs, and interests of the students. A planned cycle of presentation of content areas ensures that necessary topics will be included and will receive appropriate emphasis at each grade level.

A cycle plan helps eliminate useless repetition and ensures that topics are covered to the depth necessary for a particular grade. A cycle plan also prepares children for the subject matter awaiting them in their remaining educational experiences.

Developing Scope and Sequence

Content areas must not only be identified, they must also be ordered and organized. That is, the scope and sequence of the health education curriculum must be determined. **Scope** refers to the depth or difficulty of the material—the "what" to teach. **Sequence** refers to the order in which the material is to be covered—the "when" to teach it. Here again the state department of education health guide or the local city or country guide can be of great use. Such guides usually spell out the scope and sequence of health education for each grade level. They may also indicate what competencies a child should possess after completing the course of study.

Planned health instruction should attempt to ensure that each previous learning experience provides the basis for new learning. Topics should build on one another and not be presented as isolated bits of information. Concepts within each lesson should relate to each other, lessons within a unit should relate to each other, and units within the course should relate to each other. In this way, students will see health education as a whole rather than as seemingly unrelated fragments.

Scope also refers to the arrangement of the curriculum from kindergarten through senior high school. As such, it serves as a reminder that everything done in the classroom should be built on what has been previously accomplished so that initial learning becomes the basis for subsequent learning.

The seven National Health Education Standards can be found in the pages that follow. These standards should serve as the foundation for curriculum development and instruction in health education. These standards are a framework for health educators in the United States. The goal is to create an instructional program that will enable students to experience comprehensive health education, which in turn will enable them to become/remain healthy and to achieve academic success (AAHE 1995, 1; Joint Committee on National Health Standards 1995).

Determining What to Teach

Although state health education guidelines are helpful in determining the scope and sequence of the health curriculum, they should not be the sole planning aid. In developing the curriculum, other factors, such as the social mores of the community, student interest, and student health needs, must be considered. Curriculum needs may vary according to community, state, or region.

SOCIAL MORES

The curriculum that is developed must be acceptable to the community in which it is located. Ascertaining the social mores of the community demands careful judgment. Teachers have an advantage if they are well acquainted with the community. However, it may be difficult to assess feelings within the community about how best to teach certain health topics, such as substance abuse or sexuality education. Controversial topics should be discussed with administrators before any course of instruction is implemented.

Another community influence on curriculum development comes from special interest groups, which may be national, state, or local. Their charge is to promote or protect their own philosophy or special interests. Most of these groups are sincere about bringing beneficial services to the children in a community, but such groups can also have a detrimental influence on curriculum development. For example, groups that form to stop sexuality education can be formidable opponents to the development of a comprehensive health education program. Regardless of content area, it is wise to be familiar with local and state guides and recommendations for teaching health education.

Each state has its own set of guidelines or standards for teaching health education, and many states also have curriculum guides that can aid teachers and school districts in the selection of content. These sources should be consulted, reviewed, understood, and implemented when creating a health education curriculum.

STUDENT INTEREST

Children are interested in some health topics more than others, depending on their age. For example, younger children are likely to be more interested in the parts and functions of their bodies than are older children. Also, because primary age children are more self-centered, they are less concerned about social topics than are upper elementary age children.

Questionnaires, checklists, and direct questioning can all aid in determining student interest in the classroom. In fact, there is no substitute for interacting directly with a class to gauge interest in various topics. Familiarity with professional literature on the subject is equally important. There are basic health interests common to all students, regardless of location or socioeconomic class.

Later in elementary school, children's abstract reasoning becomes better developed, and students are capable of dealing with more than immediate life situations. Then increasingly abstract health concepts, such as pollution or aging, can be taught. Reasoning and insight into causal relationships also develop.

HEALTH NEEDS

All children, regardless of community, have certain basic health needs. These include the need for love and nurturing, sound nutrition, intellectual stimulation, proper dental care, and safety. However, specific health needs vary from community to community, and the curriculum that you plan should take into account these specific needs. For example, inner-city children may need emphasized instruction about the dangers of lead poisoning, as many inner-city dwellings still contain lead-based paint. Similarly, the safety instruction provided may vary, depending on whether the community is rural or urban.

TEXTBOOKS AND COURSES OF STUDY

Most elementary health textbooks contain detailed suggestions for developing curricula. The teachers' editions of these texts provide outlines and units for teaching health and identify major concepts to be taught at a given grade level. Like state health guidelines, however, textbooks cannot provide a course of study tailored to a specific community and a specific classroom. Because textbooks are developed for national use, they may lack sufficient depth of coverage on topics of particular relevance to a given setting.

To supplement the textbook you use, you will probably wish to obtain pamphlets, videos, Web site addresses, CD-ROMs, and other learning aids from government or private health-related agencies such as the U.S. Department of Agriculture or the National Safety Council. Most health-related agencies will make classroom materials available free of charge or at a nominal cost. Be sure, however, to screen all materials before classroom use to determine their appropriateness, currency, and possible biases.

Teaching for Values

Values give direction to life and determine behavior. Members of our society share many of the same values. However, each community, family, and individual has a more specific set of values. Values are closely linked with personal feelings and must be carefully considered when planning health instruction.

Failure to do so can result in the blocking of effective learning and opposition from parents and community organizations. Values are learned through a variety of experiences and interactions with the environment. The family, peer group, school, church, and media all influence personal value formation. In other words, value formation is a continual process. Yet many parents become concerned when formal teaching about values takes place in the schools. There is concern that values contrary to the parents' values will be taught. Any recommendation or point of emphasis by a teacher can be construed as the imposition of values. Conversely, to take no stand at all can imply an anything-goes attitude.

Therefore, in planning health instruction, it must be made clear how values will be a part of the teaching. A teacher's job is not to impose his or her values; it is to help children develop their own values by making wise decisions about health-related matters. Children will form values with or without their teacher's assistance, but their teacher can help them make positive decisions that will lead to high-level wellness by providing factual knowledge about health and by allowing children to clarify their own feelings.

Attitudes and behavior are intertwined. If a balance between knowledge and attitudes toward health education is to be achieved, student feelings must be addressed in teaching. In other words, the study of health must be personalized if it is to have an impact. By providing opportunities for children to identify feelings and personalize health information, teachers can help them understand how information, attitudes, and behavior affect quality of life. In doing so, children become better equipped to deal with peer pressure, communicate more effectively, and develop sound decision-making skills.

Each person must weigh the importance or value of a decision against perceived rewards and costs involved. To brush one's teeth regularly, to smoke, to have regular physical examinations, and to experiment with drugs are all examples of decisions that affect health. Decisions must be made by the individual; consequently, teachers must make a planned effort to help children think through the possible consequences of health-related decisions.

Curriculum Approaches

Many helpful resources are available to assist teachers in planning a course of health education for the classroom. As noted, these resources include the state health education guidelines, commercial health education textbook series, and materials from government and private health-related agencies. There are also numerous Web sites that offer content and strategy suggestions. The discussion that follows includes resources approved by the National Diffusion Network and potential commercial sources. Most of the mentioned materials have Web sites that provide greater detail about the nature of the resource. The Web sites usually contain information on the training necessary to use the material, the philosophy of the curriculum approach, and the type(s) of information the curriculum provides.

Health Highlight

THE NATIONAL HEALTH EDUCATION STANDARDS
Health Education Standard 1:
Students will comprehend concepts related to health promotion and disease prevention.

Rationale

Basic to health education is a foundation of knowledge about the interrelationship of behavior and health, interactions within the human body, and the prevention of diseases and other health problems. Experiencing physical, mental, emotional, and social changes as one grows and develops provides a self-contained "learning laboratory." Comprehension of health promotion strategies and disease prevention concepts enables students to become health-literate, self-directed learners, which establishes a foundation for leading healthy and productive lives.

Performance Indicators

As a result of health instruction in grades K–4, students will

1. describe relationships between personal health behaviors and individual well-being
2. identify indicators of mental, emotional, social, and physical health during childhood
3. describe the basic structure and functions of the human body systems
4. describe how the family influences personal health
5. describe how physical, social, and emotional environments influence personal health
6. identify common health problems of children

7. identify health problems that should be detected and treated early
8. explain how childhood injuries and illnesses can be prevented or treated

As a result of health instruction in grades 5–8, students will

1. explain the relationship between positive health behaviors and the prevention of injury, illness, disease, and premature death
2. describe the interrelationship of mental, emotional, social, and physical health during adolescence
3. explain how health is influenced by the interaction of body systems
4. describe how family and peers influence the health of adolescents
5. analyze how environment and personal health are interrelated
6. describe ways to reduce risks related to adolescent health problems
7. explain how appropriate health care can prevent premature death and disability
8. describe how lifestyle, pathogens, family history, and other risk factors are related to the cause or prevention of disease and other health problems

SOURCE: Joint Committee on National Health Education Standards 1995

THE NATIONAL DIFFUSION NETWORK

There are many approaches to health education at the national, state, and local level. There are so many that it is difficult for teachers to determine what is an excellent, good, or (sometimes) a poor program. State and local districts often have their own plans for curriculum, but teachers who are asked to review or select a new program may find it a difficult task based on the overwhelming number of plans available.

One of the best ways to approach the task is by becoming familiar with the **National Diffusion Network (NDN).** This federally funded program is designed to improve educational opportunities and achievement for all levels of education. The philosophy of NDN is to identify exemplary programs from their

Planning for Health Instruction   **45**

Health Highlight

THE NATIONAL HEALTH EDUCATION STANDARDS
Health Education Standard 2:
Students will demonstrate the ability to access valid health information and health-promoting products and services.

Rationale

Accessing valid health information and health-promoting products and services is important in the prevention, early detection, and treatment of most health problems. Critical thinking involves the ability to identify valid health information and to analyze, select, and access health-promoting services and products. Applying skills of information analysis, organization, comparison, synthesis, and evaluation to health issues provides a foundation for individuals to move toward becoming health-literate and responsible, productive citizens.

Performance Indicators

As a result of health instruction in grades K–4, students will

1. identify characteristics of valid health information and health-promoting products and services

2. demonstrate the ability to locate resources from home, school, and community that provide valid health information

3. explain how media influences the selection of health information, products, and services

4. demonstrate the ability to locate school and community health helpers

As a result of health instruction in grades 5–8, students will

1. analyze the validity of health information, products, and services

2. demonstrate the ability to utilize resources from home, school, and community that provide valid health information

3. analyze how media influences the selection of health information and products

4. demonstrate the ability to locate health products and services

5. compare the costs and validity of health products

6. describe situations requiring professional health services

SOURCE: Joint Committee on National Health Education Standards 1995

---

development sites and transfer them to other educational settings. NDN provides educational institutions with a wide array of offerings from which to select those that best meet their respective philosophies, needs, and resources. Limited funds are also available to help create awareness of outstanding programs, help with adoption decisions, and provide in-service training and follow-up assistance. Some funds are also available for the purchase of teaching aids.

To be classified as an "exemplary program," a program must be reviewed by the Program Effectiveness Panel (PEP), which represents the U.S. Department of Education. Approval by PEP means that the panel has examined objective evidence of effectiveness submitted by the developers of the program. The panel must be convinced that the program has met its stated objectives at the developmental site. In addition, the developers must prove that the program will meet the educational needs of others in similar locations (NDN 1995, 9). Approved programs are eligible for NDN funds or from other federal funding programs.

To help public and private schools identify NDN programs, the U.S. Department of Education supports facilitators' projects in every state, the District of

Health Highlight

THE NATIONAL HEALTH EDUCATION STANDARDS
Health Education Standard 3:
*Students will demonstrate the ability to practice
health-enhancing behaviors and reduce health risks.*

Rationale

Research confirms that many diseases and injuries can be prevented by reducing harmful and risk-taking behaviors. More importantly, recognizing and practicing health-enhancing behaviors can contribute to a positive quality of life. Strategies used to maintain and improve positive health behaviors will utilize knowledge and skills that help students become critical thinkers and problem solvers. By accepting responsibility for personal health, students will have a foundation for living a healthy, productive life.

Performance Indicators

As a result of health instruction in grades K–4, students will

1. identify responsible health behaviors
2. identify personal health needs
3. compare behaviors that are safe to those that are risky or harmful
4. demonstrate strategies to improve or maintain personal health

5. develop injury prevention and management strategies for personal health
6. demonstrate ways to avoid and reduce threatening situations.
7. apply skills to manage stress

As a result of health instruction in grades 5–8, students will

1. explain the importance of assuming responsibility for personal health behaviors
2. analyze a personal health assessment to determine health strengths and risks
3. distinguish between safe and risky or harmful behaviors in relationships
4. demonstrate strategies to improve or maintain personal and family health
5. develop injury prevention and management strategies for personal and family health
6. demonstrate ways to avoid and reduce threatening situations
7. demonstrate strategies to manage stress

SOURCE: Joint Committee on National Health Education Standards 1995

Columbia, and several territories worldwide. These facilitators help schools determine their problems and needs and select NDN programs appropriate for their situation. The facilitators can aid in providing training and follow-up in either monitoring or evaluating the program(s) selected by the schools. Limited funds also are available to support travel to demonstration sites.

HEALTH PROGRAMS APPROVED BY NDN

Although programs are certified and recertified for NDN exemplary program status, the 1995 edition of *Education Programs That Work* lists the following elementary health programs: (1) Healthy for Life, (2) Know Your Body School Health Promotion Program, (3) Me-Me Drug and Alcohol Prevention Education Program, (4) Growing Healthy, (5) Project CHOICE, and (6) Social Decision Making and Problem Solving. All descriptions of the programs are those provided by NDN in the 1995 edition of *Education Programs That Work,* pages 9–2 to 9–11.

Health Highlight

THE NATIONAL HEALTH EDUCATION STANDARDS
Health Education Standard 4:
Students will analyze the influence of culture, media, technology, and other factors on health.

Rationale

Health is influenced by a variety of factors that coexist within society. These include the cultural context as well as media and technology. A critical thinker and problem solver is able to analyze, evaluate, and interpret the influence of these factors on health. The health-literate, responsible, and productive citizen draws on the contributions of culture, media, technology, and other factors to strengthen individual, family, and community health.

Performance Indicators

As a result of health instruction in grades K–4, students will

1. describe how culture influences personal health behaviors

2. explain how media influences thoughts, feelings, and health behaviors

3. describe ways technology can influence personal health

4. explain how information from school and family influences health

As a result of health instruction in grades 5–8, students will

1. describe the influence of cultural beliefs on health behaviors and the use of health services

2. analyze how messages from media and other sources influence health behaviors

3. analyze the influence of technology on personal and family health

4. analyze how information from peers influences health

SOURCE: Joint Committee on National Health Education Standards 1995

Healthy for Life. The Healthy for Life (HFL) program is designed to help students in grades 6 through 8 manage situations that are high risk. The program seeks to improve health behaviors in nutrition; tobacco, alcohol, and marijuana use; and sexuality.

Description. HFL is a comprehensive program consisting of four components: (1) **curriculum** that is cumulative, sequenced, and focused on health promotion lessons, activities, and teaching strategies; (2) **peer leadership** to employ students to teach through their words and actions; (3) **family** to facilitate communication between the adolescent and one significant family member or other adult; and (4) **community** to enlist community people actively working to reinforce the behavioral messages of the curriculum and launch an attack on the pervasive double messages about the target behaviors that most communities transmit. Games, role plays, videos, cooperative learning activities, and hands-on demonstrations keep students engaged and participating. Homework, which involves students "interviewing" parents, encourages the sharing of family values and rules. Fifty-eight lessons are given in sequence every day for four weeks, first to one cohort of sixth graders and then to the same cohort as seventh and eighth graders. In this version, topics are addressed when they are most salient in the adolescent's life, and students build on their skills and

Health Highlight

THE NATIONAL HEALTH EDUCATION STANDARDS
Health Education Standard 5:
Students will demonstrate the ability to use interpersonal communication skills to enhance health.

Rationale

Personal, family, and community health are enhanced through effective communication. A responsible individual will use verbal and nonverbal skills in developing and maintaining healthy personal relationships. Ability to organize and to convey information, beliefs, opinions, and feelings are skills that strengthen interactions and can reduce or avoid conflict. When communicating, individuals who are health literate demonstrate care, consideration, and respect of self and others.

Performance Indicators

As a result of health instruction in grades K–4, students will

1. distinguish between verbal and nonverbal communication
2. describe characteristics needed to be a responsible friend and family member
3. demonstrate healthy ways to express needs, wants, and feelings
4. demonstrate ways to communicate care, consideration, and respect of self and others
5. demonstrate attentive listening skills to build and maintain healthy relationships
6. demonstrate refusal skills to enhance health

7. differentiate between negative and positive behaviors used in conflict situations
8. demonstrate nonviolent strategies to resolve conflicts

As a result of health instruction in grades 5–8, students will

1. demonstrate effective verbal and nonverbal communication skills to enhance health
2. describe how the behavior of family and peers affects interpersonal communication
3. demonstrate healthy ways to express needs, wants, and feelings
4. demonstrate ways to communicate care, consideration, and respect of self and others
5. demonstrate communication skills to build and maintain healthy relationships
6. demonstrate refusal and negotiation skills to enhance health
7. analyze the possible causes of conflict among youth in schools and communities
8. demonstrate strategies to manage conflict in healthy ways

SOURCE: Joint Committee on National Health Education Standards 1995

experiences in previous grades. The intensive version delivers the lessons in one sequential, twelve-week block to an entire cohort of seventh graders.

Know Your Body School Health Promotion Program. A multicomponent comprehensive school health promotion program for students in grades K through 6, the Know Your Body (KYB) program has the goal of empowering students with the skills they need to make their own positive health choices.

Description. The KYB School Health Promotion Program consists of five basic components: (1) skills-based health education curriculum, (2) teacher/coordinator training, (3) biomedical screening, (4) extracurricular activities, and (5) program evaluation.

The curriculum and the teacher/coordinator training are considered the "core" components of the program, while the others are considered optional

Health Highlight

THE NATIONAL HEALTH EDUCATION STANDARDS
Health Education Standard 6:
*Students will demonstrate the ability to use goal-setting and
decision-making skills to enhance health.*

Rationale

Decision making and goal setting are essential lifelong skills needed in order to implement and sustain health-enhancing behaviors. These skills make it possible for individuals to transfer health knowledge into healthy lifestyles. When applied to health issues, decision-making and goal-setting skills will enable individuals to collaborate with others to improve the quality of life in their families, schools, and communities.

Performance Indicators

As a result of health instruction in grades K–4, students will

1. demonstrate the ability to apply a decision-making process to health issues and problems

2. explain when to ask for assistance in making health-related decisions and setting health goals

3. predict outcomes of positive health decisions

4. set a personal health goal and track progress toward its achievement

As a result of health instruction in grades 5–8, students will

1. demonstrate the ability to apply a decision-making process to health issues and problems individually and collaboratively

2. analyze how health-related decisions are influenced by individuals, family, and community values

3. predict how decisions regarding health behaviors have consequences for self and others

4. apply strategies and skills needed to attain personal health goals

5. describe how personal health goals are influenced by changing information, abilities, priorities, and responsibilities

6. develop a plan that addresses personal strengths, needs, and health risks

SOURCE: Joint Committee on National Health Education Standards 1995

components or "enhancements." Although implementation of the full KYB program is recommended, the program may be effectively implemented without the additional components. The American Health Foundation will assist schools in customizing a program that best suits their needs, goals, philosophies, and capacities.

KYB curriculum materials include age-appropriate teacher's guides (grades K through 6), student master sheets (grades K through 3); student activity books (grades 4 through 6); a class Big Book (grade 1); and puppet sets (grades K through 3). A comprehensive user's guide (*Coordinator's Guide*) is also available and provides detailed instructions for implementing all of KYB's program components.

The program stresses individual responsibility for health and provides the basis for making health-promoting and disease-preventing decisions. Behavioral goals are geared toward outcomes that children of this age can realistically affect, such as breakfast and snack choices, and asking adults not to smoke in their presence.

Health Highlight

THE NATIONAL HEALTH EDUCATION STANDARDS
Health Education Standard 7:
*Students will demonstrate the ability to advocate for
personal, family, and community health.*

Rationale

Quality of life is dependent on an environment that protects and promotes the health of individuals, families, and communities. Responsible citizens, who are health literate, are characterized by advocating and communicating for positive health in their communities. A variety of health advocacy skills are critical to these activities.

Performance Indicators

As a result of health instruction in grades K–4, students will

1. describe a variety of methods to convey accurate health information and ideas

2. express information and opinions about health issues

3. identify community agencies that advocate for healthy individuals, families, and communities

4. demonstrate the ability to influence and support others in making positive health choices

As a result of health instruction in grades 5–8, students will

1. analyze various communication methods to accurately express health information and ideas

2. express information and opinions about health issues

3. identify barriers to effective communication of information, ideas, feelings, and opinions about health issues

4. demonstrate the ability to influence and support others in making positive health choices

5. demonstrate the ability to work cooperatively when advocating for healthy individuals, families, and schools

SOURCE: Joint Committee on National Health Education Standards 1995

It is recommended that the KYB program be taught for a minimum of forty minutes per week. Most teachers are able to use the program much more often because of its interdisciplinary approach.

The KYB program addresses the National Goals for Education in several ways. Through its substance use prevention, healthy relationship, and skill modules, the program can help reduce drug use and violence (goal seven). As part of the KYB training, program coordinators learn how to improve their school food service programs as well as how to achieve a smoke-free campus, thereby creating an "environment conducive to learning."

Me-Me Drug and Alcohol Prevention Education Program. This is a school-based, multidisciplinary, year-long prevention program for grades 1 through 6 that helps improve children's self-esteem, improve their ability to solve problems and make responsible decisions, and increase their knowledge about the dangers of all drugs.

Description. The Me-Me Drug and Alcohol Prevention Education Program was developed to improve low self-esteem and other conditions found to be evident in most young people and adults who abuse drugs and alcohol. The program places great emphasis on enhancing the self-esteem of children during their formative years when most of their learning and self-identify development takes place. Children learn to make responsible decisions by learning how to predict the consequences of their choices and by recognizing and resisting negative peer influences. They receive the most up-to-date information about the dangers of all drugs—including prescription and over-the-counter medicines, and alcohol. The Me-Me Program meets the National Goals for Education that pertain to (1) student achievement and citizenship and (2) safe, disciplined, drug-free schools. All classroom teachers (K through 6) are responsible for implementing the program and coordinating their teaching styles with the program's goals. Activities are incorporated into all areas of the curriculum as well as into noncurriculum areas. An entirely new curriculum has been written and expanded to include other areas of concern. For example, a parent component for each area of emphasis has been added that includes areas not previously explored in other programs. All teachers must attend a six-hour training conducted at their site. Program expenses include manuals for each teacher and travel, lodging, and meal expenses for the trainer. Everything used in the program is found in the manuals. Technical assistance is available. General information about the program is available at no cost, and program staff are available to conduct awareness sessions.

Growing Healthy. Growing Healthy is a comprehensive health education program designed for grades K through 6 to foster student competencies to make decisions enhancing their health and lives.

Description. Growing Healthy includes a planned sequential curriculum, a variety of teaching methods, a teacher training program, and strategies for eliciting community support for school health education. Through group and individual activities, children learn about themselves by learning about their bodies. There is one eight- to twelve-week unit for each of the grades K through 6. Each grade studies a separate unit specifically designed for their age group. The units include an introduction of the five senses, feelings, caring for health, wellness, and general health habits; the senses of taste, touch, and smell and their roles in communicating health information; the emotions and communication methods with regard to sight and hearing; the skeletal and muscular systems; the digestive system; the respiratory system; the circulatory system; and the nervous system. Throughout all grades, health information about safety, nutrition, environment, drugs and alcohol, hygiene, fitness, mental health, disease prevention, consumer health, wellness, and lifestyle is explored and reinforced. Access to a variety of learning resources, including audiovisuals, models, community health workers, and reading materials, is provided. The curriculum is designed to integrate with the lives and personality development of children by providing situations in which they may assume responsibility, research ideas, share knowledge, discuss values, make decisions, and create activities to illustrate their comprehension and internalization of concepts, attitudes, and feelings. The curriculum has been developed to enhance other school subjects such as reading, writing, arithmetic, physical education, science, and the creative arts. Twenty-four separate studies, including a ten-year longitudinal study, indicate that Growing Healthy is effective in increasing health-related knowledge and providing positive health-related attitudes. Growing Healthy requires a school team composed of two classroom teachers, the principal, and one or more curriculum support persons to receive training in the grade level being adopted.

Project CHOICE. This is a cancer prevention program for students grades K through 12.

Description. Project CHOICE lessons are taught during a two-week time period at each grade level. The Project CHOICE curriculum consists of comprehensive, sequential units that promote three primary learning goals: (1) Students will learn cancer information and components of cancer risk, (2) students will learn a rational process of information evaluation and decision making, and (3) students will assume the locus of responsibility for behaviors leading to cancer risk reduction and wellness.

The curriculum kits include original filmstrips, experiments, decision-making scenarios, group work, classroom reports, debates, and discussions. The overall program emphasis is on positive health promotion, personal responsibility for health, the role of health professionals, and an understanding of risk and risk reduction concepts. The lesson themes attempt to replace a fear of cancer with a positive and active approach to maintaining health. At different grade levels, the units deal with seven broad areas of cancer risk: host factors; drugs, including alcohol and tobacco; occupational hazards; stress; environmental factors, including radiation exposure; nutrition; and sun exposure.

Not all cancers can or will be eliminated by cancer risk reduction practices; therefore, students are taught to understand and recognize cancer warning signs, methods of early detection, appropriate treatment, and unproven methods of cancer treatment. By developing their own personal cancer risk reduction plans, students enhance their awareness of their own responsibility for their health. Teachers are provided with complete lesson plans, student learning objectives, a *Cancer Resource Guide* with information that corresponds to lesson content, and all teaching materials.

Social Decision Making and Problem Solving. This program teaches children to "think clearly" under stress. The program is curriculum-based and occurs in three developmental phases. The readiness phase targets self-control, group participation, and social awareness skills. The instructional phase teaches an eight-step social decision-making strategy to students. The application phase teaches children to use these skills in real-life interpersonal and academic situations.

Description. Social Decision Making and Problem Solving works by training educators and parents to equip children with skills in self-control and group participation, the use of an eight-step social decision-making strategy, and the practical knowledge regarding the use of these skills in real life and academic areas.

The primary objective is to teach children a set of heuristic social decision-making steps. Lessons are taught to the children on a regular basis by their classroom teacher. Extensive guided practice and role playing are used, as is skill modeling and the use of hypothetical social problem situations. Facilitative questioning and dialogue stimulate the integration of the techniques. And cooperative group projects and writing assignments further advance that process. The Social Decision Making program targets the National Goals for Education, which address substance abuse and violence, the rights and responsibilities of citizenship, productive employment, and the critical thinking skills inherent in all aspects of academic and social learning.

OTHER TEACHING MATERIALS

Agencies such as the American Cancer Society, American Heart Association, March of Dimes, American Red Cross, American Dental Association, and American Dairy Association provide free and inexpensive materials through their local affiliates.

Developing a Health Curriculum

A health curriculum is a comprehensive plan for kindergarten through twelfth grade, designed to encompass pertinent health concerns and provide learning experiences throughout the school years. Such a plan should help promote responsible decisions and practices regarding personal, family, and community health. A comprehensive school health education plan should be prepared for each local school district and then developed for the individual schools within the district. Although a district may elect to use a state-developed or other existing curriculum, in some cases, the decision may be made to develop a new curriculum approach.

There are numerous commercial programs that have potential for inclusion in an elementary or middle school health education curriculum. The Centers for Disease Control and Prevention (CDC) has a Web site (*www.cdc.gov/nccdphp/dash/atc/index.html*) working on a new process that will help meet the needs of state and local schools in identifying appropriate health risk reduction programs for elementary, middle, and secondary schools. At the time of this publication, the process for helping the state and local agencies has not been fully identified. However, information concerning curricula that were endorsed as being effective under the old *Programs That Work* can still be obtained by calling CDC DASH information services at 1-888-231-6405.

THE MICHIGAN MODEL—A STATE MODEL

Although there is not an officially mandated national curriculum, several models have been suggested as possibilities. An excellent model that several states have adopted is the Michigan Model for Comprehensive School Health Education. The model was a result of a coalition of eight state agencies that included the Department of Education, Department of Public Health, Department of Social Services, Department of Mental Health, Department of State Police, Office of Substance Abuse Services, Office of Health and Medical Affairs, and Office of

Table 3.1 *Content Areas and Grade-Level Concerns of the Michigan Model*

	K	1	2	3	4	5	6	7	8
Sexual behavior						■	■	■	■
■ HIV	■	■	■	■	■	■	■	■	■
■ Other STIs					■	■		■	■
■ Teen pregnancy							■	■	■
Tobacco Use									
■ Smoking	■	■	■	■	■	■	■	■	■
■ Smokeless			■			■			■
Substance abuse	■	■	■	■	■	■	■	■	■
Injury prevention	■	■	■	■	■	■	■	■	■
Suicide prevention								■	■
Nutrition	■	■	■	■	■	■	■	■	■
Physical activity	■	■	■	■	■	■	■	■	■

Highway Safety Planning. In addition, over 120 voluntary and professional groups agreed to promote comprehensive health education.

Currently, 85 percent of Michigan's public schools have implemented the model. The model also is being implemented in 129 of Michigan's private schools. Throughout the United States other public and private school systems have also adopted the program. Over one million students have been reached through implementation of the Michigan Model. The parent/family involvement component of the curriculum has been expanded to include a magazine that is available to parents, community groups, physcians, and youth-serving groups to inform people concerning the content of school and community resources. In addition, a series of videos are designed to be watched by families and to inform parents on health and parenting topics. Table 3.1 contains the scope and sequence plan for the content areas offered through the Michigan Model. Table 3.2 lists the classroom time required at each grade level.

TEACHING UNITS

A **teaching unit** is an organized method for developing lesson plans for a particular group of students and thus can be tailored to each classroom. The resource unit serves as a guide, whereas the teaching unit is the plan for student learning. Unlike the resource unit, which is prepared by a curriculum committee, the teaching unit is developed by the classroom teacher. It is specific; the resource unit is general. The teacher selects the specific concepts to be studied, as well as the objectives, content, learning strategies, evaluation methods, and references that will be used in class. Given a well-developed resource unit that identifies major concepts, creating a teaching unit is fairly easy. In addition to the resource unit, the state health education guidelines, the teacher's edition of the classroom textbook, and various materials from health-related agencies can all be used to develop the teaching unit. In preparing a teaching unit, a variety of

Table 3.2	Classroom Time Required at Each Grade for the Michigan Model Curriculum	
	Average Minutes per Session	Number of Sessions per Year
K	30	39
1	30	40
2	30	37
3	40	40
4	40	39
5	40	44
6	40	40
7	50	59
8	50	63

formats can be used, depending on individual preference. The Teaching in Action box on the following page illustrates a typical format.

LESSON PLANNING—SELECTED STRATEGIES

Once the teaching unit has been developed, plans are made for how to teach the unit. This is done by creating daily lesson plans that provide a logical progression of the unit from start to finish. Each lesson plan must be based on concepts taught in previous lessons so that learning builds on the established base.

The Teaching in Action box on page 58 shows a typical daily lesson plan for grade 3. Notice that the format of this lesson plan parallels the format used for the teaching unit. A conceptual statement and performance indicator are stated for that day. (**Performance indicators** are the expectations of what the students will demonstrate if the intended instruction and learning have taken place.) The content outline provides a summary of the main topics to be covered. The strategies are the heart of the lesson plan. They should be described in detail and listed in the order in which they are to be used.

As shown in the daily lesson plan example, each strategy should be followed by an evaluation activity ("Closure for Strategies"). Through this activity, the teacher will be able to judge to some extent how well the students have learned the concept presented. Because the strategy is a performance in nature, it can also be used to determine how well the objectives have been achieved.

Deciding Student Outcomes

Keeping with the philosophy of focusing on individual health behaviors that represent at least half the causes of premature death and illness, health educators have moved away from the traditional concept of behavioral objectives to

TEACHING IN ACTION *Typical Unit Format*

Title of Unit: <u>Eating for Good Health</u>   Grade Level: <u>K-4</u>

Performance Indicator: <u>The student will demonstrate the ability to apply decision making in food selection</u>
<u>and eating patterns.</u>

Instructional Objectives: Student will	Content	Strategies/ Learning Activites	Evaluation Strategies	References: A. Student B. Teacher
Place foods that are found on the food pyramid in their proper category	I. Food Groups A. Milk, yogurt & cheese: cheese, ice cream, cottage cheese B. Meat, poultry, fish, dry beans, eggs, & nuts pork, fish, dry beans, beef C. Fruits: oranges, apples, peaches, pears D. Vegetables: corn, green beans, beets, squash E. Bread, cereal, rice and pasta rice, bread, whole grains II. Serving Sizes A. Milk, yogurt, & cheese B. Meat, poultry, fish C. Fruits D. Vegetables E. Bread, cereal, rice & pasta	1. Discuss the four food groups, why they are important, and what foods are in each group. 2. Have students play grocery store with empty cartons, cans, etc., and place one food from each of the food groups in their sack. 3. By using wrappers from a fast-food restaurant, the students pretend that they are at a fast-food hamburger restaurant and they choose one food from each of the basic food groups to form a nutritious meal. Follow up with a field trip to a hamburger restaurant.	1. List four foods for each group. 2. From a group of pictures, ask the students to choose a food from each food group to form a nutritious menu for a day.	A. Student FILMSTRIPS The Fruits and Vegetables, Encyclopedia Britannica Educational Corporation. 1997 Foods from Grains, Coronet BOOKS Richmond, et al., <u>You and Your Health, II.</u> 1997. Scott Foresman Fodor, et al., <u>Being Healthy,</u> 1996. Laidlaw Bisc, Chapter 6. B. Teacher BOOKS <u>You and Your Health II,</u> 1997. Scott Foresman, Chapter 3. Fodor, et al., <u>Being Healthy,</u> 1996. Laidlaw Bisc, Chapter 6.

TEACHING IN ACTION *Daily Lesson Plan*

Lesson Title: <u>Mental Health——Getting to Know Me</u>

Date: <u>February 19, 2001</u>   Time: <u>10:00 am</u>   Grade: <u>Three</u>   Teacher: <u>Avery</u>

Instructional Objective: <u>Students will identify several emotions & state acceptable ways to express them.</u>

Teacher Needs: <u>Pictures of people expressing emotions, crayons, paper. Write role-playing situations.</u>

Content (Progression)

Emotion——the way we feel

A. Anger

B. Love

C. Sadness

D. Fear

E. Excitement

Expressing Emotions

A. Facial expression
  1) Smile
  2) Frown
  3) Tears
  4) Eyes

B. Talking
  1) Soft voice
  2) Loud voice
  3) Excited voice
  4) Fast voice
  5) Slow voice

C. Body language
  1) Using arms
  2) Kissing
  3) Clapping

Strategies (Full Description)

1. Discuss what feelings are and list on the board. Show pictures of people displaying different emotions. Use several pictures that reflect certain emotions.

2. Discuss ways we express emotions. Ask students to give ways that are acceptable/unacceptable means of expressing feelings. Have students role-play these ways to express the various emotions.

Closure for Strategies

1. Give children crayons & have them draw a face of the emotion requested.
   <u>Processing Questions</u>
   A. How many of you have used one of the emotions drawn?
   B. What are some of the reasons we express an emotion?

2. Give the children a situation that illustrates an expression of a particular emotion. Have them role-play an acceptable way to express the emotion.
   <u>Processing Questions</u>
   A. What ways are best for expressing our emotions?
   B. What are some ways we should not express our emotions?
   C. Is it "OK" to get angry? Cry? Hit someone?

Teacher evaluation

1. Keep the lesson as taught? yes _____   no _____

2. What I need to improve _____

3. Next time make sure _____

4. Strengths of lesson _____

what the Joint Committee on National Health Standards (1995) refer to as performance indicators. These are a series of specific concepts and skills students should know and be able to do in order to achieve each of the National Health Educations Standards.

From these writers' perspective, an excellent way of measuring performance indicators is through the development of sound instructional objectives. In particular, broad-scope measurable objectives are most helpful in assessing fulfillment. Performance indicators can help identify potential assessment areas, particularly when viewed within the three areas of framework found in Bloom's Taxonomies of Educational Objectives (Bloom 1956). The three domains are cognitive or knowledge; affective or attitudes/values; and behavioral, which focuses on skills or behavior. The problem in using this framework is that the emphasis may be only on the cognitive or knowledge component. However, it is imperative in the teaching of health education to recognize that learning is reflected in other ways than simply in recalling the content of health education. The ability to think, judge, evaluate, and act on the information is more important than simple recall of facts. Nonetheless, instructional objectives can provide a framework for performance indicators, as mentioned in Chapter 5. What is important to remember is students must not only have a correct knowledge base, but they must also be able to evaluate and clarify their values/feelings if they are to select behaviors conducive to optimal health. Experiences must enable students to examine their beliefs and facilitate the skills of decision making, resulting in the potential for a positive lifestyle.

WRITING INSTRUCTIONAL OBJECTIVES

To consider important only what can be measured results in the trivialization of instruction. What can be accomplished through well-planned instructional objectives is exposure to all three domains so that students can make decisions that have the potential to enhance the overall quality of health throughout life. Children can be helped to internalize information so that it helps them make decisions that lead to positive health behaviors. The use of instructional objectives is a start in the right direction.

It is useful to think of instructional objectives as having five components. Definitions and examples of these components follow.

1. **Who**—the student or the one who is to exhibit the knowledge, attitude, or behavior as the result of the teaching/learning process.

2. **Behavior expected**—what the student will do to show that learning has taken place.

3. **Learning requirement**—what the student will know, feel, or do when the learning is completed. For example, "the student will label the diagram." It is generally a good idea to keep the verb as action-oriented as possible. However, the preciseness demanded by many educators has been replaced by the concept that the objective should be as broad in scope as possible, salient, and measurable (Popham 1995). An example of a broad-scope objective might be as follows: "After reading a selected article on the social and physiological effects of alcohol, the student will

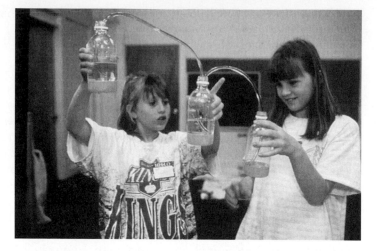

Learning activities help children internalize the content and form concepts. The teacher must select the activities that are best suited to each class.

compose a critical essay on the potential dangers of alcohol use associated with their personal use."

4. **Conditions**—the specific conditions under which the student will be expected to do the activity; for example, on a test, orally, or working in a group.

5. **Standard of performance**—the minimum level of achievement, either quantitative or qualitative, that will be accepted as meeting the requirements for demonstrating successful achievement; for example, 80 percent correct, writing a critical essay, constructing an exhibit, judged acceptable by a group of peers (peer evaluation).

In using instructional objectives, the teacher should strive to develop a reasonable number of manageable, broad, yet measurable objectives that will help in assessing whether students have achieved the desired performance level. Attempting to become too precise in stating the objective may limit or obscure other valid indicators of a skill or ability. Instructional objectives should be viewed as starting points; they are not the totality of quality education. An alternate behavior exhibited by the student at the end of instruction may be an equally valid indicator that learning has taken place. With performance-based evaluation (see Chapter 5), the use of many different indicators of learning and behavior is now being fully recognized and appreciated.

Summary

- Teachers must recognize the complexity of life and seek to incorporate the dimensions of wellness into the teaching of health education.

- Content must be organized to ensure comprehensive coverage of grades K through 12.

- Scope and sequence must be considered when developing curriculum.
- The National Health Education Standards provide the foundation for curriculum development and instruction.
- Health topics should be based on the needs, interests, and comprehension ability of the students.
- Health literacy is the ability of the student to obtain, interpret, and understand basic health information and services and the competence to use information and services in ways that enhance health.
- Effective health education requires a balance between factual information and the attitude or valuing component.
- Time must be allotted for examining values and for practicing critical thinking skills.
- Many useful curriculum approaches are offered through the NDN, the CDC, and state departments of education.
- The Michigan Model is an excellent example of a curriculum plan that used a coalition of state and voluntary agencies to develop a comprehensive approach to health education.
- Outcome-based education as measured using performance indicators is the direction in which health education is currently moving.

DISCUSSION QUESTIONS

1. What determines the nature of the content for a given grade level?
2. What is meant by the "scope and sequence" of health education?
3. Why are the National Health Education Standards important?
4. What are some barriers to quality health education?
5. Describe what is meant by the phrase "teaching for values."
6. What is the NDN?
7. What types of standards, curriculum guides, etc. are available from your state to help provide guidelines for teaching health education?
8. How does your state curriculum model for health education compare with the Michigan Model?
9. What purpose do objectives fulfill in the educational process?
10. What is outcome-based education?

CRITICAL THINKING QUESTIONS

1. Review the National Health Education Standards. Do they reflect what a "health-educated" child needs to know, value, and do to live a quality life that maximizes his or her potential? Are there modifications or additions you would make to better express the needs of the K through 8 child?
2. Review the *Programs That Work* from the CDC Web site and evaluate them as to whether they meet the criteria suggested in the textbook by the NDN. What

(if anything) do the commercial programs need to meet the criteria established by the NDN? You may wish to compare a curriculum suggested by your instructor rather than one found in the text.

WEB SITE ACTIVITY

Select one of the Web sites listed below and search for position papers on various health education concerns. Review one of the position papers to determine if the way health is currently taught is reflected in the position paper.

WEB SITES OF INTEREST

American Association for Health Education
www.aahperd.org/aahe/aahe-main.html

American Medical Association: *www.ama-assn.org*

American School Health Association: *www.ashaweb.org*

CDC's Comprehensive School Activities
www.cdc.gov/nccdphd/dash/rtc/index.htm

Children's Defense Fund: *www.childrendefense.org*

National Center for Health Education, Growing Healthy curriculum
www.nche.org

Youth Risk Behavior Surveillance System: *www.cdc.gov/nccdphp/dash/yrbs*

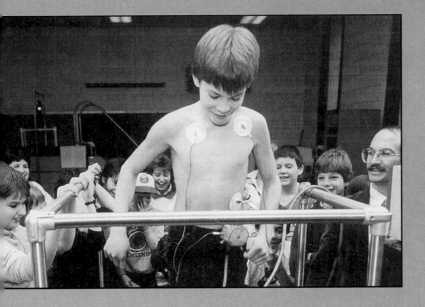

CHAPTER FOUR

Strategies for Implementing Health Instruction

School health programs offer the opportunity for us to provide the services and knowledge necessary to enable children to be productive learners and to develop the skills to make healthy decisions for the rest of their lives.

—National School Boards Association et al. (1995)

VALUED OUTCOMES

After reading this chapter, you should be able to:

- list the factors that affect teaching strategy selection
- describe the elements of an effective decision-making model
- list reasons why developing refusal skills is important
- discuss the various styles of learning
- describe the implications of multiple intelligence on teaching
- discuss the salient points to consider when selecting strategies for the various learning styles
- describe the various forms of clarifying strategies

- describe the effective use of decision stories
- describe how to effectively use role-playing in the classroom
- discuss ways to use technology in the classroom
- identify different strategies that enhance learning for the different styles

REFLECTIONS

As you read through this chapter, try to think of situations in which students might use the various strategies. This helps students personalize the information and formulate their feelings about the material presented. Think in terms of what learning styles might be best suited to the plethora of possibilities for developing a knowledge base and for personalizing information. Develop several scenarios for and various strategies to address each learning style.

The Relationship of Strategies to Learning

Learning strategies are things that make content and objectives come alive. This enlivening involves selecting strategies and techniques that make learning exciting and motivating. Carrying this out is the direct responsibility of teachers, who, having established a working knowledge of the many strategies available in health education, are limited only by their own creativity.

A **strategy** is any activity or experience that teachers use to interpret, illustrate, or facilitate learning. Foder and Dalis (1989) view a strategy as anything used with or on students to accomplish the objectives of the program. For the most effective learning to take place, teachers should seek strategies that are student-centered and provide for group involvement. Additionally, they should use more than one strategy or activity for each major concept so that their instruction more fully encompasses the variety of student abilities and aptitudes.

The teacher must remember that selecting a variety of strategies does not ensure learning. Several other factors influence effective learning and must be considered, such as a relationship with the students that is conducive to learning. Treating students fairly is the first step in facilitating learning and creating a proper classroom atmosphere. Many techniques to help promote creative learning are available. With proper preparation, the following strategies can be useful:

audiocassettes	CD-ROMs	demonstrations/
brainstorming	charts/maps	experiments
bulletin boards	computers	dramatization
buzz groups	cooperative	DVDs
case studies/	learning	exhibits
committee work	debates	field trips

magazines	resource speakers	transparencies
newspapers	role-playing	values clarification
panel discussion	self-appraisals	videotapes
peer helpers	slides	word searches/
posters	specimens/models	crosswords
puppet shows	storytelling	
radio	television	

FACTORS AFFECTING STRATEGIES

When selecting strategies to provide learning experiences, keep the following criteria in mind:

Select strategies that contribute to total learning. Some activities lend themselves to acquiring knowledge, whereas others are better suited to attitude assessment and decision making. Ideally, the strategies selected should help the student develop the ability to reason and assess the information being presented. Any strategy selected should involve the students as participants in the activity.

The more complex the concept, the more activities are needed to develop the concept. As a general rule, for each concept, two strategies or activities should be employed. If the material being studied is difficult, more than two strategies or activities should be used. Another reason for using more than one strategy is that students learn in a variety of ways and through different means. Thus, a variety of strategies will help all students to grasp the concept under examination.

The strategies selected should begin with the simple and move to the more complex. Once the teacher has prepared the class for the activity through a proper introduction, the students should become part of the learning activity. With simple activities, students should be able to learn by means of group involvement, self-assessment, and class–teacher interaction. As the students become better able to deal with more difficult topics, more complex strategies can be used that require self-discovery or analysis of materials and conclusions.

Audiovisual aids should be included whenever possible. These can include models, classroom exhibits, videos, DVDs, CD-ROMs, and so forth. Audiovisual aids add another dimension to teaching concepts and are excellent for reinforcing learning.

Strategies can be classified into many different categories. Some authorities distinguish between strategies, media, and instructional materials, whereas others group all three into one category. Classification is unimportant as long as you can identify the strengths and weaknesses of each available technique. Your objective should be to select strategies that are appropriate and effective with your class and that are based on the learning styles of the students.

In the strategy chapters that follow, suggested grade levels are provided for which the various activities are best suited. It is important to remember that with minor changes, most activities would be appropriate for use at other grade levels and can be used in combinations to optimize the desired mix of learning styles.

LEARNING STYLES AND STRATEGIES SELECTION

Having insight into the different types of learning styles is useful for many reasons. When planning a health lesson, it is most important to employ a variety of strategies that appeal to the three basic learning styles: through sight (visual), sound (auditory), and touch/doing (kinesthetic).

It is impossible to address the many different theories of learning styles within the context of this book. Fortunately, most theories are similar in concept. Children—like all people—learn new information in different ways. Using a strategy that does not "fit" with a particular child's learning style will result in an inability to successfully process information. Thus, having a basic understanding of differences in learning styles and planning strategies can contribute to successful learning, assessment, and, ultimately, behavior change.

As learners we perceive information differently. Some of us are "feelers," others are "thinkers." Feelers absorb life experiences through their senses; for them, learning is a form of intuition. These experiential learners learn best in situations where their emotions are used, or where they can interact with someone who has experienced previously. A "feeler" is more likely than a thinker to be affected by hearing someone talk about a personal perspective.

Thinkers perceive reality by thinking about it. They are analytical by nature, approach new information logically, and look at data objectively. Thinkers respond to data they can analyze and from which they can draw conclusions. Lists, statistics, and facts appeal to this type of learner (McCarthy 1987).

The following list explains the differences between the psychological types:

Feelers—validate events and perceptions based on emotions, tend to be very aware of other people and their feelings, are people-oriented and sympathetic, and need love and harmony

Thinkers—arrange life events into rational categories, do not readily show emotion, judge categories and their content, and make decisions impersonally

Sensors—consciously perceive events but do not categorize them, do things in established ways, are good at precise work, work steadily, and are patient with details

Intuitors—apprehend instinctively, like solving problems, reach conclusions quickly, work in bursts of energy with slack time in between, and are patient in complicated situations

We also process information in different ways—by doing or by watching/ listening. Combinations of how people perceive (feelers or thinkers) and how they process (by doing or watching/listening) can reflect, therefore, four different styles of processing (see Figure 4.1). People who take in information by feeling and process it by watching are said to learn by "reflective observation"

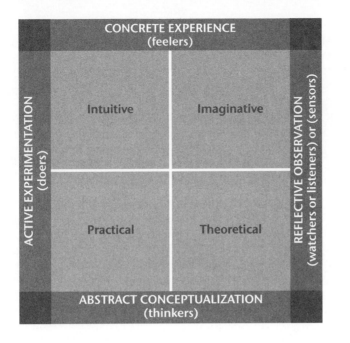

Figure 4.1
Learning Styles

(watchers). People who perceive by thinking rationally and process by watching are described as "abstract conceptualization" learners (thinkers). People who take in information by analysis and then process it through action are said to use "active experimentation" (doers), and those who perceive through their feelings and act according to what they feel are designated "concrete experience" learners (feelers) (Jung 1976, 150).

Learners "learn" when issues are addressed using the basic concepts to which they respond best. The concrete experience learners (feelers) are interested in personal meaning. They want to have a reason to learn new information or adapt new behaviors. They like to discuss. They want to know "why." Reflective observers (sensors) are most interested in data. They want to use facts to provide them with a deeper understanding of what needs to be done and how to do it. Abstract conceptualizers (thinkers) will want to try new things. They want to think about what needs to be done and then have the opportunity to do it. Active experimenters (intuitives) want the opportunity for self-discovery. They want to "feel" the experience by interacting with others. Most children will tend toward a particular learning type but will have some characteristics of other learning styles from time to time.

It is important for teachers to build in various strategies that will appeal to the various learning styles. One problem is that teachers unconsciously tend to select the strategies they use themselves. Teachers must constantly remind themselves to use a variety of approaches to facilitate knowledge assimilation, assessment of information, and influence behavior change.

An inventory developed by G. Price and R. Dunn (see Table 4.1) was the first comprehensive approach to the assessment of student learning styles. The inventory, called the Learning Style Inventory (LSI), is designed for grades 3

Table 4.1 *Environmental, Instructional, Social Groupings, and Motivating Factors That Maximize Individual Learning*

Area	Student Preference
Noise level	Does the child prefer quiet or sound when learning?
Light	Does the student work best under bright lights or need dim or indirect light?
Temperature	Does the child concentrate best in a warm or cool environment?
Design	Does the student learn best in a formal environment, such as the classroom, or an informal environment, such as on a lounge chair, bed, or floor?
Unmotivated/self-motivated	Does the child do well to please him- or herself?
Not persistent/persistent	What is the student's inclination to complete tasks: to complete the task once begun or to take intermittent breaks?
Not responsible/responsible	What is the student's desire to do what he or she thinks ought to be done? Students with low responsibility scores usually are nonconforming.
Structure	Does the student need specific directions or explanations when doing a task or prefer doing an assignment his or her own way?
Learning alone/peer-oriented learner	Does the student prefer to study alone or with a friend/group?
Authority figures present	Does the student feel more comfortable when someone with authority or special knowledge is present?
Prefers learning in several ways	Does the child need a variety of learning situations as opposed to routines for learning?
Auditory preferences	Does the child learn best listening to verbal instructions?
Visual preferences	Does the child learn visually? An example is a child who can close her eyes and visually recall what she has read or seen earlier.
Tactile Preferences	Does the student need to underline while reading, take notes when listening, or keep his or her hands busy?
Kinesthetic preferences	Does the child require whole-body movement and/or real life experiences to best retain material?
Requires intake	Does the student seem to eat, drink, chew, or bite objects while concentrating, or learn best with no such intake?
Functions best in evening/morning	What time of day does the student prefer to learn?
Functions best in late morning	Does the child prefer to learn during the late morning? The energy curve for these students is highest in late morning around 10 A.M.
Functions best in afternoon	Does the child prefer to learn during the afternoon? Energy level higher after lunch hour.
Mobility	How long can the child sit?
Parent figure–motivated	Does the individual want to do well to please the parent(s)?
Teacher-motivated	Does the student want to learn and complete tasks to please the teacher?

SOURCE: *Learning Style Inventory* (LSI). Price Systems, Box 1818, Lawrence, KS 66044. Reprinted by permission.

through 12. The LSI seeks to provide those elements that are imperative to children learning. What is unique about the LSI is that it identifies the type of environment, instructional activities, social grouping(s), and motivating factors that maximize individual learning (Price and Dunn 1997, 5). The LSI surveys each student's preferences in each of twenty-two different areas, and it provides information as to how children prefer to function, learn, concentrate, and perform during educational strategies.

This scheme of learning may seem a bit overwhelming, but teachers must have a conceptualization of what strategies to employ in the classroom if their students are to learn best. Teachers can use the awareness provided by the LSI to build in a variety of learning situations and environments and thus enhance the learning potential of their students.

MULTIPLE INTELLIGENCE— IMPLICATIONS FOR HEALTH EDUCATION

In 1993, Howard Gardner, a professor of psychology at Harvard University, defined seven types of intelligence. Since this initial group of seven, two other types have been added for a total of nine types. The nine types of intelligence that have been identified are shown in the Health Highlight box on page 70.

According to multiple intelligences theory, all humans possess—in varying amounts—the nine identified types. Each person has different intellectual compositions. From the perspective of health education, the concept of multiple intelligences provides several thoughts concerning the planning of strategies for successful teaching. Many of these concepts have already been pointed out in the preceding sections of this chapter. However, the keys to multiple intelligences theory are successful strategy planning and implementation in the classroom. The guidelines below reflect the essential items for lesson planning that address multiple inteligences theory (Concept to Classroom: Tapping into Multiple Intelligence—Implementation 2002).

Teach subject matter through a variety of activities and projects. The classroom should be filled with engaging activities that evoke a range of intelligences. Students should be encouraged to work collaboratively as well as individually to support both their interpersonal and intrapersonal intelligences.

Assessments should be integrated into learning. Students need to play an active role in their assessments. Students should be offered a number of choices for "showing what they know" about a topic. In addition to traditional paper-and-pencil tests the student should be given opportunities to create meaningful projects and authentic presentations.

All students have all intelligences. These should be nurtured throughout the whole spectrum of types to foster their learning and strengthen their entire intelligence.

THE NINE MULTIPLE INTELLIGENCES

1. **Verbal-Linguistic**—well-developed verbal skills and sensitivity to the sounds, meaning and rhythms of words. A child whose strength is in this area enjoys language arts, that is, speaking, writing, reading, and listening. This child will do well in the traditional classroom.

2. **Mathematical-Logical**—ability to think conceptually and abstractly and has the capacity to discern logical or numerical patterns. Children with this strength have an aptitude for numbers, reasoning, and problem solving. These children will also do well in the traditional classroom, where teaching is logically sequenced and students are asked to conform.

3. **Musical Intelligence**—ability to produce and appreciate rhythm, pitch, and timber. These children learn well through songs, patterns, rhythms, instruments, and musical expression.

4. **Visual-Spatial**—capacity to think in images and pictures, to visualize accurately and abstractly. These children learn best through visuals and spatial organization. They like to see what you are talking about in order to understand. They enjoy charts, graphs, maps, tables, illustrations, art, and puzzles.

5. **Bodily–Kinesthetic**—ability to control one's body movements and to handle objects skillfully. These children learn best through activities like games, movement, and hands-on tasks such as building something. They may be labeled "overly active" in traditional classrooms where they are told to sit and be still.

6. **Interpersonal**—capacity to detect and respond appropriately to the moods, motivations, and desires of others. This child is people-oriented and outgoing and does his or her learning cooperatively in groups or with a partner. He or she may be labeled as "talkative" or "too concerned about being social."

7. **Intrapersonal**—capacity to be self-aware and in tune with inner feelings, values, beliefs, and thinking processes. These children are especially in touch with their own feelings, values, and ideas. They may appear to be reserved but are quite intuitive about what they learn and how it relates to themselves.

8. **Naturalist**—ability to recognize and categorize plants, animals, and other objects in nature. These children love the outdoors, animals, and field trips. They also like to pick up on subtle differences in meanings.

9. **Existential**—sensitivity and capacity to tackle deep questions about human existence, such as what is the meaning of life, why do we die, and how did we get here. These children learn in the context of where humankind stands in the "big picture" of existence. They ask "Why are we here?" and "What is our role in the world?"

SOURCE: Adapted from McKenzie 1999

Decision Making and Health Strategies

As you have seen, it is important for students to have an opportunity to personalize information and make decisions relative to their health. They also must have a model that helps them assess the possibilities and consequences of their potential actions. If students are to make positive health decisions, the process of how to make intelligent decisions is crucial. These skills must be taught and utilized throughout the educational experience, and students must practice making decisions and enhance their decision-making skills. This practice goes beyond the model and helps them feel good about themselves (self-esteem), see that they can have control of their behavior (locus of control), and believe in their own decision-making skills (self-efficacy). See Chapter 6 for more information on self-esteem.

Several models can be utilized. A good model should have the characteristics described below.

1. It helps the student identify and define exactly what the problem/decision is.

2. It provides the opportunity to identify possible actions. It helps prepare the student to respond immediately to a situation and to formulate strategies for dealing with problems that do not require an immediate response.

3. It provides the opportunity to evaluate each of the possible actions the student might take to deal with the problem. Many alternative ways of dealing with the problem/situation should be identified—the more ideas the better.

4. The model must also provide a way to assess the possible results of the various potential decisions previously identified. Questions that might be asked during this time include the following:

   ■ What has worked in a similar situation?

   ■ What might work that has not been tried before?

   ■ What does the law say concerning the potential solution?

   ■ Would my parents be proud of the decision?

   ■ What are the pros and cons of each alternative solution?

   ■ What are my fears concerning each alternative?

   ■ What are my feelings concerning each alternative?

5. It provides the opportunity to share the information with several people if time warrants. Make sure one of the people is a responsible adult—preferably it would be a parent.

6. The model should help select the most appropriate action to be taken. Eliminate alternatives that are dangerous to oneself or others or are illegal. The model should help determine the following questions:

   ■ Does my decision contribute to my health and welfare?

   ■ Does my decision contribute to others' health and welfare?

   ■ Does my decision violate any laws or rules?

   ■ Does my decision show respect for myself?

   ■ Does my decision follow what responsible adults would do?

7. The model should help decide what steps must be taken to put the decision into action. Questions might include:

   ■ What do you need to do?

   ■ Where do you need help to enact your decision?

   ■ What is the timetable for enacting your decision?

8. Once the action has been taken, the model should help to reflect, evaluate, and revise the decision. Questions might include:

- How do I feel about the decision?
- Did it work out the way I wanted?
- What would I do differently?
- Would another alternative have worked better?

THE POWER MODEL FOR DECISION MAKING

Included in the Michigan Model for Comprehensive School Health Education is The POWER Model (reprinted by permission). It is an excellent example of a decision-making model that fulfills the above criteria. The POWER model, shown in the Teaching in Action box, can be used at all grade levels with minor modifications. For grades that have not yet developed their writing and reading skills, the teacher may have to read the headings and list the responses on an overhead or on the board. The important point is to introduce the steps for making wise decisions early in children's educational experience. As their skills improve, they can use the model in written form. Then they will have a framework for making decisions as their choices and consequences become more difficult. The model will probably have to be used in a group situation in early elementary grades but can be used in individual or group work for the later grades. An example demonstrating how the model works is given below.

Situation/Problem: Beth is a good friend of yours. She borrowed your favorite CD last week and has failed to return it. She has promised to bring it to school every day for the last several days but always says she forgot it. You are feeling very angry because you want to listen to the CD.

P: What's the PROBLEM?

The situation is:	My friend Beth borrowed my CD and hasn't returned it.
The facts are:	I loaned it to her last week, and she keeps promising to return it but hasn't. I want my CD back.
My feelings are:	I'm angry because Beth keeps breaking her promise. I'm disappointed because I thought I could trust her.
I think (concerning the situation):	I think I should not have loaned her the CD.
My friends think/ feel:	Some understand my feelings, others think I'm being stingy.
My problem is:	Beth has not returned my CD as she promised, and I want it back.

P: What's the PROBLEM?

The situation is: _____

The facts are: _____

My feelings are: _____

I think (concerning the situation): _____

My friends think/feel: _____

My problem is: _____

O: What are the OPTIONS?

The outcome I want is: _____

My options for reaching my outcome are:

    1. _____

    2. _____

    3. _____

    4. _____

    5. _____

W: WHAT'S BEST to do?

Try out the three best options:

1. If I did this:	**Possible Good Results**	**Possible Bad Results**
_____	_____	_____
_____	_____	_____

2. If I did this:	**Possible Good Results**	**Possible Bad Results**
_____	_____	_____
_____	_____	_____

3. If I did this:	**Possible Good Results**	**Possible Bad Results**
_____	_____	_____
_____	_____	_____

The option I chose: _____

E: ENACT your Plan

The steps I need to take are:

Task	*Who Does It*	*By When*
1. _____	_____	_____
2. _____	_____	_____
3. _____	_____	_____
4. _____	_____	_____
5. _____	_____	_____

I could get help from: _____

R: REFLECT on the outcome and REVISE your strategy (if necessary)

Now that the decision has been carried out:

I think _____

I feel _____

I achieved/did not achieve what I wanted because _____

and it turned out _____

I learned I _____

I learned that others _____

Next time I'll _____

O: What are the OPTIONS?

The outcome I want is: For Beth to return my CD and to keep her friendship.

My options for reaching my outcome are:

1. Ask Beth again.
2. Tell Beth how important the CD is to me.
3. Tell Beth she will not be my friend if she doesn't return the CD.
4. Talk to my parents.
5. Tomorrow call Beth's parents.

W: WHAT'S BEST to do?

Try out the three best options:

1. *If I did this:* Called Beth's parents

Possible Good Results	Possible Bad Results
Now: I'll get my CD back.	Beth could be in trouble.
Later: They might get Beth her own CD.	Beth would not be my friend.

2. *If I did this:* Told Beth how important the CD is to me

Possible Good Results	Possible Bad Results
Now: She might understand and give the CD back.	She'll just laugh at me.

3. *If I did this:* Talked to my parents

Possible Good Results	Possible Bad Results
Now: They would buy me a new CD.	My parents would be mad.

The option I chose: Tell Beth how important the CD is to me. I'll offer to call her in the morning to remind her to bring it to school.

E: ENACT your Plan

The steps I need to take are:

Task	Who Does It	By When
1. Find time to talk to Beth.	Me	After school
2. Ask Beth if I can talk with her.	Me	At lunch
3. Think about what I want to say.	Me	During study hall
4. Meet and talk with Beth.	Me	After school

I could get help from: My parents, my brother, Beth's parents

R: REFLECT on the outcome and REVISE strategy (if necessary)

Now that the decision has been carried out:

I think	telling people the truth works pretty well.
I feel	good that I confronted her.
I achieved/did not achieve what I wanted because	I got my CD back and I got it without hard feelings on the part of Beth—
and it turned out	well for me and Beth was not mad at me.
I learned I	do not have to allow a friend to take advantage of me.
I learned that others	will respond to a reasonable request.
Next time I'll	be more careful who I loan my things to and establish how long they can keep them.

It is suggested that you take the other four options formulated as possible solutions and work through the potential good and bad results of these. What option are *you* most comfortable with?

DEVELOPING REFUSAL SKILLS

Refusal skills are part of good decision making. We need good refusal skills when it is necessary to say "No" to an action or to leave a potentially harmful situation. Any situation that threatens personal safety (emotionally or physically) or health, tempts students to break the law, detracts from personal character, asks students to disobey parental rules, or results in loss of self-respect calls for strong refusal skills. The following rules teach students to develop good refusal skills.

Employ assertive behavior. Acting assertively is being honest with what you are thinking and feeling. It lets others know that you are in control of your behavior and the situation. You say "No" clearly and firmly while looking directly at the person you are addressing.

Use body language that matches your assertive verbal behavior. Your body language must indicate that you are sincere without being aggressive or disrespectful. It's also important to make sure your body language does not say "I would like to, but I don't think I can." Make it totally clear that you do not desire the drink, drug, or physical advances of the person with whom you are talking.

Don't get involved in potentially harmful/dangerous situations. Think ahead concerning potentially dangerous situations. Avoid allowing yourself to be in a place where you might be pressured or tempted.

Be a positive role model. Attempt to act and talk in a manner that commands respect and reflects your personal value system. You have a responsibility to protect yourself, obey the laws, and demonstrate good character. Your reputation is important, and the people you associate with should be known for their own good character.

You don't have to say "No, thank you." In a situation where you are feeling pressured there is no need to be polite. You are telling a person you do not appreciate his or her thought or action. You are being very emphatic that you want no part.

Each of the strategies chapters includes opportunities for children to practice both the decision-making skills and refusal skills. Only through practice and being prepared can children make decisions and be prepared to resist the many pressures they face during the formative years.

A Positive Climate for Learning

Regardless of the strategy employed, the teacher must strive to create a classroom environment that is conducive to learning. Students should look forward to class, feel emotionally/intellectually unthreatened, and realize that they will be supported in their learning efforts. There are several things a teacher can do to facilitate a positive learning climate.

- Identify appropriate instructional goals and discuss them with the student so that the intent is clear concerning what is expected.
- Insist that work be completed satisfactorily to mutually determined standards.
- Refuse to accept excuses for poor work.
- Communicate acceptance of imperfect initial performance when students struggle to achieve new learning.
- Convey confidence in the student's ability to do well.
- Display a "can do" attitude that generates student excitement and self-confidence.
- Avoid comparative evaluations, especially of lower-ability students, that might have them conclude they cannot meet expectations (Evertson et al. 1997, 123).

CLARIFYING ACTIVITIES

To personalize health concepts, students must relate to health instruction from the affective domain or attitudinal level. An excellent strategy for achieving this end is through the use of valuing strategies activities. By examining and clarifying values, children can learn positive health behavior. As mentioned earlier, however, the use of values clarification techniques is not without some controversy. Values cannot and should not be avoided when teaching health education, but the teacher must be adequately prepared to do the job correctly.

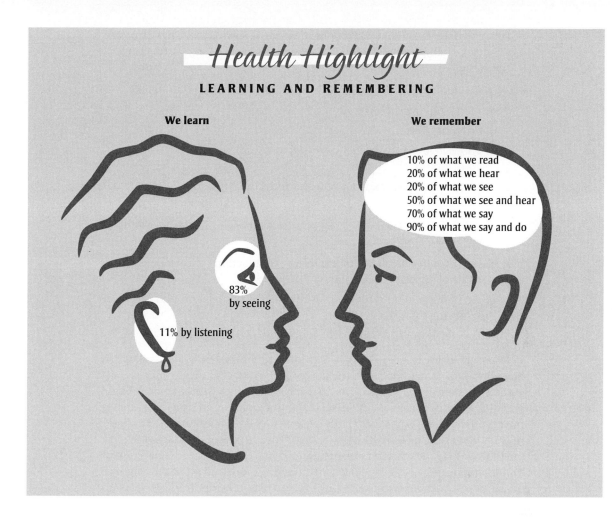

Health Highlight
LEARNING AND REMEMBERING

We learn

83% by seeing

11% by listening

We remember

10% of what we read
20% of what we hear
20% of what we see
50% of what we see and hear
70% of what we say
90% of what we say and do

Begin by recognizing that values are relative, personal, and often situational. You should not attempt to teach your own personal values or the "correct" values; instead, your goal should be to assist students in assessing and developing their own values so that these values lead to positive health behavior. It is essential that any value judgment made by the students be made through their own cognitive process. According to Hochbaum, Rosenstock, and Kegeles (1960), for a value judgment or health practice to evolve, the following criteria must apply:

- Students must perceive the issue as being important.
- Students must believe that they are susceptible to the problem.
- Students must believe that the problem is serious.
- The intensity of the threat and resultant anxiety must not be so great as to paralyze the ability to act.
- There must be an action to take that the individual believes will be effective.

For students to function effectively when using clarifying strategies, they also must be prepared. Greenberg (1989, 43) states that the following are requisites of learner-centered instruction:

1. familiarity with and trust of other program participants (students)
2. friendship with at least one other participant
3. listening skills
4. knowledge of and experience with roles assumed by members and leaders of groups
5. knowledge of and experience with the decision-making process
6. cooperation and participation among all members of the program
7. an understanding and appreciation of both one's own feelings and the feelings of others
8. open communication among disagreeing factions and empathy with those of opposing viewpoints
9. recognition of unfulfilled needs of program participants and means of satisfying those needs
10. appreciation of individual differences and unique potential

When engaging in any values clarification activity, the teacher must allot sufficient time for students to assess their own feelings about the issue under examination. Students must also feel free to assess their values without fear of being ridiculed or being forced to pay lip service to the opinions of others, including the teacher. Keep in mind that clarifying activities do not lead to one "correct" solution to a problem; they are open-ended. (The purpose of these activities is to open the doors to additional assessment.) Also, as a teacher you are a participant in the activities and a role model for the students. Every student has the right to decline from speaking, without having to give a reason for declining. Respect individual feelings, and keep the activity nonthreatening.

Many instructional devices are available for incorporating clarification activities into the health curriculum. The ones you choose should be appropriate for the developmental level of the students. As already discussed, young children are not capable of dealing with highly abstract issues. Further, they do not have the experiential background to deal knowingly with topics far removed from their everyday world. Therefore, it is not realistic to attempt to grapple with such values-related issues as euthanasia or world hunger at the primary level.

SIMPLE VALUES-RELATED STRATEGIES

One of the simplest and most appropriate activities for younger students involves what is known as a shield activity, which is excellent for teaching children the ten prerequisites suggested by Greenberg. The major objective of this activity is to assist children in identifying values they have. The activity consists of filling in each segment of the shield with a values-related response, either in words or with drawings. A typical shield is illustrated in the Teaching in Action box on the facing page. Each child is given a copy of this box to complete . For younger children, you should read the instructions aloud.

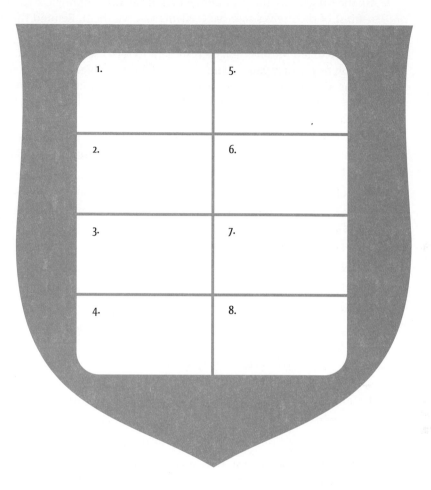

1.	5.
2.	6.
3.	7.
4.	8.

1. Name or draw something that you do well.

2. Name or draw something that you are trying to get better at.

3. Write down a feeling that would be very hard for you to change.

4. Write the thing that you are most proud of having done.

5. Tell about a happy thing that happened to you.

6. Tell about a sad thing that happened to you.

7. Tell what you want to do with your life.

8. Write three words that best tell about who you are.

The following steps may be used to help children work through the activity.

1. After students have filled out the shield, ask them to cross out any area of the shield they are unwilling to discuss.

2. Ask the students to move about the room in silence, holding the shield in front of themselves so other students can see them. Remind them that they should not talk.

3. After five to ten minutes, ask each student to select someone standing close by, or you may pair students. Tell students to sit together to discuss the shield. The process begins with the first student asking the other a question concerning his or her shield. After answering the question, the second student asks a question. The process continues until all the areas in the shield have been covered. This usually takes five to ten minutes.

4. Ask the students who were paired to introduce one another as each feels his or her partner would want to be introduced.

5. To bring closure, you might ask the children the following questions:

   - How many of you knew the name of your partner before beginning the activity?
   - Did you introduce yourself?
   - Did you find some things that you shared with your partner?
   - Did you find some things that were different from your partner?
   - How did you feel about your introduction of the other student?
   - What would you change about the introduction your partner made about you?
   - Did you feel you were a good listener when your partner answered your questions?
   - Can you write down one thing you learned about yourself?
   - Can you write down one thing you learned about your partner?
   - Can you write down one thing you learned about the entire group?

In presenting such an activity, it is essential that you thoroughly introduce, carry out, and summarize the experience. If this is not done, the activity becomes nothing more than a game. Through careful introduction, a psychological set is established so that the activity will be meaningful and the students will understand why they are doing it. By careful summation, you can help students assess their feelings and clarify existing values.

DECISION STORIES

Decision stories are open-ended vignettes that describe a values-related dilemma that asks students to suggest a course of action. The stories should reflect real-life circumstances and should be appropriate to the age level of the children. No easy answer should suggest itself in the story, but viable courses of action must be possible for the activity to be meaningful. If only unacceptable or repugnant alternatives seem possible, children will be unable to incorporate positive decision-making skills into their own behavioral repertoires. A decision story that children can identify with and relate to can provide an excellent springboard for values discussion. A good decision story not only encourages students to sort out opinions, values, and feelings, but also requires students to think about them, test them, and try them out. The real test of the importance of values comes with application.

In preparing decision stories, keep in mind that the story should be between 50 and 150 words in length. It should include enough detail to establish realism and character, but it should not be so long as to obscure the central issue. Establish a focus on the main issue with relevant supportive facts and events. Be careful to not slant the story so that only one solution or course of action is implied. Remember to provide a descriptive title, and end with a focus question that asks each student to suggest a course of action. This question is also the basis for discussion of the issue. (Hamrick, Anspaugh, and Smith 1980, 455). Following are examples of decision stories.

Pressure. Jim and Paul are fifth graders in the same classroom. In the past few weeks, they have become friends. One day while walking home from school, Jim and Paul meet some of Paul's other friends by the park. Paul's friends are all smoking. They offer Paul a cigarette. He takes it and lights up. Paul's friends also offer Jim a cigarette, but he says no. The boys start to make fun of him and call him a chicken. Even Paul is laughing at his friend.

Focus Question: What should Jim do?

Hot Spot. Mary's fourth-grade class is taking an important arithmetic test. Mary has studied hard for the test. In the seat next to her is her friend Julia. Julia is worried that she will not pass the test. The teacher leaves the room for a minute. While she is gone, Julia asks Mary for some of the test answers. The other students see and hear this. The teacher will be back in the room soon.

Focus Question: What should Mary do?

Students are an excellent source for developing such decision stories. After being exposed to a few models that you have written or located in values-clarification materials, students are usually eager to write vignettes of their own. This should be encouraged, as student-developed stories are highly relevant and motivating to the students themselves.

Presenting Decision Stories in Class. Begin by setting the stage for the story to motivate the class for the activity and to focus the inquiry. Discuss the title of the story and ask the children what it suggests to them. Stimulate the students' curiosity and get them involved from the start. For decision stories to be effective, students must be participants and not merely passive listeners. After a few minutes of this warm-up phase, present the story itself. Most of the stories can be read aloud. However, in some circumstances, it may help to give copies of the stories to the students, so they can consider the details of the presentation.

Have the students offer individual responses to the focus question: What course of action do you think is most appropriate? Encourage thought and reflection on the matter, but do not force any student to respond unwillingly.

A good way to get students thinking is to have each write a response on paper. The writing process facilitates thinking through the situation that has been presented. This process could be structured in a manner that requires students to begin by defining the problem. Below the definition, the options or choices can be listed, along with the possible consequences of each action. Consequences can be either positive or negative or a combination of the two. Writing also requires each student to make a commitment based on the information presented. It should be made clear, however, that the written responses need not be shared with the class at this point.

Pooling Ideas. Next, generate a list of all possible solutions to the decision story dilemma by asking students to share their responses with the class. This should be done on a volunteer basis. The teacher should not provide feedback to the students such as "That's good" or "I'm not sure that is such a good idea." Attempt to remain noncommittal. Respond with such phrases as "Thank you for sharing that idea with us," or by simply paraphrasing their responses. Then collect the responses and compile a list of solutions on the chalkboard without revealing which student offered any particular solution. You should also add possible solutions to the list that the students have overlooked.

Consider all the ideas put forth. Do not be judgmental, and do not reject any solution out of hand. Remember that the teacher's role is to help students clarify their own values, not to impose values on them.

Now divide the class into small groups and have each group discuss the possible solutions to the dilemma. Allow time for each group to reach a consensus on the preferred solution. Encourage the students to offer reasons for their choices.

Discussion and Reappraisal. After each small group has come to some sort of agreement, have them present the results of their discussions to the whole class. Different groups will probably opt for different solutions. Ask individual students why one solution seems better than another. Again, refrain from being judgmental and display neutrality. Instead of commenting, "So you think that Mary should just pretend that she didn't hear Julia," you might ask, "How could Mary have responded to Julia?" Finally, have each student reconsider the decision story in light of the class discussion (Smith, Hamrick, and Anspaugh 1981, 637). Some children will want to change their minds at this point. Others may modify their approach to the problem. Again have each student write down his or her solution to the problem along with reasons why the solution seems best. Have the students reflect on the ramifications of their decisions. Without necessarily requiring verbal responses, ask questions such as the following:

Have you ever been in a situation like the one in the story?

Did you come to the same solution then?

Did you or would you carry out your planned decision?

What happened or what do you think would happen if you tried out this decision?

How did this decision affect your own values? How were you affected by the decision? How were others affected?

Would you always make a similar decision?

Table 4.2	*Guidelines for Effective Role-Playing*

Select role-players or ask for volunteers.

Set the scene. Describe the situation carefully but briefly.

Give brief, clear instructions.

End the situation if it becomes stalemated or repetitive.

Provide time to discuss:

■ What happened?

■ Why did it turn out the way it did?

■ Did it turn out as desired?

■ Who would have had to do what to make it turn out differently?

SOURCE: Barth 1996

Using this structured approach to decision stories will help students develop decision-making skills. It will also assist them in applying rational thought to everyday problems involving values.

ROLE-PLAYING

Role-playing is an excellent strategy for helping establish what students are feeling, determining how others might feel in a given situation, or helping to decide how they might handle a given situation or event. Students may either act out roles identified by the teacher or (after becoming comfortable with the technique) write their own roles. To facilitate an effective role-playing situation, the students should be given a basic description of the situation and the role(s). The actual role-playing should be done with little or no rehearsal. A typical role-play should have a time limit of one to three minutes, followed by class discussion. Potential discussion questions include: Why did the role-players react to the situation in a particular way? What are some other potential solutions/suggestions for dealing with the situation? How might the role-play situation be done differently? Table 4.2 lists some guidelines for effective role-playing.

Other Verbal and Discussion-Oriented Strategies

Values clarification activities rely to a large extent on discussion, as do many other classroom strategies. Discussion is a useful technique, but it must be structured. Always keep in mind your objective in employing any particular discussion strategy so that you do not lose the focus. Several other discussion-oriented strategies that have proven effective in health instruction are presented below.

BRAINSTORMING

Like valuing strategies activities, brainstorming can be used to improve decision-making skills by having students generate many possible ideas concerning an issue. Freedom of expression and creativity are also encouraged. This strategy can be employed by all age groups and can foster a higher level of thinking. It is imperative that precise instructions be given about "how" and "what" is to be brainstormed. Possible topics for brainstorming sessions include:

How can you get students to follow safety rules?

How can you encourage students to eat nutritious snacks instead of junk food?

How can we make our physical environment more healthful and more pleasant?

In conducting a brainstorming session, it is very important to follow these four rules:

1. The problem to be brainstormed must be well defined.

2. Any and all ideas must be accepted.

3. Criticism of any idea put forth is not allowed.

4. All ideas should be evaluated objectively when the session is over.

Brainstorming can be used effectively in the lower as well as upper elementary grades. The biggest drawback is that, in a large class, not all children will have the opportunity to express their thoughts. Nonetheless, the activity can be quite productive. By encouraging and accepting all opinions, new or novel possible solutions to a problem may be found. Even impractical suggestions can lead to new ways of thinking about an issue.

Follow-up is important. In the follow-up session, ask children to elaborate on their ideas. Present additional information that will be useful in making suggestions more practical or realistic. In doing so, emphasize to the class how the free-wheeling brainstorming session led to many approaches to the problem.

BUZZ GROUPS

Akin to brainstorming, buzz groups are an effective strategy for examining a specific problem. Generally, this technique is productive if students are mature enough to use the format. It permits student participation in an atmosphere conducive to discussion. The buzz group strategy should not be overused, however, because too much small-group work can lessen student enthusiasm.

To use this approach, divide the class into groups of three to five students. Avoid putting friends in the same group or the discussion may tend to stray to issues besides the assigned task. Have each group focus on a specific problem that you have introduced and discussed so that the children will have a knowledge base for their discussion. Each group should choose a chairperson and a recording secretary. The chairperson must keep the discussion on the topic, and the secretary records important points. Walk from group to group to help maintain the focus of each group.

Allow three to fifteen minutes for buzz group discussion. Suitable topics for this strategy include how an accident victim should be handled, how children can get along better with brothers and sisters, what can be done to educate children to the dangers of smoking, and what can be done about vandalism.

After the discussion time is over, ask the recording secretary for each group to present the results of that group's discussion. The more controversial the topic, the more likely it will be that many diverse opinions will be aired. In the summary discussion, encourage objective consideration of all approaches put forth.

CASE STUDIES

Case studies are actual events that you can use in class for discussion. The decision story format (see pages 80–83) lends itself well to the case study strategy—just substitute the actual event for the hypothetical one. Good sources for case study materials are health journals, newspapers, news magazines, and television programs.

COOPERATIVE LEARNING

An excellent strategy for fostering cohesiveness in the classroom is cooperative learning. This technique involves having students work together to solve an identified problem or to work toward some common goal. Divide the class into small groups and instruct each to arrive at a conclusion on a particular problem or situation. This strategy allows students to work together, and each child can provide input to the conclusions. Above all, one or two students should not be allowed to dominate any group. This problem can be overcome by the teacher listening carefully to the group discussions and refocusing them when needed. It is difficult to assign grades for cooperative learning since contribution to solving the problem or arriving at the solution is not easily determined on an individual basis. Topics such as those suggested for the brainstorming or buzz group activities lend themselves to cooperative learning.

CRITICAL ESSAYS

The teacher asks the students to write their evaluation or judgment concerning an issue, product, or concept. This strategy is an excellent way to help students determine their feelings, how they would react, or their perspective on a situation or issue. Critical essays allow the students to express their own personal learning experiences. Teachers might ask the students to write why they feel a certain way, by what path they arrived at their feelings, or what effect the information, insight, or feeling will have on their behavior. This technique allows information gathered to be personalized in such a fashion that it has potential to develop attitudes and change/reinforce behavior.

DEBATE

Debate focuses on the merits and problems associated with a proposed solution to an issue. Through the use of this technique, you can ensure that both sides of the issue are presented. Although debate can be used in the lower elementary grades, the strategy is more effective when used with older children, who are more articulate and better able to organize their thoughts for oral presentation. Students must also be able to work individually as well as cooperatively in groups.

Topics suitable for debate include the use of nuclear power or its alternatives, the supposed merits of organic foods versus genetically engineered food products, and the use of laboratory animals in medical experiments. Environmental issues are also good debate topics.

Thorough preparation for a debate is essential. Students who volunteer to be part of a debate team should be given ample time to become knowledgeable about the issue they will discuss. The whole class should engage in this preparation so that students not on the debate teams are prepared to deal with the pros and cons of the arguments objectively.

In selecting students for debate teams, be sure that both sides are well balanced in ability. The teacher's role is that of moderator. The moderator should keep both debate teams on the topic and also guard against emotions becoming too extreme during and after the debate.

COMMITTEE WORK

This technique allows small groups of children to research a topic of interest. Each group member has an opportunity to do in-depth research on the topic. For elementary school children, the work must be closely supervised and structured. It is very important that each member of the group contribute to the project if it is to be successful. Projects that lend themselves well to committee work include investigating different types of pollution, collecting newspaper and magazine articles on a recent medical discovery or health approach, or researching types of foods used in different cultures as sources of essential nutrients.

Results of the committee work are presented orally. Encourage committee members to use exhibits and multimedia aids to reinforce their presentations. This strategy can also be used on an individual basis. In such an instance, each student makes a presentation of the research done.

LECTURE, GROUP, AND PANEL DISCUSSION

Discussion, in one form or another, is probably the most common technique used in education. Lecture discussion is usually thought of as a lecture delivered by the teacher. However, this strategy should not be limited to one-way communication. Lecture discussion can be from teacher to student, student to teacher, or student to student. The technique should be a means for achieving two-way communication.

For group discussion to be effective, the teacher must develop an atmosphere of freedom in the classroom. Without this atmosphere, students will not state their true feelings. And the discussion must be kept on course. Curtis and Papenfuss (1980, 139) offer the following suggestions for conducting group discussion.

- Present a discussion topic or legitimize an appropriate student-formulated topic.
- Establish and maintain an atmosphere of thoughtful communication without injecting teacher value judgments.
- Make the ground rules for the discussion clear and enforce them.
- Try to understand what students are attempting to say, but do not badger or cross-examine.

Panel discussion offers an opportunity for three to five students to investigate and report on a particular health topic. This strategy is similar to committee work, but it allows more give-and-take between the participating students. Usually fifteen minutes is sufficient time for a panel discussion. Adjust the time allotted to the attention span and developmental level of the class. When using this strategy, be sure that the students who will be panel members have a precise theme to explore. A prepared outline is also necessary so that the presentation is organized.

All three of these discussion techniques encourage the exchange of information and ideas between students. In this way, children are involved in the teaching/learning process. Discussion techniques also help students develop respect and understanding for the feelings and opinions of others.

To be successful, discussion must be guided. Stone, O'Reilley, and Brown (1980, 281) note six elements that must be addressed when preparing for a discussion.

1. Choose a topic that the students can discuss and have opinions on, such as violence.

2. Introduce the topic and motivate the class about it. For example, write the word *violence* on the board and ask the students, "What is this word? Can you give me some examples of violence? Where have you seen violence in your own life? Have you ever been in a fight? Have you ever hit anyone? Have you ever thrown something at someone with the intention of hitting them? All of these are acts of violence."

3. Prepare key questions that generate discussion; for example, "If you have been in a fight or hit someone, do you think it was appropriate or necessary? If someone hits you, should you hit back? If not, what should you do? Is it ever necessary or the best option to hit someone else? When might those times be? If not, what course of action can be followed?"

4. Provide structure to the discussion by keeping it going in a predetermined direction. The focus of this topic for each student is to develop his or her own concept of the appropriateness or inappropriateness of violence. The emphasis needs to remain on these issues, even if the specifics get diverse.

5. Develop closure on the topic discussed. As an activity, students can write a paragraph describing their personal outlook on violence.

6. Summarize and reinforce the key points. After writing the paragraphs, the class members can review the issues discussed. For example, the

teacher can write on the board, "We have decided that violence involves these kinds of activities...." and list them, along with "We think violence is appropriate/not appropriate in the following situations...."

RESOURCE SPEAKERS

Speakers can enrich many areas of health instruction. Possible resource speakers include doctors, nurses, police and fire department personnel, nutritionists, and health researchers. When contacting a resource speaker, be sure to provide that person with information about your class, including grade and developmental level. In this way, a speaker is less likely to talk down to or over the heads of the children. You should also politely emphasize that the speaker stick to the specific topic to be examined because some speakers are apt to digress to a favorite cause or concern not in keeping with your instructional objectives. Suggest that the speaker use multimedia aids if appropriate, as this will heighten student interest. Also, ask the speaker to allow time for a question-and-answer session.

Before the speaker addresses the class, be sure that adequate instruction has been provided, so the students are not introduced to the topic cold. Also, provide information about the position and background of the resource speaker. For example, what exactly is a nutritionist? What does a nutritionist do, and for whom does the person work? Resource speakers can be very instructive, especially if the students are properly prepared and the speaker uses multimedia aids to keep the students' interest.

Action-Oriented Strategies

A variety of action-oriented or student-centered strategies can be used to enliven health instruction. These range from seatwork activities to field trips. Whenever possible, any strategy selected should help students discover concepts through action-oriented means. Strategies that incorporate at least two of the senses can greatly facilitate learning. Listening is fine, but listening plus seeing, tasting, smelling, touching, feeling, and doing is better.

DRAMATIZATIONS

Plays, skits, and puppet shows are all effective dramatization techniques. Each of these strategies is an excellent way of allowing students to express their feelings. Thorough preparation and follow-up are essential, however, lest these activities be seen merely as fun, with the point of the exercise being missed.

Presenting a play involves use of a script and props. You can use a commercial script or have students write their own. A skit is much more informal. Only an outline for the story needs to be prepared, not an actual script. Each character speaks extemporaneously. Props are not required. Nonetheless, plays and skits are both quite time-consuming.

Puppet shows are great motivators for health behavior and attitude development. They are especially effective in the lower grades. Commercial puppets may be used, or children can make their own. Puppets can be used for plays, skits, or role playing (Timmreck 1978, 140).

STORYTELLING

As a strategy, storytelling is similar to dramatization. However, the teacher is the active participant, and the children are onlookers. This is nonetheless an effective strategy for helping students identify positive health habits and for shaping attitudes. Using a flip chart or other visual aid can heighten the impact of storytelling, although no props are needed for many stories.

FLANNEL, FELT, AND MAGNETIC BOARDS

Flannel or felt boards are made by stretching a piece of either material over a large board or easel. Objects that will cling to the fabric can be placed on the board. Such boards are quite useful as aids in telling a story or developing a concept, because objects can be added or taken off during the presentation. These boards can also be used by the students in developing their own stories or presentations.

Magnetic boards serve the same purpose as flannel and felt boards. A magnetic board is simply a sheet of metal to which objects can be attached by means of small magnets. Chalk or special markers can also be used to write directly on many magnetic boards.

CROSSWORD PUZZLES

Crossword puzzles are useful seatwork devices for building vocabulary and reinforcing concepts. They can be developed by the teacher, the students, or a computer-generated program. Commercial materials are also available. Crossword puzzles for younger children must be kept relatively simple. This technique is best employed with children in grade 3 and above. The Teaching in Action box on page 90 shows an example of a crossword puzzle concerning milk and milk products.

DEMONSTRATIONS AND EXPERIMENTS

Demonstrations and experiments help make verbal explanations more meaningful to students because they involve other senses, such as sight or touch. In a demonstration, the outcome should always be the same; in an experiment, the predicted outcome may vary. Otherwise, the two terms mean much the same. These techniques are especially good for use with elementary school children. Students are always interested in demonstrations and experiments because these strategies help clarify what they have learned. Appropriate areas for demonstrations and experiments include typing blood, feeding animals, determining the starch content of food, and brushing and flossing teeth.

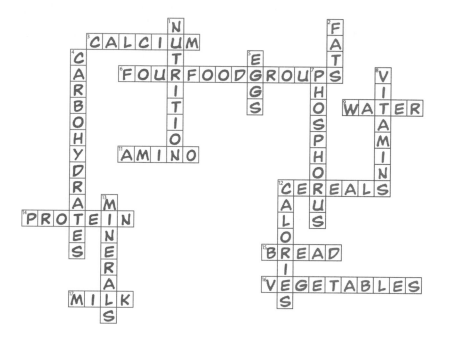

Across

3. A mineral in milk that builds strong bones and teeth.

6. A useful guide for eating daily (three words).

9. Helps regulate body temperature.

11. Parts of protein, called _____ acids.

12. Foods rich in carbohydrates. Oatmeal is an example.

14. A nutrient that builds and repairs body tissue.

15. A food product rich in carbohydrates. Good for making sandwiches.

16. Lettuce and carrots are examples. Can be eaten fresh or cooked.

17. Beverage from cows that is rich in protein.

Down

1. The science of food as it relates to optimal health and performance.

2. Food substances that do not dissolve in water.

4. Nutrients found in many foods, especially in the Bread and Cereal Group; a source of energy.

5. Product of chickens that is popular for breakfast. Contains plenty of protein.

7. Helps build strong bones and teeth.

8. A group of nutrients that help other nutrients do their job. Known by letter names.

12. Measure energy provided by food. Dieters count them.

13. Sometimes called the "structural framework" of the body.

SOURCE: Developed by the Memphis Nutritional Center, Memphis City Schools.

When you consider either a demonstration or an experiment, careful planning is essential to make sure that it will actually work. All equipment should be set up ahead of time, and it is wise to have a rehearsal before the class actually views the procedure. Introduce the procedure to the class and explain what you plan to do. All students should be able to see the activity. Encourage them to ask questions as you go, and be sure to explain what is happening at each stage. After the activity, reinforce the learning by writing important points on the chalkboard.

EXHIBITS

Exhibits allow students to view, examine, and touch health-related materials. Exhibits are most effective when the children help in the design and construction. Careful planning is essential, as is a central theme. Always ask yourself: What is the point of the proposed exhibit? Your answer will provide a focus for the children, too.

Examples of appropriate exhibits include X rays of broken and healed bones, safety equipment used in different types of sports, dental instruments, and samples of raw foods, such as cereal grains. If the actual objects are unavailable or impractical for classroom display, pictures can be substituted, although they are not as effective.

Everything in an exhibit should be clearly labeled. If sound and motion can be added, student interest will be increased. Use your imagination to make the exhibit as visually appealing and interest-provoking as you can.

FIELD TRIPS

Field trips can provide rich learning experiences. This strategy must be used sparingly, however, because field trips are time consuming and often expensive. Further, parents and administrators must give their approval for any activity outside the school, and liability must be considered.

A field trip should always be a culminating activity rather than an introductory one. Children should be well prepared for the experience through prior classroom instruction. If the field trip is to be of value, the students must be able to understand what they will be seeing.

Good places for health-related field trips away from the school include the local health department, a dairy farm, a food-processing plant, or a sewage treatment facility. There are also many opportunities for field trips within the school grounds. These are often quite effective as learning experiences for younger children. Although the places themselves are familiar, you can add a new dimension to them by explaining the structure and planning behind the situation. Examples of on-site field trips include visits to the school cafeteria, to a crosswalk area, or to the playground. For instance, at the crosswalk area you can ask children how the crosswalk is planned for safety. Are there school speed limit signs to slow traffic during school hours? Are crosswalk lines painted on the street? Do crossing guards supervise the crossing? These and other questions will help the students see the area in a new light.

GAMES

Games can stimulate interest while providing a review of concepts learned through other strategies. They are also sometimes a welcome relief from the normal classroom routine. In addition, games particularly help younger children understand the importance of following rules and provide useful experience in socialization. Many commercially available games, such as bingo, can be adapted to health-related topics, or you may wish to develop your own games if you have the time.

When using games as part of health instruction, be sure that the fun of the activity does not overshadow the health-related content of the game. Also, keep the game from becoming too competitive so that no player feels inferior.

MODELS AND SPECIMENS

Models and specimens allow students to have multisensory experience of health-related topics. The value of models and specimens lies in their degree of accuracy. Many excellent models of body parts are available commercially. These include models of the human eye, heart, lungs, and other organs. Another useful model is Resuscitation Annie/Andy, a functional model used to teach mouth-to-mouth resuscitation.

Specimens can be obtained from biological supply houses. These include tissue samples, animal eyes, and so forth. Commercial slaughterhouses can also supply some of these items. Exercise discretion in the use of specimens. For some children, such exhibits can be too grisly, and models are better employed.

PEER HELPERS

Peer-helper programs have proven successful in a number of informal settings. Peer helpers are children who have been trained to listen, support, offer assistance, and serve as models in a variety of roles, such as class monitors, tutors, big brothers/sisters, and playground helpers. Peer helpers can serve as excellent conduits between the children and teachers.

The children selected to serve as peer helpers are usually a grade or two ahead of the groups they help. The key to a successful program is the training and supervision peer helpers receive. In the school setting, peer helpers can occasionally help to lead discussions or to work one-on-one with other children. They should be trained to help children think about a situation and develop a solution to or attitude about it. Peer helpers have been successful in helping to prevent smoking, drug and alcohol use, and eating disorders.

These ingredients must be present for a successful peer-helper program:

Well-qualified adult leaders: Leaders must be knowledgeable in all aspects of program development, maintenance, and evaluation. National certifications and training workshops are available to help adults develop the skills for training the children.

Well-established goals: A needs assessment must be done to determine what the needs are of the school, community, and children. The identified needs should be stated as goals, with the school and community aware of the goals and purposes of the program.

Effective recruitment and selection process: Some programs will accept everyone who applies for training. Others may find it necessary to screen the students through interviews, letters of intent, and input from teachers. The program should represent all the social and ethnic groups in the school community. If a child is not selected, he or she should be informed tactfully about the reasons for not having been selected and, whenever possible, used in some other aspect of the program.

Training: Training should be adequate and appropriate. Typically it should include an introduction to the issue or topic based on the students' needs and a skill-building activity designed to help practice, receive coaching, and build on their natural abilities. It is not unusual for the training to require a time framework of twenty-five to thirty hours.

Peer-helper involvement: The ways that peer helpers become involved will depend on the needs of the school. Even if some of the peer helpers have no formal duties, they can act as natural helpers in their own classrooms. The school should have some way to recognize peer helpers.

Supervision: A most critical element of an effective peer program is supervision. Weekly feedback and contact should be provided. Training should be a continuous process to help provide support and skill development for the peer helpers. The ability of the supervisor(s) to model the use of skills in real-life situations is a crucial ingredient.

Evaluation: Evaluation should be in terms of the program goals. It should describe how well the program has met its goals and point to possible changes (Carr 1992, 4).

SELF-APPRAISALS

There are many inventories that children can be given to help them assess their health status or feelings concerning an important issue. These instruments may be teacher developed or commercially prepared. Unfortunately these assessments may not be appropriate for very young children or may provide a false sense of security. There is always the risk that the children will not accurately report their true feelings. For example, a child may state that he does not smoke, realizing that to correctly report that he does would indicate a poor health habit. The strength of such inventories and assessments is that they help make children aware of potentially harmful behaviors and help to provide insight into positive health behaviors.

The Use of Media in Health Instruction

Educational media include everything from videotape to computers. For the present purposes, the term will be defined as any nonprint vehicle used for instructional intent. Such media include computers, television, DVDs, videotapes, slides, overhead transparencies, and audiotapes.

COMPUTER-ASSISTED INSTRUCTION

Advances in technology and the decreased cost of computers and CD-ROMs in the last few years have led to more widespread use of computers in the classroom. In fact, many children today come from homes where personal computers are used for a variety of purposes, from keeping business records to playing video games. There will be an increased use of computers in health instruction.

Today most schools have access to a vast array of information through the **Internet,** a global network that can be linked to schools through the **World Wide Web (WWW).** The Web makes extensive use of multimedia, incorporating not only printed matter, but pictures, graphics, animation, and sound. Unfortunately, the Web has become host to much commercial advertising, but it remains a source of increasing health-related information that can be used in school. The computer holds great potential for a variety of activities. Some suggestions for student use in the classroom include helping students manage large volumes of electronic information stores, developing skills that help students identify information that is essential and related to the task at hand, and developing information acquisition skills. In this regard the student should be able to analyze information, apply information gathered, and evaluate the information acquired (Rivard 1997, 21).

Further benefits of using the computer include active involvement of students and the ability both to see knowledge in relational ways to carry out higher-level thinking by selecting and evaluating information and to delve deeply into subjects and concepts while working either alone or in groups. The use of computers provides an excellent tie-in with outcome- or performance-based evaluation. For example, in both performance-based evaluation and in the use of computers the student must prepare, practice, experiment, and evaluate. As a result, students are expected to create a product and demonstrate competence before or among others. In addition, when there are several participants, performance can be interactive, enabling students to learn the impact of their actions through immediate feedback. Finally, outcome-based evaluation is promoted by the ability of peers to provide commentary on how to improve performance (Wagner et al.1997).

As shown in Table 4.3, computer instructional programs tend to follow one of six types. Computers have great potential in the classroom. However, there are potential concerns of which teachers must be aware. Obviously, the high cost of purchasing sufficient quantities of computer hardware and software for the classroom, as well as the incompatibility of different systems are problems. Gold (1991) also expressed concern at the possibility of dehumanizing the health education process. However, with the advent of outcome-based evaluation, this seems less of a problem, because teachers must assist in developing objectives for the project, serve as overseer, and interact with the student as the work progresses. The abundance of software programs makes choosing quality software more of a challenge, and because of limited school budgets, anything purchased generally must be used for a long time. Nevertheless, computer instruction is here to stay. New technology is coming online everyday and is adding to the potential that computers have in the classroom.

Table 4.3   *Six Types of Computer Instructional Programs*

1. Drill and practice.

In drill and practice, students are presented a series of questions to be answered or problems to be solved. The microcomputer immediately checks the responses and provides feedback to the student. Although drill-and-practice programs are one of the most common educational applications of computers, they can be unnecessarily boring for students and tend to promote rote learning. This strategy is most often used to reinforce or review material learned elsewhere.

2. Tutorial.

The objective of the tutorial is to teach concrete concepts. The microcomputer presents new information to the student, and then it poses a series of questions. Based on the responses provided by the student, the program either presents additional information or reviews the previous lesson. Users of this strategy should ensure that the software does not overwhelm the student with screen after screen of text. This repetition can quickly lead to learner fatigue.

3. Demonstrations.

Demonstration programs allow students to observe a functioning model or situation. By observation, the student learns how systems work. For example, one commercial program demonstrates the effect of exercise on a graphic representation of a human heart, and another illustrates how nerve impulses travel through the nervous system of a human body.

4. Simulations.

Simulation programs imitate real or imaginary systems based on a modeler's theory of the operation of that system. Students test hypothetical courses of action by manipulating variables and observing the impact of these changes. This process allows the student to formulate realistic projections based on sound theory. Simulations can be used to make defined concepts more understandable. Programs currently available can simulate such things as a nuclear reactor, the human circulatory system, various ecosystems, and a malaria epidemic.

5. Instructional games.

Games often use one or more of the strategies previously described. Instructional games, unlike arcade games, are designed to meet well-defined instructional objectives. Instructional games have explicit rules and winners, but educational concepts and information must be mastered for the player to become successful. For example, a commercially available game requires a knowledge of human anatomy and physiology to successfully complete a voyage through the human body.

6. Problem solving.

Many advocates of computer-assisted instruction view the area of problem solving as one of the most powerful for the computer. Research has not indicated that using a computer is a significantly better way to teach problem solving than other strategies because the limited programming environment doesn't automatically guarantee transfer to real life. However, a new kind of problem-solving program has recently been introduced. This strategy is to confront learners with original situations that require the use of already acquired knowledge in new circumstances. Because the computer provides both prompts as needed and immediate responses, the computer manages this type of activity well. Make sure that the educational strategy employed by the instructional program is appropriate for the content area and the students' abilities. Most important, consider whether the program being reviewed is superior to other strategies of teaching the same content.

TELEVISION, VIDEOTAPE, AND DVD

It is probably safe to state that every school in the United States has access to television and VCRs (videocassette recorders), and an increasing number of schools have DVD (digital videodisk) players. Many fine health-related programs, designed with the elementary school child in mind, are available. Both the Public Broadcasting Service (PBS) and National Educational Television (NET) regularly provide programs that can be used in health education. The commercial networks also occasionally produce suitable programs.

In addition to scheduled broadcasts, public and commercial agencies also make many programs available on videotape or DVD. The Best Foundation for a Drug-Free Tomorrow distributes two programs through the Agency for Instructional Technology in Bloomington, Indiana. The programs are Just for Me (1992), and My Best (1993). Just for Me is designed for grades 2, 3, and 4. This series of six fifteen-minute video programs consists of a teacher component, peer component, and home component. The emphasis is on positive skills for dealing with stress, peer and media pressure, self-esteem, and self-responsibility. A teachers' guide, informational video, and community component are included in the package. The second program, My Best, is designed for grades 7 and 8. This series of six videos deals with the same issues covered in the Your Choice Our Chance series.

Making your own videotapes for health instruction is also a useful approach although an expensive one because of the equipment involved. If your school has the equipment, however, you should consider using it. Record class plays, skits, and sociodramas. For example, suggest that students produce their own health public service messages or commercials for use in conjunction with consumer health discussions.

CHOOSING VIDEOTAPES, CD-ROMS, OR DVDS

Some classrooms still may use 16-mm films, but this type of media has been largely replaced with videotape and DVD. In considering videotape or DVD as instructional devices, keep in mind that they should not serve as the sole basis of instruction and that every video must be carefully chosen and previewed. The following questions should be considered when selecting either videotapes or DVDs for use in the classroom.

- Is the contained material interesting and appropriate to the age and grade level?

- Does the contained material convey the desired facts and concepts, and is it likely to contribute to the formation of positive health attitudes or behavior?

- Is the information accurate and up-to-date?

- Can the information be correlated with and integrated into the course of study at the required grade level?

- Is the language suited to the intended audience?

- Does it meet reasonable standards of technical excellence in terms of quality, sound, and acting?

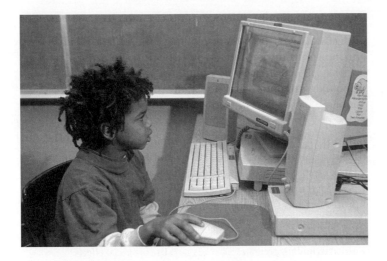

Computers can serve as excellent motivational tools for students.

- Is the videotape or disk of appropriate length?
- Are there commercial overtones that are distasteful and detract from the educational message?

Keep a file of all audiovisuals you preview. An example of a typical file entry is shown in the Teaching in Action box on page 98. Such recordkeeping will help you build an index of especially useful films and will alert you to inappropriate ones.

SLIDES

Another fairly inexpensive medium is 35-mm slides. These can be purchased from commercial sources, or you can make them yourself if you have a 35-mm camera and a bit of photographic skill. Slides are colorful and easy to store. Depending on the kind of projector system you have, one slide tray will hold from 40 to more than 100 two-by-two-inch slides.

If you make your own slides, the subject matter could include class activities and field trips, health fairs, environmental problems in the community, and class projects. An advantage to using slides is that you can delete or add slides to the sequence as you desire. In this way, you can keep your slide collection current.

OVERHEAD TRANSPARENCIES

Used with an overhead projector, transparencies are extremely popular as teaching tools. Photocopy your material onto an acetate that is compatible with a photocopying machine. Overheads can also be made directly from a computer utilizing an appropriate printer.

One unique feature of using a transparency is the ability to show a progression by using a series of overlays. Overlays can be employed to show the position of organs within the body or to add or remove captions for informal quizzes.

TEACHING IN ACTION *A Checklist for Audiovisuals and Instructional Software*

Title _____ Date Reviewed _____

Distributor _____ Rent _____ Cost _____

Loan _____ Purchase _____ Cost _____

Media Type   □ Videotape   □ 35-mm slides   □ Filmstrip   □ CD-ROM
                □ DVD   □ Audio tape   □ Computer software   □ Other

Evaluation Instructions

Below are criteria that can be used to rate audiovisuals, CD-ROMs , and other media. Not all sections are appropriate for all types of media. A four-point scale is provided for evaluating the various media.

     4 = Excellent   3 = Good   2 = Average   1 = Poor

Content/Format

____ 1. Is the production technically accurate?   ____ 7. Use of special effects

____ 2. Accuracy of content   ____ 8. Length of production

____ 3. Grammar/spelling   ____ 9. Music, background, dress

____ 4. Multicultured   ____ 10. Sound quality

____ 5. Viewer appeal   ____ 11. Creative production

____ 6. Exude or elicit biases   ____ 12. Reference or user's guide

Overall Rating   48–43 = Excellent content/format   36–31 = Average content/format

                  42–37 = Good content/format   30 and below = Poor content/format

Appropriate for intended audience(s)?   □ Yes   □ No

Useful for special projects?   □ Yes   □ No

Comments _____

_____

_____

Computer Software/CD-ROM

Title _____

Distributor _____ Phone _____

License _____ Costs _____

Compatible with what hardware   □ Mac   □ Windows   □ Other
                              Version _____   □ Updates available

Needs for operation   □ RAM   □ Memory   □ Modem   □ Hard Drive   □ CD-ROM

Grade level _____   **Computer skill level required:**   □ Beginner   □ Intermediate   □ Advanced

Technical information   □ Graphics   □ Help screens   □ Personalize database   □ Pulldown menu
                □ Information display   Help hotline (   ) ____-_____   □ Assessments available

Output of individual student data   □ Yes   □ No   Classroom data output   □ Yes   □ No

Manuals provided   □ Teacher   □ Student   □ Technical

Comments _____

_____

_____

Reviewed by _____ Date _____

Recommended purchase   □ Yes   □ No

AUDIOTAPES

Selectively used, audiotapes can be valuable teaching tools. They are inexpensive and can be stopped as needed for discussion. Finding useful tapes may take some work on your part, however, because relatively few are available that relate directly to health instruction.

Tape recordings are in some ways more versatile than visuals. You can easily make recordings of radio and television programs, for example, or of interviews with health officials, classroom guest speakers, and so forth. Recording commercials for classroom use can be useful when teaching consumer health.

SELECTING APPROPRIATE SOFTWARE

Initially, most educational software consisted of drill-and-practice exercises that were marginally useful in the classroom, and teachers were often disappointed with the results of using software. Today, computers are no longer a novelty, but an important part of the instructional strategies for promoting learning. The selection of software should be taken as seriously as the selection of any media, technology, or textbook. Several guidelines have been established to ensure a successful selection process (Komoski and Plotnick 1995).

Analyze needs—Is the computer the most appropriate medium to satisfy the goals and objectives of the instructional process?

Specify requirements—Factors to consider include:

- Will the school require multiple copies?
- Will a site license be required?
- Is the software compatible with the hardware available?
- Is the software user friendly?
- Is there technical support via a toll-free number?
- Does the software meet the goals and objectives of the needs analysis?

Identify promising software—Join an Internet listserv and read catalogs and reviews to find out what other teachers and professionals think of the software.

Preview software—The most effective way to judge software is to personally review the material and to observe students as they utilize the program(s). If you cannot preview the software, do not use it in your classroom.

Get post-use feedback—Create a written record with a quantitative scale for rating the software. After using the software, review this record to determine if the software helped meet the goals and objectives of the instructional effort.

Health Highlight

EXAMPLES OF SOFTWARE/CD-ROMS FOR CLASSROOM USE

A.D.A.M. Essentials: (Grades 5–9)
School Edition

4,000 identification labels in approximately 100 layers. Detailed overviews of 13 anatomical systems with classroom activities and animation summaries for each system. Lists of key terminology and student activity sheet. Includes a teacher's guide.

Forest Biomes   (Grades 5–9)

The forest ecosystem is explored with live action video. Study the balanced network of plant and animal relationships that make up the food chain.

Scholastic's *The Magic School*   (Grades 1–4)
Bus Explores the Human Body

Students travel aboard a bus into a human body to learn about the parts of the body and how organs and systems work.

3-D Body Adventures   (Grades 2–8)

CD-ROM in which students use 1950s-style 3-D glasses to fly through organs, examining them from every angle and in cross sections of actual human tissue. Students hear complete descriptions of anatomy and systems. "Emergency Room" players can cure patients based on their symptoms and medical history. This aspect provides a great test of what was learned in using the material.

Grab a Byte   (Grades 6–8)

Consists of three separate programs: (1) Restaurant—students enter their height and weight and choose foods for their meal(s). Nutritional values, calories, vitamins, etc. are provided; (2) Grab a Grape—three levels of difficulty in six nutritional areas. Examples are food and sports, and weight management; (3) Nutrition Sleuth—clues are provided to nutritional mysteries.

The Body Awareness   (Grades 6–7)
Resource Network (BARN)

Primarily for adolescents, the program can be used for grades 6–7. Program includes information on physical activity, alcohol, drugs and smoking, family communication, and stress management.

Health Watch   (Grades 4–6)

Provides information concerning six categories of wellness. Incorporates simulation gaming to make points and provide information. A system developed by Comp Tech Systems Design which incorporates simulation gaming concerning fitness, nutrition, and dental hygiene.

Keeping Safe   (Grades K–6)

Simulation is used to help elementary children make safe decisions concerning abuse.

Healthy Decisions   (Grades 4–6)

Developed by the American Cancer Society. Requires that students use decision-making skills to make decisions that influence their health. A take-home guide contains information that can be used for parental involvement.

Heart Medley   (Grades 4–6)

Developed by the American Heart Association. Contains a five-part package that teaches how the heart functions, the role of genetics, nutrition, and lifestyle. Utilizes gaming strategies.

Friend C.H.I.P.   (Grades 4–6)

Focuses on fitness, nutrition, self-esteem, and peer relationships. Uses responses to paper-and-pencil test. Plethora of teacher materials. Produced by Campbell Soup Company.

Summary

- A strategy is an activity or experience that the teacher uses to interpret, illustrate, or facilitate learning.
- Proper selection of strategies helps provide interest, motivation, and reinforcement of learning.

- Strategies should contribute to total learning. More complex concepts should have several strategies, proceed from the simple to the complex, include audio-visual aids, and be based on the learning styles of the students.

- Regardless of the strategy, an environment that is conducive for learning must be developed and maintained.

- Values-clarification activities help students to determine their feelings concerning issues and concepts.

- An effective model to facilitate good decision making must provide opportunities to practice decision-making skills.

- When selecting strategies, learning styles are an important consideration.

- Multiple intelligence provides insight into why implementation of a variety of strategies is essential to quality learning.

- Role-playing is an important tool that aids in decision making and helps determine feelings about situations or events.

- Verbal and discussion-oriented strategies include brainstorming, buzz groups, case studies, cooperative learning, critical essays, committee work, debates, panel discussion, and resource speakers.

- Action-oriented strategies include dramatizations; storytelling; flannel, felt, and magnetic boards; crossword puzzles; demonstrations/experiments; exhibits; field trips; games; and model/specimens.

- Peer-helper programs are an excellent strategy for offering other children assistance and serving as role models. Peer helpers must be trained.

- Instructional media are not strategies in themselves, but they do serve as valuable approaches for involving students in the learning process. Examples include computers, television, videotapes, DVDs, overhead transparencies, and audio tapes.

- The decision to use any strategy should be based on how effective it will be in facilitating learning.

- A strategy should be chosen because it offers some teaching advantage, not simply novelty.

DISCUSSION QUESTIONS

1. What factors should you keep in mind when selecting strategies for classroom use?

2. What elements should an effective decision-making model contain?

3. List and discuss the types of learning styles.

4. What is meant by the concept of multiple intelligence? What are the implications for health education?

5. Discuss the strengths and weaknesses of clarifying techniques.

6. What are the guidelines for developing effective role-playing situations?

7. Describe the process for using decision stories in the classroom, from preparation of the stories to discussion and follow-up activities.

8. Select three types of discussion-oriented strategies, such as brainstorming and debate, and discuss the strengths and weaknesses of each approach.

9. Select three types of action-oriented strategies, such as dramatizations and field trips, and discuss the strengths and weaknesses of each.

10. Why must discussion-oriented strategies be structured for greatest effectiveness?

11. What are the criteria for selecting software for the classroom?

12. Select three types of media, such as computers and television, and discuss the strengths and weaknesses of each.

CRITICAL THINKING QUESTIONS

1. In the real-world classroom, how much consideration is given to attempting to incorporate some theory of learning style? What examples can you cite in relationship to your position? What do you think teachers could do to better incorporate learning-style theory into classroom instruction?

2. If you were given three days to plan what you would consider the most exciting, motivating classroom for teaching health education, what would that class be like in terms of atmosphere, strategies, student involvement, and technology? Realistically can your plan be implemented in today's schools? Why? Why not?

WEB SITE ACTIVITY

Visit one of the Web sites listed below. Determine the types of lesson plans and teaching that pertain to the various content areas of health education. Would they prove useful in a variety of situations? What are the strengths and weaknesses of the lesson plans and teaching strategies presented on the Web site?

WEB SITES OF INTEREST

Price Systems, Inc.: *www.learningstyle.com*
  Information on learning styles. Discusses the theory behind learning styles and allows visitors to assess their own learning styles.

Schrock Family Home Page: *www.schrockguide.com/index.html*
  Internet site lists materials, lesson plans, etc., for enhancing curriculum and teacher professional growth. Updated daily.

The Gateway: *www.thegateway.org*
  Resources for teaching grades K through 12. Includes health and physical education.

LetsNet: *http://commtechlab.msu.edu/sites/letsnet*
  Learning exchange for teachers and students through the Internet. Michigan State University helps teachers experience the potential of the World Wide Web.

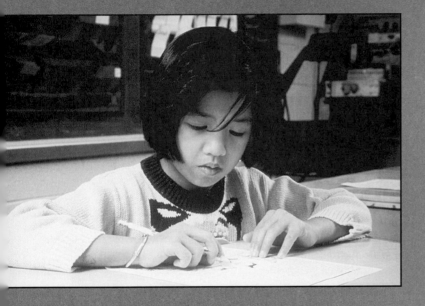

CHAPTER FIVE

Measurement and Evaluation of Health Education

We are seeking the best methods possible to measure a student's success in school.

—Hamilton County (Tennessee) Department of Education (2002)

VALUED OUTCOMES

After reading this chapter, you should be able to:

- explain the difference between measurement and evaluation
- list the teacher skills needed to be competent in measuring and evaluating student progress
- discuss the steps necessary for developing a teacher-designed test
- identify alternative methods of assessment of student progress
- discuss the use of benchmarks and standards in grading

The ultimate goal of measurement and evaluation is to determine how well the teacher has taught and the student has learned. As you read through this chapter, reflect on how you can most effectively use the concepts related to measurement and evaluation to enhance the success of your teaching and your students' learning.

Measurement and Evaluation

Every instructional effort should be evaluated to determine how successful it has been. Both student learning and teacher effectiveness must be determined. The emphasis in recent years on teacher accountability has made evaluation more important than ever.

In the education process, perhaps no terms are misused more often than *measurement* and *evaluation*. **Measurement** is the collection of information on which a decision is based. The purpose of measurement is to collect information for evaluation, such as tests. The measurement process is the first step in evaluation; improved measurement leads to accurate evaluation (Baumgartner and Jackson 1999, 4). Measurement generally results in quantitative data in numerical form. The various types of tests, rating scales, attitude scales, checklists, and observation techniques used in the elementary school are all forms of measurement. The resulting raw data, however, must be evaluated before the effectiveness of the instruction can be assessed. Data are not information; they are only the basis for information. They answer the question of "How much?"

Evaluation is the use of measurement in making decisions. For example, information gathered through measurements is interpreted according to established standards so that decisions about student progress can be made (Baumgartner and Jackson 1999, 4). Uses for evaluation and grading include the following (Morrow et al. 1994, 124):

- motivation and guidance of the learning of students
- communication to students and parents about students' progress
- appraisal of students for use by the school itself in tailoring education to student needs and interests
- evaluating the effectiveness of teaching methods

Evaluation can be either objective or subjective. It is a judgment of what the numerical measurement data actually mean. For example, if all the students in a class get a perfect score on a test, has the instruction been successful? Perhaps not. The test might have simply measured what was known before any instruction. Or the test might have been so poorly constructed that the correct answers were obvious, whether instruction had been provided or not.

More importantly, evaluation is now seeking to provide more than a score to determine successful learning. Techniques include performance-based evaluation, narrative grading, portfolio evaluation, group projects, individual exhibits, and critical thinking essays.

Two different forms of evaluation of student progress are formative and summative evaluation. **Formative evaluation** is gathering data for the purpose of improving specific aspects of a teaching/learning process. **Summative evaluation** is that evaluation conducted at the end of a unit of instruction. An example is the use of a written test. Measurement and evaluation help teachers to:

Assess the effectiveness of the learning activities. Measurement and evaluation will help determine whether learning activities that have been designed and employed have increased knowledge, helped clarify values or determined attitudes, and promoted decision-making skills. If not, the activities must be revised or replaced.

Motivate the student. Tests help students recognize how much learning has taken place. Pretests are useful for introducing the scope of a topic and making students aware of the material that will be covered. Posttests then are used to chart actual student progress.

Help develop the scope and sequence of teaching. Measurement and evaluation can help determine the level of teaching and the order in which it should occur. For example, if the knowledge level of a class is high, a simple review of the factual material may be all that is necessary before moving on to new subject matter. Or, if the factual material is known, the decision may be to work next on developing attitudes toward this knowledge.

Teacher Skills Needed for Competent Measurement and Evaluation

Becoming competent in measurement and evaluation does not happen overnight. Developing the skills that will be needed occurs in education classes, in educational psychology classes, and during student teaching. As a teacher gains professional experience, these skills will be sharpened. To be competent at measuring and evaluating, the National Council on Measurement in Education (2002) notes that a teacher should be skilled in the seven areas described below.

Choosing assessment strategies. They can describe the nature and use of different types of formal and informal assessments, including questionnaires, checklists, interviews, inventories, tests, observations, surveys, and performance assessments.

Identifying, accessing, and evaluating the most commonly used assessment instruments. They know which assessment instruments are most commonly used in school settings to assess achievement, including computer-assisted versions and other alternate formats.

The techniques of administration and methods of scoring assessment instruments. They can implement appropriate administration procedures, including administration using computers. They can standardize administration of assessments when interpretation is in relation to external norms.

Interpreting and reporting assessment results. They can explain scores that are commonly reported, such as percentile ranks, standard scores, and grade equivalents. They are skilled in communicating assessment information to others, including teachers, administrators, students, parents, and the community.

Using assessment results in decision making. They recognize the limitations of using a single score in making an educational decision and know how to obtain multiple sources of information to improve such decisions.

Interpreting and presenting statistical information about assessment results. They can describe data (for example, test scores, grades, and demographic information). They can compare a score from an assessment instrument with an existing distribution, describe the placement of a score within a normal distribution, and draw appropriate inferences.

Conducting and interpreting evaluations of programs. They understand and appreciate the role that evaluation plays in the program development process throughout the life of a program. They can describe the purposes of an evaluation and the types of decisions to be based on evaluation information. They can identify and evaluate possibilities for unintended outcomes and possible impacts of one program on other programs.

In health education, measurement and evaluation cannot be limited to the cognitive domain but must also be vitally concerned with the formation of attitudes and behavior patterns among students. The emphasis in testing instruments is on quantitative measures, but these measures must also be employed to gain insight into qualitative areas. Selection of an instrument is not simply a matter of locating a test on specific content. It is important to select the best test available, *best* being defined in terms of most appropriate for specific objectives and for specific students. If one test fails to measure what the teacher wants it to measure, another one needs to be developed. Tests for assessing knowledge, attitudes, and practices are used to assess the impact of education on children.

Teacher-Designed Tests

Teacher-designed tests can be tailored to specific purposes and groups of students. This is a primary advantage. On the negative side, teacher-designed tests may lack validity and reliability. However, with experience, the tests that teachers develop should become increasingly good indicators of student learning and change.

In constructing tests, each of the following six areas must be included.

Validity. Does the test measure what it is supposed to measure? If the desire is to determine changes in student attitudes, for example, a test that asks students for factual information will not fulfill this intent. Validity is a matter of degree, not a characteristic that is absent or present. A test that is currently valid may not necessarily be so in the future. Because tests are designed for a variety of purposes, and because validity can be viewed only in terms of purpose, it is not surprising that there are several types of validity. **Content validity** is defined as the degree to which a test measures an intended content area. **Construct validity** is the degree to which a test measures a hypothetical construct, such as intelligence. **Concurrent validity** is the degree to which the scores on a given test are related to the scores on another test. **Predictive validity** is the degree to which a test can predict how well a student will do in a particular situation.

Reliability. A reliable test must provide consistent measurements. For example, if a student whose knowledge has not changed is measured twice with a perfectly reliable test, the two scores will be identical (Baumgartner and Jackson 1999, 96). Other factors that can affect the reliability of a test include inappropriate test items, the way the test is administered to the students, how the test is scored and interpreted, and the physical condition of the test environment.

Objectivity. Is the test fair to the students? For example, if the readability level is too high, students may be unable to supply correct answers even if they understand the concept being tested. If there is more than one possible correct answer, students should not be penalized for providing reasonable alternatives.

Discrimination. Does the test differentiate among good, average, and poor students?

Comprehensiveness. Is the test long enough to cover the material? Keep in mind that a fifty-item test may be no more comprehensive than a ten-item test if the items tap only certain areas while neglecting others.

Administration and Scoring. Is the test easy to give, use, and score? Keep in mind that the easiest test to administer and score may not be the best test for assessing the area. For example, an essay test, which is more difficult to score, may provide a better assessment of certain concepts than an easier-to-score true/false test.

Developing Tests

Developing good tests is a difficult task. The starting point is to establish a table of specifications. This table serves as the blueprint for the test. The purpose of the table of specifications is to ensure that all the objectives for a unit or lesson

Table 5.1 *Specifications for Unit on Substance Abuse*

Valued Outcome:

The learner will . . .	Content	Percentage of items
Define what constitutes substance abuse.	What substance abuse is; what can result from abuse; what some symptoms are	15%
List the various substances that can be abused.	Depressants (types); cocaine; marijuana; designer drugs; hallucinogens	35%
Discuss why people use drugs.	Reasons for drug use	15%
List where to get help for substance abuse.	Agencies; organizations; professionals	10%
Develop techniques for avoiding substance abuse.	How to say no to substance abuse	25%

are covered on the test. By developing the table, the teacher can ensure that the proper percentage of test items appears in relationship to the emphasis placed on each objective (see Table 5.1). The process of developing a test should involve the following steps:

1. Prepare the table of specifications based on the unit objectives.
2. Draft the test items.
3. Decide on the length of the test.
4. Select and edit the final items.
5. Rate the items in terms of difficulty.
6. Arrange the items in order of difficulty from easiest to most difficult.
7. Prepare the instructions for the test.
8. Prepare the answer key and decide the rules for scoring.
9. Produce the test.

The next area of concern is developing the various types of test items. Several types of test items can be used for assessment purposes. Some teachers may wish to use a variety of types, while others may prefer one or two types. It is wise to employ at least two types of test items because some students don't always do well on a particular type of test item. For example, some students do well on essay tests, while others do better on multiple choice.

Another important consideration is the order in which the test items appear. Most important, all similar items should be grouped together. This helps to simplify directions, makes it easier for students to maintain the same psychological set throughout each section, and makes the scoring of the test easier. Test items should proceed from the simpler items to more complex ones. The following order is suggested for sections of test items:

1. **True/false.** Consists of declaratory statements that are either true or false.

   Examples:

   _T_   **A.** Drugs are harmful if they are abused.

   _F_   **B.** A burn on the skin should be bandaged tightly.

2. **Matching.** Answers in one column to be paired with the correct item in another column. A form of multiple-choice test, except that the number of choices is compounded.

   Example:

   _a_   **1.** compensation   **a.** covering faults by trying to excel in another area

   _c_   **2.** regression   **b.** creating make-believe events

   _d_   **3.** rationalization   **c.** acting in an immature way

       d. making an excuse for a mistake or failure

3. **Multiple choice.** Requires the student to recognize which of several suggested responses is the best answer. This kind of test provides an opportunity to develop thought-provoking questions. It is considered the best short-answer test format.

   Example:

   _c_   **1.** Which of these nutrients helps repair the body?

       a. carbohydrates

       b. fats

       c. proteins

       d. vitamins

4. **Short answer.** Includes a variety of types of questions ranging from fill- in- the- blank to listing.

   Examples:

   A. List the four chambers of the heart.

   Right atrium
   Left atrium
   Right ventricle
   Left ventricle

   B. The iris controls the amount of __*light*__ going to the lens.

5. **Essay.** Requires the student to organize information in a systematic fashion. Allows the teacher to gain insight into the amount of understanding students have developed.

   Example:

   What has been the most influential factor in shaping your perceptions of yourself? Do you feel some of these perceptions are correct?

Regardless of the type of item employed, each item should be evaluated as to that item's effectiveness (Linn and Gronlund 1999, 230).

Measuring Health Attitudes

Because attitudes are so important in health behavior, they are frequently measured in health education and health promotion programs. Without favorable attitudes toward a health behavior, the student is not likely to be sufficiently motivated to continue or change a behavior (Simons-Morton, Greene, and Gottlieb 1995, 171). An attitude involves feelings, values, and appreciations. An attitude can also be described as a predisposition to actions.

Because one of the goals in teaching health is the development of positive health attitudes, it is essential to attempt to assess student attitudes. This is no easy matter, because attitudes are not within the cognitive domain and are not thus readily tapped by most kinds of tests. Many tests that attempt to measure attitudes are not constructed in a scientific manner, and offer only limited information to the teacher (Morrow et al. 1995, 323). Even those that are designed for this purpose often lack validity, as students may respond with answers they think the teacher will favor rather than state their true feelings or predispositions. Thus, it is important to supplement such testing instruments with other means of assessment, such as self-inventories, questionnaires, checklists, observation, informal conferences, small-group discussion, and anecdotal record-keeping. These strategies produce subjective indications of what the child's attitudes may be. With these limitations in mind, we now examine some of the more common written measures for assessing student attitudes.

ATTITUDE SCALES

A scale is a testing instrument that requires the student to choose between alternatives on a continuum. Two polar choices, such as yes/no or agree/disagree, may be offered, or a range of choices may be provided.

The Teaching in Action box below shows a **forced-choice scale,** one that provides only two options about each statement being considered. This kind of attitude scale is appropriate for use with younger children, who lack the developmental ability to handle more complicated attitude scales.

TEACHING IN ACTION *Example of a Forced-Choice Attitude Scale*

Rating Myself: How I Feel

	Agree	Disagree
1. My overall physical health is excellent.	_____	_____
2. I have a positive attitude toward most things.	_____	_____
3. I have the ability to make my life work.	_____	_____
4. I relate well to other people.	_____	_____
5. I have control of my life.	_____	_____

TEACHING IN ACTION *A Likert Scale with a Five-Choice Spread*

Feelings about Exercise

	Strongly Agree	Agree	Not Sure	Disagree	Strongly Disagree
1. Exercise is healthy for a person.	_____	_____	_____	_____	_____
2. I like to run and jump.	_____	_____	_____	_____	_____
3. I would rather watch TV than engage in exercise.	_____	_____	_____	_____	_____
4. I feel relaxed after exercising.	_____	_____	_____	_____	_____
5. Playing sports is fun.	_____	_____	_____	_____	_____
6. I cannot work on exercise.	_____	_____	_____	_____	_____
7. Playing sports and games is too much work to program into my daily schedule.	_____	_____	_____	_____	_____
8. I would rather watch sports than play them.	_____	_____	_____	_____	_____
9. Exercise helps keep me healthy.	_____	_____	_____	_____	_____

The major disadvantage of the forced-choice scale test is that students can readily perceive what the "correct" response should be. They will respond accordingly, even if the answer does not reflect their actual attitude toward the issue. This problem can be overcome to a certain degree by establishing an atmosphere in the classroom of warmth, trust, and rapport.

A **Likert scale** is a more sophisticated attitude scale that provides a range of choices about each attitudinal issue. The more choices that are offered, the more discrimination a student must have to complete the scale. The Teaching in Action box above provides an example of a Likert scale.

Scoring may be done in a variety of ways, depending on how the statements in the scale are phrased. For example, the continuum of responses may be weighted from 1 to 5, with the lowest score for a *strongly disagree* statement and the highest score for a *strongly agree* statement. Thus, if a student checks *strongly agree* to the statement, "Being stoned all the time is no way to live," the score would be a 5. An *undecided* response would rate a 3, and a *strongly disagree* would rate a 1. Note that the scoring rank must be reversed for oppositely worded statements, such as "Experimenting with drugs is not really very risky." In this case, a *strongly disagree* response would score as a 5.

The total numerical score derived from adding the individual response scores offers a measure of how firmly opinions and attitudes are held about the issues examined in the scale. However, this measure, despite its seeming quantitative preciseness, is only a rough indicator of attitude. Bear in mind that the scoring system is arbitrary; that even with five options, students are still making forced choices; and that students may respond with "correct" answers that do not actually reflect their true attitudes. Instruments used for attitude assessment should not be used for purposes of grading, because this will further bias the students' responses.

OBSERVATION

As mentioned earlier, the use of attitude scales to assess children's feelings and values has its limitations. The results of such scales are often inconclusive. Scales or other measurement devices, such as checklists or student surveys, should be augmented with other techniques, including observation and anecdotal recordkeeping.

Observation is an excellent way of assessing behavior. Because observation can be done on an ongoing, daily basis, it can provide important clues as to attitudes and predispositions to actions. A major disadvantage of observation is that it is time-consuming. Further, discretion must be exercised so as not to violate student and parent privacy.

Teachers can structure activities in order to observe students' attitudes toward various health issues. For example, the teacher can mark several spots throughout the classroom with *Strongly Agree* and *Strongly Disagree* labels. As a teacher calls out a specific issue, e.g., "A family member should always tell a terminal patient about his or her illness," the students can walk to the spot that best reflects their attitude toward the statement. This type of activity enables the students to take a public stand regarding the issue; however the teacher should use caution in including controversial issues in such a public forum. Also, some students might be too embarrassed to declare their values publicly and might go to the spot occupied by friends or the majority of the class.

TEACHING IN ACTION *Observation Checklist for Assessing Respect for Others*

Name _____ Date of Assessment _____

Observation _____

Observer _____

Directions: Listed below are characteristics related to "Respect for Others." For the student listed, check those characteristics that are appropriate.

_____ Respects views and opinions of others

_____ Is sensitive to needs of others

_____ Is sensitive to problems of others

_____ Respects the property of others

_____ Works cooperatively with others

_____ Addresses others in a respectful manner

In assessing student health attitudes, an attempt to remain neutral in observations should be made. Variations in personal health attitudes and behaviors are not necessarily a cause for concern. Children are still forming their attitudes about health-related issues. They should not be expected to have completely made up their minds about health practices. If they have, there would be far less point to the job of teaching.

Further, attitude formation is a gradual process. Instant changes in behavior patterns are not necessarily going to occur. The teacher's efforts can make a difference. With these thoughts in mind, one method to use in assessing attitudes is the checklist. The checklist allows the observer to note quickly and effectively whether a trait or characteristic is present. Checklists can be useful in evaluating learning activities or some aspects of personal-social interaction. The Teaching in Action box on page 112 is a sample checklist for evaluating student behavior after a unit on respect for others.

As has been noted, measuring attitudes is difficult. Any technique used to measure and evaluate attitudes or health practices should be done carefully and with student input if it is to be part of the grading process. If this is done, students will be more likely to reveal their true feelings or their actual practices. Alternatively, the evaluation can be used to plan for future instruction and to help students understand their current level of development. The more aware students become about themselves, the more likely it is that they will use this awareness to make conscious decisions about future behavior.

Traditional Grading Strategies

Grades serve to inform students, parents, teachers, and administrators about the progress and work efficiency of the student. Ideally, grades should not be an end in themselves. Instead, they should act as motivators for students to do their best and as guides for the students to future courses of study. For parents, student grades identify the child's strengths and weaknesses and also help clarify the goals of the school. If parents gain insight through grades as to what the school is attempting to accomplish, they will be in a better position to cooperate with the teacher in enhancing the child's educational process. Administrators can use grades to see how effective the curriculum is and to step in to provide extra help for students who need it by means of special programs, counseling, and so forth.

Each school district has its own approach to grading. Teachers should become familiar with the system used in their district in order to apply the standards objectively and fairly.

THE PERCENTAGE METHOD

This grading method is based on 100 percent. It assumes more precision than can actually exist and essentially reduces the range of scores that might fall between 70 and 100 percent if other grading methods are used. Any student falling below 70 percent correct responses on a given test fails. Many school districts that employ this method use a scale similar to the following:

A = 93–100%

B = 85–92%

C = 78–84%

D = 70–77%

F = Below 70%

THE A TO F COMBINATION METHOD

The A to F combination method system of grading is a combination of the percentage method and other descriptors that indicate student performance. With this method, students can be rated in relation to both the group norm and personal development. The A to F combination method better enables students and parents to know whether learning and work are being accomplished at peak capacity. For example, it is possible for students to make a C grade and still have them appreciate that they are working near maximum effort. A typical example of how this method is structured is as follows:

A = excellent work and working at or near capacity; 95–100%

B = good work and working at or near capacity; 85–94%

C = average work or all that should be expected; 77–84%

D = much less than should be expected; 70–76%

F = no noticeable progress; less than 70%

1 = above grade level

2 = at grade level

3 = below grade level

The numbers can be used in conjunction with the letter grades. For example, a child who receives a grade of B-2 is performing near capacity at grade level, whereas a child who receives a grade of B-3 is performing near capacity but below grade level.

PASS/FAIL

Some of the symbols used to indicate achievement are O, S, and U for *outstanding, satisfactory,* and *unsatisfactory.* The symbols P and F are also used to indicate *pass* or *fail.* Others may use E, S, N, or U for *excellent, satisfactory, not satisfactory,* and *unsatisfactory.*

Unfortunately, any course using these symbols may be viewed as less important than those courses receiving the traditional A to F grades. Certainly, in the case of health education, this connotation must be avoided because the knowledge, attitudes, and behaviors developed have the potential to be life enhancing, and, in some cases, lifesaving.

There are no easy answers in choosing a grading system. The best method is really a combination of systems. Each teacher and school system must weigh the advantages of each type of grading and select the one that best informs students and parents of progress.

PERFORMANCE-BASED EVALUATION

In addition to traditional cognitive testing, which generally involves the use of paper-and-pencil tests, teachers must now seek to base their evaluation of students "upon the values, diversity, and ability to make environmentally sound and healthy personal choices" (Read 1997, 148). Most evaluation specialists refer to these types of evaluation as **performance-based evaluation.** Performance-based evaluation is not contingent on what the students recall, but on how they show what they have learned. Several techniques lend to this type of evaluation. Examples include portfolios, exhibitions, group projects, and critical thinking essays.

Portfolios are defined as a purposeful collection of student work that exhibits effort, progress, and achievement. This effort must include the student's participation in selecting the content, how the material will be assessed, and what will provide evidence of student self-reflection (Woolfolk 1995). To ensure that portfolios will serve as useful tools, the following guidelines should be kept in mind:

1. There must be student involvement in selecting the components that will constitute the portfolio.

2. Students should include information that allows them to self-reflect and self-criticize.

3. Student activities should be reflected in projects, writing, and drawing and result from the student's learning goals.

4. The portfolio should reflect the growth of the student in progress toward achieving insight and attitude/behavior development. It should reflect the feelings and thinking of the student.

5. Evaluation should be based on each student's established standards, not on comparisons with other students in the class.

Exhibitions are considered a performance test or demonstration of learning that is presented before an audience and takes extended time to prepare (Woolfolk 1995). Examples of exhibits might include developing displays, writing skits or plays, or designing bulletin boards.

Critical thinking essays can be defined as a cognitive writing activity that allows the student to analyze or synthesize information in order to make a decision (McCown, Driscoll, and Roop 1996, 382). An excellent way to promote critical thinking in elementary students is to provide the student with what King (1990) referred to as *reciprocal questioning* by having the students work in pairs or small groups to answer questions concerning the health topic such as:

How would you use . . . to . . . ?

What is a new example of . . . ?

How are . . . and . . . similar?

What are the strengths and weaknesses of . . . ?

Performance-based evaluation is a very important concept in health education, because attitude and ultimately behavior are the culminating factors. Obviously, in the case of both portfolios and exhibitions, group work and critical essays may be an extensive part of the process. Certainly when using this type of evaluation, it is difficult to tell where instruction stops and assessment starts because of the interwoven nature of the two in performance-based evaluation. The goal should be to help students focus on what they have learned, how they have changed, and what they have achieved as a result of the process. What better way to do this than to allow the student to have input on what will constitute learning and evaluation? Perhaps the greatest advantage of performance-based evaluation is that, if done properly, children can learn, achieve, and progress in a fashion that does not label or negatively affect their self-esteem.

PEER EVALUATION

A trend in the current rethinking of how evaluation should occur is to involve students in the process. One strategy for accomplishing this is through peer evaluation. Peer evaluation occurs when students evaluate each other's work (McCown, Driscoll, and Roop 1996, 457).

Peer evaluation happens all the time on an informal basis when students look at one another's work for comparison with their own efforts. For peer evaluation to be effective, students should work together to establish the criteria or standards used for judging their work. By setting the standards for judgment, students have established their own goals, which they expect their work to reflect. Assessment can be done through the use of checklists or questionnaires.

NARRATIVE GRADING

Narrative grading has been defined as "serious dialogue between student and teacher about the quality of the work" (Shor 1992). The dialogue should be student generated and should reflect creative options as well as critical thinking. The facts should not be isolated from the student's experience. Effort should be made to help the student personalize the information to ensure positive health-related behavior. The advantage of this type of grading is that, once verbalized, ownership of the concept(s) is more likely to occur. This strategy also enables students to assess their feeling on particular topics. The biggest disadvantage is that the process can be very time consuming when working with a large group.

NATIONAL HEALTH STANDARDS AND GRADING

A curriculum based on the National Health Education Standards requires teachers to rely heavily on assessment strategies through which students contribute to a process and, in many cases, create a product or participate in a performance. To help schools and teachers assess students' performance on competencies set out in the national standards, the Council of Chief State School Officers (2002) coordinated the Health Education State Collaborative on Assessment and Student Standards (SCASS) project to develop an assessment system. These assessments include selected response items and performance-based assessments, such as tasks, events, and student portfolios, with rubrics that are consistent with the national standards (Marx and Wooley 1998, 52).

The **rubric** is an authentic assessment tool that is particularly useful in assessing complex and subjective criteria. Authentic assessment is geared toward assessment methods that closely correspond to real world experience and applies such evaluations to all areas of the curriculum. It was originally developed in the arts and apprenticeship systems, where assessment has always been based on performance. The instructor observes the student in the process of working on real-life problems, provides feedback, monitors the student's use of the feedback, and adjusts instruction and evaluation accordingly.

The rubric is a formative type of assessment because it becomes an ongoing part of the whole teaching and learning process. Students are involved in the assessment process through both peer and self-assessment. As students become familiar with rubrics, they can assist in the rubric design process. This involvement empowers the students and, as a result, their learning becomes more focused and self-directed. Authentic assessment, therefore, blurs the lines between teaching, learning, and assessment.

The advantages of using rubrics in assessment are that they: allow assessment to be more objective and consistent; focus the teacher to clarify his or her criteria in specific terms; clearly show the student how his or her work will be evaluated and what is expected; promote student awareness of which criteria to use in assessing peer performance; provide useful feedback regarding the effectiveness of the instruction; and provide benchmarks against which to measure and document progress.

Rubrics can be created in a variety of forms and levels of complexity; however, they all contain common features that focus on measuring a stated objective (performance, behavior, or quality), use a range to rate performance, and contain specific performance characteristics arranged in levels indicating the degree to which a standard has been met.

Some states are working together currently to develop the actual assessment standards and measures related to the National Health Standards. States are invited to join one or more of the projects that develop standards and student assessments through pooled resources and effort. (These projects will be linked to the emerging national health standards and new ideas about appropriate assessment methods.) One such project is the Health Education Assessment Project, in which the group has developed assessment measures, performance tasks, and performance events, plus a portfolio assessment model to measure this area. Member states will have sufficient assessment resources to conduct assessment at the state and local levels. Professional development materials are also being developed (San Diego State University 2002).

Using Benchmarks and Standards to Assess Student Progress

In the last several years, school systems have turned to content standards and benchmarks to guide the teaching and learning that takes place in the classrooms. Many, if not most, educators are unaware of the impact the very discussion of standards, let alone the reorganization of schools around standards, has had on American education. Educators and administrators consider the standards movement one of the most controversial issues in school reform.

Standards and benchmarks are used to help the teacher understand what students are expected to know and to be able to do in each subject. These methods are used in assessing students' progress in learning, and as an attempt to raise the performance of all students. The theory behind this concept of evaluating student progess is that when students know and are able to do what is expected, they will rise to the challenge and perform at higher levels. Grading systems which use content standards and benchmarks use several assessment tools along with tradtional ones. Usually a school system implements standards and benchmarks in the early stages, and classroom management is not very different from the traditional classroom. Teachers are given the freedom to use a variety of teaching methods to enable children to reach standards at different paces (Marzano and Kendall 1996).

CONTENT STANDARDS

Content standards describe the knowledge and skills expected of students at certain stages in their education. Implementing content standards means that every school in a particular school system has the same expectations for all students in key subjects, although there is enough flexibility to allow individual schools and teachers to help students meet the standards in different ways. For example, schools may use various materials, and teachers may teach differently. But the goal is the same: clear learning expectations and high levels of achievement for all.

Often, a school system will create **performance tasks** that determine if a student has reached the content standards. These tasks include hands-on demonstrations, written projects, and portfolios of student work, as discussed earlier in this chapter. Typically, these new methods of assessing student work supplement the traditional ones. Teachers often use these performance tasks and scoring guides to describe a student's expected level of performance. Since all students do not test well, a well-rounded series of assessments will give students a variety of opportunities to demonstrate what they have learned.

BENCHMARKS

Benchmarks are set at various grade levels (similar to the National Health Standards in Chapter 4—i.e., fourth, eighth, and twelfth grades). Benchmarks are used to ensure that students are progressing appropriately. For example,

Health Highlight

EXAMPLE OF HEALTH CURRICULUM GUIDE

FROM TENNESSEE DEPARTMENT OF EDUCATION
Standards for Healthful Living

Personal Health and Wellness: K–2

Domain Description: Personal health and wellness is influenced by individual heredity and involves a lifelong process of choices and behaviors that lead to healthful living and disease prevention.

Standard 1: The student will understand the role of personal hygiene practices as related to healthful living.

Learning Expectations:

The student will:

1. demonstrate appropriate personal hygiene practices;
2. identify the effects of poor personal hygiene practices.

Performance Indicators:

At Level 1, the student will be able to:

- identify proper hygiene skills (e.g. handwashing, shampooing, flossing, toothbrushing, and bathing);
- identify basic signs and symptoms of head lice.

At Level 2, the student will be able to:

- apply proper hygiene practices (e.g. handwashing, shampooing, flossing, toothbrushing, bathing);
- identify consequences of poor oral hygiene (e.g. cavities, gum disease, and tooth loss);

- identify consequences of poor personal hygiene (e.g. body odor, illness, and poor self image);
- practice prevention of head lice.

At Level 3, the student will be able to:

- demonstrate proper hygiene practices;
- explain the importance of proper hygiene practices;
- identify signs and symptoms of head lice.

Teacher Assessment Indicators (examples):

The teacher may:

- apply cooking oil and ground cinnamon to the students' hands. Students rub their own hands together, see the sediment and think it is dirt, wash hands as normally do. Observe that oil and cinnamon are still evident. Students then apply soap and use proper handwashing techniques as taught by the teacher;
- provide a dental mold for students to demonstrate proper toothbrushing techniques (invite dental professional if needed);
- have the students demonstrate the practices of prevention of head lice (e.g. not sharing mats, hats, combs, and headphones).

Curriculum Integration: N/A

SOURCE: Tennessee.gov

National Health Standard 2 says that all "students will demonstrate the ability to access valid health information and health-promoting products and services." The benchmarks for that standard would be more specific. A fourth grade benchmark, for example, might say that students must recall main ideas and details, put events in order, predict outcomes, and draw conclusions. By the eighth grade, students must be able to understand the techniques used by the author and the author's purpose. By the twelfth grade, students must read to determine goals and beliefs and to take positions on issues. Not all students will reach benchmarks at the same time. Some students may need more assistance. For example, a school system might provide before and after-school tutoring, summer school, or Saturday school as opportunities for students.

Summary

- The purpose of measurement and evaluation is to determine whether instructional objectives have been fulfilled.
- Measurement involves the construction, administration, and scoring of tests.
- Evaluation is the process of interpreting, analyzing, and assessing the data gathered.
- Newer methods used for evaluation include performance-based evaluation, narrative grading, portfolios, group projects, individual exhibits, and critical thinking essays.
- Tests should be valid; reliable; objective; discriminate; comprehensive; and easy to give, use, and score.
- Typical test question types are true/false, matching, multiple choice, short answer, and essay.
- Measuring attitudes is difficult; examples of useful tools include attitude scales, checklists, and critical thinking essays.
- Traditional grading strategies include the percentage method, the A to F combination, and the pass/fail or satisfactory/unsatisfactory method.
- Newer methods include performance-based evaluation, critical thinking essays, peer review, and group projects.
- Benchmarks and standards are now used to guide teaching and learning.

DISCUSSION QUESTIONS

1. Differentiate between measurement and evaluation.
2. Discuss the purposes of measurement and evaluation, and explain how you can achieve these purposes.
3. Why is a table of specifications necessary when developing a test?
4. Discuss some of the techniques used to assess attitudes in health education. What are the shortcomings of these techniques?
5. What purposes does grading serve in health education?
6. Discuss some of the common methods of grading used in the elementary school. Explain how they changed in the 1990s.
7. Explain what content standards and benchmarks are, and describe the implications of their use in schools throughout the country.

CRITICAL THINKING QUESTIONS

1. In what ways can you as a teacher reduce the "adversarial relationship" between student and teacher sometimes caused by the grading process?
2. How can you as a teacher help your students enjoy learning for the sake of learning instead of learning just to make a grade?

3. What skills do you possess that will enable you to be a competent evaluator of student progress? What skills do you need to develop?

4. Explain your feelings about the relative importance of measuring attitudes in a health education class.

5. Your principal has suggested to you that health education should be graded on a pass/fail basis. How would you justify using a grading scale similar to other core subjects?

WEB SITE ACTIVITY

Go to *www.ascd.org/handbook* and find the Association for Supervision and Curriculum Development's Curriculum Handbook. Then click Demo Version for Non-Subscribers. Click Standard Version—Using Frames. Click Open the Curriculum Handbook. Then find the Overview for Health Education. Comment on the Implications of the National Health Standards.

WEB SITES OF INTEREST

Association for Supervision and Curriculum Development (ASCD):
   www.ascd.org
ASCD is a unique international, nonprofit, nonpartisan association of professional educators whose jobs cross all grade levels and subject areas.

Council of Chief State School Officers: *www.ccsso.org/scass.html*
The State Collaborative on Assessment and Student Standards is designed to assist states in developing needed student standards and assessments in conjunction with other states expressing similar needs.

National Council on Measurement and Evaluation (NCME): *www.ncme.org*
NCME is an organization that is incorporated exclusively for scientific, educational, literary, and charitable purposes. Its purposes include encouragement of scholarly efforts.

National Education Association (NEA): *www.nea.org*
America's oldest and largest organization committed to advancing the cause of public education. NEA proudly claims over 2.3 million members who work at every level of education, from preschool to university.

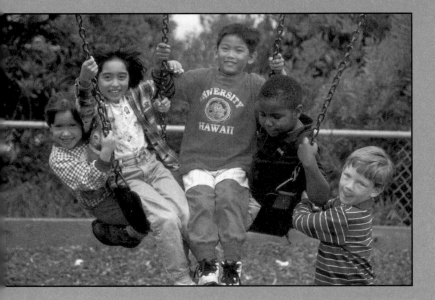

CHAPTER SIX

Mental Health and Stress Reduction

Dwell upon the brightest
parts in every prospect . . .
and strive to be pleased with
the present circumstance.

—Abraham Tucker (1774)

VALUED OUTCOMES

After reading this chapter, you should be able to:

- define mental health
- identify the characteristics of the emotionally healthy individual
- describe how psychosocial factors contribute to mental health
- describe the importance of self-esteem and the development of positive mental health
- discuss strategies of enhancing the self-esteem of children
- discuss the indicators of major psychiatric problems
- identify the factors that lead to obsessive-compulsive behaviors

- discuss panic disorder in students
- discuss problems associated with latchkey children or children from separated/divorced families
- identify the means of dealing with students who have experienced the death of a pet, grandparent, parent, or sibling
- define the terms *stress* and *stressor*

- describe the detrimental health effects of prolonged stress
- briefly discuss each of the rules for fostering good mental health
- identify strategies for dealing with stress
- discuss the role of the family in maintaining a child's emotional health

REFLECTIONS

There was a folk singer by the name of Jimmy Rogers who recorded a song called "Child of Clay." One of the lines in that recording was "bended, molded, and shaped into what we are today." As you read this chapter, reflect on the many factors that influence student's perceptions of self and ultimately their mental health. What are significant influences in children's lives? What potential impacts (both negative and positive) do these events, people, and institutions have? What can teachers do to positively influence the children under their tutelage?

The Importance of Mental Health

There is probably no area more vital than that of helping students to develop sound mental health practices. We need only look at the rates of alcohol and drug use among our nation's youth, the suicide rates for adolescents, the reported depression among youth, the number of school-age children who run away from home each year, or the violence that occurs in our schools to realize the importance of helping students achieve and maintain good mental and emotional health. Without the sense of inner peace and balance that comes with good mental health, no individual can be considered completely healthy. The links between mental and physical health are clear. Yet the goal of good mental health is in many ways more elusive than that of good physical health. If an individual receives proper nutrition, exercises on a regular basis, gets plenty of relaxation and sleep, and follows good personal health practices, he or she has a high probability of remaining physically fit. Unfortunately, there is no easy prescription for good mental health. There are, however, identifiable characteristics of people who are mentally healthy. Experts have defined **mental health** as the ability to perceive reality as it is, to respond to its challenges, and to develop rational strategies for living (Hales 1992, 25). A component of mental health is **emotional health,** or the ability to deal constructively with reality, regardless of whether the actual situation is good or bad (Greenberg and Dintiman 1992, 20).

Implied in these two definitions is the concept that emotionally healthy people are in touch with their feelings and can express those feelings in a proper fashion. This chapter provides information about mental health principles that will help your students develop sound mental health. Topics discussed include human needs and the development of self-esteem, behavior and the expression of emotions, stress and its relationship to mental health, values and patterns of decision making, and the role of the family in the development of mental health.

Characteristics of the Emotionally Healthy Individual

If mental health is defined as the ability to perceive reality and to respond to the challenges of life, then what are the characteristics of an emotionally healthy individual? Maslow has conceptualized emotional happiness in what he calls self-actualized people. There are individuals who seemed to live, or be living, at their fullest. Maslow goes on to suggest that a self-actualized person has five important qualities (Maslow 1983).

A sense of realism—the ability to deal with the world as it is and not demand that it be otherwise.

A sense of acceptance—the ability to accept themselves and others.

A sense of autonomy—the ability to direct themselves, acting independently of their environments. They are not afraid to be themselves. They are inner-directed people who find guidance from within their own values and feelings.

A sense of creativity—a sense of appreciation for what goes on around them. They are open to new experiences and do not fear the unknown.

A capacity for intimacy—the ability to be open to the pleasure of intimate physical contacts and the risks/satisfaction of being close to others in a caring, sensitive way.

Payne and Hahn (2002) expand upon the concept of an emotionally healthy person by listing the following characteristics. Healthy people:

- feel comfortable about themselves
- are capable of experiencing the full range of human emotions
- are not overwhelmed by their emotions—either negative or positive
- accept life's disappointments
- feel comfortable with others
- receive and give love easily
- feel concern for others when appropriate
- establish short-term and long-term goals
- function autonomously where and when appropriate

Health Highlight
SENSITIVITY TO MULTICULTURAL DIVERSITY

In society today there is a wide diversity of people and cultures. These differences have arisen because of the need to accommodate unique physical, demographic, and economic situations (Garcia 1991). The elementary teacher must strive to view all children of various cultures from students' perspectives rather than from his or her own cultural perspective. This means the classroom facilitates a climate of understanding and sensitivity to diverse cultures, ethnicities, and races.

To understand multicultural sensitivity and diversity, several terms must first be understood. Page and Page (2000, 91) define *culture* as a set of values, attitudes, and practices held in common by a group of people, usually identified by ancestry, language, and geography. *Ethnicity* refers to a portion of a population or subgroup having a

common cultural heritage. *Race* denotes a population distinguished by genetically determined physical traits, such as hair texture or color, skin color, eye shape, and body shape.

The elementary teacher can develop multicultural sensitivity in several ways. He or she should strive to develop personal skills, such as showing warmth, respect, sincerity, concern, and caring for people of all cultures. It is imperative that the teacher understand the communities from which the children come. In addition the teacher must be culturally sensitive to how different ethnic groups learn and solve problems. Part of this is understanding learning style; communication patterns; and such factors as eye contact, body language, and physical closeness.

- generally trust others
- lead a health-enhancing lifestyle that includes regular exercise, sound nutrition, and adequate sleep

There is no one ideal for emotional health. Certainly the lack of any one characteristic does not indicate an emotionally unhealthy person. Probably no one has all these characteristics, and most of us fall short at some time, but the lists can provide a benchmark for how well we are achieving or moving toward being emotionally healthy.

This process of achieving mental wellness is a lifelong process and begins the moment we are born. How we interact with our siblings, how our parents relate and interact with us, and our perceptions throughout life influence our mental wellness. The experiences each child undergoes while in the elementary school are very important. The perceptions of success, feelings of acceptance by peers and teachers, and the supportive emotional climate in the classroom all contribute to the emotional well-being and development of the child's self-esteem. The process begins when the child enters school each morning and continues until he or she leaves in the afternoon. The information learned each day, each year, year after year, eventually shapes self-perception and molds us into what we perceive ourselves to be. The home, family, and other institutions also help develop our perceptions, but none impacts as strongly as each teacher with whom we have contact during our elementary school years. The elementary

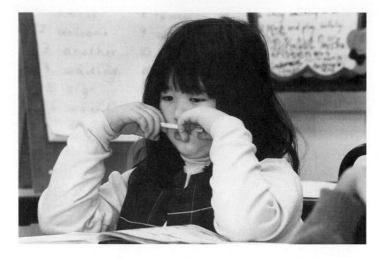

Teachers must be aware of possible depression in children.

teacher can provide confidence, appreciation, praise, fairness, security, approval, friendship, and acceptance. Through modeling, developing decision-making skills, and being in a success-oriented situation, the children learn to accept themselves and others.

What Children Need to Achieve Emotional Health

The fulfillment of basic emotional needs such as love, affection, acceptance, and a feeling of importance are essential to children developing a self-identity and their self-esteem. All people need to receive love and affection. Everyone needs to feel a sense of acceptance and importance from others. If these basic needs can be fostered, the child's potential for successfully interacting with others, meeting individual needs for independence and self-expression, and resolving personal and social conflicts are clearly enhanced. The child is freer to pursue higher human goals, culminating with what Maslow calls *self-actualization needs* (Hamrick, Anspaugh, and Ezell 1986). Maslow's hierarchy of human needs (shown in Figure 6.1) applies throughout our lives and certainly in the early developmental years of the elementary child.

W. Edward Deming, noted statistician and the father of quality management, offered the following points in an essay entitled "A System of Profound Knowledge" (Deming 1994). These points seem most relevant to keep in mind when discussing the mental health of children. (In this excerpt, we have substituted the term *children* for *people,* which was originally used in the essay). Deming stated:

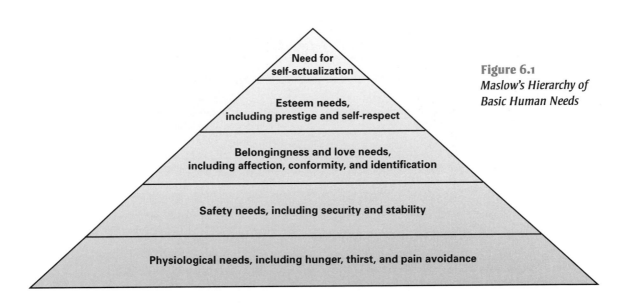

Figure 6.1
*Maslow's Hierarchy of
Basic Human Needs*

Need for
self-actualization

Esteem needs,
including prestige and self-respect

Belongingness and love needs,
including affection, conformity, and identification

Safety needs, including security and stability

Physiological needs, including hunger, thirst, and pain avoidance

- Children are different from one another.
- Children learn in different ways and at different speeds.
- Children are born with a need for relationships with other people and with the need to be loved and esteemed by others. There is an innate need for self-esteem and respect.
- Circumstances provide some children with dignity and self-esteem. Circumstances deny other children these advantages.
- No one can enjoy learning if he or she must constantly be concerned about grading and gold stars for performance.
- Extrinsic motivation is submission to external forces that neutralize intrinsic motivation.
- Under extrinsic motivation children are ruled by external forces.
- Leaders (teachers), by virtue of their authority, have an obligation to make changes in the system of management that will bring improvement. (The authors believe that Deming means preparing teachers to facilitate within the school and each individual classroom an atmosphere that helps each child feel respected and successful.)

Self-Esteem and the Development of Emotional Health

Many health educators and mental health authorities believe that self-esteem is the foundation of emotional health. **Self-esteem** can be defined as a combination of self-confidence and self-respect—the feeling that one is capable of

Health Highlight

FOSTERING A POSITIVE CLASSROOM ATMOSPHERE

Here are several guidelines developed by Page and Page (2000) for fostering an emotional climate conducive to mental wellness.

1. Quickly learn the names of students, call them by name, become familiar with their interests and talents, and show respect for each student.

2. Be well prepared and enthusiastic. Make learning fun and subject matter relevant and challenging to students.

3. Begin each class promptly. Develop and maintain routines for taking attendance, opening class, and so on.

4. Remember the three Fs of good discipline: *Firm, Fair,* and *Friendly*.

5. Expect no problems: don't be looking for them. Expect students to be competent, capable, and eager to learn. It is better to be proven wrong than to have students live up to negative expectations.

6. When problems arise, handle them immediately and consistently before they escalate into larger ones. Don't use "major artillery" for minor infractions.

7. Avoid sarcasm, ridicule, and belittling remarks, and help students do likewise.

8. Avoid all suggestions of criticism, anger, or frustration. It is better to make personal corrections in private conferences with students.

9. Be alert for indications of latent skills and interests in students and encourage them in their development.

10. Listen nonjudgmentally to student comments, and create an atmosphere where students feel at ease.

11. Arrange for a high ratio of successes to failures in academic tasks.

12. Involve students in the setting of individual academic goals.

13. Avoid encouraging competitiveness between students in your grading practices and learning activities.

14. Demonstrate the characteristics of effective teachers: warmth, friendliness, fairness, a good sense of humor, enthusiasm, empathy, openness, spontaneity, adaptability, and a governing style that is more democratic than autocratic.

coping with life's challenges and is worthy of happiness. In other words, self-esteem is how people perceive themselves. People with high self-esteem have confidence in themselves; have the ability to solve problems rather than just worry about them; have the ability to confront or eliminate the things that frighten them; have the ability to take reasonable risks; and are able to nurture themselves (Martin and Martin 2002).

In the early years of children's lives, self-esteem is based largely on their perceptions of how the important adults in their lives judge them. The extent to which children believe they have the characteristics valued by the adults and peers in their lives determines greatly their perception of self. Families, communities, and ethnic groups may vary in the criteria on which self-esteem is based. Some groups may emphasize athletic ability, others physical appearance; others evaluate boys and girls differently. Factors such as stereotyping, prejudice, and discrimination may also contribute to low self-esteem among children (Katz 2002).

Bean (1992) says four conditions are important if children are to develop and maintain high self-esteem:

1. **A sense of connectiveness**—children must feel a part of something; feel related in important ways to specific people, places, or things; identify with a group of people; feel something important belongs to them (a sense of ownership); and feel they belong to something or someone.

2. **A sense of uniqueness**—children must feel that they have special qualities; are valued for who they are; and can do things that no one else knows or can do. They must feel that they can express themselves in their own unique way; feel creative and imaginative; feel respect for themselves; feel enjoyment for their differences or uniqueness; and feel that they are affirmed for what they are rather than what they are not.

3. **A sense of power**—children must believe in themselves; feel competent; feel comfortable with responsibility; feel in control of themselves despite pressures experienced; feel comfortable when they have responsibility to fulfill; feel confident they can make decisions to solve problems; be able to use skills they have learned; are comfortable about learning new skills; and feel others can't make them do things they really don't want to do.

4. **A sense of models**—children have the ability to tell right from wrong; have people in their lives who are worthy of being emulated; have a consistent set of values and beliefs to guide their actions; can depend on past experiences to help avoid problems or be intimidated by new ones; have a sense of purpose; are able to make sense of their lives and of the circumstances in which they live; know the standards being used to judge them; are able to organize their environment to accomplish tasks; and experience satisfaction from learning.

Some general ways to improve self-esteem in the classroom are (Rinholm 1999):

1. **Build a sense of security**—children need to feel safe and know what is expected. Discuss the rules in the class and the advantages of having them, follow predictable routines, make the class a safe environment (emotionally and physically), make the classroom a positive and comfortable place to be.

2. **Build the child's sense of identity**—this concept refers to feeling unique and helping students know their strengths/weaknesses. Activities include collages, pictures, reports on their interests, likes, dislikes, and experiences.

3. **Enhance the child's sense of belonging**—it is important for children to feel part of a larger group and that they are accepted. Activities such as those that help the students learn about one another, opportunities for group work, and how to handle social situations—such as dealing with conflict or knowing what to do or say when given a compliment.

4. **Build a child's sense of purpose**—children must have goals and be actively working toward them. Activities that support this notion include helping children set their daily/weekly goals and helping them identify individuals they admire.

5. **Build a child's sense of competence**—help children to develop the belief that they can meet goals and achieve success. Help children see their strengths and the progress they have made; teach them to praise themselves for their successes.

A most important point for teachers to keep in mind is the axiom from medical practice that states "First, do no harm." As teachers, our words can weigh heavily on the children we teach. We are role model, parent, and authority figure, and children pay close attention to our attitudes and interactions with them. Every day we should find something positive to say to each child and give each child a special moment in the classroom.

Self-esteem is necessary for developing self-expression and independence. A person with a feeling of self-worth is also better equipped emotionally to show concern for others. As the individual begins to develop meaningful relationships with others who recognize and reward his or her unique qualities of expression, independent thinking flourishes. A strong sense of self-worth permits open and honest communication with others because rejection or disapproval are not feared as great risks. The establishment of self-esteem is a lifelong process. This lifelong quest is more easily attainable if the nurturing of emotional and social well-being has been emphasized in infancy and childhood, thus promoting a sense of security, identity, autonomy, and intimacy early in life.

Self-esteem is the result of three factors: (1) how children perceive themselves, (2) how they want to be, and (3) what expectations they perceive others have for them. The foundation of positive self-esteem is shaped in early childhood, primarily by interactions with parents and other family members. Positive comments and attitudes toward the child contribute to his or her sense of competency and shape the perception of self.

R. Weissberg has stated "We all know that social and emotional factors affect learning and preparedness to learn. If a kid is feeling unhappy, it's hard for him or her to focus on school work. If a kid is feeling stressed, or is pressured by peers not to perform well, this can reduce academic learning" (Kuersten 1999). Kuersten goes on to say that there are many ways that schools can address childrens' emotional needs. They can offer a coordinated, systematic social and emotional education curriculum and a supportive, safe environment in which the teacher nurtures students' personal development; schools also can do much to establish a network of supportive programs and individuals in the community. In essence what Kuersten is suggesting is the necessity of a coordinated school health program (see Chapter 1).

When children enter school, teachers should help them to develop positive self-esteem by providing a positive emotional climate in the classroom. Teachers also can help children view themselves realistically and as being unique and lovable. Children need to know they are valued and accepted regardless of intellect, appearance, dress, or other social criteria.

Values and Patterns of Decision Making

Central to the establishment of self-esteem, the expression of emotions and resulting behavior, and the ability to cope effectively with distress are the decision-making patterns that children learn in order to make life adjustments in harmony with their value system. When decisions about a particular issue reflect actions and attitudes that are in agreement with strongly held values, a person is left intact emotionally because personal behaviors and values remain compatible. If decisions produce behaviors that contradict a person's value system, self-esteem is diminished, emotions are exhibited in an unhealthy fashion resulting from lack of resolution over inner conflicts, and stress increases. Decision-making patterns can serve as valuable clues to the way individuals perceive themselves, their relationships with others, and the world around them. Children's actions tell much about their underlying value system, which in turn mediates many of the decisions made about life adjustments. Learning to make decisions following clarification and consideration of values can help each child sustain and enhance self-esteem and the emotional balance crucial to good mental health.

Behavior and the Expression of Emotions

The most obvious indicator of a child's emotional health status is behavior. Psychologists state that there is always a reason for behavior. The reasons may not be immediately apparent either to the child or to others; nevertheless, there are underlying motives for all behavior. Much of a child's conscious and subconscious behavior is centered around fulfilling basic emotional needs. Such behavior patterns are often shaped by the ways in which these needs were satisfied or reinforced early in life. Thus, if a change in behavior is desired, the child must learn new, and perhaps healthier, ways of fulfilling basic needs. Everyone experiences feelings of sadness, anger, joy, fear, depression, and apprehension, but the way in which these emotions are expressed varies from person to person. Usually the emotional expression of these feelings becomes labeled as the individual's "behavior." Therefore, a better understanding of emotions may lead to greater understanding of a child's behavior and overall emotional health.

The way in which a child expresses his or her feelings is largely determined by the way the child perceives, either consciously or subconsciously, the situation that triggers the feeling. In other words, two students who are exposed to the same situation—say, disagreement with a teacher over an answer to a test question—may react quite differently, based on different individual assessments of the situation. Such assessments are based in part on how the situation affects fulfillment of basic needs or efforts aimed at attaining autonomy, identity, or other personal goals. In many cases, the situation is perceived as having little impact and therefore elicits minimal emotional expression. Situations that are perceived as having great influence tend to elicit stronger, more overt expression. Thus, emotions are displayed in varying modes of expression as well as varying degrees of intensity. A child is considered more emotionally healthy when emotions are exhibited in a positive way and with an intensity proportional to the situation's impact. Children who consistently display either minimal emotional expression about circumstances generally viewed as having major importance (intimacy with others, successful completion of a difficult task, death of a family member or pet) or intense emotional expression about events that are not generally viewed as having major importance (having to redo a homework assignment, misplacing an article of clothing, losing a football game) are considered less emotionally well adjusted.

Emotion itself does not determines mentally healthy or unhealthy behavior, but rather the degree and frequency of the emotion expressed. All children on occasion have allowed their emotions to run out of control or be expressed in ways that were not as appropriate, positive, or desirable as they could have been. This type of behavior is a problem only when it becomes a consistent pattern. Often such a pattern of emotional outburst is a result of inner anxiety due to stress originating from conflicts between unconscious drives or needs and conscious values that have been imposed. All people (adults as well as children) share the same emotions. A feeling or emotion is not inherently "good" or "bad," but can be expressed in ways that either promote well-being or detract from it. Mentally healthy behavior largely stems from an individual's ability to recognize, analyze, interpret, and communicate feelings in a consistent, balanced, and positive manner.

Defense Mechanisms

A **defense mechanism** is any behavior a person uses to avoid confronting a situation or problem. Children learn and use various mechanisms early in their elementary school years. Although defense mechanisms can be helpful in dealing with the stresses of life, some children can use them to the extreme. When defense mechanisms are used inappropriately, they can hinder a child's emotional health. Examples of common defense mechanisms are provided in Table 6.1.

Children and Major Psychiatric Disorders

A child who has a major psychiatric disorder has a very serious illness that may affect the life of the child for many years. Some of the signs that a child may need to be examined by a psychiatrist include:

Table 6.1   *Common Defense Mechanisms*

Defense Mechanism	Definition
Compensation	Making up for weakness in one area by emphasizing strengths in another area. *Example:* A child is unsuccessful as an athlete but is a musician; consequently, emphasis is placed on music.
Daydreaming	Escaping from frustrations, boredom, or unpleasant situations through fantasy. *Example:* Faced with a divorce of the father and mother, a child creates a mental image of the perfect family.
Displacement	Transferring feelings concerning one situation or person to another object, situation, or person. *Example:* Unable to respond with anger toward a parent, the child goes home and abuses a younger child.
Idealization	Holding someone or something in such high esteem that it becomes perfect or godlike in the eyes of the child. *Example:* A star athlete who is held in such high regard that his or her human characteristics or shortcomings are overlooked.
Identification	Taking on the quality of someone who is admired. *Example:* Performers are often so admired that children attempt to talk, walk, and act as they perceive their idol to do.
Projection	Shifting the responsibility of one's behavior onto someone else. *Example:* The child blames the teacher because a test grade was poor rather than accept the responsibility for not studying sufficiently.
Rationalization	Providing plausible reasons for behavior that are not the real reasons. *Example:* A child states she does not like birthday parties and refuses to attend when she really just feels insecure.
Regression	Childish, inappropriate behavior by an adult or a return to former, less mature behavior when under stress. *Example:* Becoming extremely angry when unable to attend a movie or social event. A regressive response may be to cry or throw something.
Repression	Attempting to bury or repress unpleasant or upsetting thoughts. *Example:* The child is unable to remember a psychologically painful event, such as the death of a grandparent.
Sublimation	Turning unacceptable thought or actions into socially acceptable behaviors. *Example:* An aggressive child turns to athletics to redirect his or her energies.

- failure to look or smile at parents or other caregivers
- very strange actions or appearance
- lack of movement or facial expression
- odd way of speaking or use of private language that no one else understands
- strange conversations with self
- strange, odd, or repetitive movements such as spinning, hand-flapping, or head banging
- panic in response to a change in surroundings

Teachers and parents should remain alert to any of these behaviors. A comprehensive evaluation will involve a psychiatrist, parents, teachers, pediatricians, and neurologists, and the administration of a broad array of developmental and psychological tests. Partly because of the tremendous changes that occur in children as they grow, diagnosis of major psychiatric disorders in children is one of the most difficult areas of medicine. According to the American Academy of Child and Adolescent Psychiatry (AACAP), no sign should be ignored: the earlier severe mental problems can be identified, the better the prognosis (AACAP 2002).

Obsessive-Compulsive Disorder in Children

As many as 1 in 200 children and adolescents may have **obsessive-compulsive disorder (OCD).** OCD is characterized by recurrent obsessions or compulsions, impulses, or images that are unwanted. They are not simple worries or preoccupations. The obsessions and compulsions cause significant distress and anxiety and interfere with daily routine, relationships, social functioning, and academic performance.

A younger child with OCD may fear that harm can occur as a result of an intruder entering an unlocked door or window. As a result, the child may check all doors and windows in an attempt to relieve anxiety. Children may develop rituals such as compulsive hand-washing.

Researchers have demonstrated that OCD is a brain disorder and tends to run in families, although this does not mean a child will automatically develop symptoms. Recently, studies have shown that OCD may develop or worsen after a strep infection. A child may develop OCD with no previous family history (AACAP 1999a). Most children can be treated with a combination of psychotherapy and medications such as the serotonin reuptake inhibitors. Family, school, and teacher cooperation are central to successful treatment.

Panic Disorder in Children

Children with **panic disorder** have unexpected and repeated periods of intense fear or discomfort, accompanied by racing heartbeat and shortness of breath. General panic disorders typically begin in adolescence, although they may begin in childhood.

The attack may last from a few minutes to hours. They occur without warning, and the symptoms include intense fearfulness; racing or pounding of the heart; dizziness/lightheadedness; trembling or shaking; sense of unreality; and fear of dying, losing control, or going crazy (AACAP 1999d). In severe cases, the child may be afraid to leave home and may become depressed, at risk for use of drugs and alcohol, or even prone to suicidal behavior. Treatments for the disorder are quite effective. Psychotherapy can help the child and family learn ways to reduce stress or conflict that cause an attack. Medications stop the panic attacks.

Depression and Children

Depression in children parallels that in adults with minor differences due to developmental considerations (Magg and Forness 1991). A condition characterized by loss of interest and feelings of extreme or overwhelming sorrow, sadness, and debility, **depression** is a symptom of underlying conflict, tension, or anxiety and may be exhibited in varying degrees for varying lengths of time. The same criteria used to identify depression in adults are used for diagnosing the condition in children. The American Psychiatric Association (APA) and AACAP have stated the following criteria that need to be present for a diagnosis of depression (APA 1999, AACAP 1999c). According to the APA, at least five of these criteria must be present for a diagnosis of depression to be made (APA 1987):

- depressed mood
- loss of interest or pleasure in all or almost all activities
- significant weight loss or weight gain
- insomnia or excessive sleeping
- psychomotor agitation or retardation
- fatigue or loss of energy
- feelings of worthlessness or excessive or inappropriate guilt
- diminished ability to think or concentrate; indecisiveness
- thoughts of suicide or suicide attempts

THE CAUSES OF DEPRESSION

There are no simple answers to why children become depressed. The APA (1999) estimates that three million to six million children and adolescents suffer from depression in the United States. They also state that most children with depression go untreated. Most experts now believe there are multiple reasons for depression. Obviously, not all the reasons apply to children, but some of the situations presented hold implications for the development of depression in children. Some possible factors include the following (Chandler and Kolander 1989, 4–5; APA 1999):

Heredity—studies show some depressive disorders are hereditary. For example, bipolar disorder has been linked, in some cases, to a genetic defect.

Environment—environment can also contribute to the onset of a depressive disorder. Research has shown that stressful life events,

Health Highlight

DEALING WITH TERRORISM

In the wake of the terrorist attacks on the World Trade Center in New York City and the Pentagon in Washington, DC, our lives and those of our children changed forever. The Psychological Trauma Center has identified several important issues to be aware of when helping children cope with the magnitude of the events of September 11, 2001, and those that may follow as the result of the actions of extremist groups throughout the world.

The issue of war

Children will not understand the War on Terrorism. Children need to have explained that this a very different kind of war. They will see pictures of the military and military action taking place on television. They will see the devastation of suicide bombers and the carnage of the war. Some may have a family member called to serve his or her country. Children must be given an opportunity to talk about what they are seeing, hearing, and feeling concerning the threat(s) to our country.

Expressing anger toward a different culture or ethnic group

Children must realize that the terrorists who attacked the World Trade Center and the Pentagon were a group of people who have very different ideas about the world in which we live. These individuals performed an evil act. This does not mean that other people of the same cultural background share the same beliefs. Rather, they too may be feeling angry and sad about what has happened.

All questions may not be answerable

Children want their questions answered. The Psychological Trauma Center suggests that we answer the question of "why" by explaining that *"Bad people in this world who wanted to make a statement are behind the events of September 11 (and the events that will occur in the future). The way they went about making their statement was hurtful to many people. The government is looking for them for the bad things they did."* It is fine to say we don't have an answer. It may be necessary to say, "I don't know" or "I'll try to find out."

Blaming

Some children may express fear and anxiety toward children of other nationalities, feeling someone from their country was responsible for acts of terrorism. Children need to be taught how to deal with their feelings without blaming others.

SOURCE: Adapted from Psychological Trauma Center 2000

---

especially those involving a loss or threatened loss, often precede episodes of depressive illness. Examples include the death of a loved one, a divorce, the loss of a job, a move to a new home, physical illness, the breakup of an important relationship, or financial problems. In most instances the loss induces feelings of sadness and anxiety and often guilt or shame. Less commonly, depression follows the achievement of a desired position—the so-called success depression. In this case, the loss typically associated with depression is the loss of a future goal.

Background and personality—people with certain psychological backgrounds or personality characteristics appear to be more vulnerable to depression. Many specialists believe that some depressive disorders can be traced to a troubled childhood; they attach particular importance to disturbed relationships between a child and his or her parents. Also, people who have low self-esteem, who consistently view themselves and the world with pessimism, or who become easily overwhelmed by stress tend to be more prone to depression.

Biochemical factors—some types of depression may result from abnormal chemical activity within the brain. These chemicals play a role in the transmission of electrical impulses from one nerve cell (neuron) to another. These chemical "messengers," called *neurotransmitters,* set in motion the complex interactions that control moods, feelings, and behaviors. They also regulate pain, learning, and memory as well as the desire to eat, drink, and sleep. Three neurotransmitters—dopamine, norepinephrine, and serotonin—have been associated with depressive illnesses. Research suggests that episodes of depression or mania may be related to an improper balance of neurotransmitters. Do biochemical factors cause depression, or does depression cause the biochemical disturbance? No one knows with certainty. Some experts theorize that a genetic vulnerability combined with prolonged stress, physical illness, or some other environmental condition or event may bring about the chemical imbalance that results in depression.

Physical illness—people with chronic medical illnesses are at high risk of psychiatric illness, especially depression. Some diseases, such as hypothyroidism (underactive thyroid gland) or arthritis can bring on a depressive reaction. Depression also may follow a heart attack or stroke. It may be an early sign of a serious underlying disease such as cancer of the pancreas, a brain tumor, parkinsonism, multiple sclerosis, or Cushing's disease, among others. Also, depression can be an undesirable side effect of certain prescription medications—especially steroids (cortisone-like drugs), some antihypertensive medicines, antiparkinsonian agents, and, less commonly, oral contraceptives.

As stated previously, not all of the above causes are considerations for depression in children. However, Patros and Shamoo (1989) have identified several indicators of childhood depression, as shown in Table 6.2 on page 138.

Suicide in Children and Adolescents

Each year, more than 5,000 young people between the ages of fifteen and twenty-four kill themselves. Each day, over 1,000 people in this age group attempt suicide. For every individual who is successful at committing suicide, 100 more will attempt the act and fail. Statistics also reveal that children as young as five or six are committing suicide (Grollman 1988). Suicide is the sixth leading cause of death for children five to fourteen years of age (AACAP 2002). Children and adolescents who commit suicide feel cut off, alienated, and isolated. They truly believe that living is useless and more than they can tolerate.

Although the overall rate of suicide in the United States has remained fairly constant in recent years, the rate of suicide among young children has increased. The numbers might even be higher if the current social stigma against

Table 6.2   *Indicators of Childhood Depression*

Indicator	Response in Child
Lack of interest	daydreams, withdrawn, poor schoolwork, disruptive
Change in appetite	picks at food, gives away food, increase in appetite
Changes in sleep pattern	falls asleep in class, listless, tardy, poor attention in class
Loss of energy	tired or restless behavior
Blaming self inappropriately	self-critical, cries quickly, upset by surprises or changes
Negative feelings of self-worth	critical of others, socially withdrawn, doesn't stand up for herself/himself
Feelings of sadness, hopelessness, and worry	sad, unhappy, feels defeated, withdrawn, acts frightened, poor peer relationships
Morbid thoughts	talks or writes about death, overreacts to someone's death
Aggressive or negative behavior	picks on others, talks back, easily frustrated
Increased agitation	cannot sit still, short attention span, makes noise, talks under breath
Increased psychosomatic complaints	frequently complains of headaches, stomachaches, or vague physical symptoms
Decreased academic performance	drop in grades, poor concentration, messy work area, poor test performance
Poor attention and concentration	cannot stay on task, frequently interrupts, disruptive behavior, appears not to listen.

suicide did not cause many adolescent suicide cases to go unreported. Ten percent of the children in any public classroom may be considered suicidal (DeSpelder and Strickland 1987).

Adolescents are most likely to commit suicide when they experience overcrowded conditions; a broken family; or feelings of rejection, hopelessness, or loss. Some wish to escape from a difficult situation, gain attention, or punish people who caused them to have negative feelings; therefore, they may view death as an acceptable alternative. Further, an adolescent is at higher risk for suicide if a significant adult role model attempts or commits suicide or if violence is commonplace in the child's environment, either in the home or through the media (DeSpelder and Strickland 1987).

Nelson and Crawford (1991) found that elementary students who experienced thoughts of suicide reported that family problems were significant contributors. Such things as divorce, separation, and parental alcoholism were the main factors. Peer acceptance and academic pressures also contribute to elementary children's suicide attempts.

Most childhood suicides are preceded by changes in behavior, some subtle and some more overt. They may lose interest in school and friends, experience an increase of illnesses, become very sad for increasing periods of time, and quit eating or sleeping well. Other observable signs of suicidal behavior are:

- saying such things as "I wish I were dead" or "I'd be better off dead"
- giving away prized objects

- lacking direction or goal-setting behavior
- exhibiting depression, withdrawal, weight loss, or apathy
- showing a sudden lack of academic progress
- communicating feelings of hopelessness
- using drugs and alcohol
- withdrawing from friends, family, and normal activities
- undergoing a radical personality change
- exhibiting violent, hostile, or rebellious behavior
- revealing a preoccupation with death through a school composition
- mutilating the self
- running away from home

Other signs could probably be added to this list. Every teacher must be cognizant of these signs and symptoms if suicide is to be prevented. It is imperative that children suspected of suicidal thoughts receive help from professionals trained to deal with the situation.

Latchkey Children

The term **latchkey child** describes any child regularly left without direct adult supervision before or after school. Indications are that over seven million children under age thirteen are either left to go to school or return home without adult supervision. Kids left in these situations may be the result either of both parents working or of divorce. The end result is that many children leave home without breakfast or return home to care for themselves—with the possible consequences of fear of someone breaking into their home, fear of being alone, fear of older siblings, and greater likelihood of being lonely and bored (Stroher 1986). Fear and boredom can lead to involvement with gangs or to a greater chance of trouble resulting from the lack of adult supervision. Undersupervised children may experience significantly more personality problems and a higher incidence of depression in adolescence and adulthood (Page and Page 2000).

Obviously, latchkey children are expected to assume a great deal of responsibility for their own welfare. Stroher (1986, 16) has suggested that teachers can help latchkey children by carefully structuring homework assignments because these children do not have adults around to help them complete assignments correctly. Consider the possibility of establishing a telephone hotline to help students with homework. During the school day, allow time for children to discuss their personal concerns with the teacher. Latchkey children particularly need time to discuss or talk with adults. Also establish streamlined, workable procedures for contacting the parents in emergency situations involving the child, and develop both before- and after-school daycare programs. Children do better with continuous adult supervision in school-based programs than when left to their own resources.

Divorce and Separation: The Effects on Children

Almost half the children in the United States will spend some portion of their childhood in a single-parent situation. Over one million divorces occur each year; over 49 percent of second marriages result in divorce. In 2002, 22 percent of children lived only with their mothers, 4 percent lived only with their fathers, and 4 percent lived with neither of their parents (U.S. Department of Health and Human Services 2002). The net result is that teachers are having to deal with more emotional/psychological problems than ever before. These problems are represented by delinquency, psychological disturbance, hostility, low self-esteem, low evaluation of the family, and poor self-restraint and social adjustment.

The reactions of children may depend on age. Preschoolers may become frightened about the separation or divorce because they see themselves as being abandoned. A child of this age may not want to attend or may fear attending school. Such children may regress in their behavior, with lapses in toilet training or their ability to dress themselves (Ricci 1982). They may use dolls, teddy bears, and blankets as security objects. Among children six to eight years of age, the most common feeling is sadness. This is manifested through crying, sobbing, and a desire to be with the missing parent. Children nine to twelve are likely to respond with vigorous activity. Older children may align themselves with one parent and want little or nothing to do with the other (Wallerstein and Kelly 1981). School-age children may blame themselves for causing the divorce. Parents' ongoing commitment to the child's well-being is vital. Children do best if they understand that their mother and father will still be their parents and remain involved with them even though the marriage is ending. Long custody fights and pressure to choose one parent over the other only add to the damage the child suffers as a result of divorce. Psychotherapy for the children and divorcing parents can be helpful to all concerned (AACAP 1999b).

The teacher may be the one source of stability and security the child has in a divorce or separation. This can be emphasized by the fact "that only 45 percent of children do well after divorce; 41 percent are doing poorly, worried, underachieving, self-deprecating, and often angry; and 14 percent are strikingly uneven [in their emotional functioning]. Girls consistently adjust better to divorce than boys, both socially and academically. This would imply that boys may be suffering more from the absence of their fathers" (Stepfamily Foundation 2003). The teacher may be able to assure such children that the separation/divorce was not their fault, that they are still loved, and help them discuss their feelings of fear, anger, and guilt. Encourage the child to be honest about his or her feelings. In addition, be watchful for signs of academic failure, overaggressiveness, lack of concentration, nervousness, or becoming isolated from peers, which may require informing the parent or the school counselor.

Death and Children

In today's society, most children do not directly experience the trauma of death. The concept of death is alien to many children. Most children develop a sequence of understanding concerning death, beginning with total unawareness in early childhood to a developmental point where death is conceptualized as final and universal (Fredlund 1984). For many children, initial contact with death may be the result of a pet dying. Children feel significant pain and need extra support to deal with their feelings of loss and grief, even for the death of a pet. The effects of death on children and adolescents are discussed in greater detail in Chapter 23.

Rules for Developing and Maintaining Mental Health

Children should be encouraged to practice positive mental health habits in the same way they are taught to practice sound personal health habits. Just as children can take responsibility for their own physical well-being by following health "rules," they can also foster high levels of emotional well-being by following similar mental health "rules." By internalizing certain guidelines and incorporating them into daily living, each individual can promote good mental health and effective life adjustment. Positive mental health can be taught each day of every school year. Teachers must realize that they are directly responsible for establishing the emotional tone of their classrooms, as well as the foundation of student's self-worth. When each child leaves elementary school, she or he needs to have developed the positive self-esteem and perceptions of living that foster the rules outlined in the Health Highlight box on page 142.

The Role of the Teacher in Promoting Mental Health

There are many other ways in which the teacher can promote positive emotional characteristics. Each child should be treated as a unique individual. It is important for the teacher to offer personal observations or words of praise that let a child know he or she is performing well or progressing well on a given task. Encourage children to hone their individual talents by providing opportunities for them to do so during the normal course of classroom activity. The chance to work on a special project of personal interest or to contribute ideas and opinions without being ridiculed or rejected may enhance autonomy and initiative.

Health Highlight

GUIDELINES THAT FOSTER POSITIVE

SELF-ESTEEM IN CHILDREN

1. Teach the children to like themselves. Help them discover their unique qualities, skills, and talents and to be proud of who they are.

2. Teach the children to be good to themselves. Encourage them to reward themselves periodically with "strokes"—emotional or material favors.

3. Help the children learn to be introspective, to examine motives for behavior, and to be insightful about their own conduct.

4. Help each child accept her or his limitations. Think in terms of competency levels rather than in terms of "success" or "failure."

5. Help the children deal with a problem or crisis as it arises rather than allowing pressures to mount by worrying about "what if's."

6. Help each child establish realistic goals, both short term and long term, and work toward accomplishing them.

7. Help the children express their emotions in terms of how the emotion makes them feel rather than in terms of how others make them feel. "I feel angry for having to do a homework assignment over the weekend" is healthier than "Ms. Barnes, you make me angry. You shouldn't assign a homework assignment over the weekend."

8. Encourage the children to involve themselves in diversified activities and cultivate many interests. Encourage them to not center their life around one person, place, or activity.

9. Encourage children to develop a sense of humor. Help them learn to laugh and enjoy life.

10. Teach the children to be optimistic.

Learning experiences that both challenge and provide success will reinforce children's feelings of competency and mastery.

Teachers can provide activities that help students consider how they want to live their lives and what their goals should be. For example, a teacher can ask them to write down things they hope to accomplish in the near and in the distant future, and then help them develop ways of achieving these goals. This method of clarifying important goals will help students keep minor problems in perspective (Olsen, Redican, and Baffi 1986). Furthermore, teachers need to help sudents place their inability to meet goals in the proper perspective, so that feelings of doubt, embarrassment, or inadequacy do not result.

It is important for a teacher to become an effective listener and a skilled observer. Children regularly need opportunities that let them express their feelings and thoughts openly. A teacher can become an active listener by paraphrasing the student's comments to let the child know the message was understood. Such active listening will demonstrate to children that the teacher genuinely cares about them.

The role of the teacher in promoting student mental health is crucial. The attitudes teachers demonstrate during their daily interactions with students affect the emotional climate of the classroom. One of the best things a teacher can do to promote emotional health in students is to help them learn to accept

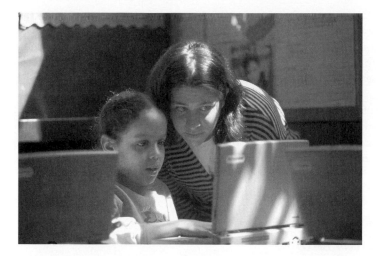

The teacher is most important in establishing a positive classroom atmosphere.

responsibility for their own behavior. A common mistake we all make is to try to shift the blame for something we did onto someone else. Students must be taught that a crucial element of emotional development is the ability to accept responsibility and live with mistakes. Further, the type of rapport that is established between teacher and student conveys many messages that influence children's perceptions about acceptance, trust, support, self-esteem, competency, and independence.

The Role of the Family in Developing Emotional Health

An individual's emotional health status can be gauged by assessing how much the basic emotional needs for love, acceptance, and support from others contribute to the individual's feelings of self-worth. It is helpful also to determine the degree of balance with which behaviors are expressed and the ways in which people face and resolve situations through decisions that are compatible with personal values. All these foundations of positive mental health are first learned and cultivated within the family. As a result, it is crucial that all teachers have some notion of how family structure, interaction, and values influence the behavior and attitudes of students in the classroom.

Single-parent families which currently exist in high numbers may greatly affect a child's view of self as well as the world in general. Some children also face the task of having to be incorporated into two different family structures that produce different sets of stepparents and stepsiblings. Teachers must be sensitive to these differences in living arrangements and family structure.

Family interaction also contributes greatly to the development of children's mental health. Communication patterns between parents, parents and their children, and between siblings are all important factors. Communication should allow for intimacy—that is, sharing of one's innermost fears and concerns—without reprisal or rejection. Interaction patterns between family members set the tone for all other social interaction. Within the family, children develop a sense about what they can do or accomplish; what their roles in life should be; and what types of behaviors are appropriate, acceptable, and desirable. Criteria for sharing, completing expected tasks, being praised or punished, and many other things are learned through family modeling and values. The family sets guidelines for all behavior by means ranging from types of discipline to ways of expressing love and affection. As a result, attitudes, habits, and emotions reflect family attitudes, habits, and emotions.

Stress and Its Relationship to Mental Health

Because of its influence on behavior and the expression of emotions that may result, the topic of stress should be included in any discussion of mental health. Everyone, young and old, is exposed to daily stress that must be accommodated to ensure emotional stability. Therefore, people of all ages must realize that many situations produce feelings of anxiety or apprehension that cause the same types of fluctuation in levels of mental wellness as those experienced in physical wellness. The key is to learn to reduce anxiety and tension as they arise so that levels of stress are more easily managed.

Stress is the nonspecific response of the body to an unanticipated or stimulating event. Stress can accompany a pleasant or unpleasant event. Hans Selye has described stress resulting from a pleasant event as **eustress.** This type of stress comes from events such as getting something new or being selected as a class officer. Although anxiety is produced, this type of stress helps us be more effective in physical, social, and psychological functioning. **Distress** is stress generated from a negative or unpleasant event. Prolonged distress can have a negative or debilitative effect on health. Unchecked distress interferes with physiological and psychological functioning (Selye 1975).

Anything that elicits a stress response is called a **stressor** (see Figure 6.2). A stressor can be an event or situation. What one person may perceive as stress may be totally nonstressful to someone else. For example, skydiving would be terrifying for many people, yet others may view it as a relaxing recreational activity. Possible sources of stress in children include:

- death of a parent or grandparent
- death of a brother or sister
- marital separation of parents
- divorce of parents
- hospitalization of a parent
- remarriage of a parent to a stepparent
- birth of a brother or sister
- loss of job by father or mother
- moving to a new city

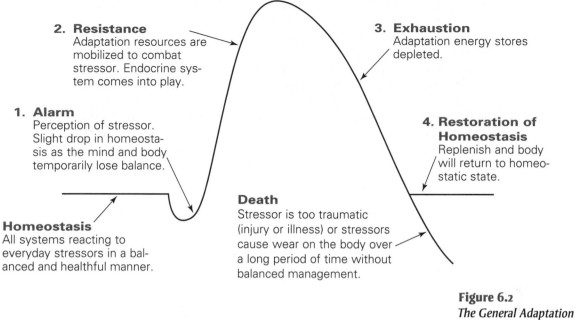

2. Resistance
Adaptation resources are mobilized to combat stressor. Endocrine system comes into play.

3. Exhaustion
Adaptation energy stores depleted.

1. Alarm
Perception of stressor. Slight drop in homeostasis as the mind and body temporarily lose balance.

4. Restoration of Homeostasis
Replenish and body will return to homeostatic state.

Homeostasis
All systems reacting to everyday stressors in a balanced and healthful manner.

Death
Stressor is too traumatic (injury or illness) or stressors cause wear on the body over a long period of time without balanced management.

Figure 6.2
The General Adaptation Syndrome

It is both impossible and undesirable to live in a stress-free environment. Stress does occur and cannot be totally avoided. From a positive perspective, stress can enhance ability, act as a motivator, and be a means of self-protection. Unfortunately many children live in highly stressful situations. Factors such as poverty, crowding, and exposure to drugs, abuse, and domestic and street violence can all contribute to stress.

The General Adaptation Syndrome

Any event or circumstance that upsets the body's physiological balance is a stressor. The body is constantly striving to maintain a physiological balance, or **homeostasis.** Regardless of the type of stress that occurs, eustress or distress, when an individual perceives a stressor, the body automatically responds with a three-stage process known as the **general adaptation syndrome (GAS)** (Selye 1975). (See Figure 6.2.)

The first phase of the general adaptation syndrome is referred to as the *alarm phase.* The brain interprets an event or situation as a stressor and immediately prepares the body to deal with it. Sometimes this initial response is called the fight-or-flight syndrome because the body literally reacts as if it is either going to stand and fight or run away. The emotional response causes physical reactions such as muscle tenseness, increased heart rate, dry mouth, or sweaty palms. The second stage of the GAS is *resistance.* During this phase the perceived stressor is dealt with through increased strength and sensory capacity. Only after meeting the demands of the stressful event can the body return to normal.

When stress is chronic, sufficiently pervasive, or traumatic enough, the third stage of *exhaustion* is reached. At this point the body must restore itself and rest or serious health problems are potentially possible. Adverse effects of mismanaged or long-term stress include heart problems, stomach problems, high blood pressure, and/or achy muscles and joints.

All the stages in the GAS are the result of chemical messages in the form of hormones. For example, during the alarm phase the pituitary gland releases a hormone (adrenocorticotropic hormone, or ACTH) that stimulates other endocrine glands to also release hormones, resulting in the fight-or-flight response. Hormonal messages increase blood volume and blood pressure. The hormones epinephrine and norepinephrine initiate a variety of physiological responses, including increased heart rate and increased metabolic rate. They also stimulate the release of other hormones called **endorphins,** which serve to diminish pain.

Obviously, the continual hormonal stimulation caused by chronic stress doesn't let the body return to homeostasis. Fortunately, the effects of most stressors can be partially or completely reversed with adequate stress management techniques. Early use of these techniques can reduce the adverse effects of stress.

Effects of Chronic Stress

Chronic stress can cause problems in several areas of a child's life. Psychosomatic illness, such as headaches and physical injuries, may result from an abnormal response to stress. A child may withdraw emotionally from others and experience feelings of worthlessness, apathy, loneliness, anger, hostility, and low self-esteem. Behavior problems such as hyperactivity, accident susceptibility, truancy, substance abuse, and low academic achievement may also result from stress. Low self-esteem and anxiety may lead to a lack of concentration and a disrupted capacity to process information (Jones 1985).

Other behaviors that could indicate that children are under too much stress include the following:

- frequent headaches
- sighing
- diarrhea/ constipation
- nausea
- faintness
- hair twirling
- clenched fists

- nervous cough
- fast or excessive talking
- fingernail biting
- back-and-forth rocking
- depression
- anger

- continual boredom
- lip biting
- crying
- proneness to errors
- nightmares
- persistent (compulsive) itching

Dealing with Stress

It is important to determine which sources of stress arise from intrinsic stimuli, such as being inwardly driven to reach a goal, and which ones arise from extrinsic stimuli, such as pressure from a teacher to turn in a homework assignment, parental separation, or death of a grandparent. It is also beneficial to attempt to determine whether the source is regular, routine, or consistent, as in the case of a daily conflict or being self-conscious with peers. Sources of stress that are regular, routine, or consistent generally have a greater potential for creating long-term negative effects because they wear on the individual constantly and may therefore demand more time to resolve. Sudden, isolated sources of stress tend to be crisis situations that first require a return to some degree of normalcy and may later involve a more lengthy process of conflict resolution.

Putting the stress-producing situation in realistic perspective is helpful in objectively evaluating its impact. To do this, the teacher should help the student mentally classify events as they arise and to decide which situations can be personally handled after careful consideration of the possible alternatives. Those events involving either deeper inner conflict or interaction with others may require the assistance of a third party or outside expert. After putting the cause of the stress into perspective and outlining possible courses of action, students should be helped to select the course of action that seems likely to produce the most healthful, positive, or desirable results. The student should then be aided in carrying out the course of action and evaluating its effectiveness to determine whether similar courses of action should be repeated for similar circumstances or whether modifications need to be considered.

Stress Management in Children

Stress management and stress reduction skills can help children cope with life's stresses and increase their potential for reaching and maintaining high levels of emotional health throughout life. There are a variety of healthful ways to reduce the adverse effects of stress. Examples include exercise, relaxation techniques, and deep-breathing exercises. Some children can use hobbies, arts and crafts, and reading activities as alternative forms of stress reduction.

EXERCISE

One of the most natural methods of relieving the body of the effects of stress is exercise. Aerobic exercise activates the hormones, fatigues the tense muscles, and allows the stressed student to return to a pleasantly tired, but relaxed, state. Activities such as walking, jogging, cycling, and swimming all directly reduce adverse symptoms of stress.

RELAXATION TECHNIQUES

Several kinds of relaxation techniques may be used to combat the ill effects associated with stress. These techniques include, but are not limited to, progressive relaxation, meditation, and creative visualization. A child who is able to relax under very trying circumstances will experience fewer of the physical symptoms associated with poor stress management.

Progressive relaxation is one method that is especially useful for children. Progressive relaxation requires a quiet room and the space to assume a comfortable position. Instructions can be given on an audiotape or verbally by a teacher/facilitator in a classroom situation.

The key to progressive relaxation is to tense each muscle group as the command is given (typically for about ten to fifteen seconds); then when the signal is given, relax that muscle group immediately and completely (for approximately ten to fifteen seconds). This is a procedure that needs to be practiced, but once the method is learned, it can certainly help to reduce stress.

Deep-breathing exercises are very similar to natural relaxation. In fact, deep breathing uses the body's natural relaxation response. Students can be reminded that they often use deep breathing (sighing) when under stress without being aware of it. Deep-breathing exercises done in regular patterns can further help the student relax when experiencing stress.

Meditation can be approached from several perspectives. The purpose of the technique is to help the student temporarily "tune out" the world while evoking the relaxation response. During a meditation session, a word or phrase is concentrated on to help eliminate all outside distractions. While in a comfortable position on a couch, chair, or bed, the participant breathes deeply, slowly inhaling and exhaling. The word or phrase is focused on with each breath. This format can best be learned from an instructor or tape that can provide instruction.

Visualization (creative imagery) is a form of relaxation that makes use of the imagination. This is an excellent method to teach students. To use this technique, a comfortable position is assumed, the eyes are closed, and several deep breaths are taken. There are several variations of visualization that an individual can use. For example, a tranquil scene such as a beach or forest can serve as the focal point for the visualization. Visualization can be used to envision a goal or behavior change. There are a variety of tapes available that can aid the teaching of this technique.

Biofeedback is based on scientific principles designed to enhance awareness of body functioning. Sensory equipment is used to create awareness of subtle body changes such as increases or decreases in body temperature, muscle contractions, or brain wave variations. As people become more sensitive to fluctuations in functioning, they can learn to evoke the relaxation response by countering their automatic stress response as it occurs. A few sessions are usually required to recognize differences and then alter physiological responses. Equipment for biofeedback ranges from relatively inexpensive to quite costly.

Health Highlight

THE MENTAL HEALTH NEEDS OF

ELEMENTARY SCHOOL CHILDREN

A study has indicated some very revealing findings about the emotional needs of elementary children. For example, the most frequent behaviors/characteristics identified by respondents as not receiving adequate attention in the schools, and thus representing unmet needs, are:

- poor decision-making/problem-solving skills
- poor self-image; negative self-statements
- low self-confidence
- inability to resolve interpersonal conflicts
- depression and unhappiness
- overly influenced by peers; poor refusal skills
- inability to concentrate; inattentiveness

About 80 percent of the causes of these behaviors were directly parent or home related, whereas school-linked problems accounted for less than 5 percent of responses. To the contrary, only about 20 percent of proposed solutions to the problems directly involved parents, whereas the majority of the proposed solutions were school based.

This is strong justification for schools, teachers, and parents to give mental health high priority.

SOURCE: Adapted from Goodwin, Goodwin, and Cantrill 1988, 282–287

OTHER RELAXATION TECHNIQUES

Other techniques that require no special equipment or training but serve to help dissipate stress symptoms are humor, music, and effective time management.

Laughing is a powerful stress-reducing agent. Laughing or humor helps us to keep things in perspective, maintain a positive attitude, and realize that life is seldom perfect. It has been found that blood pressure and heart rate can actually decrease after a good laugh. Laughing or even smiling are excellent ways to alter a negative mood. Certainly one of the things that can be promoted in a healthy classroom environment is laughter. The laughter should not be based on racial or ethnic factors or at the expense of a student, but on the funny things that occur during the school day.

Quiet music serves to soothe the autonomic nervous system by easing tensions and lessening strong emotions. It is difficult to invoke the relaxation response if the music is inappropriate or irritating to the listener. Classical music affords exposure to the artistic beauty of life as well as evoking the relaxation response.

A perceived or actual lack of time is a major contributor to stress response. In children, effective time management can be fostered by helping them to establish goals and priorities in their daily lives. By learning effective time utilization at an early age, a great deal of stress can be eliminated as the child matures. Some suggestions for effective time management include teaching children to not procrastinate, set realistic goals, establish priorities and write them down, learn to say no when necessary, build in relaxation time every day, and visualize themselves completing their priorities.

The Role of Effective Communication in Reducing Stress

People often experience a tremendous amount of stress when they feel others are controlling their lives. Anxiety results when a person feels exploited, humiliated, and/or a lack of respect. This anxiety and the accompanying stress can be reduced through a change in attitude toward oneself and through the use of effective communication skills.

Many times stress will result from children's inability to express feelings to others honestly. Individuals often refuse to express their feelings to others because they want to avoid confrontations or because they do not feel as important as the other person. Some do not wish to hurt anyone's feelings, yet this type of passive behavior causes a child to think less of himself and to be angry at the other person. Such a lack of respect for self increases stress because the person tends to store the anger internally. Conversely, aggressive behavior, in which a person physically abuses, insults, or criticizes the other person, can ruin relationships and thus increase stress.

Assertive communication—the type that communicates a respect for self as well as the other person—permits individuals to stand up for their rights without ignoring the rights of others. An important part of assertive behavior is a healthy self-concept in which people believe they are worthy individuals, capable of having their own feelings and beliefs. It also implies that people have a right to speak up if they have been treated unfairly, and they have a right to say no. Assertiveness involves making "I" statements; for example, I feel . . . I think . . . , which imply that a person takes full responsibility for his or her feelings. Assertive people are able to clearly and confidently say no and tell others what they think and feel without hurting others or putting them down. Teachers can help children learn how to communicate and be good listeners. Children can learn to speak with positive verbal and body language and yet be polite. Such communication is very effective in improving self-image and relationships with others and in dealing with stress.

Emotionally intimate communication with others also helps lessen the effects of life's stressors. This type of communication is more than just discussing the weather or other superficial topics. Teachers can facilitate such communication by allowing children to share their innermost feelings. Children should not be afraid to share their feelings with others for fear of being rejected. If a child bares his or her soul to the teacher, the teacher must sympathize with the situation and provide emotional support. If the teacher demonstrates through words or behavior an unwillingness to give emotional support, anxiety, loneliness, and rejection can result. However, if children learn they are safe in sharing their intimacies, teacher-child relationships can become much stronger. Such intimate relationships add greatly to the child's quality of life, whereas the lack of such relationships contributes to discontentment, anxiety, and stress.

Summary

- The characteristics of the emotionally healthy child include positive self-esteem, a positive sense of self-worth, a concern for others, the ability to develop meaningful relationships, and the ability to make decisions.

- Unexpressed emotions can lead to frustration, hostility, and resentment.

- Mechanisms used to deal with feelings include compensation, daydreaming, idealization, projection, rationalization, regression, and sublimation.

- Depression is the most frequently occurring emotional disorder and is a symptom of underlying conflict or tension.

- Depression can be the result of heredity, personal background, personality, biochemical factors, or physical illness.

- Depression can be a major cause of adolescent suicide.

- Students should be helped to like themselves, be good to themselves, accept their personal limitations, deal with their problems, establish realistic goals, express emotions properly, develop their sense of humor, and cultivate an optimistic attitude.

- Teachers must recognize the impact of familial socializations on the child entering the classroom and attempt to relate equally and objectively to children from diverse backgrounds and living arrangements.

- Students with special emotional health needs include the latchkey child; children of separation, divorce, or single parents; or a child experiencing loss in the form of death of a parent, grandparent, sibling, or pet.

- How students relate to emotional situations and crisis tends to depend on their age.

- Teachers need to listen and show their acceptance, support, encouragement, and concern for all children, especially for those experiencing special situations or crises.

- Stress is defined as the body's physical and/or psychological response to an unanticipated event.

- Stress can be pleasant (eustress) or unpleasant (distress); prolonged distress has a debilitating health effect.

- Anything that causes stress is called a *stressor*.

- The body goes through three stages (collectively called the general adaptation syndrome) in response to a stressful event—alarm, resistance, and exhaustion.

- Students can be taught techniques for dealing with stress, such as exercising, deep breathing, meditation, visualization, biofeedback, humor, and effective time management.

- Learning effective communication patterns is one of the best methods of protecting against negative stressful responses.

DISCUSSION QUESTIONS

1. Identify the characteristics of good emotional health.
2. Why is self-esteem so important in the development of mental health?
3. How can the teacher enhance self-esteem in the classroom?
4. What are some major concerns for severe psychiatric disorders in children?
5. Describe obsessive-compulsive disorder.
6. What can be some long-term consequences of panic attacks?
7. What are some possible signs of depression in children?
8. What is the general adaptation syndrome (GAS)?
9. What is the difference between eustress and distress?
10. How can good decision-making skills help the child deal with distress?
11. What should teachers strive to teach students for promoting emotional health?
12. What are the implications of divorce for children?
13. What potential problems may arise for latchkey children?

CRITICAL THINKING QUESTIONS

1. It has been said, "Our histories form our perceptions, which are realities of how we perceive life." What are some reasons that our perceptions may not be accurate?
2. Think about fostering a classroom that promotes optimum opportunity to facilitate learning and promotes the health and welfare of the student. Develop a written statement that reflects your basic beliefs about what type of atmosphere must exist and teacher attributes that would be conducive to facilitation of your philosophy.

WEB SITE ACTIVITY

Select one of the topics discussed in this chapter—stress in children, depression in children, suicide in children, self-esteem and children, and so on. Search the Web for a variety of perspectives on your topic, and then write a one- to two-page summary on what you found.

WEB SITES OF INTEREST

American Academy of Child and Adolescent Psychiatry: *www.aacap.org*
Contains a great deal of information on mental health. Excellent section on helping teachers boost student learning and achievement.

Education World: *www.educationworld.com*
Provides themes, pamphlets that might be useful for teaching health education. Some materials related to mental health.

Mind Tools: *www.mindtools.com*
Site is devoted to various coping skills. Deals with topics such as time management, problem solving, and general coping skills.

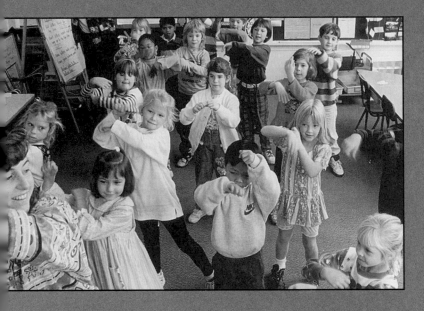

CHAPTER SEVEN

Strategies for Teaching Mental Health and Stress Reduction

We are nothing more than a
product of the decisions we
choose to make.

—Author Unknown

VALUED OUTCOMES

*After doing the activities in this chapter, the
students should be able to express and illustrate
the following guidelines:*

- Each person is unique and special, and everyone
  has many good qualities.

- All people share basic human needs for physical
  safety, love, security, emotional support, and
  acceptance from others.

- Personality development is affected by one's self-
  concept and acceptance from others.

- Mentally healthy expressions of emotion are
  consistent in frequency and intensity of the event
  that triggered the emotion.

- Open and honest communication with others is a
  necessary part of mental health.

- A stressful situation can best be minimized by identifying the situation as it arises, putting the event into perspective, and altering or eliminating the situation.

- Learning to relax and find pleasure in life activities on a day-to-day basis helps to reduce stress.

- Decisions concerning personal conduct must be compatible with a person's value system to enable emotional balance, unity, and inner peace.

- Ultimately each person must accept responsibility for his or her own behavior.

REFLECTIONS

As you review the activities in this chapter, select a strategy for grades K through 8 from the text or develop a new one that would demonstrate a personalization of the topic chosen. Be prepared to discuss how your strategies at each grade level would enhance the conceptualization of the topic at each grade level.

Mental Health: An Integral Part of Life

Mental health is a very significant part of our overall health. Sometimes our mental health is more difficult to maintain than our physical health. As teachers, we can enhance our students' mental health through the ways in which we interact with them. An open, accepting demeanor on the part of the teacher in a classroom can determine the effectiveness of the learning environment. Conversely, a regimented, pressure-filled atmosphere in the classroom will stifle students' creativity and interfere with their ability to learn. One of the most important aspects of mental health to teach elementary students is the acceptance of others. Teachers should emphasize that each individual is unique and that differences among individuals should make life more interesting, not more difficult. This concept of uniqueness is especially important to teach when a greater number of special students are mainstreamed into the "normal" classroom.

Another vital lesson to be taught in emotional health is the relationship between freedom and responsibilities. Elementary children struggle with ambivalent feelings toward dependence and independence. Sometimes they get angry when their parents treat them like little children, yet they are reluctant to accept the additional chores and responsibilities that accompany growing older. Students need to understand that growing older can mean greater freedom, in that they are allowed to do things younger children cannot do, but with the additional freedom comes the expectation to act prudently and responsibly.

Good relationships with others often begin with a healthy image of ourselves; therefore, a major goal in teaching mental health and stress reduction should be to foster self-esteem in children and to help them understand that in order to love others, they must accept themselves. Healthy self-esteem can enhance effective communication with others, which in turn helps build good relationships and resolve conflicts with family and friends. Further, an important part of a relationship is being able to communicate assertively and listen effectively. Building good mental health must begin in infancy and early childhood. By the time children enter school, their mental health has been strongly influenced by family and peers. But effective learning strategies are also a powerful shaping influence. By helping children build feelings of positive self-esteem, develop good decision-making skills in harmony with their values, and learn to cope with the stressors in life, the teacher can guide children toward emotional well-being.

Shown to the right of each activity in this chapter is the suggested grade level(s) for which the activity might be appropriate. However, many of the suggested activities could be modified for use at various grade levels.

Value-Based Activities

Value-based activities are designed to help children develop their critical thinking skills, personalize information, and establish concepts conducive to high-quality wellness. Teachers can design a variety of activities that are value based, depending on the content being discussed. Some suggestions follow.

VALUED POSSESSIONS   Grades (4–8)

Valued Outcome: The students will be able to identify what is really important to them and their well-being.

Description of Strategy: This activity is designed to help children determine what is important to them and understand that what we are expressing in our decisions are values or feelings concerning the type of life we wish to lead.

Materials Needed: paper, pencils

Value Question: Pretend that you are going on a trip in a spaceship. What three things would you take with you and why?

Processing Questions:
1. Why did you choose those three particular items?
2. Do these represent something you value?
3. How would you describe a value?
4. Do values reflect what we do and the decisions we make? Why/how?

SPECIAL ME   Grades (PK–3)

Valued Outcome: The students will realize they are special and unique at all stages of their lives.

Description of Strategy: This strategy is designed to help students feel good about themselves and enhance their self-esteem. Ask the students to list five things they are good at or that they have accomplished. Have the students draw, color, and label each event or accomplishment. Compile the drawings in a folder and have the students decorate the front of the folder (some students may choose to use photographs). Emphasize that everyone has special talents and abilities, with different accomplishments throughout their lifetimes.

Materials Needed: construction paper or colored paper, glue or tape, markers or crayons, folders, photographs (optional)

Processing Questions:

1. What are the things that make you feel good about yourself?
2. What are your talents?
3. How can we help other people feel good about themselves?
4. Should we always believe everything someone says about our performance or actions? Why or why not?

LOOKING AT ME   Grades (4–6)

Valued Outcome: The students will be able to understand that everyone has strengths and weaknesses.

Description of Strategy: Have the students make a list of five to ten things they consider to be their strengths and weaknesses. It is helpful if the teacher will also compile a personal list to be shared with the class. Allow time for discussion and sharing so students will realize that nobody is perfect. Follow up the discussion by having the students select a famous person and research what they think were that person's strengths and weaknesses. After reviewing the famous people, ask the students how that person could have improved his or her weaknesses. Then ask students to look at their own weaknesses and to suggest ways they could overcome or deal with what they consider a weakness. Emphasize that no one is perfect.

Materials Needed: pen or pencil, paper, references on famous people

Processing Questions:

1. What strengths did you identify?
2. What weaknesses did you identify?
3. Does everyone have strengths and weaknesses?
4. Do even people who are famous or whom you admire have some weaknesses? What are some examples?
5. Is it okay that we are not always perfect?

HELPING OTHERS   Grades (K–6)

Valued Outcome: The students will realize that we can help others feel good about themselves through our encouragement and kindness.

Description of Strategy: Divide the class into small groups. Have the students share ways that others make them feel good about themselves (compliments, encouraging words, and so on). Following the small group discussion, ask the class to share each group's thoughts. Write the class responses on a large sheet of paper. Ask each person in the various small groups to provide a compliment to every person in his or her group. Make sure the comments are sincere and that everyone has nice things said about him or her. Emphasize that in order to feel good about ourselves, it is important to not always think about ourselves, but to encourage others and be kind in our comments to each other.

Materials Needed: marker, butcher paper

Processing Questions:

1. Can we help others feel good about themselves?
2. How do we sometimes make others feel bad about themselves?
3. Why is it important to consider others' feelings and not always our own?

SETTING MY SAILS   Grades (4–8)

Valued Outcome: The students will realize that setting realistic personal goals and accomplishing these goals can help them to have higher self-esteem.

Description of Strategy: Explain/review to the students what goals are. Ask them to write down two short-term and two long-term goals. Ask each student to list the things they have to do to accomplish their goals. Inform them that over the next couple of weeks they will be asked to list things that they have done to accomplish their short-term goals. Emphasize that one way to feel good about ourselves is to set goals and attempt to accomplish them. During the discussion, ask the students what they think the following saying means: "Aim at the stars—even if you don't hit them, you will land pretty anyhow."

Materials Needed: pen or pencil, paper

Processing Questions:

1. Why do you think having goals is important?
2. Do you think we can always achieve every goal we set for ourselves?
3. Why might we not achieve our goals?
4. Why does accomplishing our goals make us feel good?

VOTING QUESTIONS   Grades (4–6)

Valued Outcome: The students will examine their feelings for the various topics presented.

Description of Strategy: Voting questions are another way to help students establish their feelings on various topics. The teacher can develop a variety of questions that lend themselves to a particular topic. The questions should be read aloud. Ask students to raise their thumbs up if they agree with the question, thumbs down if they disagree, and to fold their arms if they are unsure or undecided. Some examples of potential questions: How many of you find it difficult to talk with your parents? feel scared to speak in a large group? have a friend to discuss problems? wish others would listen to you better?

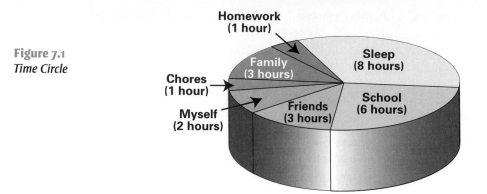

Figure 7.1
Time Circle

Materials Needed: teacher- or student-prepared voting questions

Processing Questions:

1. What seem to be the areas that represent the biggest problems?
2. What are some ways we can deal with these problems?

THE TIME OF MY LIFE   Grades (7–8)

Valued Outcome: The students will be able to identify how they spend the hours of each day.

Description of Strategy: For this activity, have each student draw a circle and divide it into four sections on a piece of paper (see Figure 7.1). The circle represents a twenty-four-hour time span, with each quadrant equaling approximately six hours. From the categories shown, ask each student to divide the circle according to the amount of time that he or she thinks should be spent on these activities: with friends, with family, learning at school, for homework, for sleeping.

Materials Needed: paper to draw circle (or a prepared form), pencils

Processing Questions:

1. How do you like your time schedule?
2. Is there anything you need to change?
3. Why is how we use our time important?
4. Why do we tend to do those things we like best?

NAME TAG DESCRIPTORS   Grades (4–6)

Valued Outcome: The students will be able to name ways in which they are unique.

Description of Strategy: Each student should be provided with a piece of paper and crayons. Discuss how each person is unique. Instruct the student to make a name tag with a drawing that will show one of his or her interests. Cut the name tag out, and write the child's name on the tag. The class can then guess each person's interests.

Materials Needed: paper or name tags, crayons or colored pencils

Processing Questions:

1. How do the activities we like to do differ?
2. Is it okay that we all like different activities?
3. What are some ways that all of us are alike?
4. What are really important characteristics that we should all have?

FRIENDS SHOULD BE . . .   Grades (4–8)

Valued Outcome: The students will be able to name ways in which they are unique.

Description of Strategy: Using the following list, ask each student to rank-order within each grouping the characteristics most important to look for in a friend. Then group the students by gender and ask them to decide, by consensus, rankings that are shared with all other groups.

A	B	C
_____ Smart	_____ Honest	_____ Loyal
_____ Popular	_____ Dependable	_____ Conscientious
_____ Funny	_____ Dedicated	_____ Trustworthy

D	E	F
_____ Open	_____ Quiet	_____ Healthy
_____ Discreet	_____ Bubbly	_____ Happy
_____ Closed	_____ Talkative	_____ Successful

Materials Needed: above list (may be expanded by the teacher/student), pencils

Processing Questions:

1. What common characteristics did the various groups identify?
2. Were there differences between the boys' and the girls' choices of important characteristics?
3. What other characteristics would be important to you in a friend?
4. Of the important characteristics identified, do you feel you portray those characteristics?

RELATIONSHIP COLLAGE   Grades (4–8)

Valued Outcome: The students will develop insight into the many people who influence their lives.

Description of Strategy: This activity is designed to help students see the influence of relationships they have with peers, family, teachers, coaches, and so on.

Have the students make a collage of their relationships. A picture of the student should be in the center of a piece of posterboard. Around his or her picture, the student puts other pictures or drawings that represent the many people he or she associates with.

Materials Needed: paper, colored pencils, pictures or drawings of students and individuals with whom they interact

Processing Questions:

1. Who are the most important people in your life?
2. What do these people do for you?
3. How do they influence you and your behavior?
4. Are there any negative influences from these people?
5. What can you do about the negative influences?

Decision Stories

Follow the procedure discussed in Chapter 4 (pages 80–83) for presenting decision stories such as the following.

WHERE DID I PUT THEM?   Grades (4–6)

Sally is getting ready for school. She cannot remember where she put her shoes. She looked under the bed, under the chair, and behind the door. Sally begins to cry because she thinks she will be late.

Focus Questions: What could have been done to keep Sally from getting upset? What should Sally do now?

A NASTY NOTE   Grades (7–8)

Juan was going to the lunchroom when he saw Fred sticking something in Peggy's locker. Later, Juan sees Peggy crying because she found the note, which made fun of her family.

Focus Questions: What should Juan do to help? How does Peggy feel?

I DARE YOU   Grades (4–6)

Ling is new in her neighborhood and wants to make new friends. Jill asks her to take an unsafe dare in order to be accepted by the others in the neighborhood.

Focus Questions: What should Ling do? Is it worth placing yourself at risk to be accepted? How can Ling decide which is more important?

NEW GIRL IN SCHOOL

Grades (4–6)

Betty notices that the new student in class is being ridiculed by two of Betty's friends because the new student is the only one in class wearing glasses. They are talking with other girls and writing notes.

Focus Question: What should Betty do?

HANDLING STRESS

Grades (K–3)

José has just invited his friend, Leroy, to play, but Leroy replied, "I don't want to play with you anymore." José feels angry, frustrated, and rejected.

Focus Question: How can José handle the stress caused by this situation?

Other Strategies for Learning

GUESS MY TRAIT

Grades (4–6)

Valued Outcome: The students will be able to express a specific personality trait through role-play.

Description of Strategy: Ask several children to role-play a personality trait that you have whispered to them. One child will act out the personality trait, and the rest of the class will guess the personality trait. Both positive and negative traits can be role-played.

Materials Needed: none

Processing Questions:

1. What is one of your own personality traits?
2. Were all the traits demonstrated in the role-play situations desirable ones?
3. Differentiate between the desirable and the undesirable personality traits.

TRUTH AND CONSEQUENCES

Grades (4–6)

Valued Outcome: The students will observe, discuss, and role-play consequences that result from taking specific actions.

Description of Strategy: Have a small group of volunteer students role-play the following situations and the resulting consequences:

1. A student decides not to do his homework.
2. A man speeds on the highway because he is late.
3. A girl receives a birthday gift and refuses to thank the person she received it from.

   Afterward, discuss these questions: Did the person accept the responsibility involved? What results would occur if he or she had acted differently?

Materials Needed: none

Processing Questions:

1. What are the consequences of not doing your homework?

2. What are the consequences of disobeying laws or rules?

3. What action would you expect the girl who received a birthday gift to demonstrate?

APPROPRIATE PERSONALITY TRAITS   Grades (K–3)

Valued Outcome: The students will be able to demonstrate healthy ways to react to specific feelings.

Description of Strategy: Have class members role-play the following situations to illustrate healthy personality traits appropriate to the situation.

  1. getting a poor grade on a test

  2. losing your favorite toy

  3. accidentally damaging someone else's property

Materials Needed: none

Processing Questions:

1. Is it okay to get angry? Why or why not?

2. What is one good way to handle anger?

3. Think of a situation in which you got angry. What did you do? How could you have reacted differently?

BODY LANGUAGE   Grades (4–8)

Valued Outcome: The students will be able to identify ways in which a listener's positive or negative body language affects the speaker.

Description of Strategy: Group the class into pairs. One person is the listener, and the other is the speaker. The speaker talks about a teacher-selected topic, such as "My most embarrassing moment" or "What I want to do this summer." The listener responds nonverbally with positive body language, for example, nodding the head, eye contact, erect posture. This activity can be repeated with the listener displaying negative body language such as anger, sadness, rejection, or superiority. Afterward, the class discusses the effects of positive and negative body language on the speaker.

Materials Needed: none

Processing Questions:

1. Name two ways to demonstrate positive body language when listening.

2. Name two ways to demonstrate negative body language when listening.

3. Describe one way the speaker reacts to each type of body language.

EMOTIONAL REACTIONS   Grades (4–8)

Valued Outcome: The students will be able to explain how the same emotion can be expressed in different ways.

Description of Strategy: Role-play how you would act if you felt good about yourself or if you did not feel good about yourself, for example, after being disciplined in public by parents for inappropriate behavior. Ask two or three students to do this. Note how differently they role-play these emotions.

Materials Needed: none

Processing Questions:

1. Give an example of a wrong way to handle a specific emotion.
2. What might the consequences be of handling an emotion a wrong way?
3. Which way seemed to be the best way of dealing with the emotion and why?

BODY LANGUAGE   Grades (4–6)

Valued Outcome: The students will be able to express emotions in both verbal and nonverbal ways.

Description of Strategy: Role-play how you can communicate the same thing with or without words. Have students use body language to express an emotion, and then have them verbally demonstrate the same emotion.

Materials Needed: none

Processing Questions:

1. Give an example of a verbal statement to let someone know you care about them.
2. Name a nonverbal way to let someone know you care about them.
3. Give an example of a nonverbal expression of anger.

HIDDEN MESSAGES   Grades (4–8)

Valued Outcome: The students will be able to communicate in both verbal and nonverbal ways, identifying advantages and disadvantages to both ways.

Description of Strategy: Divide students into small groups. Ask half the groups to present a play with a hidden message or moral of their choice using dialogue, and ask the remaining groups to give their presentations nonverbally. After all groups have finished, ask for identification and interpretation of the messages, and discuss the advantages and disadvantages of verbal and nonverbal communication.

Materials Needed: none

Processing Questions:

1. Name one disadvantage of nonverbal communication.
2. Name one advantage of nonverbal communication.
3. Name one advantage of verbal communication.

WORDS CAN HURT   Grades (PK–3)

Valued Outcome: The students will be able to describe and discuss both tactful and rude ways to handle specific situations.

Description of Strategy: Ask the class as a whole to devise a hypothetical, open-ended situation in which communication could take the form of being either rude or tactful. Then divide the class into two groups. Ask one group to describe several tactful ways the situation could be handled. Ask the other group to describe several rude ways the situation could be handled. Follow by leading a discussion about students' views concerning each handling of the situation.

Materials Needed: none

Processing Questions:

1. What advantage does using a tactful answer have over using a rude response?
2. What might occur if a rude comment is used in response to a situation?
3. What might occur if a tactful response is used in a situation?

THE DECISION   Grades (4–8)

Valued Outcome: The students will be able to demonstrate ways to handle emotions associated with rejection and family crisis situations.

Description of Strategy: Provide an open-ended hypothetical situation appropriate for the grade level that involves either rejection by a peer group or a family crisis. Then divide the students into three groups. Supply two of the groups with the ending they will enact. Ask the third group to devise their own scenario. Let each group dramatize its ideas and compare differences. If time and attention allow, provide additional situations and rotate tasks.

Materials Needed: none

Processing Questions:

1. What is one good way to handle rejection?
2. What is one bad way to handle rejection?
3. What is a helpful thing to do in a family crisis?

PAIRING   Grades (K–3)

Valued Outcome: The students will be able to demonstrate and discuss a variety of emotions associated with specific situations.

Description of Strategy: Divide students into pairs. Have one member of each pair draw a situation from a box full of hypothetical interactions between two people, such as making a new friend, responding to someone who has broken your favorite toy, or sharing ice cream with a playmate. Use imagination, creativity, and diversity in developing these situations, and focus on many areas of mental health. Allow each pair to act out its situation, and encourage class discussion after each enactment.

Materials Needed: box containing slips of paper with hypothetical situations listed

Processing Questions:

1. What is a good way to respond to someone who has broken your favorite toy?
2. What is a bad way to respond to someone who has broken your favorite toy?
3. How would you go about trying to make a new friend?

GIVING AND GAINING   Grades (4–8)

Valued Outcome: The students will be able to demonstrate an understanding of the necessity for compromise in specific situations.

Description of Strategy: Have several students role-play a situation where an individual's personal values must be compromised for the good of the group. Examples might include the mayor allowing an individual to make an unpopular speech or a police officer enforcing a law he or she does not agree with. Follow with a discussion of why the person made the compromise.

Materials Needed: none

Processing Questions:

1. What is a situation in which it would not be good to compromise? Why?
2. Why is compromise necessary in some situations?
3. What might happen if no one ever compromised?

GETTING TO KNOW YOU   Grades (4–6)

Valued Outcome: The students will be able to describe and discuss various aspects of their personalities.

Description of Strategy: Ask students to print the word *personality* as the heading on a sheet of notebook paper and have them write several phrases that describe their own personalities. Let volunteers share their papers with the class.

Materials Needed: paper, pencils or pens

Processing Questions:

1. What do you think is one of your most important personality characteristics, and why do you think it is important?
2. What personality trait do you find to be your least desirable?
3. If you could have any personality trait you wanted, what would you choose and why?

QUESTION BOX   Grades (4–8)

Valued Outcome: The students will be able to identify personal fears, worries, or dilemmas.

Description of Strategy: Supply a large, colorful box, and encourage students to anonymously submit questions that they want to discuss regarding personal fears, worries, or dilemmas. Set aside about thirty minutes each week to discuss as many of these as possible.

Materials Needed: question box

Processing Questions:

1. What is your worst fear and why?
2. What specific things cause you to worry?
3. Who are some people you could talk to about your worries and fears?

WHO CAN I TURN TO?   Grades (4–6)

Valued Outcome: The students will be able to identify sources of help for specific situations.

Description of Strategy: Ask students to think about whom they can talk to when they need advice. Give the class a situation (i.e., a friend is making fun of you). Let the students decide to whom they would go for help in the situation.

Materials Needed: none

Processing Questions:

1. To whom do you feel you can go about a problem you are having with peer pressure?
2. To whom do you feel you can go about a problem you are having with a friend?
3. To whom do you feel you can go about a family crisis?

UPS AND DOWNS   Grades (PK–3)

Valued Outcome: The students will be able to identify uplifting emotions and depressing emotions and associate them with specific circumstances.

Description of Strategy: Discuss emotions in terms of "ups" and "downs." What emotions make us feel up or down? Ask volunteers if they are feeling up or down today and what circumstances led to their feeling this way.

Materials Needed: none

Processing Questions:

1. Name two emotions that make you feel "up."
2. Name two emotions that make you feel "down."
3. Give an example of an event that caused you to experience emotions that made you feel "down."

WE ARE DIFFERENT PEOPLE

Grades (4–6)

Valued Outcome: The students will be able to describe how they behave differently in various relationships.

Description of Strategy: Brainstorm examples of how one person can function in several relationships at one time, such as friend, sibling, child, and student. Emphasize how we behave differently in various relationships.

Materials Needed: none

Processing Questions:

1. What is different about how you express anger at a parent and at a teacher?
2. What is different about the way you express love for a friend and for a sibling?
3. Do you think we hurt the people we care about the most? Why or why not?

PICTURE THE EMOTION

Grades (4–6)

Valued Outcome: Students will be able to identify exressions of emotions.

Description of Strategy: Photograph the students in a variety of situations. Post the photographs on a bulletin board, and ask the students to comment on the emotions being expressed in the photographs, such as happiness, love, sorrow, fear, and anxiety. This will help the students explore their emotions and the emotions of those around them.

Materials Needed: camera, bulletin board

Processing Questions:

1. What is the most common emotion depicted on the bulletin board?
2. Whose facial expression shows the most pain, and what are the circumstances surrounding this emotion?
3. Whose facial expression shows the most joy, and what are the circumstances surrounding this emotion?

CARING

Grades (K–6)

Valued Outcome: The students will be able to discuss ways in which they can help meet the needs of others by caring.

Description of Strategy: Discuss the different needs of a pet dog or cat. When the animal is hungry, we feed it. When it is lonely, we play with it and talk to it. When it is sleeping, we don't disturb it. People have needs that have to be met as well. Discuss how we can help meet the needs of others by caring.

Materials Needed: none

Processing Questions:

1. How could you help meet the needs of a sick parent?
2. How could you help meet the needs of an infant?
3. How could you help meet the needs of a grandparent in a nursing home?

LIVING BY THE RULES   Grades (4–6)

Valued Outcome: The students will be able to identify reasons for rules.

Description of Strategy: Sometimes it is hard for young children to understand why it is necessary to follow directions or obey rules. Discuss several rules or laws and the reasons for each. For example, a traffic speed limit helps to prevent accidents, injuries, and deaths. It also helps to conserve fuel. Rules for a game help make the activity fair and fun. Discuss what happens when someone doesn't follow the rules of a game.

Materials Needed: none

Processing Questions:

1. Why are traffic laws necessary?

2. Why are rules necessary in games?

3. What are some possible dangers associated with not following parents' rules?

I'M UNIQUE   Grades (K–3)

Valued Outcome: The students will be able to compare differences and similarities among individuals.

Description of Strategy: Have students trace the outlines of each other's bodies on butcher paper. Compare the similarities and differences with other students in the class to emphasize that we are alike in many ways and yet unique.

Materials Needed: butcher paper, markers or crayons

Processing Questions:

1. What are some similarities that exist among students in the class?

2. What are some differences that exist among students in the class?

3. Name some advantages to being different.

DIFFERENT PICTURES OF ME   Grades (4–8)

Valued Outcome: The students will be able to identify unique characteristics of each stage of development.

Description of Strategy: Have students bring in pictures of themselves as an infant, as a toddler, and as a child. Have them note the unique characteristics of each stage of development.

Materials Needed: students' photographs

Processing Questions:

1. What unique characteristics did you have as an infant?

2. What unique characteristics did you have as a toddler?

3. What are unique characteristics that you now possess?

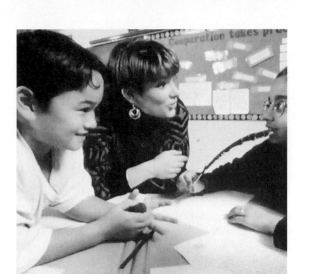

The teacher can do much to foster each student's mental health by reinforcing special talents and allowing expression of feelings.

WHICH EMOTION AM I?   Grades (K–3)

Valued Outcome: The students will be able to draw facial expressions depicting specific emotions.

Description of Strategy: Give each child a paper plate and crayons. List several emotions on the board. Assign one emotion to each child, then have each child draw his or her face reflecting that emotion.

Materials Needed: paper plates, crayons

Processing Questions:

1. Describe the face that was drawn expressing anger.
2. Describe the face that was drawn expressing joy.
3. Can you always tell what someone is feeling by his or her facial expression? Why or why not?

HAPPY OR SAD?   Grades (PK–3)

Valued Outcome: The students will be able to associate the emotions "happy" and "sad" with positive and negative situations.

Description of Strategy: Let each child draw a happy face and a sad face on a paper plate. Attach these to Popsicle sticks. The teacher will give examples of positive and negative situations, and the students will hold up the face that indicates how they would feel in each situation.

Materials Needed: paper plates, crayons, Popsicle sticks

Processing Questions:

1. Can you give an example of a situation that made you feel happy?

2. Can you give an example of a situation that made you feel sad?

3. Happy and sad are two common emotions. What are some other emotions you have felt today?

EMOTIONS BAG
Grades (7–8)

Valued Outcome: The students will be able to describe personal emotional experiences as well as reactions in those situations.

Description of Strategy: Give each student a paper bag to keep for two days. Students should keep track of their emotions for that time period by writing a description about their emotional experiences and their reactions to those situations as they happen. Students will keep each description in their bag and then share them with class.

Materials Needed: paper bags, paper, pencils

Processing Questions:

1. What was an emotion you described that made you feel bad inside? What caused this emotion?

2. What was an emotion you described that made you feel good inside? What caused this emotion?

3. Did you experience the emotion anger? If so, how did you react?

MENTAL HEALTH IN MUSIC
Grades (4–8)

Valued Outcome: The students will be able to describe characteristics of healthy living.

Description of Strategy: Have students compose songs that describe healthy living. They can bring in tapes or CDs that describe a human relationship. Discuss the feelings depicted in the music. Pay attention to the tone of the music as well as the words of the song.

Materials Needed: students' tapes or CDs, tape or CD player

Processing Questions:

1. Can you name one characteristic of a healthy relationship?

2. What feelings are mentioned in the song you wrote?

3. Besides having healthy relationships, what are some other characteristics of healthy living?

HEARING IS NOT ALWAYS LISTENING
Grades (7–8)

Valued Outcome: The students will be able to demonstrate and discuss listening and observation skills.

Description of Strategy: Set up several "listening" and "observing" demonstrations to emphasize that these are learned skills. Here are some possible examples.

- Prearrange with a student to share a hypothetical problem with several classmates during lunch or recess. They need to believe they are being told about the problem in confidence. The next day, reveal the setup to the class and ask each student involved about what he or she heard and understood to be the problem.

- Prearrange with several students to get "lost" during recess. (Have them go to the library or other supervised area.) When the rest of the class returns, ask them to help with descriptions of each missing person. Also have them indicate anything they might have overheard during recess that might give a clue to why these students are gone. After the missing students return, discuss implications of the activity.

- Tell students you are going to read a story and you want them to listen carefully. Read aloud a short story with several specific details about a main character's problem or situation and the succeeding events. Immediately following the story, ask each student to write a brief summary of the story, being as specific and accurate as possible. Let volunteers share their versions. Then read the original again. Compare listening skills.

Materials Needed: story, paper, pencils

Processing Questions:

1. What is the difference between hearing and listening?
2. How did the versions of the first scenario differ, and why do you think this occurred?
3. What is the advantage of being a good listener?

CARTOON PERSONALITIES   Grades (4–6)

Valued Outcome: The students will be able to identify personality traits of a cartoon character.

Description of Strategy: The teacher will ask the students to determine the personality traits of cartoon characters. The teacher will hold up a picture of a cartoon character and have the students describe the character's personality.

Materials Needed: pictures of cartoon characters

Processing Questions:

1. Which cartoon characters had undesirable personality traits, and what are these traits?
2. Which cartoon characters had desirable personality traits, and what are these traits?
3. Do you have any of the same personality traits as the cartoon characters? Which traits?

HUMAN SCAVENGER HUNT

Grades (4–8)

Valued Outcome: The students will be able to identify human qualities that emphasize individual uniqueness.

Description of Strategy: Have students simulate a "scavenger hunt," but have them look for various unique human qualities, such as red hair, green eyes, friendliness, or quick-temperedness. Suggest students write the names of classmates on their paper next to the appropriate quality.

Materials Needed: list of human qualities to seek, paper, pencils

Processing Questions:

1. What did you think was the most interesting quality you found in your scavenger hunt?
2. How many different qualities might one person have?
3. Do any two people have the same qualities? Why or why not?

WHO AM I?

Grades (4–6)

Valued Outcome: Students will be able to recognize the different and unique qualities of every individual.

Description of Strategy: Have students write a story and make a drawing about themselves. After they have completed the stories and drawings, collect them and read the papers aloud. Have students guess whose paper is being read.

Materials Needed: paper, pencils, crayons, or markers

Processing Questions:

1. Name as many favorite animals as you can remember that were mentioned by your classmates.
2. Name as many different hobbies as you can that were mentioned by your classmates.
3. What other interesting qualities were mentioned in your classmates' stories?

COSTUME PARTY

Grades (4–6)

Valued Outcome: The students will be able to express personality traits through costume.

Description of Strategy: Ask each student to come to class in a costume that depicts as many of his or her personality traits as possible. The class as a whole lists what traits students think are revealed. A secret ballot vote is cast for costumes that are the most accurate, inaccurate, humorous, puzzling, and eye catching.

Materials Needed: costumes from students' homes, materials for casting secret ballot (pencils, paper, box, etc.)

Processing Questions:

1. Explain why you chose the costume you were wearing.
2. Describe the costume and personality traits of your closest classmate.
3. Which classmate had the most humorous costume? Why?

SILENT STEPS   Grades (7–8)

Valued Outcome: The students will be able to identify feelings experienced through a nonverbal group effort to reconstruct a jigsaw puzzle.

Description of Strategy: Divide students into groups of five to seven. Provide each group with a sealed manilla envelope that contains a sheet of colored construction paper cut into five to seven shuffled jigsaw pieces. Each group should receive a different colored puzzle with differently shaped pieces of equal difficulty. Instruct each group member to randomly select a puzzle piece from the envelope. When you give the signal to start, students must reconstruct the pieces without saying a word. As each group completes the puzzle, have them raise their hands—they still cannot talk. When all groups have finished, allow the students to discuss their feelings during this activity.

Materials Needed: manilla envelopes with jigsaw puzzle pieces

Processing Questions:

1. What feelings can result from nonverbal communication?
2. Discuss how the puzzle would have been solved if verbal communication had been used.
3. What are the advantages to verbal communication?

STEPS TO THE TOP   Grades (4–8)

Valued Outcome: The students will be able to name a quality or rule for building mental health.

Description of Strategy: Have students trace one of their feet on construction paper. Inside the foot outline, ask each student to write a quality or rule for building mental health. These qualities can include self-love, self-respect, consideration of others, open communication, honesty, practicing what you preach, or sound decision making. Tack the footprints on a bulletin board in ascending steps to good mental health.

Materials Needed: construction paper, scissors, markers or pens, bulletin board

Processing Questions:

1. Explain how your footprint relates to building mental health.
2. Why is it important to have good mental heath?
3. What are some characteristics of poor mental health?

Stress is becoming a common cause for illness or other problems among students of all ages. Students need to be able to identify the causes of stress in their lives and their reactions to stressful events. There are several ways you can help them identify these.

1. Have the students determine stressful events that occur during the week by keeping a journal. They should record stressful events and how they coped with the events for one week.

This will help them identify the coping mechanisms they are using. Keeping a journal will also allow them to identify their physical and emotional reactions. Let the students share their journals with each other and discuss the different ways they reacted.

2. There is a very good NBC video titled, *Stressed to Kill*. This video is narrated by Connie Chung and contains experiments that explore the mind and body's response to stress.

COPING WITH STRESS   Grades (4–8)

Valued Outcome: The students will be able to identify positive ways to reduce stress.

Description of Strategy: Divide students into four groups. Ask each group to create a bulletin board that focuses on positive ways to reduce stress. Bulletin boards should be redone each week for a month so that each group's message can be seen and discussed.

Materials Needed: construction paper, scissors, stencils, bulletin board

Processing Questions:

1. Name three positive ways to reduce stress.
2. What might happen to someone who is under too much stress?
3. How often should stress reduction techniques be used and why?

FACIAL FORECASTS   Grades (PK–3)

Valued Outcome: The students will be able to draw a facial expression depicting a specific emotion.

Description of Strategy: Assign each student an emotion. Provide students with paper plates and crayons, and ask them to draw their own faces indicating the emotion. Have the students use mirrors if necessary. The plates may be used for a colorful wall display.

Materials Needed: paper plates, crayons, mirrors

Processing Questions:

1. How did your face look when you expressed anger?
2. How did your face look when you expressed happiness?
3. Do people's facial expressions always indicate how they feel? Why or why not?

REFUSAL SKILLS   Grades (4–8)

Valued Outcome: The students will be able to identify five refusal skills to use when responding to peer pressure.

Description of Strategy: Students will discuss the definition of peer pressure and how it is used by friends and others to influence their behavior. Specific techniques used by peers and others will be identified: name calling, acceptance, and so on. The teacher will solicit responses regarding the results of using poor judgment and giving in to peer pressure. The following questions will be asked:

- How will you feel about yourself if you use poor judgment?
- What kinds of trouble could you encounter as a result of your actions?
- What physical effects will your action cause?

Explain and cite examples of the following refusal steps:

1. Ask questions.
2. Name the trouble.
3. Identify consequences.
4. Suggest alternatives.
5. Leave.

Students will practice refusal steps in an activity called "The Pressure Seat." Students sit in a circle with one student in the center of the group. The student chooses a peer pressure situation strip from the can. He or she reads the situation aloud and responds in one minute. The group is then called on to discuss the situation and tell if it agrees or disagrees with the decision made by the student. The student in the pressure seat then chooses another student to take his or her place until each group member has had a chance to sit in the pressure seat.

Materials Needed: chairs to form a circle, strips of paper listing different peer pressure situations, can

Processing Questions:

1. What are the five refusal steps?
2. What are some things that might occur if you are unable to effectively deal with peer pressure?
3. How did you feel about the decisions you made in the pressure seat?

EMOTIONAL MUSICAL CHAIRS   Grades (K–6)

Valued Outcome: The students will be able to associate emotions with facial expressions.

Description of Strategy: Students will discuss specific feelings they have had on specific occasions. Tell the students that everyone's feelings are important and should be respected. Then have students participate in a game of musical chairs. Chairs are arranged in the same way as for the traditional game; however, no additional chairs are removed during the game. Before starting, place pictures, each with a face showing a different emotion, in a box. Students move around the chairs as the music plays and try to find a place to sit when the music stops. The student without a chair draws a picture out of the box and shows it to the other students. The student then tells what emotion he or she thinks the person in the picture is feeling. All of the students then tell what emotion he or she thinks the person in the picture is feeling. Have the students make faces and act out the emotion until the music starts again. The game continues until all the emotions in the box have been acted out.

Materials Needed: chairs, pictures of faces showing different emotions, box, music player, music

Processing Questions:

1. What are some of the ways you express your emotions?
2. When do you share your feelings or emotions with others?
3. Discuss a time when you made someone else happy, sad, angry, and so on.

HOW TO HANDLE PEER PRESSURE   Grades (4–8)

Valued Outcome: Each student will be able to list two positive characteristics about him- or herself.

Description of Strategy: Solicit responses to the following questions:

1. Name a situation in which you were influenced by your friends in a decision you made.
2. Why do you think friends are able to persuade you to do things you know are wrong?
3. Why is it important to avoid the negative influence of your friends?
4. How can being influenced by your friends be dangerous to yourself and others? Give specific examples.
5. What are some positive ways peers can influence one another?
6. What is unique about you?
7. List four characteristics of your two closest friends.
8. List two physical and two personality characteristics of your two closest friends and discuss these characteristics.

Emphasize the need for accepting who you are and being proud of your decisions.

Materials Needed: none

Processing Questions:

1. Why do we sometimes give in to peer pressure?
2. How is each of us different?
3. What are some dangers of peer pressure?

STATE OF MIND   Grades (4–6)

Valued Outcome: The students will be able to differentiate between positive and negative ways to express emotions.

Description of Strategy: Ask students to share with the class specific times when they felt happy, sad, mad, or some other strong emotion. Ask students to also share how they acted when they felt these emotions. Obtain copies of "Goofus and Gallant"—the cartoon series depicting two young boys, one who acts bad and one who acts good from *Highlights* magazines. Hand them out to the class. Have the class discuss why they think Goofus and Gallant acted as they did. Ask, "What will be the consequences of the good action?" Also call for a discussion of consequences of the bad action.

Materials Needed: photocopies of cartoon "Goofus and Gallant"

Processing Questions:

1. Why is sharing our emotions with others so important?
2. Give an example of healthy ways to handle anger.
3. Give an example of unhealthy ways to handle anger.

WHO AM I?   Grades (4–6)

Valued Outcome: Each student will be able to identify and discuss unique qualities of his or her own and of others.

Description of Strategy: Lead a discussion emphasizing the uniqueness of every individual. Students will receive a worksheet to fill out about themselves. The teacher will then read one aloud, and the students will guess who it is about.

Materials Needed: "Who am I?" worksheet (see the Teaching in Action box on page 26)

Processing Questions:

1. What does it mean to have a unique quality?
2. Will people have some different qualities even if they seem just alike? Explain.
3. What makes each person different?

Listed below are several questions. After you are through, we will share with the class to see if we can guess each others' identity.

1. My two favorite things to do are _____.

2. My favorite food is _____.

3. My favorite TV program is _____.

4. My best subject in school is _____.

5. What I like best about myself is _____.

6. Friends should _____.

7. If I could change one thing about me it would be _____.

8. I am special because _____.

9. I have brothers/sisters _____.

10. My favorite activity is _____.

11. Three words I would use to describe myself are _____.

UNIQUE! THAT'S ME!   Grades (K–3)

Valued Outcome: Each student will be able to identify two ways in which he or she is unique in relationship to his or her classmates.

Description of Strategy: Ask students to discuss ways in which individuals are unique. The students will play a voice-guessing game to show how everything about a person, even their voice, is unique and special. A student will sing the words, "Voices never are the same. Can you guess what is my name?" to the tune of "Twinkle, Twinkle, Little Star." The rest of the class, with eyes closed, will raise their hands to guess the voice. Repeat the activity until everyone has had a turn to sing with students relocating around the room after each turn. Students will then examine their fingers and those of their classmates with a magnifying glass. Students will be given fingerpaint ink and will make a thumb print on a paper star to be worn on their clothing.

Materials Needed: poster with song words, magnifying glasses, fingerpaint or ink, paper stars, safety pins for name tags

Processing Questions:

1. What does the word *unique* mean?

2. Is it good or bad to be unique? Explain.

3. In what ways are you a unique person?

COPING WITH AND CONTROLLING STRESS

Grades (7–8)

Valued Outcome: The students will be able to assess their stress level and use relaxation and self-management techniques in response to stressful situations.

Description of Strategy: Ask students to list three things they find stressful and want to discuss. List the responses on the board. Ask, "Why are peer pressure, grades, and the need for acceptance such common stressors?" Lead a discussion on effectively dealing with these stressors, and explain the following techniques for handling stressful situations: quiet reflection, biofeedback, progressive muscle relaxation, and visualization. Obtain a copy of a stress test and have students take it to determine their current level of stress. Explain to students that they are to maintain a daily journal listing all stressful situations they encounter, how they react, and if there could be a better way to handle the stressor.

Materials Needed: stress test, paper and pencils for journal

Processing Questions:

1. What areas of your life create the most stress for you?
2. Describe one effective way of handling a stressor.
3. What are some advantages and disadvantages of stress?

MUSICAL COMPLIMENTS

Grades (4–8)

Valued Outcome: Each student will be able to write positive statements about other students and will describe feelings in response to positive statements made about her or him.

Description of Strategy: Lead a discussion about self-esteem, asking the following questions:

1. How does it make you feel when someone says something nice about you?
2. Do you make it a point to compliment people when they do something good?
3. Do you try to note the good things about a person, even when there are things about them that you dislike?
4. Have you ever thought about your own good qualities and why people like to be around you?

Give each student a piece of paper cut into one of various shapes, such as a child, a musical note, or a heart. Have students write their names on the cutout they receive and pass them around the room while you play music. When the music stops, each child will write something positive about the person whose cutout they receive. Continue this until the students have written on several different cutouts. Give students a few minutes to sit quietly and read the comments written about them. Then ask students to write a paragraph telling how this activity made them feel.

Materials Needed: cutouts, markers, music player, music, paper, pens or pencils

Processing Questions:

1. Which comment on your card made you feel particularly special, and why?
2. How did it make you feel to write something nice about someone else?
3. Give an example of a compliment.

FEELINGS AND FACES   Grades (K–3)

Valued Outcome: The students will be able to associate emotions with facial expressions.

Description of Strategy: Hand out duplicated sheets of stylized emotions to the students (see the Teaching in Action box, Worksheet for Emotions and Me). Have each student identify and label the emotion depicted on each face. Follow this activity with a class discussion.

Materials Needed: worksheet showing facial expressions depicting specific emotions

Processing Questions:

1. Which emotions are not showing a smiling face?
2. Which emotions are not showing frowns?
3. How do the eyes look on the face that shows surprise?

EMOTIONS AND ME   Grades (K–3)

Valued Outcome: The students will be able to match facial expressions with emotions, identify emotions associated with specific situations, and discuss reasons for having specific feelings.

Description of Strategy: Ask who in the class is happy, sad, or angry, and why. Explain the importance of expressing emotions and understanding behaviors associated with specific emotions. Give students a worksheet showing different faces with different expressions (see the Teaching in Action box, Worksheet for Emotions and Me). The worksheet will ask the students to match a word from the top of the sheet with its expression. Help students with this, asking what types of situations made the student feel each emotion. Students will then role-play different situations and discuss why the situation made them react the way they did.

Materials Needed: worksheet with faces and emotions, role-playing cards

Processing Questions:

1. What feelings make us feel good inside?
2. What feelings make us feel bad inside?
3. Why is it important to be able to express your feelings?

Emotions: Under each face, write the name of the emotion shown. The emotions are happiness, sadness, anger, excitement, kindness, and fear.

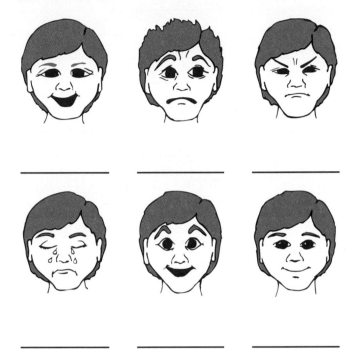

HOW DO I SEE MYSELF?

Grades (K–6)

Valued Outcome: Each student will be able to describe and discuss differences and similarities between her- or himself and others.

Description of Strategy: Lead a discussion regarding differences and similarities among individuals, pointing out that many things that are similar have different qualities. For example, "fruit" includes all fruit, but a pear is not like an apple. Animals have many varieties, as do plants. Give students paper and crayons, and ask them to make their own name tags with drawings of things that describe them.

Materials Needed: visual aids of different fruits, animals, and plants; construction paper; crayons; safety pins for name tags

Processing Questions:

1. What are some positive aspects of individual differences?

2. What type of attitude should we have regarding other peoples' differences?

3. In what ways do you treat others the way you would like to be treated?

Name _____ Date _____

Stress Event: _____

What Occurred: _____

_____

_____

Time of Day: _____

How I Handled the Event: _____

_____

_____

_____

_____

_____

STRESS FEELINGS   Grades (7–8)

Valued Outcomes: The students will be able to define stress, identify five feelings they have that cause stress, and be able to use one breathing exercise to reduce stress.

Description of Strategy: Define stress, and lead students to think of times when stress has affected them. Discuss the advantages and disadvantages of stress. The students will list times when they have felt stress. Ask students to discuss the feelings and physical symptoms they have had in association with stressors. Demonstrate a breathing exercise effective in reducing stress. Hand out copies of the Stress Worksheet provided in the Teacing in Action box above. Have students keep a record of stressful events that occur at home and bring them back to class for discussion.

Materials Needed: poster showing common symptoms of stress, paper and pencils, stress worksheets

Processing Questions:

1. Name two physical symptoms of stress.
2. Name two feelings that might be associated with stress.
3. Why do you think the breathing exercise demonstrated in class helps to reduce stress?

DEEP DIAPHRAGMATIC BREATHING FOR RELAXATION

Deep breathing is the most basic technique used in relaxation and is often the foundation for other methods of relaxation and stress reduction. The primary benefit of this technique is that it can be done anywhere and anytime. The methodology consists of completely filling the lungs when breathing and exhaling very slowly. This type of breathing necessitates a conscious decision to re-direct attention to the basic physiological function of breathing. There are four phases to the process.

Phase I: Inspiration—Taking the air into your lungs through your mouth. Completely fill your lungs.

Phase II: Slight pause before exhaling.

Phase III: Exhalation—Release the air from the lungs very slowly through the mouth.

Phase IV: Another very slight pause after completely releasing all air in the lungs and then begin the next inhalation.

Focus on your breathing and notice how relaxed your whole body becomes during the breathing exercise, especially the chest, shoulders, and abdominal areas.

"ME" POSTER   Grades (4–6)

Valued Outcome: Each students will be able to identify personal interests, characteristics, relationships, goals, and other important aspects of his or her life.

Description of Strategy: The students will draw, bring in pictures, or write about their lives. They will then place items—possibly including baby pictures, birthday pictures, a list of future goals, family members' pictures, or other important mementos—on a poster to be displayed in the classroom. Set aside class time for the children to tell about their posters.

Materials Needed: glue, scissors, poster boards, essays, drawings, magazines, personal mementos, photographs

Processing Questions:

1. Which things in your life make you feel most proud?
2. What has been the most important event in your life and why?
3. Who are the most important people in your life and why?

FACIAL FORECASTS   Grades (K–6)

Valued Outcome: The students will be able to identify signs, symptoms, and causes of stress and be able to describe effective coping mechanisms and resources for dealing with stress.

Description of Strategy: Lead a discussion about stress, including information dealing with signs, symptoms, and causes of stress. Students will use a mirror to observe their own facial expressions when they are under stress. Pass out paper plates and markers or crayons so they can draw their impressions of themselves under stress.

Materials Needed: photocopied pages of common stressors among children, danger signs of stress, ways of coping with stress, mirror, paper plates, markers, crayons

Processing Questions:

1. What are some signs of stress?
2. What is one thing you can do when faced with a stressor?
3. Who are people you can talk to about stressful events in your life?

WEB SITE ACTIVITY

Review one of the Web sites listed below for new ideas on fostering mental health and self-esteem. Share your findings with the class.

WEB SITES OF INTEREST

Community Learning Network: *www.cln.org/themes/self_esteem.htm*
Provides resources and lesson plans for grades K–6 on activities and lesson plans for building self-esteem.

Education World: *www.educationworld.com*
Activities, articles, lesson plans for developing mental health and self-esteem.

American Psychological Association: *www.apa.org*
Provides information on a wide variety of mental health issues and conditions, many of which are of direct concern to teachers.

American Medical Association: *www.ama-assn.org*
Provides information on a variety of conditions, including mental health.

Resources

BOOKS

Bean R. 2000. *The four conditions of self-esteem.* Santa Cruz, CA: ETR Associates.

Canfield, J., and F. Siccone. 1995. *101 ways to develop student self-esteem and responsibility.* Boston: Allyn & Bacon.

Canfield, J., and H. C. Wells. 1999. *101 ways to develop student self-esteem and responsibility.* 2d ed. Boston: Allyn & Bacon.

Herod, L. 1999. *Discovering me—A guide to teaching health and building adolescents' self-esteem.* Boston: Allyn & Bacon.

Johnson, M. D. 1996. *Caring, sharing and getting along.* Santa Cruz, CA: ETR Associates.

Quirez, H. C. 1997. *Think, choose, act healthy.* Santa Cruz, CA: ETR Associates.

Rice, P. L. 1992. *Stress and health.* Monterey, CA: Brooks/Cole Publishing Company.

Tillman, K. G., and P. R. Toner. 1990. *How to survive teaching health.* West Nyack, NY: Parker.

PAMPHLETS

Feeling great! Self-esteem for kids. Santa Cruz, CA: ETR Associates.
Encourages positive attitude and explains that a positive attitude is essential for believing in one-self. Grades 4–6.

Our children's self-esteem—Thoughts for parents and teachers. Santa Cruz, CA: ETR Associates.
Provides important information about self-esteem and how it relates to children's abilities to develop a positive self-identity. Grades 5–8.

Self-esteem and mental health. Santa Cruz, CA: ETR Associates.
Provides overview of the development of self-esteem. Grades 6–9.

Self-esteem—The ABC's. Santa Cruz, CA: ETR Associates.
Encourages positive attitudes and direction of developing healthy life skills. Grades 6–9.

VIDEOS

Anger, rage, and you (Grades 5–9)
Teaches students how to deal with anger before it gets out of control. Helps students to identify and handle misplaced and suppressed anger. Available from Sunburst Communications, 101 Castleton Street, Pleasantville, NY 10570-0040. (23 minutes)

Everybody makes mistakes (Grades K–2)
Helps students understand that everyone makes mistakes, that you can learn from a mistake, and that mistakes can be corrected. Available from Sunburst Communications, 101 Castleton Street, Pleasantville, NY 10570-0040. (16 minutes)

I'm telling—A tattler's tale (Grades K–2)
Helps students understand the difference between appropriate telling and inappropriate tattling. Available from Sunburst Communications, 101 Castleton Street, Pleasantville, NY 10570-0040. (14 minutes)

I know how to listen (Grades PK–2)
Introduces children to paying attention, asking questions, and listening for feelings at school, at home, and at play. Available from Sunburst Communications, 101 Castleton Street, Pleasantville, NY 10570-0040. (15 minutes)

Kids and stress (Grades 5–8)
Looks at how stress affects kids. Discusses eating and sleeping disturbances, drug and alcohol use, mental illness, depression, and suicide. Available from Films for the Humanities and Sciences, P. O. Box 2053, Princeton, NJ 08543-2053. (28 minutes)

CHAPTER EIGHT

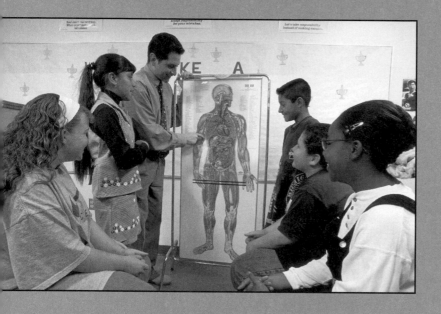

We are fearfully and
wonderfully made.

—Psalm 139:14

VALUED OUTCOMES

After reading this chapter, you should be able to:

- explain the different roles of the cerebrum and the cerebellum

- discuss the function of selected components (structures) of the nervous system

- describe the functions of selected glands and the hormones associated with the endocrine system

- discuss the role of each component of the respiratory system in the breathing process

- trace a drop of blood through the circulatory and pulmonary systems

- describe the major function of the red blood cells

- explain the function of white blood corpuscles in fighting off infection
- describe how food travels through the body
- describe the function of the skeletal system

- describe how liquid and solid wastes are filtered in the body
- differentiate between voluntary and involuntary muscles

REFLECTIONS

All the organs and systems of the body are dependent on each other. When one part is not functioning properly, it sometimes affects several other parts. As you read this chapter, note the many ways in which the various body systems are interdependent.

A Unique Machine

The human body is an efficient functional organism, an amazing and well-organized machine. If cared for properly, it will generally perform well.

At conception, individuals are given the capacity for growth, development, and functioning through genetic factors. However, environmental factors—especially health-related behaviors—determine what actually occurs.

Health and health enhancement cannot be achieved without keeping the body and its systems in good condition. This chapter and the next will provide you with information you can use to help children learn about their bodies and how to care for them. A brief outline and description of several of the major systems of the body are presented here with a discussion of how these systems function.

The Nervous System

Because all physiological functions and many psychological ones are controlled in one way or another by the brain, discussion of the nervous system and its anatomy is a logical and appropriate beginning. The nervous system is composed of two major divisions—the central nervous system and the autonomic nervous system. The central nervous system includes the brain and the spinal cord. The autonomic nervous system includes the peripheral portions of the outlying nerves and nerve pathways not directly connected to the central nervous system.

THE CENTRAL NERVOUS SYSTEM

The central nervous system is divided into two major parts: the brain and the spinal cord (see Figure 8.1). The brain contains about 100 billion nerve cells

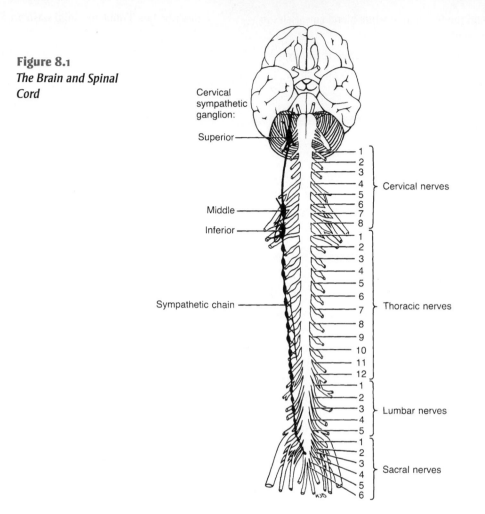

Figure 8.1
The Brain and Spinal Cord

Cervical sympathetic ganglion:

Superior

Middle

Inferior

Sympathetic chain

Cervical nerves

Thoracic nerves

Lumbar nerves

Sacral nerves

(neurons) and trillions of support cells called glia. The spinal cord is 42–45 cm long, and it weighs about 35–40 g. The vertebral column, the collection of articulated bones (back bone) that houses the spinal cord, is about 61–71 cm long—much longer than the spinal cord.

The Brain: An Overview. The average human brain weighs about 1,400 g (3 lb). When the brain is removed from the skull, it looks a bit like a large pinkish-gray walnut. The brain is composed of four parts: the cerebrum (seat of consciousness), the diencephalon, the cerebellum, and the brainstem.

The *cerebrum* governs intelligence and reasoning, learning, and memory. Within the cell, learning involves change in gene regulation and increased ability to secrete transmitters.

The *diencephalon* includes the hypothalamus and thalamus. The *hypothalamus* regulates homeostasis. It has regulatory areas for thirst, hunger, body temperature, water balance, and blood pressure, and links the nervous system to the

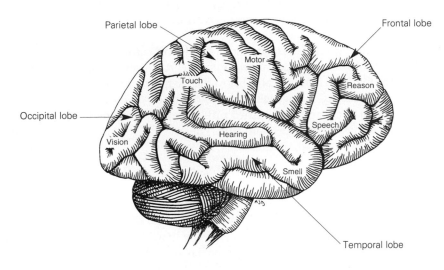

Figure 8.2
The Control Centers and Lobes of the Brain

endocrine system. The *thalamus* serves as a central relay point for incoming nerve messages.

The *cerebellum* is the second largest part of the brain, after the cerebrum. It functions in muscle coordination and maintains normal muscle tone and posture. The cerebellum coordinates balance.

The *brainstem* has three parts: the medulla oblongata, pons, and midbrain. The *medulla oblongata* is closest to the spinal cord and is involved with the regulation of heartbeat; breathing; vasoconstriction (blood pressure); and reflex centers for vomiting, coughing, sneezing, swallowing, and hiccuping. The *midbrain* and *pons* are also part of the unconscious brain and largely act as relay stations for neural information.

The Cerebrum and Lobes of the Brain. The cerebrum, the largest part of the human brain, is divided into left and right cerebral hemispheres connected to each other by bundles of nerve fibers, the most obvious of which is the corpus callosum. The cerebral hemispheres are covered by a thin layer of gray matter known as the cerebral cortex. The word *cortex* comes from the Latin word for tree bark, thus the cortex is a sheet of tissue that makes up the outer layer of the brain. The cortex in each hemisphere of the cerebrum is between 2 and 4 mm thick.

The surface of the cerebral cortex is covered with bumps, or bulges, called *gyri* (singular *gyrus*), and grooves called *sulci* (singular *sulcus*). In higher mammals, such as humans, there are many gyri and sulci; lower mammals like rats and mice have very few gyri and sulci.

The folding of the cerebral cortex produced by these structures increases the amount of cerebral cortex that can fit in the skull. (In fact, the total surface area of the human cerebral cortex is about 324 square inches—about the size of a page of newspaper!) Although most people have the same patterns of gyri and sulci on the cerebral cortex, no two brains are exactly alike.

The various sulci and gyri divide each outer hemisphere of the cerebral cortex into four lobes: occipital, temporal, parietal, and frontal (see Figure 8.2).

(A fifth lobe is actually located deep within the cortex.) No region of the brain functions alone, although major functions of various parts of the lobes have been determined.

The frontal lobe is located in front of the central sulcus and is concerned with reasoning, planning, parts of speech and movement (motor cortex), emotions, and problem solving. The temporal lobe is located below the lateral fissure and is concerned with hearing, processing of language, and memory. The parietal lobe is located behind the central sulcus and is concerned with perception of stimuli related to touch, taste, pressure, temperature, and pain. The occipital lobe is at the base of the skull and processes visual information.

The Diencephalon. Two major structures of the diencephalon are the thalamus and hypothalamus. The thalamus acts as a switching center for nerve messages. The thalamus receives sensory information and relays this information to the cerebral cortex. The cerebral cortex also sends information to the thalamus, which then transmits this information to other areas of the brain and spinal cord. The hypothalamus is a major homeostatic center having both nervous and endocrine functions.

The Cerebellum. The cerebellum, along with the pons and medulla, is part of the hindbrain, but it is not considered part of the brainstem. The word *cerebellum* comes from the Latin word for "little brain." The cerebellum is located behind the brainstem. In some ways, the cerebellum is a bit like the cerebral cortex: the cerebellum is divided into hemispheres and has a cortex that surrounds these hemispheres. Functions of the cerebellum include fine motor coordination and body movement, posture, and balance.

The Brainstem. The brainstem is a general term for the area of the brain between the thalamus and spinal cord. Structures within the brainstem include the midbrain, pons, and medulla oblongata, which is continuous with the spinal cord. The brainstem is the smallest and most primitive part of the brain, so it controls the most basic bodily functions. For example, the medulla oblongata and pons control heart rate, constriction of blood vessels (and thereby blood pressure), digestion, and respiration; the reticular formation, which runs through the entire brainstem, controls level of consciousness; and the colliculi of the midbrain are involved with reflexes that coordinate head and eye movements and mediate the startle reflex (turning the head toward a sound).

The Spinal Cord. The spinal cord runs along the dorsal side of the body and links the brain to the rest of the body. The spinal cords of vertebrates are encased in a series of (usually) bony vertebrae that comprise the vertebral, or spinal, column. The gray matter of the spinal cord consists mostly of cell bodies and dendrites. The surrounding white matter is made up of bundles of interneuronal axons (tracts). Some tracts are ascending (carrying messages to the brain), others are descending (carrying messages from the brain). The spinal cord is also involved in reflexes that do not immediately involve the brain.

The spinal cord is the main pathway for information connecting the brain and peripheral nervous system (where information is received by specialized receptors and sent out to muscles and glands).The human spinal cord is protected

Health Highlight

THE LATEST RESEARCH: THE BRAIN AND LEARNING

Practice not only makes perfect, it makes the brain efficient. What has previously been seen with monkey brains now has been seen on humans. Using functional MRI, a German university has shown that when learning a motor movement such as learning to play the piano, a great deal of the motor regions of the brain are used. With experience, smaller and smaller regions of the brain are used. In professional musicians, only very tiny regions of the motor cortex are involved in their playing. Thus practice makes neural networks efficient and frees up regions of the cortex again to be used for other things (Jancke et al. 2000).

According to a study at Columbia University, teachers should praise students more for effort than for intelligence. The study showed that, in fifth graders, praising intelligence actually caused students to work less, and experience less enjoyment and persistence in tasks. Praising the students' efforts had the opposite effect (Mueller and Dweck 1998).

Smaller class size doesn't seem to make a difference in quantity of material taught, but does affect quality. A UC San Diego study shows that in smaller classes, teachers covered the same amount of material during the year, but the time spent on individual assistance, tutoring, and one-on-one help increased (Betts and Shkolnik 1999).

The University of Illinois has been studying children's tendency to ask for help. Children who have lower academic expectations for themselves tend to ask for help less often. The study found that classrooms that emphasize self-improvement rather than relative ability encourage students to ask for help. In other words, let your students focus on how well they personally have improved rather than on comparing themselves to others in the room.

SOURCE: Nunley 2003

by the bony *vertebral column,* which is made up of bones called *vertebrae.* Although the vertebral column is somewhat flexible, some of the vertebrae in the lower parts of the vertebral column become fused as the sacrum and coccyx (tailbone). The spinal cord is located within the *vertebral foramen* (central holes in the vertebrae).

THE PERIPHERAL NERVOUS SYSTEM

The peripheral nervous system connects the central nervous system with sensory receptors and organs, muscles, and glands. Twelve pairs of cranial nerves extend from various brain regions; thirty pairs of spinal nerves (eight cervical, twelve thoracic, five lumbar, and five sacral) and one coccygeal nerve arise from the spinal cord. The peripheral nervous system has two components: the somatic nervous system and the autonomic nervous system. The somatic nervous system provides the motor output to skeletal muscles that control voluntary movements of the body (see the section on muscles, page 204) and will not be discussed in detail. The autonomic nervous system, also called the involuntary or visceral motor system, innervates cardiac (heart) muscles and smooth muscles of the various organs and glands.

The Autonomic Nervous System. The organs (the *viscera*) inside our body, such as the heart, stomach, and intestines, are regulated by a part of the nervous system called the *autonomic nervous system (ANS)*. The ANS is a part of the peripheral nervous system and it controls smooth muscle of organs and glands. In most situations, we are unaware of the workings of the ANS since it functions in an involuntary, reflexive manner. For example, we do not control when blood vessels change size or when our heart beats faster.

The ANS regulates muscles in several parts of the body—for example, in the skin (smooth muscle around hair follicles and blood vessels); around blood vessels (smooth muscle); in the eye (smooth muscle controlling pupil size and lens shape); in the stomach, intestines, and bladder (smooth muscle of organ walls); and of the heart (cardiac muscle).

The autonomic nervous system is divided into two parts: the sympathetic division and the parasympathetic division. The sympathetic division activates the body's fight-or-flight response and prepares the individual to deal with stress. The parasympathetic division of the ANS has the opposite effect: it promotes calming and digestion.

The Endocrine System

Closely associated with the nervous system is the endocrine system. Both systems provide means of communication within the body, but the endocrine system is the slower of the two. This section describes some of the glands associated with the endocrine system.

The endocrine system's role is that of a regulator. Through the production and secretion of chemical-signaling substances called *hormones* from glands dispersed throughout the body, the endocrine system keeps the other body systems and processes in balanced operation. The two "controller" glands of the endocrine system are the hypothalamus and the pituitary. They secrete hormones that in turn signal other endocrine glands to activate. The hypothalamus and the posterior lobe of the pituitary gland contain neural tissue, thus establishing the close relationship between the endocrine system and the nervous system.

THE HYPOTHALAMUS

The hypothalamus is composed of several different areas and is located at the base of the brain. It is only the size of a pea (about $\frac{1}{300}$ of the total brain weight), but it is responsible for some very important behaviors. One important function of the hypothalamus is the control of body temperature. The hypothalamus acts like a thermostat by sensing changes in body temperature and then sending out signals to smooth muscle of blood vessel walls to adjust the temperature. For example, if you are too hot, the hypothalamus detects this and then sends out a signal to expand the capillaries in your skin. This causes blood to be cooled faster. The hypothalamus also controls the pituitary gland.

THE PITUITARY GLAND

The pituitary gland is actually two different lobes located in a small bony cavity at the base of the brain. The anterior lobe is made of glandular tissue and produces and secretes a number of hormones. The posterior lobe is made of neural tissue and acts as a storage unit for hormones produced by the hypothalamus. A stalk links the posterior pituitary to the hypothalamus, which controls release of pituitary hormones.

Anterior Pituitary Lobe. The anterior lobe (often called the master gland) is connected to the hypothalamus through a network of specialized vessels and secretes six different hormones. These hormones influence such functions as affecting skin pigmentation, activating the reproductive glands, regulating human growth and development as a whole, and regulating adrenal secretions.

Posterior Pituitary Lobe. The posterior pituitary stores and releases hormones into the blood. Antidiuretic hormone (ADH) and oxytocin are produced in the hypothalamus and transported by axons to the posterior pituitary where they are dumped into the blood. ADH controls water balance in the body and blood pressure. Oxytocin is a small peptide hormone that stimulates uterine contractions during childbirth.

THE THYROID GLAND

The thyroid gland is located in the neck. Follicles in the thyroid secrete thyroglobulin, a storage form of thyroid hormone. Thyroid-stimulating hormone (TSH) from the anterior pituitary causes conversion of thyroglobulin into thyroid hormones T_4 and T_3. Almost all body cells are targets of thyroid hormones.

Thyroid hormone increases the overall metabolic rate, and regulates growth and development as well as the onset of sexual maturity. Calcitonin is also secreted by large cells in the thyroid; it plays a role in regulation of calcium.

THE ADRENAL GLANDS

The adrenal glands are located above the kidneys. Each gland is divided into an inner medulla and an outer cortex. The medulla synthesizes amine hormones, the cortex secretes steroid hormones. The adrenal medulla consists of modified neurons that secrete two hormones: epinephrine (sometimes called adrenaline) and norepinephrine. Stimulation of the medulla by the sympathetic division of the ANS causes release of hormones (especially epinephrine) into the blood to initiate the short-term fight-or-flight response to stress. The adrenal cortex produces several steroid hormones in three classes: mineralocorticoids, glucocorticoids, and sex hormones. Mineralocorticoids maintain the electrolyte balance critical for proper bodily functions. Glucocorticoids produce a long-term, slow response to stress by raising blood glucose levels through the breakdown of fats and proteins; they also suppress the immune response and inhibit the inflammatory response. The sex hormones (especially testosterone) produced by the adrenal cortex are important mostly during the fetal stage and early puberty then decline in significance compared to sex hormones produced by the gonads (ovaries and testes).

THE PANCREAS

The pancreas contains exocrine cells that secrete digestive enzymes into the small intestine and clusters of endocrine cells (the pancreatic islets) that secrete the hormones insulin and glucagon. The balance between insulin and glucagon levels regulates blood glucose levels. After a meal, blood glucose levels rise, prompting the release of insulin, which causes cells to take up glucose and liver and skeletal muscle cells to form the carbohydrate glycogen. As glucose levels in the blood fall, further insulin production is inhibited. If blood glucose levels fall too far, glucagon causes the breakdown of glycogen into glucose, which in turn is released into the blood to return glucose levels to within a homeostatic range. Glucagon production is inhibited when blood glucose levels rise.

The Respiratory System

Air enters the body through the nose and is then warmed, filtered, and passed through the nasal cavity. Air moves through the pharynx, then the epiglottis (a flap that prevents food from entering the trachea) and into the trachea, or windpipe. The upper part of the trachea contains the larynx. The vocal cords are two bands of tissue that extend across the opening of the larynx. After passing the larynx, the air moves into the bronchi that carry air in and out of the lungs. Figure 8.3 illustrates the respiratory system.

The trachea and bronchi are reinforced with cartilage to prevent their collapse and are lined with ciliated epithelium and mucus-producing cells. Bronchi branch into smaller and smaller tubes known as bronchioles, which terminate in grapelike sac clusters known as alveoli. Alveoli are surrounded by a network of thin-walled capillaries. Only about 0.2 μm separate the alveoli from the capillaries due to the extremely thin walls of both structures.

The lungs are large, lobed, paired organs in the chest (also known as the thoracic cavity). Thin sheets of epithelium (pleura) separate the inside of the chest cavity from the outer surface of the lungs and reduce friction as the chest expands during breathing. The bottom of the thoracic cavity is formed by the diaphragm.

Ventilation is the mechanics of breathing in and out. When you inhale, muscles in the chest wall contract, lifting the ribs and pulling them outward. The diaphragm moves downward enlarging the chest cavity. Reduced air pressure in the lungs causes air to enter the lungs. Exhaling reverses these steps.

THE ALVEOLI AND GAS EXCHANGE

Diffusion is the movement of materials from a higher to a lower concentration. The differences between oxygen and carbon dioxide concentrations are measured by partial pressures. The greater the difference in partial pressure the greater the rate of diffusion. Respiratory pigments increase the oxygen-carrying capacity of the blood. Humans have the red-colored pigment *hemoglobin* as their

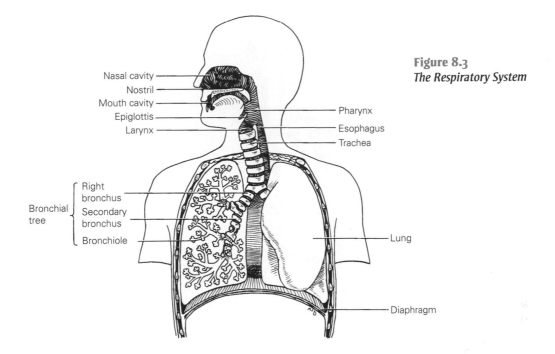

Figure 8.3
The Respiratory System

Nasal cavity
Nostril
Mouth cavity
Epiglottis
Larynx

Pharynx
Esophagus
Trachea

Right bronchus
Secondary bronchus
Bronchiole

Bronchial tree

Lung

Diaphragm

respiratory pigment. Hemoglobin increases the oxygen-carrying capacity of the blood between sixty-five and seventy times. Oxygen concentration in cells is low (when leaving the lungs, blood is 97 percent saturated with oxygen), so oxygen diffuses from the blood to the cells when it reaches the capillaries.

The Circulatory System

The heart is a two-sided, four-chambered structure with muscular walls that contract in a rhythmic pattern to pump blood. An *atrioventricular (AV) valve* separates each auricle from each ventricle. A *semilunar* (SL also known as arterial) *valve* separates each ventricle from its connecting artery. Figure 8.4 illustrates part of the circulatory system. For a discussion on the diseases that affect the cardiovascular system, see Chapter 15, pages 438–443.

THE HEART

The heart beats (or contracts) seventy times per minute. The human heart will undergo over three billion contraction cycles during a normal lifetime. The cardiac cycle consists of two parts: *systole* (contraction of the heart muscle) and *diastole* (relaxation of the heart muscle). Atria contract while ventricles relax. The pulse is a wave of contraction transmitted along the arteries. Valves in the heart open and close during the cardiac cycle. Heart muscle contraction is due to the

Figure 8.4
The Circulatory System

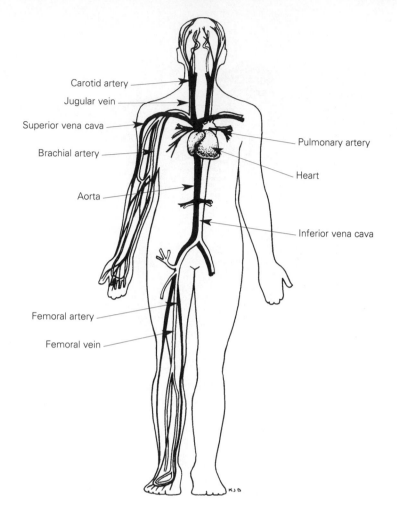

Carotid artery

Jugular vein

Superior vena cava

Brachial artery

Aorta

Pulmonary artery

Heart

Inferior vena cava

Femoral artery

Femoral vein

presence of nodal tissue in two regions of the heart: the *sinoatrial (SA) node* initiates heartbeat, and the *AV node* causes ventricles to contract. The AV node is sometimes called the pacemaker, since it keeps the heartbeat regular. Heartbeat is also controlled by the ANS.

Blood flows through the heart from veins to atria to ventricles and then out by arteries (see Figure 8.5). Heart valves limit flow to a single direction. One heartbeat, or cardiac cycle, includes atrial contraction and relaxation, ventricular contraction and relaxation, and a short pause. Normal cardiac cycles (at rest) take 0.8 seconds. Blood from the body flows into the venae cavae, which empty into the right atrium. At the same time, oxygenated blood from the lungs flows from the pulmonary vein into the left atrium. Seventy percent of the blood from the atria passively flows into the ventricles, then the muscles of both atria contract, forcing additional blood downward through each AV valve.

Diastole is the filling of the ventricles with blood. Ventricular systole opens the SL valves, forcing blood out of the ventricles through the pulmonary artery

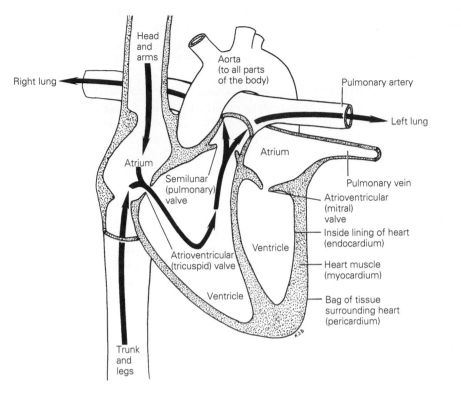

Figure 8.5
Flow of Blood through the Heart

and aorta. The sound of the heart contracting and the valves opening and closing produces a characteristic "lub-dub" sound. Lub is associated with closure of the AV valves, dub is the closing of the SL valves.

Human heartbeats originate from the SA node near the right atrium. Modified muscle cells contract, sending a signal to other muscle cells in the heart to contract. The signal spreads to the AV node, where it is relayed to cause the ventricles to contract simultaneously.

The two main routes for circulation are the pulmonary circuit (to and from the lungs) and the systemic circuit (to and from the body). Pulmonary arteries carry blood from the heart to the lungs. Blood in the pulmonary arteries is low in oxygen and high in carbon dioxide, whereas blood in the pulmonary veins is high in oxygen and low in carbon dioxide. In the lungs gas exchange occurs: oxygen diffuses into the blood, and carbon dioxide (a waste product of cellular metabolism) diffuses out of the blood. Pulmonary veins carry blood from lungs to heart. The aorta is the main artery of systemic circuit. The venae cavae are the main veins of the systemic circuit. Coronary arteries deliver oxygenated blood, food, and so on to the heart.

BLOOD

Plasma is the liquid component of the blood. Mammalian blood consists of a liquid (plasma) and a number of cellular and cell fragment components. Plasma makes up about 55 percent of blood, cells and fragments, 45 percent. Plasma has 90 percent water and 10 percent dissolved materials, including proteins, glucose, ions, hormones, and gases. Plasma contains nutrients, wastes, salts, proteins, etc. Proteins in the blood aid in transport of large molecules such as cholesterol.

Red blood cells, also known as *erythrocytes,* are flattened, doubly concave cells that carry oxygen in the cell's hemoglobin. Mature erythrocytes lack a nucleus. They are small, four million to six million cells per cubic millimeter of blood, and have 200 million hemoglobin molecules per cell. Humans have a total of 25 trillion erythrocytes, which is about a third of all the cells in the body. Red blood cells are continuously manufactured in the marrow of long bones, ribs, skull, and vertebrae. The life of an erythrocyte is only 120 days, after which it is destroyed in the liver and spleen. Iron from hemoglobin is recovered and reused in erythrocyte synthesis by red marrow. Each second, two million red blood cells are produced to replace those taken out of circulation.

White blood cells, also known as *leukocytes,* are larger than erythrocytes, have a nucleus, and lack hemoglobin. Leukocytes are less than 1 percent of the blood's volume. They are made from stem cells in bone marrow and function in the cellular immune response. There are five types of leukocytes (neutrophils, eosinophils, basophils, lymphocytes, and monocytes—one form of which is the macrophage), each with a different role in the immune system. The functions of the different leukocyte types include releasing histamine, an inflammatory chemical that dilates blood vessels and attracts other leukocytes to the inflamed site; producing antibodies to aid in protecting against infection; attacking and scavenging foreign proteins and bacteria, some fungi, viruses, parasitic worms, and antigen-antibody complexes; and moving out of the capillaries to fight infectious diseases in interstitial areas (regions between cells). Some cells inactivate inflammatory chemicals that are released during allergic reactions and attack the antigen-antibody complexes involved in allergy attacks.

Platelets result from cell fragmentation and are involved in blood clotting. They carry chemicals essential to the blood clotting process. Platelets survive for ten days before being removed by the liver and spleen. There are 150,000 to 300,000 platelets in each milliliter of blood. Platelets adhere to tears in blood vessels to temporarily plug the gap until a series of chemical events cause blood to coagulate (clot) in the area. A hemophiliac's blood cannot clot without treatment with correct proteins (clotting factors), although the use of transfusions and contaminated blood products has also led to HIV transmission. (Improved management of the blood supply has since greatly reduced this risk.)

THE LYMPHATIC SYSTEM

Water and plasma are forced from the capillaries into intracellular spaces. This interstitial fluid transports materials between cells. Most of this fluid is collected in the capillaries of a secondary circulatory system, the *lymphatic system.* Fluid in this system is known as lymph. Lymph flows from small lymph capillaries into lymph vessels (which are similar to veins in having valves that prevent backflow) and is filtered through lymph nodes and lymph organs. Lymph nodes are small irregularly shaped masses clustered in the armpits, groin, and neck. Cells of the immune system line channels through the nodes and attack bacteria and viruses traveling in the lymph. Lymph is then returned to the cardiovascular system through the thoracic duct and right lymphatic duct.

The Digestive/Excretory System

The *digestive system* contains organs for changing food chemically for absorption by body tissues. It is also responsible for processing food, breaking it down into usable protein, minerals, carbohydrates and fats, and other substances. The digestion process involves breaking food into simple soluble substances absorbable by tissues. Figure 8.6 illustrates the digestive system.

The digestion process includes both mechanical and chemical processes. The mechanical processes include chewing food to reduce it to small particles, the churning action of the stomach, and intestinal peristaltic (wavelike) action. Then three chemical reactions take place: conversion of carbohydrates into such simple sugars as glucose, breaking down of protein into such amino acids as alanine, and conversion of fats into fatty acids and glycerol. These processes are accomplished by specific enzymes.

The digestive process begins in your mouth when you start eating. The salivary glands produce secretions that are mixed with the food. The saliva breaks down starches into dextrin and maltose. Then it goes down your esophagus in peristaltic waves to the stomach. This only takes a matter of seconds. The stomach contains gastric juice, and the gastric juice contains chemicals such as

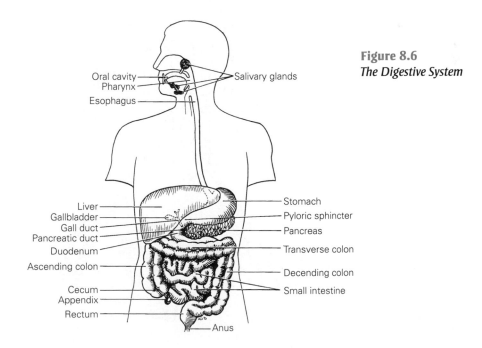

Figure 8.6
The Digestive System

Oral cavity
Pharynx
Esophagus
Salivary glands

Liver
Gallbladder
Gall duct
Pancreatic duct
Duodenum
Ascending colon
Cecum
Appendix
Rectum
Anus

Stomach
Pyloric sphincter
Pancreas
Transverse colon
Decending colon
Small intestine

hydrochloric acid and some enzymes, including pepsin. Pepsin breaks proteins into peptones and proteoses. A function of small intestine digestion is to gradually release the partially digested food (chyme) through the pyloric sphincter into the upper small intestine, where the majority of chemical digestion occurs. Two intestinal enzymes are renin (found in children) and lipase; renin separates milk into liquid and solid portions, and lipase acts on fat. The small intestine absorbs almost all the nutrients from the chyme into the bloodstream, leaving the unusable residue and some water. This passes through the colon (or large intestine) to the rectum, losing more water back to the body by absorption. The solid waste, called feces, passes out of the body through the anal canal and the anus.

THE KIDNEYS

The kidneys process blood by removing substances from it and, sometimes, by adding substances to it. The major function of the kidneys is to regulate the water content, electrolyte composition, and acidity of the body by excreting each substance in an amount adequate to achieve balance and maintain normal concentrations in the extracellular fluid. Also, the kidneys are responsible for the removal of metabolic waste products from the blood and their excretion in the urine.

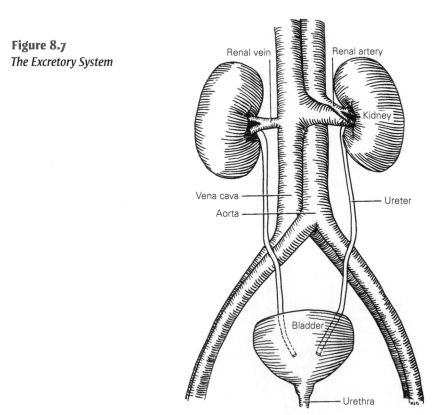

Figure 8.7
The Excretory System

Renal vein

Renal artery

Kidney

Vena cava

Aorta

Ureter

Bladder

Urethra

Nephrons (the microscopic functional units within kidneys) collect and filter waste products that have been delivered by the circulatory system through the renal artery, a major artery leading directly from the aorta to each kidney. The ureters collect the filtered fluid (urine) and pass it to the urinary bladder, where it is stored and then excreted through the urethra (see Figure 8.7).

The Skeletal/Muscular System

The body and all its organs and systems are given support, protection, and mobility by the skeletal/muscular system. More than 200 bones make up the human skeleton, and over 600 muscles attached to these bones and extending across joints allow body movement and act as a protective covering. Red blood cells are produced in the ends of the long bones of the body and in such places as the sternum (breastbone) and pelvis (hip bones) as shown in Figure 8.8.

Bones are composed of a porous, inner layer of spongy tissue surrounded by hardened outer compact bone material. In infancy, bones are elastic, flexible, and soft. Through the maturation process, with the ingestion of vitamin D and minerals (primarily calcium and phosphorus), bones become more rigid and grow thicker and longer. Throughout life, regions of bones may become thicker/stronger or thinner/weaker, depending on the degree to which the attached muscles are used; a baseball pitcher, for example, may have thicker bone attached to the muscles most frequently used to throw the baseball. The skeletal/muscular system gives overall form and shape to the human body. A characteristic feature of humans is the upright walking posture, which relies on a strong vertebral column and pelvis for support. Other major human bone structures are the skull, sternum and rib cage, pectoral girdle (shoulder), and limb bones (including the hands and feet).

The bones are connected by joints, with the degree of mobility depending on the physical needs of the location of the joint. There are three broad structural categories of joint types. **Synovial joints** have a fluid-filled cavity and are the most flexible. Examples are the hip and shoulder joints (*ball-and-socket joints,* which rotate through a wide range of motion), the junction of the skull with the top of the vertebral column, wrist bones, and the elbow and knee joints (such *hinge joints* allow motion in only one plane). **Cartilaginous joints** have the articulating surfaces covered with cartilage and permit a moderate amount of flexibility. The junctions between the ribs and vertebrae are an example, as are the epiphyseal plates (cartilaginous growth regions that connect the ends of the long limb bones to the central shaft and which elongate and eventually convert to bone as a child reaches physical maturity). **Fibrous joints** provide the least flexibility as the joints are joined together with fibrous tissue, such as that found between the teeth and their bony sockets. The sutures of the skull are relatively loose when a baby is born, which makes it easier for the baby to move through the birth canal, but will fuse together as the individual ages until the skull plates form a single unit.

Figure 8.8
The skeletal system

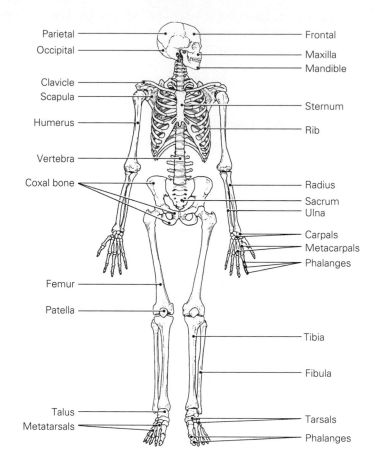

Parietal — Frontal
Occipital — Maxilla
— Mandible
Clavicle — Sternum
Scapula —
Humerus — Rib
Vertebra —
Coxal bone — Radius
— Sacrum
— Ulna
— Carpals
— Metacarpals
— Phalanges
Femur —
Patella —
— Tibia
— Fibula
Talus — Tarsals
Metatarsals — Phalanges

THE VERTEBRAL COLUMN

Composed of thirty-three bones called *vertebrae,* the vertebral column (spinal column, or backbone) extends from the base of the head down to the hip region and allows bending, twisting, and turning motions of the upper body. Because the vertebrae encase the delicate spinal cord that conducts all body messages to the brain, any injury along the spinal column is extremely serious and can lead to paralysis.

There are five divisions, or groupings, of bones in the spinal column. The first seven vertebrae are called the *cervical vertebrae* and comprise the neck. These are followed by twelve *thoracic vertebrae,* which support the upper trunk region. The five *lumbar vertebrae* extend to the waist and are followed by five fused *sacral vertebrae* in the lower back. The *coccyx*—four relatively small bones—marks the end of the spinal column and is commonly referred to as the *tailbone.* The upper twenty-four (cervical, thoracic, and lumbar) vertebrae are more flexible structures than the sacral vertebrae and coccyx because they are joined by separate disks of cartilage that cushion the impact of walking, running, jumping, and similar movements.

THE SKULL

The human skull, situated above the vertebral column, includes the cranium and the bones of the face. The cranium is a group of sixteen large, flat, hard bones that form a domelike structure surrounding and protecting the brain. The *facial bones* form protective coverings for the eyes, nasal passages, and the cheeks. These bones also make up the hinged upper and lower jawbones, the maxilla and the mandible, respectively.

STERNUM AND RIB CAGE

The sternum is a thick, flat, elongated, rigid bone that overlies the heart. Attached with cartilage to both the sternum in the front and the thoracic vertebrae in the back are ten pairs of ribs that form the *rib cage.* Two other pairs of ribs are attached to the thoracic vertebrae but are not attached to the sternum and are thus referred to as *floating ribs.* The rib cage and sternum protect the lungs and heart.

THE PELVIS

The pelvis is formed by connections of the sacral vertebrae and coccyx of the back with the hipbones in the side and front portions of the body. When joined together, these bones form a large, bowl-like structure. The pelvis helps to protect some of the organs of the reproductive system and the excretory system, as well as to support the upper part of the body and to stabilize leg motions during walking and running. The pelvis, with its ability to rotate, also aids in twisting, turning, and sitting motions.

BONES OF THE LEGS AND FEET

Extending from each side of the hip is the upper leg bone, or *femur.* It is the largest bone in the body. The femur is attached at the knee to the shin (*tibia*), which is the largest bone in the lower leg. The knee is protected by a small bony kneecap, the *patella.* To the outward side of the tibia lies the *fibula,* the other lower leg bone. Because the leg bones are porous (have a spongy bone interior rather than being solid), they are especially adapted for supporting body weight and providing mobility. Heavier, solid bones would not be suitable for these functions.

The tibia and fibula are joined to the bones of the feet at the ankles, or tarsals. Extending from the tarsals are the five long bones of the upper foot called the *metatarsals,* which are arched and joined to the fourteen bones of the toes, the *phalanges.* Because these bones are arched, they provide further support and stability for maintaining the body in an upright position.

BONES OF THE ARMS AND HANDS

Hinged to the flat, triangular shoulder blade (scapula) is the upper arm bone (*humerus*), which hangs below the collarbone (*clavicle*). The humerus is attached at the elbow to both the *ulna,* the longer lower-arm bone, and the *radius,* the shorter lower-arm bone (on the thumb side). These bones in turn connect with the eight wrist, or *carpal,* bones that provide flexibility and rotation for the hands. Attached to the carpals are the five *metacarpals* that form the palm of the hand. These are then joined to the fourteen phalanges, the bones of the fingers. Because of the multiple joints in the fingers, the hands are ideal for performing clutching and grasping motions.

THE MUSCLES

The human body contains more than 650 individual muscles, attached to the skeleton, that provide the pulling power for us to move around. The main job of the muscular system is to provide movement for the body. The muscular system consists of three different types of muscle: skeletal, cardiac, and smooth. Each of these different muscle types has the ability to contract, which allows for body movements and functions.

Muscles are either involuntary or voluntary. The muscles we control consciously are called the voluntary muscles, and the ones we cannot control consciously are the involuntary muscles. The heart (made largely of cardiac muscle) is an example of involuntary muscle.

Skeletal Muscle. Skeletal muscle makes up about 40 percent of an adult's body weight. It has stripelike markings, or striations. Skeletal muscles are composed of long muscle fibers. The nervous system controls the contraction of the muscle fibers. Many of the skeletal muscle contractions are automatic—for example, they help maintain body posture and keep the muscles toned and ready for voluntary contractions. Voluntary actions of the muscles are consciously controlled, for example, when muscle movements are desired— hence, skeletal muscle is also called voluntary muscle.

Cardiac Muscle. The cardiac muscle is the muscle of the heart. Cardiac muscle makes up the wall of the heart, called the myocardium. Like the skeletal muscles, the cardiac muscle is striated and contracts through the sliding filament method. However, it is different from other types of muscles because it forms branching fibers. Unlike the skeletal muscles, cardiac muscle cells are attached to other cardiac muscle cells instead of being attached to a bone.

Smooth Muscle. Much of our internal organs are made up of smooth muscles. They are found in the walls of the urinary bladder, gallbladder, arteries, and veins, as well as the digestive tract. Smooth muscle contractions are controlled by the autonomic nervous system and hormones. We cannot consciously control the smooth muscles, which is why they are called involuntary muscles.

Summary

- Almost every individual begins life with a sound, healthy body that requires care and maintenance.

- Knowledge of the body systems and how they interact with one another is important in building and promoting personal health and well being.

- Each body system has special roles and functions that directly or indirectly affect all other body systems.

- The brain and nervous system receive messages from all other parts of the body and act to keep both an internal and external balance between the parts (homeostasis).

- The body's internal balance depends greatly on the release and regulation of hormones from the endocrine system, which strongly influences growth, development, and reproduction.

- Oxygen, essential to all cells, is channeled into the body by the respiratory system and delivered to all tissues through the actions of the circulatory system; carbon dioxide waste is removed along the same pathway.

- The circulatory system acts as a delivery and removal system for nutrients and wastes and works with the lymphatic system to mediate the immune response.

- Other chemicals and nutrients are ingested, broken down, and made usable to cells and tissue by the digestive/excretory system so that vital processes can take place.

- The skeletal/muscular system provides physical shape and structure for the body, assists in protection, and enables movement.

DISCUSSION QUESTIONS

1. Compare and contrast the functions of the central and peripheral nervous systems, then compare and contrast the somatic and autonomic divisions of the peripheral nervous system.

2. How are the glands in the body dependent upon the hypothalamus?

3. Explain the interactive functioning of the cerebrum, the cerebellum, and the brainstem.

4. Contrast the functions of the atria and ventricles.

5. Describe the connection between the kidneys and the digestive system.

6. Compare and contrast the functions of the voluntary and involuntary muscles.

CRITICAL THINKING QUESTIONS

1. Explain the interaction of genetics, socioeconomic status, and illness with regard to their influences on personal health.

2. Describe the connection between eye problems and learning.

3. Explain the interdependence of the senses of taste and smell.

WEB SITE ACTIVITY

Using the Web site *www.lib.uchicago.edu/hw/anatomy* and the links below, try to find a written description of the five sections of the spinal vertebrae.

- Anatomy by Systemic Classification
- Nervous System
- HealthWeb: NeuroAnatomy: The Spinal Cord
- Spine Anatomy

WEB SITES OF INTEREST

American Medical Association (AMA)
  www.ama-assn.org/insight/gen_hlth/atlas/atlas.htm
Provides health information and pictures for each body system.

G. E. Corporate Research and Development: *www.crd.ge.com/cgi-bin/vw.p1*
In 1989, the National Library of Medicine (NLM) began an ambitious project to create a digital atlas of the human anatomy. The NLM Planning Panel on Electronic Image Libraries recommended a project, "The Visible Man," to create X-ray computed tomography (XRAY-CT), magnetic resonance imaging (MRI), and physical sections of a human cadaver. Another cadaver, that of a fifty-nine-year-old woman, "The Visible Woman," has just been released.

Your Health: *www.yourhealth.com*
Provides quality health-related information, including the latest health headlines, an expert question-and-answer program, "Live Online," a weekly radio-style audio program, "Studio one2one," and a large selection of health reference information.

Health A to Z: *www.healthatoz.com*
Provides personal and medical information on a variety of health topics.

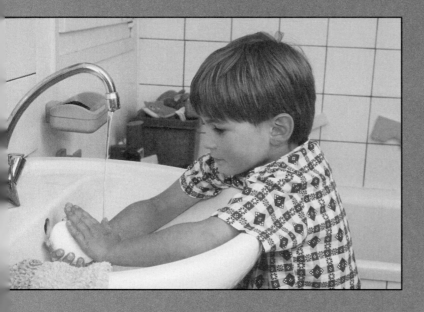

CHAPTER NINE

Personal Health

It is essential that personal
health habits be learned at an
early age.

VALUED OUTCOMES

After reading this chapter, you should be able to:

- discuss the reasons a person with acne should avoid skin creams with an oil base

- discuss the hazards of overexposing the skin to the sun

- describe proper lifting, pushing, and pulling techniques to avoid hurting the lower back muscles

- describe proper posture while sitting at a desk, walking, bending, and lifting

- list the possible behavioral indications of vision problems

- discuss the classroom adjustments a teacher should make for a student with poor vision
- list the possible behavioral indications of hearing problems

- discuss the proper health practices to prevent gum disease
- list the cardiorespiratory benefits of a regular exercise program

REFLECTIONS

There are several issues related to personal health that affect not only one's physical health, but also one's emotional health. As you read this chapter, reflect on the emotional aspects of personal health and how this can affect a student's capacity to learn.

Developing Good Habits Early

It is not enough to know about the structure and function of the human body. The human body must be given daily attention to ensure its continued performance. This attention is the responsibility of the individual. Thus, it is essential that personal health habits are learned at an early age. Inattention to personal health practices in childhood has consequences in later life.

This chapter focuses on the areas of personal health that are considered the most crucial for the elementary school child. These areas include personal appearance, care of the senses, dental health, fitness, relaxation, and sleep; disease control and prevention are described for selected topics.

Personal Appearance

A multitude of factors can influence personal appearance, including genetics, socioeconomic status, illness, and so forth. However, in this section of the chapter, only care of the skin, care of the nails, care of the hair, and the importance of posture are discussed. In addition, because of its far-reaching effects on almost all other areas of health, nutrition is presented in a separate chapter (Chapter 17).

THE SKIN

Skin is the outside covering of body tissue that protects inner cells and organs from the outside environment. The skin is the largest organ of the body, and its cells are continuously replaced as they are lost to normal wear and tear. The skin totals between twelve and twenty square feet in area and accounts for 12 percent of body weight. It is composed of two integrated layers: the **epidermis** and the **dermis**. The thickness of the epidermis and the dermis varies over different parts of the body. It is thickest on the palms of the hands and feet, where friction is needed for gripping, and it is thinnest on the eyelids, which must be light and flexible. The epidermis also grows into fingernails, toenails, and hair. The dermis, or true skin, is thick; sturdy; and rich in nerves, blood vessels, and sweat glands. It shields and repairs injured tissue. This layer consists mostly of **collagen,** which originates from cells called fibroblasts and is one of the strongest proteins found in nature. It gives skin its durability and resilience. The hypodermis is joined to the bottom of the dermis and contains **lipocytes,** which produce lipids that form a fatty layer to cushion muscles, bones, and inner organs against shocks and act as an insulator and source of energy during lean times. The skin registers sensation constantly and supports a teeming, unseen population of tiny organisms.

Skin Conditions/Diseases.

Acne. Acne is caused by inflammation of the oil glands in the skin and at the base of strands of hair. In the teenage years, hormones stimulate the growth of body hair, and the oil glands secrete more oil. The skin pores become clogged, and bacteria grow in the clogged pores. If a sebaceous gland becomes clogged, a whitehead appears; if the material oxidizes, it darkens to form a blackhead.

Ringworm (Tinea). Ringworm is an infection of the skin, hair, or nails. It gets its name from its appearance on the skin—it often looks like a ring-shaped rash. Ringworm is caused by several different types of fungi. Other names for ringworm include tinea, dermatophytosis, athlete's foot (ringworm of the feet), and jock itch (ringworm of the groin).

It is not caused by a worm! You can get ringworm from people, animals, or places. People can get it through contact with a person who has ringworm or by using items such as clothes, towels, or hairbrushes that were used by someone with a ringworm infection. Animals can carry some types of fungi on their fur or skin without showing signs of ringworm infection. Sick or carrier animals can transmit fungi to people by direct or indirect contact. Places like gyms, shower stalls, and floors can transmit the fungus if used by someone with ringworm. Other people can catch the fungus if exposed to these places. Ringworm is easily diagnosed and treated. A doctor can do some simple tests to determine whether a rash is caused by a fungus. Treatment is usually an antifungal cream applied to the site of infection or pills taken by mouth.

If you have ringworm, you can avoid spreading it to others by following your doctor's advice for proper treatment; keeping your skin, hair, and nails clean and dry; washing towels and clothing in hot water and soap to destroy the fungus; and staying away from common areas such as community pools and gyms until your infection goes away.

Ringworm can be prevented by keeping common-use areas clean; using a floor and bath cleaner that contains a fungus-killing (called "fungicidal") agent; avoiding physical contact with a person or animal who has ringworm; and not sharing clothing, towels, hair brushes, or other personal items.

Impetigo. Impetigo is a common skin infection in young children caused by streptococcal or staphylococcal bacteria. A rash appears four to ten days after exposure. The rash looks red and round and may be oozing. It can occur as small blisters containing puslike material that may break and form a flat, honey-colored crust. The rash is most commonly seen on the face and around the mouth but can occur any place on the skin and is often itchy. Impetigo is spread through direct contact with infected skin. Less commonly, it can be spread through touching articles (such as clothing, bedding, and towels) contaminated with the blisters. Topical treatments and/or antibiotics are available.

A person with impetigo should:

- wash the rash with soap and water and cover it loosely with gauze, a bandage, or clothing.
- wash hands thoroughly, especially after touching an infected area of the body.
- use separate towels and washcloths.
- avoid contact with newborn babies.
- be excluded from school or daycare until twenty-four hours after the start of treatment.
- avoid handling food until twenty-four hours after the start of treatment.

Pediculosis. Lice infestation, or pediculosis, arises when head or body lice— extremely small, parasitic insects—attach to hair shafts. They are passed from infested people through either direct contact or contact with an article of clothing or object used by the infested individual. The lice live and lay eggs in seams of clothing and come on to the skin when sucking blood. Lice were formerly responsible for the spread of typhus fever. Also, lice infestation was the major reason for physical inspections of schoolchildren during the earliest years of formal health education.

Itching results from the blood-sucking action of the lice, and a secondary infection may occur. Application of an appropriate insecticide can destroy the lice. To prevent widespread outbreaks, schoolchildren should be thoroughly inspected for lice.

Sunburn. People with fair or light complexions do not have as much protective pigment in their skin as darker people do. Therefore, lighter-skinned people should not stay in the sun for extended periods because they are more vulnerable to sunburn than others. Overexposure to the sun has been linked with skin cancer. If fair-complexioned people must be in the sun for a long time during work or exercise, they should cover the exposed areas of the skin with clothing or a good sunscreen (see Table 9.1).

Care of the Skin. Daily personal cleanliness is the best means of caring for the skin. Washing the hands, feet, and face a few times each day with warm water and soap helps remove dirt, bacteria, and oil. Although a daily shower or bath is not necessary, it is a good practice to encourage. Also, emphasize the need to wear proper clothing to suit temperature variations to protect the skin. Be sure to provide instruction concerning general skin care principles as well as information about special needs. Different skin types may require different kinds of daily care; for example, people with oily skin may need to clean their faces and wash their hair more often than people with dry skin. Allergic skin reactions to certain soaps, lotions, or creams may result, so that non-allergenic preparations may be necessary. In the event a problem arises,

Table 9.1   *Sunscreen*

The Food and Drug Administration recommends these minimum sunscreen SPF (sunscreen protective factor index) for the following skin types*:

- Always burns easily; rarely tans: SPF 20 to 30
- Always burns easily; tans minimally: SPF 2 to under 20
- Burns moderately; tans gradually: SPF 8 to under 12
- Burns minimally; always tans: SPF 4 to under 8
- Rarely burns; tans profusely: SPF 2 to under 4

*The FDA has restricted the claims that can be made about sunscreen products. The FDA has banned SPF claims over 30 and required that all products that provide greater than SPF 30 protection be labeled as SPF 30+ or "plus" regardless of their true SPF value.

SOURCE: Cosmetics, Toiletries and Fragrance Association 2000

children need to know that a dermatologist is a physician who specializes in care of the skin and skin disorders.

THE FINGERNAILS AND TOENAILS

Nails, like hair, grow from the epidermal layers of the matrix (nail base). As older cells grow out and are replaced by newer ones, they are compacted and take on a dead and hardened (keratinized) form that can be cut painlessly. The average growth rate for nails is 0.1 mm each day; individual rates depend on age, time of year, activity level, and heredity; disease, hormone imbalance, and the aging process also affect nail growth. Fingernails grow faster than toenails. Nails grow more rapidly in the summer than in the winter. Nails on a person's dominant hand (right vs. left) grow faster, and men's nails grow more quickly than women's, except possibly during pregnancy and old age (American Academy of Dermatology 1997).

Cuticles—softer than nails but nevertheless hardened skin tissue—surround fingernails and toenails and sometimes break or crack because little oil reaches them. Both the nails and cuticles protect the fingers and toes.

Care of the Nails. Due to their exposed location, nails take a lot of abuse. Nail disorders comprise about ten percent of all skin conditions. Most of us, at one time or another, have closed fingers in doors, suffered from ingrown toenails, or endured minor nail infections. Most minor nail injuries heal on their own, although they may be unsightly for a while due to the nail's slow growth rate. More serious injuries or disorders may require professional treatment. Symptoms that could signal nail (or other health) problems include color or shape changes, swelling of the skin around the nails, and pain. Additionally, the persistence of white or black lines, dents, or ridges in the nail should be reported to a dermatologist.

White spots on the nails are very common and usually recur. These small spots result from injury to the matrix of the nail, where nail cells are produced. They are not a cause for concern and will eventually grow out.

Nail biting is a common problem, especially among young children. While the habit typically disappears with age, it has been linked to anxiety with older children and adults. Not only does nail biting ruin the look of the nails, it is also a good way to transfer infectious organisms from the fingers to the mouth and vice versa. Nail biting can also damage the skin surrounding the nails, allowing infections to enter and spread. Some nail-biters are cured by applying bad tasting nail polishes or liquids to the nail.

Many nail problems are due to poor nail care. Good nail habits help keep nails healthy. The following recommendations are designed for good nail care (Medicine Net.com 1998):

- keep nails clean and dry to keep bacteria and other infectious organisms from collecting under the nails.
- soak toenails that are thick and difficult to cut in warm salt water (one teaspoon of salt to a pint of water) for 5 to 10 minutes, apply a 10 percent urea cream (available at the drug store without a prescription), and then trim the toenails.
- nails should be cut straight across and rounded only slightly at the edges. Use sharp nail scissors or clippers.
- use a "fine" textured file to keep nails shaped and free of snags.
- do not bite your nails.
- do not "dig out" ingrown toenails, especially if they are sore. Seek treatment from a doctor.
- nail changes, swelling, and pain can signal a serious problem. Report any nail irregularities to your doctor.

THE HAIR

Hair grows on almost all regions of our bodies. Males and females have the same amount of hair in the concentrated areas (such as under the arm and on the scalp), but they differ in the amount of hair on other parts of the body (such as the face). Hair growth, color, and coarseness are determined by heredity and pigment. Those with less pigment usually develop blonde or light brown hair, while those with the most pigment have black hair. Red hair typically has the coarsest texture, while blonde hair is the least coarse.

Like the nails, hair is an outgrowth of the skin itself. It originates from hair follicles in the dermis. The hair root within the follicle is composed of living cells that are nourished by blood vessels. As a result, removal of hair by its roots is painful. However, as is the case with nails, the visible hair shafts themselves are dead, keratinized tissue that can be cut painlessly. Hair shafts on the head grow from about two to six inches before they begin to fall out naturally when combed or brushed. Except in cases of inherited male pattern baldness, rare illness, or as a result of some forms of chemotherapy, hair that falls out is continually being replaced.

Hair serves a protective role. Hair on the head guards against excessive exposure of the underlying scalp to solar radiation, as does body hair to some degree.

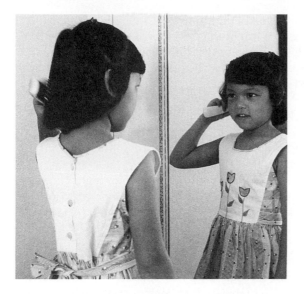

Hair should be brushed several times a day.

Denser growths of hair also act as a skin covering that helps regulate body temperature—a tremendous amount of body heat is lost when the head is uncovered in cold temperatures. The eyelashes shield the eyes from dust and other irritants.

Care of the Hair. Hair need not be washed or shampooed daily. Sebum, or oil, comes to the surface of the scalp through the hair follicle. Some people secrete more sebum than others and therefore should wash their hair more often. The hair should not be washed with extremely hot water, as this makes the hair dry and brittle. The hair should be cleaned often and brushed or combed several times a day.

Unnecessary combing, teasing, bleaching, and heat exposure should be avoided. Because dull, brittle hair, like the nails, may be a signal of underlying health problems, close attention should be paid to changes in its growth patterns and texture.

POSTURE

Posture is more than just standing or sitting straight up. The term **posture** refers to graceful, efficient movement of the body, whether walking, standing, or performing any type of motion. All parts of the body should be used correctly to maintain balance. When a person has poor posture, the muscles, instead of the bones, bear the burden of the off-center weight, and the person becomes fatigued more quickly.

Poor posture may be caused by a number of problems, including weak muscles; chronic fatigue; bone deformities; and careless habits of walking, sitting, and standing. Because students spend so much time during the school day sitting at a desk, it is important to encourage the students to sit properly. Each desk should be at an appropriate height for the individual to allow both feet to touch the floor without straining. The seat of the desk should allow the knees to be higher than the hips to remove stress from the lower back. The back of the chair should encourage the proper spinal curve when the child is seated. The tray of the desk should be slanted sufficiently so the student need not lean forward to write and read.

Posture can be positively influenced through proper nutrition for proper bone growth, exercise to tone the muscles, properly fitting clothing and shoes, well-designed furniture (including desks, chairs, and beds), lifting and carrying objects properly, and proper education.

Poor posture is most often seen in junior high and senior high school students who are self-conscious about height or breast development. However, some postural defects are skeletal in nature. For example, scoliosis, or curvature of the spine, may produce postural defects. Sometimes after an illness, injury, or infection, poor muscle tone may cause slouching or slumping. In most instances, however, these types of postural defects can be corrected under the care of an orthopedic surgeon either through surgery, body braces, various exercises, orthotic lifts in the shoes, or a combination of surgery and exercise. Ideally, these defects are discovered very early in life when correction is much easier.

The Senses

By conveying a myriad of messages to the brain each day, the sensory organs keep us in touch with our physical and emotional environments. Five major senses keep us informed about the world around us. These are vision, hearing, touch, taste, and smell.

THE SENSE OF VISION

The Eye. The eyes are the two organs of sight. They are located in the front upper part of the skull and consist of structures that focus an image onto the retina at the back of the eye; the retina is a network of nerves that converts this image into electrical impulses that are sent to the brain. The eyeball lies in pads of fat within the orbit, a bony socket that provides protection from injury. Each eyeball is moved by six delicate muscles, which are activated and coordinated by nerves in the brain stem.

The eyeball has a tough, outer coat called the **sclera,** or white part of the eye. The front, circular part is the **cornea** and is transparent. The cornea is the main lens of the eye and performs most of the light refraction (bending) to direct light toward the retina. Behind the cornea is a shallow chamber full of watery fluid, at the back of which is the **iris** (colored part) with the **pupil** (hole at the center of the iris). The pupil appears black, and its diameter changes in response to light intensity to control the amount of light which enters the eye. Immediately behind the iris and in contact with it is the crystalline **lens,** which contracts to alter its shape and permit fine focusing of an image on the retina. Behind the lens is

Health Highlight
STATE OF OHIO VISION SCREENING
OBJECTIVES AND REQUIREMENTS

Objectives

Vision screening is an efficient and effective health assessment procedure. Screening will produce both overreferrals and underreferrals; however, for the benefit of the children being screened, errors toward false positives (i.e., overreferrals) are preferred. Parents of children screened should be informed of the limitations of screening and that it does not take the place of an eye examination. Screening programs should stress that the vision screening is not an eye examination and will not detect all potential eye problems or diseases. The screening procedures required by the Ohio Department of Health are meant to aid in the detection of the following general vision disorders.

1. Observable and reportable signs and symptoms
2. Defect of visual activity
3. Ocular muscle disorders
4. Defects of binocularity
5. Color perception deficits in male

Required Screening Procedures and Frequency of Testing

1. External observation of eye signs and recording of symptoms—at all screenings
2. Distance visual activity test—at all screenings
3. Ocular muscle balance test administered at distance and near—kindergarten or at the child's initial screening

4. A test for stereopsis using random dot stereograms—kindergarten or at the child's initial screening.
5. Color perception test (males only)—in kindergarten or first grade or at the child's initial screening

Children to be Screened

■ All new and transfer students (for whom no screening record for the previous 12 months exists) must be screened during the year they enter the new school.

■ All hearing-impaired children must have their vision screened annually.

■ All teacher referrals must be screened.

■ Preschoolers enrolled in school programs shall be screened upon entrance to the program and annually thereafter.

■ All children who are untestable must be referred.

■ Failure on any one test, required or optional, will result in referral.

■ All children failing an initial screening must be rescreened as soon as possible but within 6 weeks. (Significant numbers of children will pass a second screening, reducing the over-referral rate).

■ This is a required minimum; additional grades may be screened as staff time permits.

SOURCE: Ohio Department of Health, Vision Conservation Programs for Children 2001

the main cavity of the eye, filled with a clear gel. On the inside of the back of the eye is the **retina,** a structure of nerve tissue on which the images are focused by the cornea and the lens. The retina needs a constant supply of oxygen and sugar, which are supplied by a thin network of branching blood vessels just under it called the **choroid plexus.** The eyeball is sealed off from the outside by a flexible membrane called the **conjunctiva,** which is attached to the skin at the corners of the eye and forms the inner lining of the lids. The conjunctiva's primary function is to secrete mucus that protect the eyes from damage due to dryness.

Visual Defects. The retina functions similarly to film in a camera. If light is not perfectly focused on the retina, vision will be blurred.

Astigmatism. Stigma means point. Astigma means without a point. Astigmatism occurs when light entering the eye is "split" into two separate parts instead of focusing to one, precise point on the retina. Astigmatism usually occurs because the eye's front window, the cornea, is irregularly curved. Symptoms of astigmatism include blurred vision, squinting, eyestrain, blurring of fine detail, and headache. Treatments of astigmatism may include use of corrective lenses (glasses or contact lenses) and/or refractive surgery.

Hyperopia (Farsightedness). To see clearly, light must enter the eye and come to a precise focus on the retina. Hyperopia occurs when light entering the eye is brought to a focus behind the retina. Generally most people are born farsighted, so it does not tend to develop later in life as nearsightedness often does. Symptoms of hyperopia include clearer far vision, blurred near vision, frontal headaches, and eyestrain with near work. Treatment includes glasses, contact lenses, or refractive surgery. Lenses used to correct hyperopia are called plus lenses; they are thickest in the center and get thinner toward the edge (so are convex). These lenses "pull" the eye's focus forward until it falls directly on the retina, producing clear vision. Both glasses and contact lenses use this same optical design.

Myopia (Nearsightedness). Myopia occurs when light entering the eye is focused before it reaches the retina. Symptoms of myopia include blurred distance vision, clear near vision, squinting, and poorer night vision. Treatment includes glasses, corrective lenses, contact lenses, and refractive surgery. Lenses used to correct myopia are concave, so are thinner in the center and thicker toward the edges in order to diverge the light before it enters the eye so the image will be moved backward onto the retina.

Strabismus (Crossed Eyes). Strabismus results anytime the eyes are not pointed at the same point in space. Strabismus is seen most commonly in children, where it represents a muscular misalignment between the eyes. (A total of twelve eye muscles are used to keep the eyes aligned with each other.) Contrary to popular belief, most children will not "outgrow" a crossed eye. In fact, more damage will usually result if treatment is not initiated early. Failure to treat a constantly crossed eye can lead to "lazy eye" or poor vision in the affected eye (amblyopia). Crossed eyes that occur suddenly in adults usually result in double vision and should be promptly evaluated; they are most often the result of head injury, stroke, or aneurysm. Any form of crossed eyes should be evaluated by an eye health professional. A thorough vision examination can determine the proper diagnosis and treatment plan needed to ensure a good outcome.

Care of the Eyes. The eyes are among the most sensitive and delicate organs in the body. Because they work together, an injury, infection, or impairment to one eye may result in damage to the other. Therefore, any visual abnormality should be dealt with either by a physician or optometrist.

In your instruction, emphasize individual responsibility for protecting the eyes from harmful chemicals such as dyes, bleaches, cleansing products, insecticides, and cosmetic irritants. Also stress the potential danger of playing with objects that could penetrate or damage the eye, such as air rifles, fireworks, and slingshots. Teach children to keep dirty hands, fingers, and soiled materials away from the eyes and to alert adults to any eye discomfort or visual problem. Students should never self-medicate the eyes with drops, ointments, or creams.

Eye examinations should be given at birth, followed by additional testing around the age of five, during adolescence, and every two years thereafter. More frequent eye examinations may be needed after the age of forty because the aging process usually affects vision. In addition, eye examinations often uncover many underlying health problems such as diabetes, glaucoma, high blood pressure, and systemic infections.

The teacher should make adjustments in the classroom to help alleviate some problems of students with poor vision. Have the students sit toward the front of the class so they can see the board more clearly. Some students might need a written handout if they have tremendous difficulty seeing the board.

THE SENSE OF HEARING

The sense of hearing greatly assists communication with others. It provides information about the environment in the form of sounds, both innocuous and that signal danger. The ears also contain structures that help an individual maintain a sense of balance.

The Ear. The ear is an organ for hearing and balance. It consists of three parts: the outer ear, the middle ear, and the inner ear. The outer and middle ear mostly collect and transmit sound. The inner ear converts sound waves to electrical (nervous) signals and contains an apparatus that maintains the body's balance. The outer ear is the part that is visible and is made of folds of skin and cartilage. It leads into the auditory canal, which is about one inch long in adults and is separated from the middle ear by the eardrum. The **eardrum** is a thin, fibrous circular membrane covered with a thin layer of skin; it vibrates in response to the changes in the air pressure that constitute sound. The middle ear is a small cavity that conducts sound from the eardrum to the inner ear by means of three tiny, linked, movable bones called **ossicles.** These are the smallest bones in the human body and are named for their shape: the **hammer (malleus)** connects the eardrum to the **anvil (incus)** with a broad joint; a very delicate joint connects the anvil to the **stirrup (stapes).** The base of the stirrup fills the oval window, which leads to the inner ear. The inner ear (**labyrinth**) is a very delicate series of structures deep within the bones of the skull. The front (the **cochlea**) is a tube resembling a snail's shell and is concerned with hearing. The rear part (the **semicircular canals**) is concerned with balance.

Hearing Impairments. The inability to hear can arise from a variety of causes, including congenital defects, illness, and injury. The most common hearing disability is conductive hearing loss, which can occur for a variety of reasons and is characterized by some sort of blockage or structural defect in the auditory canal or middle ear that warps or muffles the vibrations. Some conditions of conductive deafness can be corrected, and most are amenable to treatment.

Care of the Ears. The ears should be protected from loud noises, blasts, or other environmental hazards that can cause damage to the eardrum or affect frequency detection. Teach children to recognize the dangers of inserting anything into their ears as well as the importance of informing an adult of any ear discomfort. Children who continually pull on their ears or seem to have trouble with balance and equilibrium should be referred to either an otologist or an otolaryngologist, physicians specializing in care of the ears. Hearing tests should be administered at the preschool level as well as periodically throughout the school years.

Pay close attention to children who seem inattentive or unresponsive; these behaviors may signal hearing impairment rather than intellectual or emotional difficulties. The teacher should watch students for the following indications of hearing problems:

- chronic nose and throat trouble
- runny ear
- complaints of pressure, ringing, or buzzing in the ear
- frowning when trying to listen
- leaning forward or turning the head while listening
- good written work, but poor oral work

The best thing to do for a child with hearing loss is to detect the condition early and get medical attention. In the classroom, the teacher should place the child near the front of the room, look directly at the student, and speak clearly and slowly. Provide the student with a written handout to help the student keep up with any lesson that is presented orally.

THE SENSE OF TOUCH

Numerous sensory receptor cells in the skin provide the body with the sensations of pain, heat, cold, and touch (pressure). A different type of sensory receptor cell detects each of these stimuli. Heat receptors obviously trigger sensations very different from those triggered by touch receptors, for example, even though all skin sensory cells send comparable signals through the central nervous system. The difference in sensations occurs because the message from each of the four types of receptor cells is sent to a particular region of the brain. That is, heat receptors send electrical impulses to the heat centers in the brain, whereas touch receptors send their messages to the touch centers of the brain. Different areas of the skin vary in their degree of sensitivity, with the fingers being among the most sensitive due to the high concentration of receptor cells. The sense of touch arises when unequal pressure occurs between the skin and an object or material in contact with it. This unequal pressure produces a depression in the skin or moves hair follicles, and thus touch is perceived.

Care of the Sense of Touch. Problems associated with loss of sensation are neurological in nature and, as a result, are complex and varied. Therefore, very little can be done by the individual to affect the sense of touch. However, children should be aware of diminished sensation in any part of the body and should report such an occurrence.

THE SENSES OF TASTE AND SMELL

The senses of taste and smell are closely aligned because they each enhance and are enhanced by the other. These senses can affect health in many ways—for example, influencing choices of food.

Taste buds are the sensory receptor cells within the visible papillae, or bumps on the tongue. Hairlike projections on the taste buds are stimulated by food dissolving in saliva and send impulses to the brain from connecting nerves. The tongue itself contains taste centers, each of which is most sensitive to a particular taste. The tip of the tongue is receptive to food that is sweet, whereas the rear of the tongue keys into bitter-tasting food. Salty foods are more easily tasted on the sides toward the front of the tongue, whereas sour foods are more easily tasted on the sides toward the back. In addition, the tongue differentiates temperature as well as texture of foods, adding greater variety to the sense of taste.

Food is not easily tasted if nasal passages are blocked in some way, as in the case of a head cold. Food in the mouth produces odors in the form of vapors that travel through the nasal passages, where they stimulate receptor cells in the upper nasal region. If the passages are blocked, the odors do not reach these cells, and the sense of taste/smell is diminished accordingly. Nerve endings attached to these cells join to form the olfactory nerve (first cranial nerve), the nerve that sends messages concerning smell to the cerebral cortex.

Care of the Senses of Taste and Smell. As with the sense of touch, not much can be done personally to maintain the senses of taste and smell. Impairment because of blockage of the nasal cavity due to colds or infection is temporary and will abate. Impairment due to nerve damage, although rare, cannot be reversed, so loss of taste and smell may be permanent.

Dental Health

DENTAL PROBLEMS

Most oral health problems are related to dental plaque. If plaque is not removed, it begins to harden and turn into a calcified mass that is known as tartar. Plaque interacts with the foods we eat and produces acids that erode enamel and cause tooth decay (caries). Tooth decay is one of the most common human diseases. Early loss of calcium is countered by the natural tendency of saliva (which is calcium rich) to replace calcium in the enamel crystals.

The first indications of tooth decay are white spots on the enamel caused by the loss of calcium. Bacteria may invade the pulp of the tooth, causing a consistent tooth pain, especially during the night. The bacteria may also produce an abscess, and eventually the tooth must be extracted by the dentist.

When dental plaque grows, it releases toxins that irritate the gums, causing gingivitis. If left untreated it may lead to a more serious form of gum disease (periodontitis). Long-term gingivitis can cause gum recession, which exposes the tooth roots and makes teeth hypersensitive. Metabolic processes of plaque bacteria can produce organic compounds that are responsible for bad breath (halitosis). The tooth surface is susceptible to picking up stains from our diet (for example, tea) and habits (such as smoking) that cause discoloration. Problems related to the correct positioning of teeth are called orthodontic problems. These problems may be corrected by orthodontists and some dentists.

CARE OF THE TEETH

Daily flossing and brushing of the teeth, preferably after each meal but at least once a day, is the best way to maintain good dental health. Flossing should be done first, because it removes plaque from between teeth. Flossing should be done using about eighteen inches of floss wound around the middle fingers until only a few inches are left. The ends of the remaining floss section are then grasped between each thumb and forefinger and eased between the gum and tooth so that a scraping motion against the side of the tooth can occur. This procedure should be repeated with each tooth, using a new section of floss each time. Brushing removes plaque from tooth surfaces and is best accomplished by angling the brush against the gumline so that a back-and-forth (side-to-side) motion using gentle strokes can be done on the outside, inside, and biting surfaces of the teeth. A fluoridated toothpaste is recommended. Avoid brushing too hard, as this may also cause gums to recede.

In addition to daily flossing and brushing, particular attention should be paid to diet. Avoidance of sweets is recommended, and the intake of food high in vitamin D during childhood will help develop strong teeth. Regular dental examinations, preferably twice a year, from childhood through adulthood will also do much to ensure good dental health.

Fitness, Relaxation, and Sleep

FITNESS

Today, there is a growing emphasis on looking good, feeling good, and living longer. Increasingly, scientific evidence tells us that two keys to achieving these ideals are fitness and exercise. Regardless of your age, gender, or role in life, you can benefit from regular physical activity. Exercise in combination with a sensible diet can help provide an overall sense of well-being and can even help prevent chronic illness, disability, and premature death. Physical fitness in childhood has been linked to the prevention of cardiorespiratory and coronary disease in adults. The focus on fitness for youth has shifted from strenuous exercise as a prerequisite for health and fitness to physical activity and the development of an active lifestyle, with physical inactivity portrayed as hazardous to one's health (Graham, Holt-Hale, and Parker 1998, 34).

Fitness can be described as a condition that helps us look, feel, and do our best. More specifically, it is: "The ability to perform daily tasks vigorously and alertly, with energy left over for enjoying leisure-time activities and meeting emergency demands. It is the ability to endure, to bear up, to withstand stress, to

Health Highlight

EXCERPT FROM "SUMMARY OF PHYSICAL ACTIVITY AND HEALTH: A REPORT OF THE SURGEON GENERAL"

School-based interventions for youth are particularly promising, not only for their potential scope—almost all young people between the ages of 6 and 16 years attend school—but also for their potential impact. Nearly half of young people 12 to 21 years of age are not vigorously active; moreover, physical activity sharply declines during adolescence. Childhood and adolescence may thus be pivotal times for preventing sedentary behavior among adults by maintaining the habit of physical activity throughout the school years. School-based interventions have been shown to be successful in increasing physical activity levels. With evidence that success in this arena is possible, every effort should be made to encourage schools to require daily physical education in each grade and to promote physical activities that can be enjoyed throughout life.

SOURCE: Centers for Disease Control and Prevention 2000

carry on in circumstances where an unfit person could not continue, and is a major basis for good health and well-being" (President's Council on Physical Fitness and Sports 2002).

Physical fitness involves the performance of the heart, lungs, and muscles of the body. And, since what we do with our bodies also affects what we can do with our minds, fitness influences to some degree qualities such as mental alertness and emotional stability. Fitness is an individual quality that varies from person to person. It is influenced by age, sex, heredity, personal habits, exercise, and eating practices. The first three factors cannot be changed; however, one can change and improve the other factors.

Physical fitness is most easily understood by examining its components, or "parts." There is widespread agreement that these four components are basic:

1. **Cardiorespiratory endurance**—the ability to deliver oxygen and nutrients to tissues and to remove wastes over sustained periods of time. Long runs and swims are among the methods employed to measure this component.

2. **Muscular strength**—the ability of a muscle to exert force for a brief period. Upper-body strength, for example, can be measured by various weightlifting exercises.

3. **Muscular endurance**—the ability of a muscle or a group of muscles to sustain repeated contractions or to continue applying force against a fixed object. Push-ups are often used to test endurance of arm and shoulder muscles.

4. **Flexibility**—the ability to move joints and use muscles through their full range of motion. The sit-and-reach test is a good measure of flexibility of the lower back and backs of the upper legs.

Body composition is often considered a component of fitness. It refers to the makeup of the body in terms of lean mass (muscle, bone, vital tissue, and organs) and fat mass. An optimal ratio of fat to lean mass is an indication of fitness, and the right types of exercise will help you decrease body fat and increase or maintain muscle mass.

How often, how long, and how hard you exercise, and what kinds of exercises you do should be determined by what you are trying to accomplish. Your goals, your present fitness level, age, health, skills, interest, and convenience are among the factors you should consider. For example, an athlete training for high-level competition would follow a different program from a person whose goals are good health and the ability to meet work and recreational needs.

An exercise program should include something from each of the four basic fitness components described previously. Each workout should begin with a warm-up and end with a cool-down. As a general rule, space your workouts throughout the week and avoid consecutive days of hard exercise.

The amounts of activity necessary for the average healthy person to maintain a minimum level of overall fitness, according to the U.S. Surgeon General's report on physical activity and health, is as follows: "All people over the age of two years should accumulate at least 30 minutes of endurance-type physical activity of at least moderate intensity, on most—preferably all—days of the week" (Graham, Holt-Hale, and Parker 1998, 34).

Here are some of the popular exercises for each category.

> **Warm-up**—five to ten minutes of exercises such as walking, slow jogging, knee lifts, arm circles, or trunk rotations. Low-intensity movements that stimulate movements to be used in the activity can also be included in the warm-up.
>
> **Muscular strength**—a minimum of two 20-minute sessions per week that include exercises for all the major muscle groups. Lifting weights is the most effective way to increase strength.
>
> **Muscular endurance**—at least three 30-minute sessions each week that include exercises such as calisthenics, push-ups, sit-ups, pull-ups, and weight training for all the major muscle groups.
>
> **Cardiorespiratory endurance**—at least three 20-minute bouts of continuous aerobic (activity requiring oxygen) rhythmic exercise each week. Popular aerobic conditioning activities include brisk walking, jogging, swimming, cycling, rope-jumping, rowing, cross-country skiing, and some continuous action games like racquetball and handball.
>
> **Flexibility**—ten to twelve minutes of daily stretching exercises performed slowly without a bouncing motion. This can be included after a warm-up or during a cool-down.
>
> **Cool-down**—a minimum of five to ten minutes of slow walking, low-level exercise, combined with stretching.

The keys to selecting the right kinds of exercises for developing and maintaining each of the basic components of fitness are found in these principles:

Health Highlight

SOME BENEFITS OF INCREASED ACTIVITY

Improved Health
- increased efficiency of heart and lungs
- reduced cholesterol levels
- increased muscle strength
- reduced blood pressure
- reduced risk of major illnesses such as diabetes and heart disease
- weight loss

Improved Sense of Well-Being
- more energy
- less stress
- improved quality of sleep
- improved ability to cope with stress
- increased mental acuity

Improved Appearance
- weight loss
- toned muscles
- improved posture

Enhanced Social Life
- improved self-image
- increased opportunities to make new friends
- increased opportunities to share an activity with friends or family members

Increased Stamina
- increased productivity
- increased physical capabilities
- less frequent injuries
- improved immunity to minor illnesses

SOURCE: Metlife Consumer Education Center 2000

Specificity—Pick the right kind of activities to affect each component. Strength training results in specific strength changes. Also, train for the specific activity you're interested in. For example, optimal swimming performance is best achieved when the muscles involved in swimming are trained for the movements required. It does not necessarily follow that a good runner is a good swimmer.

Overload—Work hard enough, at levels that are vigorous and long enough to overload your body above its resting level, to bring about improvement.

Regularity—You can't hoard physical fitness. At least three balanced workouts a week are necessary to maintain a desirable level of fitness.

Progression—Increase the intensity, frequency, and/or duration of activity over periods of time in order to improve.

Some activities can be used to fulfill more than one of your basic exercise requirements. For example, in addition to increasing cardiorespiratory endurance, running builds muscular endurance in the legs, and swimming develops the arm, shoulder, and chest muscles. If you select the proper activities, it is possible to fit parts of your muscular endurance workout into your cardiorespiratory workout and save time (President's Council on Physical Fitness and Sports 2002).

Health Highlight

HEALTHY PEOPLE 2010 OBJECTIVES
RELATED TO FITNESS AND PHYSICAL ACTIVITY

The objectives related to fitness and physical activity are:

1. Increase the proportion of people age 18 and older who engage in any leisure time physical activity.

2. Increase the proportion of people age 18 and older who engage regularly, preferably daily, in sustained physical activity for at least 30 minutes per day.

3. Increase the proportion of people age 18 and older who engage in vigorous physical activity that promotes the development and maintenance of cardio-respiratory fitness three or more days per week for 20 or more minutes per occasion.

4. Increase the proportion of people age 18 and older who regularly perform physical activities that enhance and maintain muscular strength and endurance.

5. Increase the proportion of people age 18 and older who perform physical activities that enhance and maintain flexibility.

6. Increase the proportion of young people in grades 9 through 12 who engage in vigorous physical activity that promotes the development and maintenance of cardiorespiratory fitness three or more days per week for 20 or more minutes per occasion.

7. Increase the proportion of young people in grades 9 through 12 who engage in moderate physical activity for at least 30 minutes on five or more of the previous seven days.

8. Increase the proportion of young people in grades 9 through 12 who participate in daily school physical education.

9. Increase the proportion of the nation's public and private elementary, middle/junior high, and senior high schools that require daily physical education for all students.

10. Increase the proportion of young people in grades 9 through 12 who spend at least 50 percent of school physical education class time being physically active, preferably engaged in lifetime physical activities, at least three times per week.

11. Increase the proportion of the nation's public and private elementary, middle/junior, and senior high schools that, in addition to physical education courses, teach about physical activity in required health education courses.

12. Increase the proportion of the nation's public and private elementary, middle/junior, and senior high schools that provide access to their physical activity spaces and facilities for young people and adults outside of normal school hours.

13. Increase the proportion of worksites offering employer-sponsored physical activity and fitness programs.

14. Increase the proportion of primary and allied health care providers who routinely assess and counsel their patients regarding their physical activity.

SOURCE: U.S. Department of Health and Human Services 2002

RELAXATION

Relaxation is one of the body's most useful tools in combating fatigue, either physical, mental, or both. By learning how to relax during the day so that alert and conscious functioning continues, a person can reduce feelings of listlessness, tiredness, apathy, tension, and aches and pains.

Fatigue may be due solely to physical overexertion or to a drain of mental capabilities after engaging in such chores as reading, writing, problem solving, or studying in general. Fatigue can also be produced by adverse environmental conditions, such as improper ventilation or lighting, or by emotional stress.

Relaxation involves the releasing of physical and mental tension through varied and diverse means that can include doing nothing, meditating, watching television, listening to music, taking a hot bath, or relaxing the muscles with a massage. The ways in which an individual chooses to relax should be based on personal interests, environment, or setting, and comfort with the procedure or technique. Regardless of how achieved, relaxation needs to be incorporated into every individual's lifestyle, just as exercise does, so that stress reaction can be minimized and personal health and well-being can be maximized.

SLEEP

The body's need for sleep must be met consistently in order to maintain good personal health. Unlike exercise and relaxation, sleep is an involuntary process that does not require a planned or prescribed regimen that must be purposely enacted by the individual. In fact, scientists still cannot fully explain all the mysteries associated with sleep, including its cause and why it is needed.

The amount of sleep needed varies from individual to individual. Most adults need about eight hours of sleep in order to awaken easily and without fatigue. The amount of sleep needed decreases as age increases. Newborn infants spend a majority of their time sleeping, while most older adults sleep less than eight hours at night but may require short naps during the day. Elementary school children need eight to ten hours of sleep a night, and young adults need anywhere from six to eight hours of sleep a night (Neuropsychiatric Institute, University of California, Los Angeles 2002).

Summary

- Almost every individual begins life with a sound, healthy body that requires care and maintenance.

- Personal health, a most desired and cherished possession, is of concern to everyone.

- Without good health, the quality of life is diminished considerably and day-to-day existence becomes a burden instead of a joy.

- To ensure good personal health, each individual must assume responsibility for taking care of his or her own body so that it is kept in good condition.

- Learning to maintain and enhance one's health and well-being in early childhood through sound health practices is crucial for sustaining high levels of personal health in later life.

- It is important to teach children the elements of personal health, including an appreciation for personal appearance, the senses that allow them to relate to their environments, and good dental health.

- Children must be taught to exert purposeful, conscious action in incorporating and integrating regular intervals of exercise, relaxation, and sleep into their living patterns.

DISCUSSION QUESTIONS

1. Explain the interaction of genetics, socioeconomic status, and illness with regard to their influence on personal health.
2. Describe the connection between eye problems and learning.
3. Explain the interdependence of the senses of taste and smell.
4. Describe the effects of exercise on the major body systems.

CRITICAL THINKING QUESTIONS

1. Explain the interaction of genetics, socioeconomic status, and illness with regard to their influence on personal health.
2. Describe the connection between eye problems and learning.
3. Explain the interdependence of the senses of taste and smell.
4. Describe how to prevent the skin conditions discussed in this chapter from spreading.
5. Discuss the Healthy People 2010 Objectives that are related to Fitness and Physical Activity.

WEB SITE ACTIVITY

Using the Web site *www.medicinenet.com/Acne/article.htm,* determine the answers to the following questions about acne:

- What is acne?
- What causes acne?
- What doesn't cause acne?
- When should you start to treat acne?
- What can you do about acne on your own? (A lot!)
- What are other things you can do for acne?
- What is a good basic skin regimen?
- What can the doctor do for acne?
- How would you sum up current day treatment of acne?

WEB SITES OF INTEREST

Health A to Z: *www.healthatoz.com*
Provides personal and medical information on a variety of health topics.

Your Health: *www.yourhealth.com*
Provides quality health-related information, including the latest health headlines, expert question-and-answer program "Live Online," a weekly radio-style audio program "Studio one2one," and a large selection of health reference information.

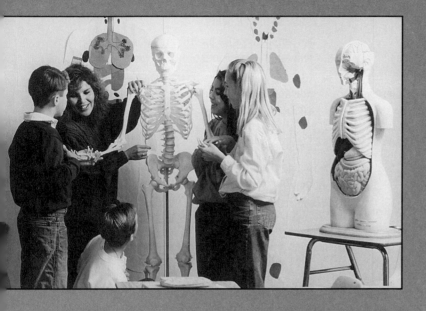

CHAPTER TEN

Strategies for Teaching Body Systems and Personal Health

A sound, healthy body is the basis for optimal personal health and well-being.

VALUED OUTCOMES: BODY SYSTEMS

After doing the activities in this chapter, the student should be able to express and illustrate the following guidelines:

- The human body is a highly organized and well-developed "machine."

- The body systems are interdependent and contribute to the healthy functioning of the body as a whole.

- There is a reciprocal relationship between growth and development.

- Growth and development as lifelong processes are enhanced by responsible behavior.

- Some growth and development characteristics are common to all living things.

- Growth and development occur at the level of the cell.

- Each person is unique in the way he or she grows and develops.

- Many factors influence physical, mental, and social growth and development.

- Daily care and maintenance of the human body and an understanding of how its systems operate serve as the foundation for personal health and well-being.

- The nervous system acts as the body's computer by receiving, interpreting, and sending messages that help direct and guide all other body systems so that the individual can make both internal and external adjustments to the environment.

- The endocrine system helps maintain balance among all body systems through the secretion of chemical substances called hormones that influence the actions of body organs and structures.

- The reproductive system is activated in puberty and creates and perpetuates human life.

- The respiratory system provides the pathway and mechanics for oxygen to enter the body and carbon dioxide to leave it.

- The circulatory system, through the heart's pumping of blood, delivers oxygen and other essential chemicals to all cells and tissues of the body.

- The digestive/excretory system is responsible for mechanically and chemically breaking down food so that it can be used for all body processes. Substances that cannot be used are eliminated from the body as waste products.

- The skeletal/muscular system provides the body and its parts with shape, support, protection, and movement.

- Although body systems operate in standard ways, personal differences in structure and physical function affect individual growth and development.

VALUED OUTCOMES: PERSONAL HEALTH

After doing the activities in this chapter, the student should be able to express and illustrate the following guidelines:

- Personal health maintenance and enhancement are essential to well-being.

- Developing positive health care habits helps maintain the body and promote overall wellness.

- Attaining personal health and well-being is an individual responsibility but can be facilitated by school, community, and social resources.

- Health care practices promote physical, mental, and social health.

- Regular visits to health care professionals are important in maintaining personal health.

- Personal health is influenced by choices made and actions taken based on individual values, attitudes, beliefs, and knowledge.

- Daily care and upkeep of our personal appearance are important components of our personal health.

- Protecting the eyes, ears, teeth, and other body parts is essential to maintaining personal health.

- Personal appearance is influenced by health habits concerning care of the skin, nails, hair, and posture.

- Preserving the five major body senses—vision, hearing, touch, taste, and smell—is essential to personal health because the senses keep us in touch with our physical and emotional environments.

- Adequate dental care may help to prevent jaw and facial deformities, speech abnormalities, and malnourishment in later life, thus safeguarding personal health.

- Consistent, routinely scheduled, prescribed exercise programs promote personal health and well-being by strengthening cardiorespiratory and muscular fitness.

- Leisure-time activities promote fitness and contribute to personal health.

- Relaxation and sleep allow bodily processes and functions to renew their energy sources, thus helping to combat physical and mental fatigue.

REFLECTIONS

As you read through this chapter, consider the interaction of the several body systems. For example, how would it affect your sense of sight if your hearing was damaged? What precautions would you have to take if a part of your endocrine system was malfunctioning?

Planning Learning Activities

A sound, healthy body is the basis for optimal personal health and well-being. From the instant of birth and throughout life, an individual strives first to meet basic physiological needs. As a result, instruction about the function and care of the human body and its interacting systems is of the utmost importance to children, especially at the elementary school level. Learning opportunities should demonstrate and emphasize health practices that ensure maintenance of body systems so that students develop positive health habits that will enhance their physiological growth and development.

Because children generally enjoy and are interested in participating in physical activity and discovering the unseen "mysteries" of their own body actions, teaching about body systems should be an exhilarating and challenging experience for you. Throughout instruction, students should be made aware of the interrelationships between all body systems and should develop a sense of "ownership" with regard to their own bodies so that personal commitment to its upkeep is fostered.

Teaching the Concept of Personal Health

Health education was formerly limited to hygienic practices. Since those days, health education has branched out to include concepts from sociology, psychology, and other disciplines; however, we must not overlook the importance of teaching children about taking care of their bodies. In teaching personal health, emphasize to your students that enhancing well-being is largely an individual responsibility. The concept of personal health is an abstract idea that young children need to learn, yet many of the practices associated with health maintenance are already familiar to them and can be used as a base for building understanding of the concept. To do this, relate daily health practices to overall well-being. In this way, students will begin to see that discrete practices, such as face washing or toothbrushing, are components of an overall approach to optimum health. That is, a person does not wash simply to clean a part of the body, and toothbrushing and flossing are not done simply to help prevent tooth decay.

Rather, these and other personal health practices are parts of an overall mainte-nance and health enhancement program. To bring this point home, note that personal body cleanliness plays an important role in the prevention of disease, just as proper dental care contributes to overall health.

The strategies described in this chapter are designed not only to teach specific health practices, but also to foster good personal health habits. Knowing how to brush one's teeth properly is of little value unless toothbrushing and allied dental care are performed on a regular basis. For this to occur, students must personalize the information you present and make decisions to develop good habits. Contin-ually emphasize that personal health is a matter of personal accountability.

Shown to the right of each activity title is the suggested grade level(s) for which the activity might be appropriate. However, many of the suggested activi-ties could be modified for use at various grade levels.

Value-Based Activities: Body Systems

VALUES VOTING   Grades (K–3)

Valued Outcome: The students will be able to clarify values regarding activities related to personal health.

Description of Strategy: The following questions can be posed by the instruc-tor, with the students voting yes or no on each. Discussion should be allowed to interrupt the voting at any time.

How many of you . . .

  use good posture when you sit, stand, and walk?

  eat foods that lead to good health?

  get regular physical examinations?

Materials Needed: none

Processing Question: What health habits most affect your personal health?

BEING GOOD TO ME   Grades (3–5)

Valued Outcome: The students will be able to discuss habits they perform to care for the body.

Description of Strategy: Divide students into small groups, and ask each group to list five routine things they do for themselves that they consider beneficial. Compare group lists to see how many items relate to care of the body. Then write on the board each item relating to body care, and ask the groups to rank them in terms of importance in maintaining body functioning. Follow with general discussion.

Materials Needed: none

Processing Question: What are the most important personal health habits necessary to maintain proper body functioning?

RANK-ORDERING HEALTH PRACTICES   Grades (4–5)

Valued Outcome: The students will be able to list in order of priority (rank-order) practices that affect each body system.

Description of Strategy: Prepare a handout from the list below that lists each body system and three health practices that affect it. Ask students to rank the practices according to the positive influence each practice has on that system, "1" being the most positive.

Examples:

Digestive/Excretory System	Skeletal/Muscular System
_____ eating fresh fruits and vegetables	_____ sitting and standing straight
_____ eating foods high in fiber	_____ getting plenty of exercise
_____ limiting sweet snacks	_____ relaxing during the day

In the class discussion that follows, indicate that all the practices are important but that some directly influence specific body systems more than others.

Materials Needed: paper and pencil, handout

Processing Question: What practices are significant in affecting the body systems?

BODY SYSTEMS POSITION STATEMENT   Grades (4–5)

Valued Outcome: The students will be able to explain the importance of each body system.

Description of Strategy: Divide the class into six groups, each representing a different body system (excluding the reproductive system). Have each group develop and present a five-minute statement that argues for the position that their system "is number one." After all the positions have been presented, have the students vote to determine a "winner." Follow with a discussion of why students voted the way they did.

Materials Needed: none

Processing Question: Is any one body system really more important than the others, or do we need the functions that each of the body systems provides?

BODY CARE COLLAGE   Grades (4–5)

Valued Outcome: The students will be able to explain how proper care of the body can influence growth and development.

Description of Strategy: Provide students with poster board, and ask them to make a collage of people with diverse body types and habits that may influence body functioning. Collages should be made from magazine pictures and newspaper clippings and should show the varying health status of the people depicted. Accompanying each collage should be a brief written description that summarizes the student's attitudes and opinions regarding how care of the body can influence growth and development.

Materials Needed: poster board for each student, magazines, newspapers

Processing Question: What are some health habits we can perform that will positively affect our growth and development?

BODY IMAGE SENTENCE COMPLETION   Grades (4–5)

Valued Outcome: The students will be able to complete sentences with their own thoughts about several statements related to body image.

Description of Strategy: Provide students with handouts containing incomplete statements such as those listed below. Have students complete the statements. Then have them share their answers with a partner.

My body is . . .	The bones of my body are . . .
I like my body because . . .	I help my muscles by . . .
I take good care of my body by . . .	When I breathe, I . . .
	When I eat, . . .

Materials Needed: pencils, handouts

Processing Question: What do you feel are the strengths and weaknesses about your body shape?

Value-Based Activities: Personal Health

HAPPY HEALTH ACTIVITIES   Grades (4–5)

Valued Outcome: The students will be able to record personal health activities.

Description of Strategy: Have children record their happy and fun activities related to personal health (such as exercises) with paint or crayons. This activity strengthens the importance of valuing health-related activities.

Materials Needed: marking instruments (such as crayons or paint), paper

Processing Question: Which personal health activities are important in enhancing one's health?

SAD AND GLAD   Grades (K–3)

Valued Outcome: The students will be able to discern which personal health behaviors they most enjoy.

Description of Strategy: Mount pictures of various personal health behaviors on large cards. With cards face down, a student chooses one and tells the group that he or she would be sad or glad to participate in this behavior. Older students may describe the activity to the class, emphasizing the sad and/or glad aspects of the behavior, and have the class guess the behavior from the student's description.

Materials Needed: pictures of people involved in health behaviors, large cards

Processing Question: In which personal health behaviors do you most enjoy participating?

EXERCISE AND SLEEP ATTITUDE SCALE   Grades (3–5)

Valued Outcome: The students will be able to clarify their attitudes toward exercise, relaxation, and sleep.

Description of Strategy: Create a handout listing the following forced-choice attitude scale to discover the students' attitudes about the concepts of exercise, relaxation, and sleep. Choose Agree or Disagree.

	Agree	Disagree
1. Exercise makes me feel good.	——	——
2. Sleep is important to my health.	——	——
3. I take time during the day to do something I enjoy.	——	——
4. I sleep eight or nine hours a night.	——	——
5. Exercise can be fun.	——	——
6. Taking time during the day to do something enjoyable keeps me healthy.	——	——
7. My body can benefit from exercise all my life.	——	——
8. I often feel tired when I awake in the morning.	——	——

After students have completed the activity, have them share their answers in a large group discussion.

Materials Needed: pencils, handout

Processing Question: How are sleep, relaxation, and exercise beneficial to you?

PERSONAL HEALTH VOTING   Grades (K–5)

Valued Outcome: The students will be able to clarify their values regarding personal health habits.

Description of Strategy: Each student will have a card with green on one side and red on the other side. Explain to the students that the green is for "agree" and the red is for "disagree." Remember that there are no right or wrong answers. When the teacher asks the question, the students hold up green cards if they agree with the question (or would answer yes) and hold up red cards if they disagree with the question (or would answer no).

How many of you . . .

> would rather go to a birthday party than keep your dental appointment?
>
> would encourage your brother or sister to clean his or her teeth?
>
> think it is funny to bump someone at the drinking fountain?
>
> feel that brushing your teeth is necessary to prevent cavities?
>
> feel that eating snacks is harmful to your teeth?
>
> would rather eat a sweet snack than fruit or a raw vegetable?
>
> go to sleep when you are very tired without brushing your teeth?

Materials Needed: cards for each student with red on one side and green on the other

Processing Question: How important are personal health habits to you?

PERSONAL WELL-BEING   Grades (3–5)

Valued Outcome The students will be able to identify what is really important to them and their well-being.

Description of Strategy: This activity is designed to help students determine what is important to them and understand that values or feelings concerning the type of life we wish to lead are being expressed in our decisions.

Tell the class the subject matter of the lesson (things we value most), and describe what a value is (things important to us that have meaning in life). Then name some of the things that you value in life and why. Select a few students to share some of their values with the class; for example, Mary may say that she values her dog.

On the board, write the following value question: Pretend you are going on a trip in a spaceship. What three things would you take with you and why? Then list the processing questions (given below) on the board, and have the students write their answers on notebook paper to turn in.

Materials Needed: pencils and paper

Processing Questions:

1. Why did you take your three choices?
2. Do these represent something you value?
3. How would you describe a value?
4. Do values reflect what we do and the decisions we make? Why/how?
5. Discuss what we learned about values today and how our values differ from one another.

SMILEY/SAD FACE   Grades (K–2)

Valued Outcome: The students will be able to differentiate between activities they like and dislike.

Description of Strategy: An activity similar to voting involves giving the students cards with a yellow circle "smiley face" on one side and a blue circle "sad face" on the other. Ask volunteer students to describe to the class an exercise they do for fun and fitness. After the student describes the exercise, have the other students hold up a smiley face if they would like to try that exercise, or a sad face if they would not. Explain that it is all right to have different preferences for exercises.

Materials Needed: cards for each student with a yellow smiley face on one side and a blue sad face on the other side

Processing Question: In what activities do you most like to participate?

DENTAL HEALTH/SELF-CONFIDENCE   Grades (3–5)

Valued Outcome: The students will be able to differentiate between good and bad dental care.

Description of Strategy: On a piece of paper, have students make two columns, one with the heading Good Dental Care and the other with Bad Dental Care. Under each heading, the students should list different ways that dental care can affect self-confidence.

Example:

Good Dental Care	Bad Dental Care
Smiles frequently	Negative self-image
Covers smile	Good first impression
Positive self-image	Poor first impression

This activity could be repeated with other personal health behaviors.

Materials Needed: paper and pencils

Processing Question: In what ways can practicing good dental health make you feel better about yourself?

GOOD HEALTH/BAD HEALTH   Grades (K–3)

Valued Outcome: The students will be able to differentiate healthy from unhealthy behaviors.

Description of Strategy: Divide the class into small groups. Distribute magazines, glue, and scissors. Each group receives a sheet of paper divided in two. One part is headed Good Health and the other Poor Health. Instruct the students to look through the magazines and find pictures that show people involved in healthy and unhealthy behaviors, and then paste the pictures under the appropriate heading. This is a team activity, and the students will have to discuss among themselves which heading would be appropriate for the behaviors.

Materials Needed: magazines, glue, paper, scissors

Processing Question: What variables make a behavior healthy or unhealthy?

BEFORE AND AFTER   Grades (K–3)

Valued Outcome: The students will be able to explain how personal appearance can be improved.

Description of Strategy: Have students either draw or cut out pictures illustrating facets of personal appearance that need improvement. These are the "before" pictures. Each student describes how he or she believes personal appearance could be improved and then draws an "after" picture to illustrate these opinions and ideas.

Materials Needed: magazines, scissors, pencils and paper

Processing Question: What are some ways in which personal appearance can be improved?

WHAT SLEEP MEANS TO ME   Grades (4–5)

Valued Outcome: The students will be able to interpret the value of sleep.

Description of Strategy: Have students sketch or paint a picture showing their interpretation of the value of sleep. Have them write a statement about their picture, such as

> I smile more when I get enough sleep.
>
> I can run faster when I get my sleep regularly.
>
> I am always tired, but I hate to go to bed.
>
> I get sleepy in school when I stay up too late.

Materials Needed: crayons or paints, paper, pencils

Processing Question: How important is sleep to one's personal health?

SELF-PORTRAIT   Grades (4–5)

Valued Outcome: The students will be able to describe their strengths in narrative and pictorial form.

Description of Strategy: Provide large pieces of paper and crayons to each student. Ask the students to draw a picture of themselves. (This may best be done at home where a mirror is available and time constraints are removed.) On the reverse side, have students list what they perceive to be their positive attributes. Also have them describe the measures they take to promote personal health.

Materials Needed: large pieces of paper, crayons

Processing Question: What are your positive attributes?

RELAXATION RANKING   Grades (3–5)

Valued Outcome: The students will be able to list ways to relax.

Description of Strategy: Prepare a list of ten ways people can relax during the day. Ask each student to rank-order the measures from most effective to least effective. Divide students into small groups, and indicate that each group must come to a consensus ranking. Record each group's ranking on the board and allow time for explanations, questions, and summarization.

Materials Needed: chalk, chalkboard, pencils, paper

Processing Question: What are the most effective ways to relax?

PERSONAL HEALTH SENTENCE COMPLETION   Grades (4–5)

Valued Outcome: The students will be able to verbalize their feelings regarding several personal health habits.

Description of Strategy: Have students provide endings to statements such as the following:

> I like the way I look because . . .
>
> Sleep is . . .
>
> I take care of my eyes by . . .
>
> If I lost my sense of hearing, . . .
>
> Sitting, standing, and walking with good posture help to . . .
>
> Lack of exercise makes me . . .

Materials Needed: none

Processing Question: How important do you think it is to take care of your personal health?

Decision Stories: Body Systems

Present decision stories such as the following to the class. Follow the procedure discussed in Chapter 4, pages 80–83, for using the stories as a values clarification activity.

RITA'S DILEMMA

Grades (5–6)

Rita comes from a large, loving family. She has three brothers and four sisters. Her family is poor, but her parents do the best they can. After studying about body systems in class, Rita is aware that it is important to have regular physical exams to make sure that the body is functioning properly. She is now in the fifth grade but hasn't seen a doctor since kindergarten. Rita knows her parents are having a hard time taking care of all the children. There never seems to be enough money to live on. Rita is feeling fine and has only missed one day of school this year (because of a cold).

Focus Question: Should she mention anything to her parents about getting a checkup?

MARY'S FATHER

Grades (K–3)

Mary's father smokes tobacco cigarettes. Mary has just learned how important the heart and lungs are for the proper functioning of the body.

Focus Question: How can Mary tell her father about the bad effects on her father's and her own body from his smoking cigarettes?

Decision Stories: Personal Health

Present decision stories such as the following, using the procedures outlined in Chapter 4, pages 80–83.

VISION PROBLEMS

Grades (K–2)

Kathy is the youngest member in her family. She has two older brothers. Both her parents and her brothers wear eyeglasses. Kathy has felt sorry for them because she thinks that glasses make people look funny, and they seem to be such a nuisance. You can't run or play games as easily because they are always falling off. Kathy has just found out that she needs glasses, too, and she is having trouble getting used to the idea.

You are a good friend of Kathy's. You have perfect vision and don't wear eyeglasses. You sense that Kathy is feeling sorry for herself and feeling jealous of your good vision.

Focus Question: What would you say to Kathy?

FITNESS DECISION STORY   Grades (3–5)

You have been invited to spend the afternoon with two different friends. You like both friends equally. One friend wants to spend the afternoon playing his new video game. The other friend wants to go rollerblading in the park.

Focus Question: Which activity do you do, and why?

TEETH AND TRUTH   Grades (K–2)

It's been over a year since Danny has been to the dentist. Danny knows that his mother forgot about his regularly scheduled dental appointment because he answered the phone when the hygienist called to remind them about the appointment. He didn't tell his mother because he didn't want to go back, but, for the last few weeks, one area of Danny's mouth has been feeling funny every time he eats. Danny hates going to the dentist. He is also afraid that he will be punished if he tells his mother what he did.

Focus Question: What should Danny do? Why?

THE CHRISTMAS PARTY   Grades (4–5)

Elizabeth's teacher has asked her to be in charge of the fifth-grade Christmas party in her classroom this year. This is really an honor for Elizabeth, and she wants to do everything just right—but Elizabeth cannot eat sugar, and most of the holiday treats are loaded with it. Elizabeth thought of maybe having a "sugarless Christmas party" with lots of vegetables and dips and other foods without sugar, but she is really worried that the other students would turn up their noses at this idea. She certainly doesn't want the party to be a flop.

Focus Question: What do you think she should do?

Dramatizations: Body Systems

Have students dramatize different body systems as if they actually were the body system in question. Be creative in developing these activities. The following examples may be helpful.

DRAMATIZING THE   Grades (4–5)
CIRCULATORY SYSTEM

Valued Outcome: The students will be able to describe the function of the circulatory system.

Description of Strategy: The students will dramatize how the heart and blood work together. Sixteen students will be required for this activity. Three students will represent the blood, four for valves, two for ventricles, two for atria, two for the venae cavae, one for the aorta, and one each for the pulmonary artery and pulmonary vein. Have the students stand in the proper position of a heart. Have the "blood" follow the proper path of blood through the heart's structure.

Materials Needed: none

SENSES ACTIVITY   Grades (4–5)

Valued Outcome: Through role-playing the students will have a better understanding of what a person without a sense or senses experiences.

Description of Strategy: Select two or three role-players by picking numbers. Describe a setting in which one of the players does not have one or two of the five senses. Give brief instructions on the situation (such as a blind person crossing a road) being reenacted in the skit. At the end of each skit, take five to ten minutes to discuss questions such as: What happened? Why did it turn out the way it did? Did it turn out the way you thought it would?

Materials Needed: none

Processing Question: What important roles do the senses play in our lives?

CIRCULATORY SYSTEM   Grades (3–5)

Valued Outcome: The students will identify the major organs of the circulatory system.

Description of Strategy: Introduce the organs of the circulatory system by showing an overhead transparency from an anatomy book and briefly describing what each one does. Divide the class by eye color and reassemble students in the form of the circulatory system of a person (lying down) using the different groups as different organs. Using red and blue beanbags to represent oxygenated and deoxygenated blood, respectively, start a rotation of the beanbags through the different groups or organs. During this process explain how each organ does its job. Rotate the groups until everyone has played all the organs of the circulatory system. Reassemble the students into their regular class formation, and ask questions about each organ and its function. Use the transparency as a guide. Make sure that everyone has answered at least one question.

Materials Needed: overhead transparency of circulatory system organs, red and blue beanbags

Processing Question: How do the organs of the circulatory system clean the blood that circulates through the human body?

SOURCE: South Carolina State University 2002

DIGESTIVE SYSTEM   Grades (3–5)

Valued Outcome: The students will identify the major organs of the digestive system.

Description of Strategy: Introduce the organs of the digestive system by showing an overhead transparency from an anatomy book and briefly describing what each one does. Divide the class by birth months and reassemble students in the basic form of the digestive system, using the transparency as a reference. Use beanbags as food particles and start a progression of the food through the system. Start with the mouth group and instruct them to pass the food on to the next organ until the food exits the body. Ask questions of each group about what their job is in the digestion process. Rotate the groups until everyone has played all the organs of the digestive system. In closing, reassemble the students into their regular class formation, and ask questions about the separate organs and their functions. Use the transparency as a guide. Make sure that everyone has answered at least one question.

Materials Needed: overhead transparency of digestive system organs, beanbags

Processing Question: How would your life be different if your digestive system did not work properly?

SOURCE: South Carolina State University 2000

EXCRETORY SYSTEM   Grades (4–5)

Valued Outcome: The students will identify the major organs of the excretory system.

Description of Strategy: Introduce the organs of the excretory system by showing an overhead transparency from an anatomy book and briefly describing what each one does. Divide the class by shirt color and them reassemble the students in the form of an excretory system using the different groups as different organs. Use colored water to represent different liquids. During this time the teacher may ask questions of the different groups pertaining to their organ's operation or contribution to the system. Rotate the groups until everyone has played all the organs of the excretory system. In closing, reassemble the students into their regular class formation, and ask questions about the separate organs and their functions. Use the transparency as a guide. Make sure that everyone has answered at least one question.

Materials Needed: overhead transparency of excretory system, different colors of water in small sealed jars

Processing Question: How do organs of the excretory system break down fluids into components that our body can consume and discard the rest in the form of waste?

SOURCE: South Carolina State University 2000

THE NERVOUS SYSTEM
Grades (4–5)

Valued Outcome: The students will be able to describe the function of the nervous system.

Description of Strategy: Tell students that they are going to act like the parts of the nervous system that send and receive information or signals. Form the class into a circle, with each student standing arm's length apart. Have them cup their hands in front of them to form a "mailbox." Drop a message in one student's pouch and have that student pass the message along to the student to his or her right, and so on. Explain that the students are acting as the sensory nerve pathways. Stop the message by tapping a student on the head. This student represents the brain. The "brain" then passes the message to the next student on his or her right, an so on. Explain that the students are acting as motor nerve pathways. Stop the message again by tapping a student on the head. This student represents an effector (muscle or gland). The student then reads the message, which gives a command such as to touch your toes or stand on one leg. Everyone follows the directions. Send additional messages, indicating that the class is functioning like the nerve pathways and brain of the nervous system.

Materials Needed: bits of paper for the nerve messages

Processing Question: What role does the nervous system play in helping our bodies function?

INSIDE-OUT
Grades (4–5)

Valued Outcome: The students will be able to illustrate, through creative writing, the functions of different body systems.

Description of Strategy: Divide the students into groups of five, and ask each group to write a fantasy play about a girl or boy who is able to travel through a human body and meet different body systems along the way. You should serve as a resource, but avoid giving too much direction, thus stifling creativity. Have the students perform their plays, with one acting as the traveler and the others representing body systems or specific organs.

Materials Needed: paper, pencils

Processing Question: How are the body systems positioned in the body?

Dramatizations: Personal Health

TANNING BOOTHS
Grades (4–5)

Valued Outcome: The students will be able to explain the hazards of tanning booths.

Description of Strategy: Instruct the students to work in small groups and write a script about tanning booths. One group could role-play a conversation between a potential customer and a tanning parlor attendant about the safety precautions practiced by the salon. Another group could enact a situation in which a customer fails to follow proper precautions in the tanning booth. A third group could role-play a person who seeks counsel from a dermatologist after several visits to the tanning booth.

Materials Needed: pencils and paper

Processing Questions:

1. What are the dangers to the skin and other body systems from exposure to tanning booths?

2. What are the proper precautions to follow when using tanning booths?

WEARING BRACES   Grades (4–5)

Valued Outcome: The students will be able to verbalize the benefits of wearing dental braces.

Description of Strategy: Have a student role-play the part of a parent who is trying to convince his or her child (another student) of the benefits of wearing dental braces. Another dramatization regarding braces could involve one student role-playing a child who wears braces to school for the first time and another student reacting to the braces with ridicule.

Materials Needed: none

Processing Questions:

1. What are the benefits of wearing braces?

2. How can a person be prepared to handle ridicule from friends when he or she is wearing braces?

IMMUNIZATION   Grades (3–5)

Valued Outcome: The students will be able to explain the importance of immunizations and will advocate getting needed immunizations.

Description of Strategy: Read and discuss the story *The Berenstain Bears Go to the Doctor* by Stan and Jan Berenstain. This book describes Sister and Brother Bears' well-patient visit to the doctor. The reason for using this book is to describe what each student may have experienced when he or she went to the doctor for a well-patient visit and to explain what an immunization shot is. After reading the story, ask questions such as "Have you ever gone to the doctor when you were not sick?" Explain that this is called a well-patient visit. Also ask, "What did the doctor do when you went for a well-patient visit?" Possible responses include that the doctor listened to the student's heart and breathing; looked at eyes, ears, and throat; weighed or measured the student; gave a shot; or did blood work. Ask students why the doctor would give a shot to someone who wasn't sick. Explain that these types of shots are called "immunizations" and they help protect people from illnesses. Point out that people used to die of different illnesses, but now doctors immunize children so that they can never get these illnesses. Also mention that sometimes it takes more than one shot to protect against an illness. Have students role-play doctor visits. Provide them with doctor kits and let them role-play well-patient visits. Be sure they include immunizations as part of the visit. Explain that the exams they role-play will be done over clothing and that nobody should remove any clothing.

Materials Needed: *The Berenstain Bears Go to the Doctor* (Berenstain and Berenstain 1981a), toy doctor kits for students, a picture of a syringe or a child getting a shot

Processing Questions:

1. What immunizations have you had?

2. What does the word *immunization* mean?

SOURCE: Health Strategies, Inc. 2002a

Discussion and Report Techniques: Body Systems

SENSE OF TOUCH   Grades (K–3)

Valued Outcome: Students will identify different ways and reasons we use our sense of touch and describe how things feel using their sense of touch.

Description of Strategy: Introduce the sense of touch by walking around the room with a rock and having the students touch it and describe what they feel. Explain to the students that they are using one of their five senses, the sense of touch. Tell them that we use our skin and hands to touch objects. Read the book *Touching and Feeling* by Henry Pluckrose. This book tells about the different textures of things, how we sometimes use our sense of touch to send messages to others, and how blind people and puppies use their sense of touch to see. This book also gives descriptive words for things we touch.

Pass out an assortment of objects (such as cotton balls, sandpaper, apples, oranges, bananas, and marshmallows). Explain that you will choose students one at a time to describe what the object in front of them feels like when they touch it. Encourage them to use the descriptive words from the book. Collect the objects from the students. Tell them that the sense of touch is important to our daily lives. Explain that it is important for them to let someone know if they cannot feel something they touch because something may be wrong.

Materials Needed: *Touching and Feeling* (Pluckrose 1998), objects that have different textures, an example of braille text

Processing Questions:

1. How do we use our sense of touch in daily life?

2. What are some words you might use to describe things we touch?

THE SENSE OF SIGHT   Grades (K–2)

Valued Outcome: The students will name the eyes as the body part related to the sense of sight.

Description of Strategy: Begin the game of "I see." Have the class move to music. Occasionally stop the music. When the music stops, students should freeze, staring straight ahead. Ask one student, "What do you see?" The student answers by describing one thing that is in his or her line of frozen vision (or what color he or she sees). The rest of the students have three tries to guess what the object is.

Materials Needed: music to accompany the game "I see," chart paper

Processing Question: How can you protect your eyesight?

SOURCE: Ezell 1992, 83–84

IDENTIFYING LEAVES (SIGHT)   Grades (3–5)

Valued Outcome: The students will be able to describe what their eyes are used for and how different life would be without sight.

Description of Strategy: The class will go outside, and each student will pick three different types of leaves off trees or bushes and bring them inside. When all the students get back in the classroom, have them spread out their leaves across their desks. Each student will then be blindfolded and will be asked to feel the leaves and try to find some differences between them. After a few minutes, the students will take off their blindfolds and write down the differences between leaves 1, 2, and 3. They will then look at each individual leaf and visually compare the differences between leaves. The students need to record on a piece of paper all of their comparisons and then present their observations to the rest of the class. After each student's presentation, ask him or her which experiment was easier to do: the one using their eyes or the one blindfolded? Record the answer of each student on a piece of paper.

Materials Needed: blindfold for each child, various leaves, pencils, and paper

Processing Question: Why are our eyes important?

SOURCE: Mace-Matluck and Hernandez 1993

LEARNING ABOUT THE FIVE SENSES   Grades (2–3)

Valued Outcome: The students will be able to identify situations that use the five senses.

Description of Strategy: In a group activity with the students sitting closely, discuss briefly the five senses: sound, sight, smell, taste, and touch. The students will go back to their seats and have a matching quiz. The quiz would be set up like this.

Word Bank

sound   sight   smell   taste

Fill in the Blank:

1. When you look at a bird, you are using your sense of _____.
2. When you bite into a sour lemon, you are using your sense of _____.
3. When you feel the roughness of a tree, you are using your sense of _____.
4. When you listen to the beat of a drum, you are using your sense of _____.
5. When you identify the scent of a candle, you are using your sense of _____.

Materials Needed: matching quiz and pencils for each student

Processing Questions:

1. How many senses do humans have?
2. Can you use all of your senses at once?

VIRTUAL BODY   Grades (4–6)

Valued Outcome: After searching the MEDtropolis Web site (*www.medtropolis. com/Vbody.asp*), students will be able to discuss each of the body systems' functions and to use various activities to demonstrate the different functions.

Description of Strategy: Have students search the Web site during class time. They will complete one group activity and make a presentation to the class. The group will create the activity, and each student must have an equal part to do. Some examples of activities they can do are making clay models of the body parts in their particular body system and explaining what that body part does. They could also play a game like Jeopardy. If four students are in a group, then three group members could be the contestants and the other group member could be the host. When presentations are finished, have two different groups get together and test each other on what they learned about the other group's body system.

Materials Needed: computers with Internet access, list of materials as compiled by students

Processing Questions:

1. What is the purpose of the respiratory system?
2. What two organs are located in the digestive system?

SOURCE: MEDtropolis 2002

REVIEW OF THE SENSES   Grades (3–5)

Valued Outcomes: The students will be able to explain what the senses do and how they work together.

Description of Strategy: Name some things that you enjoy. Have the students give examples of what they enjoy. Show the class pictures that illustrate the senses and have students recall what senses are stimulated and how they work together. Divide the class into five groups. Give each group a piece of construction paper and assign each one a sense. Have the students draw or cut out pictures from magazines then glue them on the construction paper. Tell them to write captions about the pictures. Then have each group explain the senses related to each picture and give us one way to care for and protect that sense.

Materials Needed: pictures illustrating the senses, magazines, five pieces of construction paper, markers, scissors, glue

Processing Questions:

1. How does each sense work?
2. How should you care for each of the senses?
3. How can you protect each sense?

THE FIVE SENSES   Grades (K–2)

Valued Outcome: The students will identify the five senses and the body part associated with each.

Description of Strategy: Introduce the five senses by reading to the class one of the many excellent books available on the topic. Introduce each sense by pointing to the body part that accompanies it. Point to one body part at a time and, as a group, have the students say the sense that is related to that body part. Teach the word *sense.* Display large posters of the senses throughout the room while teaching this unit. Tell the students that this week, while learning about our senses, they will put together a book of senses to put in their portfolio and take home to their parents at the end of the week.

Materials: book about the five senses; large posters of the senses

Processing Questions:

1. Which sense is involved in smelling a flower?
2. Which sense is involved in picking up a coin?
3. Which sense helps us watch the clouds?
4. Which sense helps us hear the music?
5. Which sense helps us enjoy food?

SOURCE: Ezell 1992, 81

MY FIVE SENSES

Grades (3–5)

Valued Outcome: The students will be able to describe how often they use their senses every day.

Description of Strategy: Begin by going outside to take a walk. Ask students to pick a partner to talk to about their experiences on the trip (this will help them remember more details from their trip). Walk for twenty minutes. After the walk, have the students brainstorm about their experiences with their partner on a piece of paper. Have students form into groups of four. Give each group seven minutes to brainstorm their ideas, then have each group describe one of their experiences to the rest of the class. Then have the students get back with their partners and identify the following from their original list: three experiences for sight, three for hearing, three for touch, three for smell, and three for for taste. Provide magazines and scissors, and ask students to cut out examples of people using their five senses.

Materials Needed: pencils and paper, magazines, scissors

Processing Questions: Can you name something you do every day that uses each of the five senses?

SOURCE: Mace-Matluck and Hernandez 1993

WHICH ORGAN AM I?

Grades (4–5)

Valued Outcome: The students will be able to identify the different organs of the body.

Description of Strategy: Make large cards with the names of one organ printed on each. Distribute cards to several students and have them stand in front of class wearing or holding his or her card. Have each student describe the job of his or her organ in the body. This activity could be used for just one system by naming parts of one system rather than organs.

Materials Needed: large cards with names of one organ on each

Processing Question: What are the specific jobs of each body organ?

BODY SYSTEMS MATCHING

Grades (4–5)

Valued Outcome: The students will match each body system to its function.

Description of Strategy: Prepare a worksheet from the following list and hand out copies to each student. Have students write the correct numbers of the body systems from the work bank in the blanks by the body system definitions. Tell them to use each number once and look for key words to help them.

1. skeletal system	4. urinary system	7. digestive system
2. muscular system	5. respiratory system	8. endocrine system
3. circulatory system	6. nervous system	9. reproductive system

_____ separates **liquid waste** from the blood and removes it from the body

_____ is made up of glands that make hormones that help us **grow** and **reproduce**

_____ makes **egg** cells in women and **sperm** cells in men

_____ breaks **food** down into small pieces that can move into the bloodstream

_____ carries food and oxygen to all parts of the body through the **bloodstream**

_____ **supports** and **protects** the body

_____ is made of **nerves** that carry messages throughout the body

_____ works with the bones to **move** the body

_____ contains the **lungs** that bring oxygen into the body and take carbon dioxide out of the body

Materials Needed: worksheet, pencils

Processing Questions:

1. What are the nine body systems? their functions?

2. How do the body systems work together to keep the body going?

SOURCE: National Center for Health Education 1996, 10

TRACING BODY SYSTEMS   Grades (3–5)

Valued Outcome: The students will identify, describe, and diagram parts of various body systems.

Description of Strategy: The students are divided into groups of four to five. Assign each group a body system (skeletal, digestive, respiratory, muscular, circulatory, and so on). Each group receives a six- to eight-foot piece of bulletin board paper. One student lies down on the paper while the other group members trace the outline of his or her body. Once the body is traced, the students work cooperatively to diagram their assigned body system. Groups may choose to draw directly on the paper or cut and paste parts individually. You can make this project as detailed as you wish. You may have the group write a report and/or have them make a presentation explaining functions of individual and/or specific parts to the rest of the class on their assigned body system.

Materials Needed: six- to eight-foot pieces of bulletin board paper, scissors, markers, crayons, glue, white and colored paper, resource materials with diagrams for each system

Processing Question: Why is it important to know how the body's systems work together?

HEALTHY SKIN   Grades (3–5)

Valued Outcome: The students will be able to explain why it is important to keep their skin safe and healthy.

Description of Strategy: Ask students to think of ways in which skin can be hurt or damaged. List their ideas on the board. For each item on the list, ask the students to identify one way of preventing or treating the damage (moisture cream, suntan lotion, and so on). Explain to students that they will visit a Web site to learn more about caring for their skin. Arrange students in pairs. Go to the Here's looking at you . . . Healthy Skin Web site (BioRAP 2000). Ask students to read the facts about skin damage protection, and then have them work in pairs to discuss some of the most common ways people can damage their skin.

Materials Needed: computers for accessing the Internet, board, markers

Processing Question: What are some preventive measures people can take to protect their skin?

SOURCE: BioRAP 2000

EFFECTS OF SMOKING ON THE LUNGS   Grades (3–5)

Valued Outcome: The students will discuss the negative effects of smoking cigarettes, especially the effects smoking has on the lungs.

Description of Strategy: Discuss with students the effects of cigarette smoke on human lungs. Have students find statistics of smoking related to the human body. Show the students pictures of human lungs damaged by cigarette smoke and pictures of healthy human lungs of nonsmokers. Have the students divide into small groups and make a list of positive and negative effects of smoking. The students then will discuss and compare their lists with the rest of the class.

Materials Needed: paper, pencils, resource material and statistics on smoking, pictures comparing lungs of a smoker and a nonsmoker

Processing Questions:

1. What is the job of our lungs?
2. What are the effects of smoking cigarettes?
3. What will happen to a person who smokes over a long period?

HOW DOES THE HEART WORK?   Grades (K–2)

Valued Outcome: The students will understand the concept of circulation: Blood is pumped through tubes (blood vessels) through the body and back to the heart, and the heart beats faster when you exercise.

Description of Strategy: On the board or on chart paper, draw a picture of a train with an engine and at least two cars. Draw tracks under the train, extending in both directions. Ask students to identify the picture and describe what a train does. Explain that a train's job is to transport. It picks up things at one place, carries them along a route, and delivers them to another place. Write the word *blood* on one train car. Ask the students, "How is the circulatory system like a railroad?" Tell them to imagine that the train is the blood. Encourage students to extend the analogy. The tracks are the blood vessels; the stations along the route are the heart, lungs, and body. The circulatory system carries and delivers blood to all parts of the body following a particular route, just as the train carries and delivers goods to stations along its route. Display a poster of heart anatomy (available from the American Heart Association). Explain that the blood follows a certain route each time it returns to the heart. Point to and name the four chambers of the heart as you describe the route that the blood travels: right atrium, right ventricle, lungs, left atrium, left ventricle, rest of body. Encourage students to say the names with you.

Then give students a handout with a picture of the heart on it (found on page 197). Have them use the poster to help trace the route that the blood travels as it passes through the heart. Ask the students why oxygen is important. Ask them what carries oxygen all around the body. Also, ask them what happens to the heart if it needs more oxygen. Show the students how to place a stethoscope to listen to their own hearts. Then ask them to work with a partner to listen to each other's hearts. Have partners take turns using the stethoscope, counting the number of beats in one minute. Have them listen to their own hearts, count the beats in one minute, and write the number down.

Next, have the students jump up and down for one minute. Have them listen to their own hearts, count the number of heartbeats in one minute, and write down the number.

Materials Needed: board or chart paper, drawing utensil, large picture of the heart anatomy, handout with a picture of the heart for each student, stethoscopes, clock or a watch with a timer

Processing Questions:

1. Why is oxygen important?
2. What happened to your heart rate when you exercised?
3. What happened to your heart rate when you ate or after walking?

SOURCE: American Heart Association 1996, 39

TRACING THE BLOOD FLOW   Grades (4–5)

Valued Outcomes: The students will be able to describe the path of blood through the heart, the parts of the heart, and how to care for the circulatory system.

Description of Strategy: Instruct the students on the path of blood through the heart. Provide them with a copy of the diagram of the heart found on page 197 to help them understand the pathway of the blood in the heart. On this worksheet, have students trace the pathway with their fingers; they should be able to say what part of the heart the blood flows through as they trace the pathway. Then have them label the parts of the heart. Have them shade blue the sections of the heart that transport blood carrying carbon dioxide (deoxygenated blood) to the lungs and shade red the sections that carry blood with a fresh supply of oxygen (oxygenated blood) from the lungs to the body.

Materials Needed: diagram of the heart

Processing Questions:

1. What is the main job of the circulatory system?
2. What are the main components of the blood?
3. What are the main structures of the circulatory system?

MUSCULAR SYSTEM DEBATE   Grades (4–5)

Valued Outcome: The students will identify the importance of voluntary and involuntary muscles and be able to give examples of each kind of muscle.

Description of Strategy: Divide the class into two groups for a debate. One group will argue that voluntary muscles are the most important to the human body, and the other group will contend the involuntary muscles are most important. Each group should have several minutes to get its arguments ready and should be able to support its particular muscle group with specific examples of a muscle and its function. After the debate, provide time for a rebuttal from the other group.

Materials Needed: paper, pencils

Processing Question: How does the importance of voluntary muscles compare with involuntary muscles?

VOLUNTARY HEALTH   Grades (4–5)
ORGANIZATION PANEL

Valued Outcome: The students will identify organizational purposes and duties of such voluntary health organizations as the American Heart Association, the Kidney Foundation, and the American Lung Association.

Description of Strategy: Invite representatives from several voluntary health organizations that deal with a specific organ or body system, such as the Heart Association, Kidney Association, and Lung Association, to address the class. Their presentations should be geared to the age of the students and should include facts about each organization's founding, purpose, and projects. Use a panel discussion format.

Materials Needed: none

Processing Question: How do voluntary health organizations help promote our health?

Discussion and Report Techniques: Personal Health

PRESENTATION BY HEALTH PROFESSIONALS

Grades (K–5)

Valued Outcome: The students will be able to identify the duties of various health professionals.

Description of Strategy: Invite various health professionals (such as a dentist, orthodontist, optometrist, ophthalmologist, or audiologist) to address the class, describe their occupation, and inform students about sound personal health practices in their field.

Materials Needed: none

Processing Question: How do health professionals help promote our health?

SCREENING PROCEDURES

Grades (4–5)

Valued Outcome: The students will list and describe a screening procedure used in school systems.

Description of Strategy: Prepare an outline of the various screening procedures that are commonly used in school systems. Include screening measures that may not be available in your school but are used widely. Ask each student to choose one procedure and write a report about it. Collect the reports and collate them into a screening procedure booklet that can be used as a resource.

Materials Needed: outlines of screening procedures to hand out to students

Processing Questions:

1. What screening procedures are used in your school?
2. What occurs during each screening procedure?

HEALTH RISKS FROM NOT RELAXING

Grades (1–3)

Valued Outcome: The students will identify the health risks involved with not relaxing.

Description of Strategy: Ask the students if they remember learning anything about relaxation. Allow a few students to answer. Say, "We've learned about what happens if you do relax, and we've also practiced ways to relax. Now, we'll learn about what happens if you do *not* relax. These things are called 'risks.'"

Write "trouble sleeping" on the board. Explain that if people are tense, their body can't relax enough to fall asleep. Some people have a hard time sleeping because they can't stop thinking about their problems. Explain different situations in which sleeping could be difficult, such as if parents are fighting or a favorite animal has just died.

Write "getting upset for little or no reason" on the board. Remind the students that if you don't get rid of stress in a healthy way, such as deep breathing, it will build up. This stress buildup may make us angry or upset, and we yell at people we love and hurt their feelings. Point out that sometimes parents have a stressful day at work. When they come home it's easy for them to act upset at their child, forgetting that it's not their child's fault they had a stressful day.

Write "can lead to drugs" on the board. Explain that when people don't know how to relax, they sometimes turn to drugs. Drugs may make them feel better for a while, but won't fix their problems. Sometimes these people begin to take more drugs, which can lead to an addiction.

Write "bad health" on the board. Explain that when your body is under a lot of stress, it has to work harder. If that stress is rarely released, it can cause the body to wear out more quickly, like a car. If people do not take care of their cars and fix them when they break down, then the cars wear out more quickly.

Reread each phrase on the board. Ask the students if they have any questions. Close by saying "Everybody has stress in their lives. The reason we have been learning about it is so that you can deal with it in a healthy way and avoid the risks we talked about."

Materials Needed: board or overhead projector, writing utensils

Processing Questions:

1. What are some different ways that people respond to unreleased stress?

2. Why is relaxing an excellent way to relieve stress?

SOURCE: Dauer and Pangrazi 1998, 290–291

SLEEPING AND RELAXING   Grades (3–5)

Valued Outcome: The students will be able to describe how sleep and relaxing affects their personal health.

Description of Strategy: Describe what happens to the body during sleep—activity decreases, the muscles relax, and the heart beat slows down. To illustrate this, have students count their own heart beat. Then have them lay down and relax for ten minutes in complete silence. After ten minutes have passed, have the students count their heart beat again. Discuss the difference between the two heat rates and how important rest and sleep are for the body. Explain that sleep restores energy to to keep their bodies healthy, and helps control muscles. Explain how those who go without sleep can lose energy, be quick tempered, easily distracted, and make many mistakes. Finally, have students write a paragraph on how sleep affects their health.

Materials Needed: clock, pencils and paper for each student

Processing Questions:

1. Why is sleep necessary?

2. Describe what happens to the body if deprived of sleep.

3. What happens to the body during sleep?

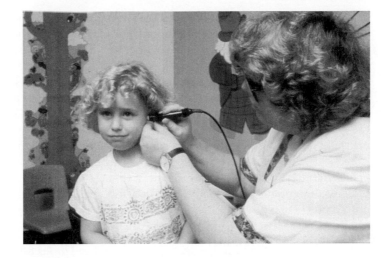

Periodic health screening will aid a child's ability to learn.

GOALS FOR PERSONAL APPEARANCE   Grades (3–5)

Valued Outcome: The students will be able to describe what they should do every day to keep their personal appearance at its best.

Description of Strategy: Have each student write "Goals for my personal appearance" at the top of a piece of paper. Then have them list ten things they should do to improve or maintain their personal appearance. Tell the students to hang their lists somewhere in their homes so they can read them every day.

Materials Needed: paper and pencils

Processing Questions:

1. Why is it important to set goals?
2. What are the most important things you should do every day for your personal appearance?

CARE OF EYES AND EARS   Grades (4–5)

Valued Outcome: The students will explain why it is important to take care of the eyes and ears and identify ways to take care of them.

Description of Strategy: Discuss sight and hearing. Have students write a paragraph on each of the following topics: why sight is important, what they would miss if they couldn't see, why hearing is important, and what they would miss if they couldn't hear. Ask students to share their responses. Identify and discuss ways to care for the eyes and ears. Explain that they should not touch the eyes with unclean hands, they should wear sunglasses with both UVA and UVB protection when outdoors, they should wear protective glasses when playing certain sports, and they should avoid loud sounds for long periods of time. Explain that noise is loud if you have to shout to make yourself heard above it. Also explain that damage can occur after as little as 15 minutes of exposure to loud noises so it is important to wear earplugs when exposed to loud sounds for long periods of time. If possible, have an audiologist or optometrist visit the class to test students' sight or hearing.

Write the words Hearing and Sight on the board; make sure to leave enough room for the students to list aids in each column. Ask the students to brainstorm things that help people with sight or hearing problems. Possible responses for the eyes may include braille, Seeing Eye dogs, eyeglasses, contact lenses, or beeping traffic signals, and for the ears may include hearing aids, sign language, or icons on traffic signals. If possible, give the students a chance to experience braille and sign language. Display a chart of the sign language alphabet. Teach students to sign something simple, such as "I love you," or their name. Distribute samples of braille writing. Darken the room, or have the students close their eyes and feel the letters.

Materials Needed: paper and pencils, board or overhead projector and markers, a chart of the braille alphabet and some samples of braille writing, a chart of the sign language alphabet

Processing Questions:

1. Why is it important to get a vision test and a hearing test?

2. How can blindness occur?

3. How can deafness be prevented?

SOURCE: Health Strategies Inc. 2002c

DENTAL HEALTH   Grades (1–2)

Valued Outcome: Students will be able to describe the experience of losing their first tooth.

Description of Strategy: Start by reading the book, *Franklin and the Tooth Fairy* by Paulette Bourgeois. (Franklin is a turtle who loses his first tooth and meets the tooth fairy.) Talk about how Franklin felt when he lost his first tooth, and what it might be like if the students lose a tooth. Ask the students who has had a visit from the tooth fairy.

Make necklaces for students who lose their teeth at school. Have the students write the words "I lost my tooth today" on tooth-shaped white construction paper, then hole punch the top of the tooth and string a ribbon through it. Collect the necklaces; throughout the year if a student loses a tooth, have him or her wear the necklace for the day.

Materials Needed: *Franklin and the Tooth Fairy* (Bourgeois 1996), construction paper cut into the shape of a tooth, hole punch, ribbon

Processing Questions:

1. What were your feelings when you lost your first tooth?

2. Describe our parents' reaction to your first lost tooth?

SOURCE: Johnson 1997, 15–22

Valued Outcome: The students will be able to explain the importance of a wellness lifestyle and will also be able to name some things they can do to develop this type of lifestyle.

Description of Strategy: Talk to the students about how a healthy lifestyle will improve their lives. Give examples of how their diet affects their health and examples of how their exercise habits affect their health. Hand out all materials to the students. Have each student cut out a heart shape from red or pink poster board, write his or her name on it, and use yarn to tie the heart shape from the center of the top wire on a wire clothes hanger. Have each student cut out a long rectangle that will hang directly from the bottom wire of the hanger. On this piece have students write "My Wellness Lifestyle." The students will cut shapes from remaining poster board. On each shape they will write what they can do to develop their wellness lifestyle (for example, walking, eating fruits). Each student will share his or her mobile with the rest of the group and tell what options he or she used. When all students have shared, hang the mobiles in the classroom as a reminder of the things they can do to improve their health.

Materials Needed: wire clothes hanger, colored yarn, colored poster board (at least seven different colors, including red or pink), markers, scissors, hole-punch

Processing Question: What behaviors can you incorporate in your lifestyle to improve your health?

Experiments and Demonstrations: Body Systems

BODY DRAWINGS   Grades (3–5)

Valued Outcome: The students will trace the outline of their bodies on a large sheet of paper and label the internal body systems. The students will weigh and measure their bodies.

Description of Strategy: Have the students work in pairs, and have the first student trace around the second student's body while the second student is lying down on a large sheet of paper. Then switch and repeat the process. Each student may then draw and label the internal body systems. On the reverse side, under each body system heading, have the students list at least two reasons why the system is important to general health. You may also wish to weigh and measure the students, and let them use the body drawings to keep up with these measurements throughout the school year. Tack the completed body drawings on the wall, interspersing the body parts side of some with the written side of others.

Materials Needed: butcher paper, markers, scale, measuring tapes, pencils

Processing Questions:

1. How is body weight determined?
2. How tall is each individual?
3. What is the relative significance of each body system?

BODY SYSTEMS BEING   Grades (3–5)

Valued Outcome: The students will participate in the construction of a "body systems being" to demonstrate an understanding of how each body system works and how they work together to maintain a healthy body.

Description of Strategy: An outline of a human form should be traced on a piece of butcher paper and pinned up so that the class can see it. This should be about the size of an average person in the class. Introduce the activity by explaining the following project goals to the class:

1. The class will construct an entire human model during the next nine class periods (or time modifications you need to make).
2. This model will have all the body systems.
3. All the body systems will be made out of construction paper and will fit inside the outline of the human form.
4. The organs should be shaped like the actual organs and placed properly in the form.
5. The class will be divided into groups, and each group will be responsible for constructing one body system.
6. Each group will conduct research on its appointed body system. Resources should be available in the classroom, and students should be encouraged to do research outside of class as well.
7. Each group also will be responsible for creating a detailed presentation to the class about the body system. This should include how the system works, what it does, details about each organ in the system, and some interesting facts discovered during the research.
8. The final product should be a life-size model of the human body with all the systems placed over each other inside the form.
9. Each group will be responsible for deciding among its members all tasks necessary to construct the system and prepare the presentation for class.
10. Each of the groups will name its model, which will be on display in the room during and after construction.
11. A plan explaining how the group tasks will be divided should be agreed on during the first group meeting.

12. At the beginning of each class period, the class will meet as a whole during the first two to five minutes. During this time, the teacher will appoint a day leader for each group. Then each group will meet to discuss tasks for the day. During the last five to seven minutes of the class period, materials should be cleaned up and resources put back.

13. Each group member should report his or her progress to the day leader, who will record progress in the group activity log. A poster entitled "Duties of the Day Leader" should be posted and referred to daily and includes the following:

- to write down each of the group members and what they will be doing that day in the log
- to keep group members on task
- to report progress at the end of the period in the group activity log
- to submit the group log to the teacher at the end of the period
- to make sure the group has cleaned up well

Divide the class into seven groups with approximately the same number of participants per group. Assign each group a body system and appoint a day leader each day. Each group will be given a notebook to use as a group activity log. (This activity is an excellent way to incorporate cooperative learning in the classroom.)

Materials Needed: a large piece of butcher paper (approximately three feet by six feet), several reference books about the body systems, construction paper in a variety of colors, colored markers, scissors, glue, tape, poster of "Duties of the Day Leader"

Processing Questions:

1. What are two ways the body systems work together to maintain a healthy body?

2. Choose two organs, and describe how they work.

3. Which body system did your group present? What was one new thing you learned about that body system?

SOURCE: Bentley 1995, 245–247

BONE TRANSFORMATION   Grades (4–5)

Valued Outcome: The students will familiarize themselves with the bones and how they are used.

Description of Strategy: To begin this activity, discuss the shapes of the bones and the purpose of those shapes, using real bones. Hand out a copy of a drawing of a bone to each student and have him or her cut it out and place it in any position on a piece of paper. Working in groups of of three or four, have the students discuss and list many different and unusual things bones could become. Each student illustrates a bone development or bone growth on his or her own piece of paper. When the students are done with their transformations, have them discuss and share them with class.

Materials Needed: real bones for examples, copies of a drawing of a bone for each student, pencils, crayons, drawing paper

Processing Questions:

1. Why do bones have to be certain shapes to perform their functions?
2. Why is the shape of the bone important?

BRAIN VIEWING   Grades (4–5)

Valued Outcome: The students will compare the parts of an animal brain to that of a human brain.

Description of Strategy: Obtain the brain of a sheep or cow. Have students compare the parts of the animal brain to those of a human brain, using a model of the human brain for the comparison.

Materials Needed: sheep or cow brain, model of human brain

Processing Question: Compare the animal's brain to the human brain with regard to size and shape.

NERVE MESSAGES   Grades (4–5)

Valued Outcome: The students will demonstrate how nerve impulses work.

Description of Strategy: Have students rub their finger across coarse sandpaper, then explain how the nerves in the fingers send messages to the brain and the limbs.

Materials Needed: sandpaper

Processing Question: How does the nerve send messages to the brain and then to the limbs?

JOINT EXPERIMENT   Grades (4–5)

Valued Outcome: The students will be able to differentiate between the types of joints in the skeletal system.

Description of Strategy: This will introduce joints into the lesson. There will be six stations that will be completed in order. Each station has a simple experiment and questions.

> **Station 1: Hinge joints**—Have the students open and close the classroom door or a closet door. They must watch the hinges closely. Have them name a part of their body that moves like a hinge.

Station 2: Ball-and-socket joints—Have the students hold a tennis ball against the concave bottom rim of a cup (or even the top rim as long as it has a smaller diameter than the ball). Rotate the cup over the ball's surface. Have them name a part of their body that works like a ball-and-socket joint.

Station 3: Sliding joints—There will be a zipper at this station (at least twelve to eighteen inches long). Have the students bend the zipper and move it in curving patterns. (Do not unzip the zipper.) A sliding joint works with several bones bending together. Have them name a sliding joint area.

Station 4: Pivot joints—A globe will be at this station. Instruct the students to spin the globe. A pivot joint rotates around an axis. Can the students think of an area of their body that pivots?

Station 5: Fixed joints—This station will have two pieces of paper glued together. These papers do not move or slide. There are bones in our body that do not move; they are fixed in one place. Have the students name one.

Station 6: No joints—Have the students walk without bending their legs. Have them write their names without bending their fingers. What other things would be hard to do without joints?

Materials Needed: access to a hinged door, cup, zipper, globe, paper glued together

Processing Question: What would happen to our bodies if we didn't have joints?

SOURCE: Calvert County Public Schools 2002

EARS HELP US HEAR   Grades (4–5)

Valued Outcome: The students will be able to explain the importance of hearing.

Description of Strategy: Explain the structure of the ear using a visual (model, poster, etc.) of the ear. Take the students outside and listen to the sounds. Record the sounds heard outside, and brainstorm other sounds. Shake two tin cans, one with only one or two marbles in it and one with several marbles in it. Have students listen and identify which one has more marbles and why. Have students complete a short essay on their favorite sound.

Materials Needed: an ear visual (model, poster, etc.), tape recorder, marbles, two tin cans

Processing Question: Explain the importance of hearing in your everyday life.

SEEING IS IMPORTANT   Grades (K–5)

Valued Outcome: The students will be able to analyze the importance of sight and experience blindness.

Description of Strategy: Explain the structure of the eye using a visual aid (model, poster, etc.). Pass out individual mirrors and have the students look at their eyes. Have students draw the color of their eyes. Have each student place the frames from a pair of glasses on their eyes and look at himself or herself in the mirror.

Discuss taking care of your eyes. How did it feel to wear glasses? Discuss eye exams. Discuss what it is like to be blind. Place the students in groups of two; one student wears a blindfold while the other student leads him or her around the classroom.

Materials Needed: an eye visual (model, poster, etc.), mirrors, paper, crayons or markers, eyeglass frames, blindfolds

Processing Question: If you were blind, how would your life be different?

PROPERTIES OF SKIN   Grades (K–3)

Valued Outcome: The students will examine the skin of the foot and its properties.

Description of Strategy: Ask students to take off a shoe and a sock so that one of the feet is bare and one is covered with a sock. Have them feel the difference between their skin and the sock covering the other foot. Let them notice the cooling reaction and why one foot feels cooler than the other does. Ask them to pull on the skin covering their foot and feel if some places are more sensitive than others.

Have each student trace his or her foot on a white sheet of paper and mark with a red marker which places are more sensitive. On the back of the paper, have each student write why they think one foot is cooler than the other.

Materials Needed: red markers, white paper, pencils

Processing Question: Why is it important to keep the hands and feet covered in cold weather?

FOLLOW YOUR NOSE   Grades (K–5)

Valued Outcome: The students will be able to describe the importance of smell.

Description of Strategy: Place four film containers on a table. Put a cotton ball with a different scent in each container. Have the students smell each container. The students guess what each smell is by selecting the correct picture (lemon, cinnamon, or peppermint).

Materials Needed: film containers; cotton balls; scented extracts such as lemon, cinnamon, or peppermint; pictures of items the extracts are derived from

Processing Question: How does the nose help us smell?

TOUCH—HANDS ONLY

Grades (K–5)

Valued Outcome: The students will be able to identify sensory descriptors, including smooth, rough, hard, soft, cold, and warm.

Description of Strategy: Provide objects with various textures and have students handle them. Then ask them if all the objects feel the same. Ask the class to give some examples of what the different objects feel like. Introduce the words *rough, smooth, soft, hard, hot,* and *cold,* and give examples of each so that students can begin to associate words with concrete examples. Divide the class into three groups, and place each group at a station. At each station, have every student touch the objects or substance there. The three stations are:

> **Station 1: Mystery boxes**—Place three or four mystery boxes on a table with smocks for students to wear. Each box should have the lid on with a hole cut out of the side of the box so that students can put their hands in the box without seeing inside it. Have the students put their hands in as many of the boxes as they want and then describe what it feels like inside the box. If students want to make a guess about what each item is, allow them to do so.

> **Station 2: Hot and cold**—Put cold water in a bucket, lukewarm water in a second bucket, and hot water (but not too hot) in a third. Have students put one hand in one bucket and one hand in another bucket and then describe how each feels and how it compares with the other. Have the students use different combinations of buckets.

> **Station 3: Textured paper**—Place various kinds of paper or fabric on a table so that students can pick up each and feel the texture of it. Have enough different examples so that everyone in the group will be able to participate without having to wait. Ask students to describe how each feels, and how it compares to it and the others.

Once all the students have been to each station, give them paper and crayons to make a page on touch. Encourage students to include things they just touched at one of the stations and to think of a word that describes what they felt like when they touched it.

Materials Needed: shoe boxes to be used as "mystery boxes"; items to go in the mystery boxes, such as wet noodles, whipped cream, Jell-O, or peanut butter; three small buckets, large enough for students to put one hand in; smocks; various kinds of textured paper or fabric with smooth and rough surfaces, such as wallpaper scraps, sand paper, or scraps of velvet or satin; construction paper; crayons

Processing Question: How do our hands help us feel?

SOURCE: University of Richmond 2000

Experiments and Demonstrations: Personal Health

TEETH PROBLEMS   Grades (4–5)

Valued Outcome: The students will demonstrate proper dental hygiene.

Description of Strategy: Discuss with students the various problems (such as cavities, root canals, loss of enamel, false teeth, and so on) that could occur from not taking care of their teeth. Discuss and list on the board or on an overhead transparency the proper steps for taking care of their teeth:

- Brush teeth after every meal.
- Use dental floss after brushing teeth.
- Rinse mouth with mouthwash.
- Take regular trips to the dentist.
- Limit the amount of sugar you consume.

Have each student copy these steps as a reminder of the proper dental hygiene procedures. Distribute toothpaste and a toothbrush to each student. Invite a dentist or dental hygienist to demonstrate the proper techniques for brushing teeth.

Materials Needed: board or overhead projector, markers, paper, pencil, toothpaste, and a toothbrush for each student

Processing Question: What are the proper steps for good dental hygiene?

TEETH AND DIGESTION   Grades (4–5)

Valued Outcome: The students will identify the roles that teeth, saliva, and digestive enzymes play in chewing.

Description of Strategy: Give students a saltine. Have them chew it without swallowing and note what happens. Explain that teeth grind food. At the same time, saliva and digestive enzymes in the mouth act on the food. Students should note how the taste of the cracker sweetens as this happens. The chewed cracker is being changed to a moist bolus so that it can be swallowed easily.

Materials Needed: saltine crackers

Processing Question: What significant part do the teeth play in digestion?

SHADOW PLAY   Grades (3–5)

Valued Outcome: The students will demonstrate the difference between proper and improper posture.

Description of Strategy: The purpose is to gain an understanding of various postural defects and practice posture improvement. The materials you will need are a shadow screen (a bedsheet may be used), lights, and equipment necessary for holding up the sheet. This is an excellent way for students to compare and dramatize good and bad posture. Act as the narrator and discuss various aspects of maintaining good posture while standing, sitting, walking, and reading. As you discuss each posture, one student standing behind the screen will demonstrate poor posture while another demonstrates proper posture. The roles of the shadow casters can be changed so that all students participate.

Materials Needed: shadow screen (bedsheet), lights, equipment to hang shadow screen (clothes pins, wire, etc.)

Processing Questions:

1. What part does posture play in overall personal health?
2. How does poor posture affect the function of internal organs?

FINGERPRINTS   Grades (K–5)

Valued Outcome: The students will compare fingerprints and recognize the different configurations of each.

Description of Strategy: Provide students with white paper and a stamp pad. Have them press their fingertips on the stamp pad and then on the paper. Ask students to label the resulting fingerprints with their names. Then let them compare each other's prints to see that no two patterns are exactly the same. Discuss the anatomy of the skin ridges that form fingerprints (and footprints).

Materials Needed: stamp pad, white paper

Processing Questions:

1. Why do we have ridges on the fingertips?
2. Why do we each have unique fingerprints?

PUPIL DILATION AND CONSTRICTION   Grades (3–5)

Valued Outcome: The students will describe the difference light plays on the dilation and constriction of the pupil of the eye.

Description of Strategy: Pair students and have them face one another so they can see their partner's eyes. Tell them to look at their partner's pupils for a few seconds and observe their pupil size. Then, at your signal, ask all students to close their eyes and not to reopen them until you tell them. Explain that on your signal, they are to open their eyes and look quickly at their partner's pupils. Give the signal after about forty-five seconds, and have the students note the constriction of the pupils on being exposed to light.

Materials Needed: none

Processing Question: What is the purpose of the dilation of the pupil?

SOUND LOCALIZATION   Grades (3–5)

Valued Outcome: The students will understand that having two ears, one on each side of the head, helps us perceive sound direction more accurately than if we only had one ear.

Description of Strategy: Pair students. One student is blindfolded and sits in a chair. The other student, who acts as the "tester," stands nearby and taps a pencil against a glass. The blindfolded student points to the direction he or she believes the sound is coming from. Have the tester move to several locations throughout the room, sometimes holding the glass high above the floor and sometimes holding it low. Repeat this with several other students to note differences. Also do the experiment with several blindfolded students who have one ear plugged, to note differences in sound localization ability.

Materials Needed: blindfolds, glass jars or drinking glasses, pencils

Processing Questions:

1. How does sight enable the sense of hearing?
2. How does sound enhance the quality of our lives?

SLEEP NEEDS   Grades (4–5)

Valued Outcome: The students will identify different needs for sleep with regard to age groups.

Description of Strategy: To demonstrate the varying needs for sleep at different ages, have students interview several people of different ages (such as siblings, peers, parents, grandparents). Instruct them to write down the names and ages in chronological order by age. Have them report on the different needs for sleep for people of different ages.

Materials Needed: paper, pencils

Processing Questions:

1. How much sleep does the student need?
2. Why do sleep needs vary at different stages of life?

HEALTH HABITS   Grades (3–5)

Valued Outcome: Students will identify four simple health habits, explain the need to stay healthy, and demonstrate simple health habits.

Description of Strategy: Demonstrate the proper care of teeth, skin, hair, and nails. For the care of teeth, show how to properly brush and floss. For the skin, show how to use soap and water to wash the hands. For the hair, show how to brush or comb the hair. For the nails, demonstrate how to use a nailbrush to scrub underneath the nails and how to use fingernail clippers. After demonstrating each technique to the class, introduce the idea of a health fair to students and allow them to suggest what they need to plan for one. Have the students set up the health fair in the classroom. Possible suggestions include labeling and setting up four separate areas with signs and providing items needed for care of teeth, skin, hair, and nails (have parents help out with the health fair and see what the children have learned about how they can take care of themselves). Tell the students that in order to prevent the spread of communicable diseases they should not share their toothbrushes, chewing gum, comb, or brush. The students should go to each station and properly demonstrate the particular technique for that station.

Materials Needed:

> **Teeth station**—cups (paper or plastic), water, toothpaste, a mirror, and a basin. Bring extra *new* toothbrushes so that each student can have his or her own to practice the activity.
>
> **Skin station**—a basin of water, mild soap, and paper towels.
>
> **Hair station**—a mirror. Students with their own comb or brush could use this area. Make sure to have a pack of *new* combs to pass out to the students who forgot to bring their own.
>
> **Nails station**—have a basin of water, soap, nail cutter, and nailbrush.

Processing Questions:

1. What do we do to take care of our bodies?
2. What health habits can prevent the spread of communicable diseases?

SOURCE: Bajah and IICBA Organization 2002

COVERING SNEEZES AND COUGHS   Grades (K–1)

Valued Outcome: The students will identify the importance of covering sneezes and coughs and will demonstrate how to avoid spreading germs when they cough or sneeze.

Description of Strategy: Discuss germs. Explain that certain germs in our body may make us sick. Tell students that germs are too tiny to see, but they can be spread from one person to another. Discuss how to care for people with illness and the importance of preventing illness from spreading. Some discussion points should be that medicine helps to fight off germs so people feel better and that it is important to try not to let the germs go to anyone else's body.

Discuss the ways germs spread. Ask students to brainstorm some ways that germs can get from one body to another. Possible responses include breathing on someone, coughing on someone, sneezing on someone, or touching someone after they have touched something with germs on it. Demonstrate how germs may travel. Put warm water in a spray bottle set to very fine mist. Stand back from the class and spray the air above students to show how far a sneeze or cough can reach. Ask students to raise their hands if they felt any water. Tell students that is how far germs can go when someone sneezes or coughs.

Some discussion points should be to instruct the students to feel the area around them. Ask the students if the water only landed on them. The answer should be no. Ask the students if their hands got wet. Ask what would happen if, instead of water in a spray bottle, that was a real sneeze or cough. Possible answers include "we would get covered in germs" or "the area around us would get covered in germs." Another point of discussion should include how students can keep their sneezes and coughs from reaching other people. Discuss ways to avoid spreading germs. Discuss the steps to take if you have to sneeze or cough. Have students practice these steps. First, get a tissue; second, cover your mouth or nose; third, cough or sneeze; and finally, throw the tissue away. Teach the students this rhyme and have them act out each step as they say it: "May I have a tissue, please, to cover my mouth and nose? I need to cough or sneeze, and then, away it goes!"

Materials Needed: facial tissues, spray bottle filled with warm water

Processing Questions:

1. What should you do to avoid spreading germs when you cough or sneeze? Why is this important?

2. What are some ways to spread germs other than coughing or sneezing?

3. Why is it important to wash our hands after using the restroom?

SOURCE: Health Strategies Inc. 2002b

DAILY WATER INTAKE   Grades (K–5)

Valued Outcome: The students will be able to describe how much water they should drink each day (one quart).

Description of Strategy: Make the following statements about water and the ways it helps your body:

- Water in blood helps it flow through the body, carrying nutrients and oxygen.
- Water helps cool our bodies when we sweat.
- Water helps our bodies remove wastes.
- Our bodies need at least a quart of water each day to replace water that it uses.

Place the students in pairs. Each pair needs either a 4-ounce glass, an 8-ounce bottle of water, a 32-ounce pitcher of water, or a 16-ounce thermos. Each group also needs a quart-size container filled with water. Have the groups measure out how many of their containers equal one quart of water. Record their answers on a worksheet. Have four groups work together to complete the worksheet. Display a picture of bottled water, watermelon, fruit juice, celery, lettuce, and a tomato. Ask students which foods are sources of water (all of them). Have students cut out pictures of foods that are sources of water. Have each student make a collage.

Materials Needed: one quart of water for every two students, worksheet; 4-ounce water glasses, 8-ounce bottles, 32-ounce pitchers, and 16-ounce thermos for each group of eight students; picture of bottled water, watermelon, fruit juice, celery, lettuce, and a tomato; magazines, scissors, and construction paper for collages

Processing Questions:

1. What is the value of drinking water instead of other drinks?
2. How do you know if you are drinking enough water each day?

SOURCE: Health Strategies, Inc. 2002c

GERMS   Grades (K–2)

Valued Outcome: The students will be able to explain that germs are smaller than the eye can see but are still destructive.

Description of Strategy: Ask the students, "What is a germ? Why is it important to wash your hands?" Divide the class into three groups. Have each student put a small amount of hand lotion on his or her hands and rub them together. Have each student sprinkle a small amount of glitter into their hands while holding them over a bucket. Tell them to spread the glitter over their hands. Let the students know that the glitter represents the germs. Have the first group try to rub the glitter off with a dry towel. Have the second group wash the glitter off with cold water only, and the last group wash their hands with warm soapy water. Then have everyone wash his or her hands in warm soapy water. Explain to the students that if they wash their hands every hour, they can prevent illnesses and bacterial infections.

Materials Needed: glitter, paper towels, hand lotion, bucket, hand soap, access to sinks or to tubs of warm soapy water and cold water

Processing Questions:

1. What was the best method for getting the germs (glitter) off?
2. Why is it important to properly wash your hands?

SOURCE: A to Z Teacher Stuff 2002a

AEROBIC AND ANAEROBIC ACTIVITIES   Grades (3–5)

Valued Outcome: The students will be able to distinguish between aerobic and anaerobic activities so that they can participate in those activities that would benefit their endurance.

Description of Strategy: Review the meaning of *aerobic* (something you can do for a long time), *anaerobic* (something that makes you out of breath), and *couch potato* (nonintellectual, sitting activities). Give each student a picture of a sport or activity (indicate on the picture whether it is aerobic, anaerobic, or couch potato), and a three-column handout labeled with each category. Designate three places around the room with signs that say "aerobic," "anaerobic," and "couch potato." Have each student get up and act out the activity; the other students guess the activity by raising their hands and allowing the demonstrator to call on them. After the students guess the activity, say "Go," and have the students stand under the sign that they think best represents the type of activity. Have the demonstrator say what kind of activity it is, and give each student who is in the correct place a sticker to put on his or her handout under the correct heading. Many of the activities could be aerobic or anaerobic based on the intensity of the activity. Explain this to the students. If a student can explain why he or she chose aerobic over anaerobic (or visa versa), let him or her also have a sticker.

Materials Needed: pictures of activities (one for each student in your room); large signs with the words *aerobic, anaerobic, couch potato;* stickers; three-column handout with anaerobic, aerobic, and couch potato headings for each student

Processing Questions:

1. Can you distinguish between activity types?
2. Which activities are better for your health?

FLOSSING TEETH   Grades (K–5)

Valued Outcome: The students will be able to explain why dental flossing is important in the care of their teeth and use yarn or twine to show how to hold dental floss as they pretend to floss their teeth.

Description of Strategy: Show students different kinds of dental floss. Explain that flossing is important to keep gums and teeth healthy and to remove food that gets trapped between teeth. Tell them that they should floss their teeth at least once a day. Give each student a piece of yarn. Compare the yarn to the floss by listing similarities and differences (size, color, shape, etc.). Show students how to wrap it around their fingers, and have them pretend to floss their teeth with it. Be sure to tell them that at home they should have an adult helping them.

Materials Needed: different kinds of dental floss, yarn, or twine cut into twelve to fourteen inch lengths

Processing Questions:

1. What do you need to do to take care of your teeth and gums?
2. What adults can help you take care of your teeth?

FOUR KINDS OF TEETH   Grades (K-2)

Valued Outcome: The students will be able to name the four kinds of teeth (incisors, cuspids, bicuspids, and molars) and describe the purpose for each type.

Description of Strategy: Create worksheets for each of the four types of teeth and label them. Hand out one set of worksheets and four pieces of paper to each student. Explain that there are different types of teeth, each one with a name and a job to do. Have students hold up the incisors worksheet. Explain that the incisors are located in front of the mouth and have sharp, chisel-shaped crowns that cut food. Have them cut a sheet of paper with scissors, simulating what their incisors do to food. Next, have them hold up the cuspids worksheet and explain that there is one cuspid next to each incisor. Cuspids are pointed to help tear food and are sometimes called canine teeth; have the students tear the paper. Next, have students hold up the bicuspids worksheet and explain that there is one bicuspid (or premolar) located next to each cuspid. Bicuspids crush and tear food; have the students act like they are crushing and tearing the paper. Have the students hold up the molars worksheet. Explain that molars grind food; have the students act out the molars' job by grinding and smashing the paper.

Materials Needed: four tooth cutouts per child, four pieces of paper and one pair of scissors for each child

Processing Questions:

1. What role do the cuspids play in eating?
2. What role do the biscuspids play in eating?

SOURCE: Sevaly 1997, 83–98

AIRBORNE SUBSTANCES AND ALLERGENS   Grades (4–5)

Valued Outcome: The students will identify airborne substances that can affect people and will be able to explain how allergens affect the body.

Description of Strategy: Fold paper plates in half and make them into the shape of a chick. Tell the students that each chick went on a picnic and many of them feel sick. Have students decorate the paper plate to look like a chick. Then spread petroleum jelly over all the chicks and put them on the floor. Using green glitter and a blow-dryer, blow "pollen" (the green glitter) onto the chicks. Observe which of the chicks that went on the picnic are suffering from allergies; those chicks will be the ones with "pollen" all over them. Have the students guess which chicks suffered the most from the pollen.

Materials Needed: paper plates, scissors, construction paper, green glitter, petroleum jelly, blow-dryer, crayons

Processing Questions:

1. Why are some people allergic to foods and other people are not?
2. What does the word *allergic* mean?

SOURCE: Santiago 2002

DENTAL HYGIENE   Grades (2–3)

Valued Outcome: The students will be able to describe what is good and bad for your teeth.

Description of Strategy: Ask the students about their first visit to the dentist and how they felt about it. Ask if they felt scared and nervous. Talk about what they think is good and bad for their teeth, and ask them what they think will happen if they do not brush their teeth, and how they can keep their teeth in good shape. Read the book *Berenstain Bears Visit the Dentist* by Stan Berenstain and Jan Berenstain and talk about Brother and Sister Bears' visit. What happened to them? What did the dentist say about their report on their teeth.

Explain to the students that they will be doing an experiment. Tell them that the hard-boiled egg represents their teeth. The soda in the cup represents all the bad things for their teeth. Have each student drop his or her "tooth" into the soda. Ask them what they think will happen if the tooth is left in the soda overnight. Have the students write a sentence or two about the first time they went to the dentist. Have them illustrate their sentences so they can hang the drawings around the room. Tell the students that tomorrow they will see what has happened to their tooth. Distribute toothbrushes and toothpaste to each student.

Materials Needed: *Berenstain Bears Visit the Dentist* (Berenstain and Berenstain 1981b), one hard-boiled egg for each student, toothbrushes for each student, toothpaste, a cup for each student, paper and pencils, dark soda

Processing Questions:

1. Is it normal to be scared and nervous on the first visit to the dentist?
2. What will happen if you do not brush your teeth?

SOURCE: A to Z Teacher Stuff 2002b

DEMONSTRATION OF CORRECT BRUSHING

Grades (3–5)

Valued Outcome: The students will demonstrate, in front of the class, the importance of brushing their teeth.

Description of Strategy: Define plaque as a type of tooth germ. Use a mouth model and "invisible" (clear plastic) plaque tiles to demonstrate how plaque builds up after eating without brushing and flossing. Tell the students that these plaque germs damage teeth by making holes called cavities. Use the mouth model, toothbrush, floss, and plaque tiles to demonstrate that brushing and flossing will rid teeth of plaque. Instruct the students to take turns brushing and flossing the mouth model. Have the students explain how brushing removes plaque from teeth.

Have students chew the red "plaque" tablets that show where plaque is on teeth and, looking in a classroom mirror, observe where the darkest red stains are on their teeth. Pass out a toothbrush and a trial size toothpaste to take home for practice.

Materials Needed: large model of set of teeth, large toothbrush, dental floss or colored yarn, toothbrushes and toothpaste for each child, plaque tiles (clear plastic), red "plaque" tablets

Processing Questions:

1. What is the correct way to brush your teeth?
2. Why is it necessary to brush regularly and correctly?

SOURCE: Merritt 2002; Smoak 2002

Puzzles and Games: Body Systems

BODY PARTS PUZZLE
Grades (4–5)

Valued Outcome: The students will correctly put together a puzzle of organs of the different body systems.

Description of Strategy: Divide the students into groups. Provide each group with a sealed package containing body parts made of construction paper and a large piece of paper that has the outline of the human body on it. At your signal, the groups open their packets and place the body parts where they should be on the paper. Record the amount of time it takes each group to complete its puzzle. With the same groups, repeat this activity a few days later and record the time again. Have students compare their timed results to see if they improved.

Materials Needed: construction paper cut into shapes of organs of different body systems, butcher paper with outline of human body, timer or clock, paper and pencil for teacher

Processing Question: What is the correct placement of body parts within the body?

THE SOUND MATCHING GAME
Grades (K–5)

Valued Outcome: The class will play a game to help them understand that many different sounds can sometimes sound a lot alike.

Description of Strategy: Fill two film containers with rice, two with beans, two with water, and so on for all the materials listed under Materials Needed. Place them on a table so that pairs are not next to each other. Explain how we use our ears. Then have the students shake the containers and listen carefully to the sound. Ask them to match up pairs that sound the same. Once the children have played the game, they can peek inside the containers to see if their answers are correct.

Materials Needed: twenty film containers, rice, beans, water, popcorn, dry cereal, sand, gravel, crumbled dried leaves, marbles, paper clips

Processing Question: What is the most important function of our ears?

I SEE
Grades (3–5)

Valued Outcome: The students will be able to describe the sense of sight and explain how to protect the eyes from injury.

Description of Strategy: Begin with a game of "I See." The class moves to music. When the music stops, the students freeze and stare straight ahead. Point at something and ask a student to describe what he or she sees without actually naming it. Have the other students guess what the object is (give them three guesses). Repeat this a few times; try asking them to describe a color. Gather the students; discuss why we have eyes and ways they keep us safe—for example, seeing oncoming traffic. Make a chart of ways to protect the eyes from injury. Include the fact that the eyes have eyelashes, eyelids, and tears for protection.

Materials Needed: CD music, CD player, chart paper, markers

Processing Question: How many ways do our eyes and our sense of sight help us in everyday life?

BODY ORGANS GAME   Grades (4–5)

Valued Outcome: The students will be able to describe the organs of the body and their functions.

Description of Strategy: Have students study the organs in a human body and focus on their functions. Then conduct a game similar to a spelling bee. The students stand as you go around the room in order. Each student is given the name of a body organ and asked to tell the function, or vice versa. If the answer is wrong, the student sits. The game ends when one person is left standing.

Materials Needed: none

Processing Question: What are the major body organs and their functions?

MEMORY GAME   Grades (4–5)

Valued Outcome: The students will repeat a sequence of movements to test their memory skills.

Description of Strategy: This game allows the students to see how the brain can store and use information. Divide the class into teams. Read several body actions, such as "touch your nose," "touch your toes," and "clap your hands." Each team takes turns to see how many actions can be followed in the sequence you read before members of the team become disorganized.

Materials Needed: list of sequences of body actions

Processing Question: How does the brain store information?

BEAN BAG TOSS   Grades (4–5)

Valued Outcome: The students will identify endocrine glands and their hormones while tossing a bean bag through holes in a cardboard box.

Description of Strategy: Cut several holes in the bottom of a large cardboard box. Label each hole with the name of a different endocrine gland and secure the box against the wall. Each student has three chances at tossing a bean bag through the holes. Score one point for getting the bag into the hole and two points if the student can name one function of the gland or one of the hormones it secretes. Each function or hormone may be identified only one time. Tally scores and announce the winners. Repeat this game periodically; make sure to change the order so that students who were first during the previous game have to go last, and vice versa.

Materials Needed: cardboard box, bean bags, scissors, marker

Processing Questions:

1. What is the function of each gland in the endocrine system?

2. What is the function of the each of the hormones secreted by these glands?

BLOOD JEOPARDY   Grades (3–5)

Valued Outcome: The students will play a game by matching parts of the blood with statements about the circulatory system.

Description of Strategy: Using an overhead projector and transparencies, write short statements about various parts of the blood and/or circulatory system. Divide students into teams and have them guess which part of the blood to which the statement applies. Various numbers of points can be awarded according to the difficulty of the statement.

Materials Needed: overhead projector, transparencies, overhead markers

Processing Question: What are the various functions of the blood?

Puzzles and Games: Personal Health

TAKE TIME FOR PERSONAL HEALTH   Grades (4–5)

Valued Outcome: The students will list different roles, functions, and health practices associated with various components of personal health.

Description of Strategy: Divide students into groups, and assign each group a different component of personal health, such as care of the hair, skin, teeth, eyes, or ears, and the need for exercise, sleep, and relaxation. Allow the groups two minutes to list as many roles, functions, or health practices associated with that component as they can. Read each list for accuracy and determine which group won the round by having the most accurate statements. Play several more rounds; explain that each time listings must be different. See not only which group can list the most per round, but also which group is able to list the most at the end of the game.

Materials Needed: none

Processing Questions:

1. What are the roles and functions of the hair, skin, teeth, eyes, and ears?

2. What are the personal health habits needed for each of these organs in order for the body to work efficiently?

Other Ideas: Body Systems

RESPIRATORY SYSTEM TRAVELOGUE   Grades (4–5)

Valued Outcome: The students will learn the parts of the respiratory system by being guided through an imaginary trip of that system.

Description of Strategy: Draw a diagram of the respiratory system on a chart or overhead transparency. Take the class on an imaginary trip through the respiratory system. You are the tour guide. Use props and tour guide dialogue. This activity can be used for any body system.

Materials Needed: chart or overhead transparency with writing utensils, various props to represent the lungs and organs of other body systems

Processing Question: How does the respiratory system move air through the body?

BODY BUILDERS   Grades (K–3)

Valued Outcome: The students will construct Popsicle-stick figures simulating bones, muscle, and skin.

Description of Strategy: Have each student make a character with "bones," "muscles," and "skin." Popsicle sticks provide the frame; yarn wrapped around sticks represents muscles; and cloth scraps serve as skin. Additional features can be added to give each model some unique characteristics.

Materials Needed: Popsicle sticks, yarn, cloth scraps

Processing Question: How do the bones, muscles, and skin work together to make the body more efficient?

Other Ideas: Personal Health

DRESSING FOR THE WEATHER   Grades (K–2)

Valued Outcome: The students will understand that dressing appropriately for the weather can prevent illness.

Description of Strategy: Make an extra-large boy paper doll and an extra-large girl paper doll along with an accompanying and varied wardrobe for all kinds of weather. Let the students take turns each day dressing the dolls appropriately for the day's weather or for different seasons.

Materials Needed: paper dolls, doll clothes

Processing Question: How can we dress appropriately for weather in order to prevent illness and/or discomfort?

IMMUNIZATION RECORD   Grades (4–5)

Valued Outcome: The students will list their immunization records.

Description of Strategy: Have each student make a chart listing his or her immunization record. Suggest that students should be proud to know that they have contributed to their own health by undergoing these immunizations.

Materials Needed: paper, pencils

Processing Questions:

1. Why is it important to maintain an immunization record?
2. Why is it important to get immunizations?

Resources

BOOKS

Archambault, J., B. Martin, and T. Rand. 1991. *Here are my hands.* New York: Henry Holt.

Armstrong, B. 1999. *Squeaky clean hygiene.* Huntington Beach, CA: Creative Teaching Press, Inc.

Balestrino, P., and T. Kelley. 1989. *The skeleton inside you (Let's read and find out).* New York: Harper Trophy.

Berger, M., and P. Meisel. 2002. *Why I sneeze, shiver, hiccup, and yawn.* New York: Harper-Collins Children's Books.

Brewer, S. 1996. *DK pockets: Body facts.* New York: DK Publishing.

Brown, D. 1991. *The visual dictionary of the human body (Eyewitness visual dictionaries).* New York: DK Publishing.

Cole, J. and B. Degen. 1990. *The magic school bus: Inside the human body.* New York: Scholastic Trade.

Dacey, J., and L. Fiore. 2001. *Your anxious child: How parents and teachers can relieve anxiety in children.* Hoboken, NJ: John Wiley & Sons.

Demuth, P., and M. Smith. 1997. *Achool: All about colds.* Parsippany, NJ: Scott Foresman.

Ely, L. 2001. *Healthy food unit study: A guide for nutrition and wellness (Grades K–5).* Milwaukee: Champion Press, Ltd.

Greene, C., and P. Danny. 1998. *At the dentist: Field trip series.* Chanhassen, MN: Child's World.

Just the facts: The human body—major systems and organs. 2001. Goldhil Home Media.

Mayer, G., and M. Mayer. 1998. *This is my body: Little golden book (Little critter).* Golden Books.

Moses, A., and M. Moses. 1997. *At the hospital: Field trip series.* Chanhassen, MN: Child's World.

Nanao, J., T. Hasegawa, and A. Stinchecum. 1995. *Contemplating your bellybutton.* La Jolla, CA: Kane/Miller.

O'Brien, M., and F. Lee. 1999. *Healthy me: Fun ways to develop good health and safety habits: Activities for children 5–8.* Chicago: Chicago Review Press.

Ostrow, W., V. Ostrow, R. Sims, and A. Astrow. 1993. *All about asthma.* Morton Grove, IL: Albert Whitman & Co.

Pollock, M., and K. Middleton. 1994. *Elementary schools health instruction.* St. Louis: Mosby-Year Book.

Richard, D. 1997. *My whole food ABCs.* Ridgefield, CT: Vital Health Publishing.

Rosoff, I., S. Awan, and H. Melville. 2000. *My first body board book.* New York: DK Publishing.

Tudor, T. 1991. *First delights: A book about the five senses.* New York: Penguin Putnam.

Yagyu, G., and A. Stinchecum. 1998. *All about scabs.* La Jolla, CA: Kane/Miller.

continued

WEB SITES

General Health

About Health: *www.abouthealth.com*

Adolescence Directory OnLine (ADOL): *education.indiana.edu/cas/adol/adol.html.* See particularly the Adolescent Health Links *www.ama-assn.org/adolhlth/gapslink/gapslnk2.htm #ADOL*

Adolescent Health On-Line *www.ama-assn.org/adolhlth/adolhlth.htm*

American Cancer Society: *www.cancer.org*

CDC Prevention Guidelines Database *www.wonder.cdc.gov/wonder/prevguid/prevguid.htm*

Health Education Forum *www.libertynet.org/~lion/forum-health.html*

Kathy Schrock's Guide for Educators *www.capecod.net/Wixon/health/fitness.htm*

The Life Education Network: *www.lec.org*

PE Central *www.infoserver.etl.vt.edu/~/PE.Central/PEC2.html*

Physical Activity and Health: A Report of the Surgeon General *www.cdc.gov/nccdphp/sgr/sgr.htm*

Resources for School Health Educators *www.indiana.edu/~aphs/hlthk-12.html*

Exercise/Physical Fitness

CDC National Center for Chronic Disease Prevention and Health Promotion *www.cdc.gov/nccdphp/nccdhome.htm*

Fitness Issues: *www.inect.co.uk/nsmi/*

Fitness Links to the Internet *www.fitnesslink.com/links.htm*

Fitness World *www.fitnessworld.com/fitnews/news.html*

The Physical Activity and Health Network (PAHNet) *www.pitt.edu/~pahnet/*

Physical Education

American Alliance for Health, Physical Education, Recreation, and Dance (AAHPERD) *www.aahperd.org*

Educational and Community-Based Programs

CDC National Center for Chronic Disease Prevention and Health Promotion *www.cdc.gov/nccdphp/nccdhome.htm*

Health Resources and Services Administration *www.hrsa.dhhs.gov*

Healthy Cities Online: *www.healthycities.org*

Office of Minority Health Resource Center, Washington State Department of Health *www.doh.wa.gov*

Oral Health

American Dental Association: *www.ada.org*

CDC National Center for Chronic Disease Prevention and Health Promotion *www.cdc.gov/nccdphp/nccdhome.htm*

NIH National Institute of Dental Research *www.nidr.nih.gov*

Surveillance and Data Systems

Agency for Health Care Policy and Research Data and Methods *www.ahcpr.gov:80/data*

CDC National Center for Health Statistics *www.cdc.gov/nchswww/nchshome.htm*

CDC Scientific, Surveillance, and Health Statistics, and Laboratory Information *www.cdc.gov/scientific.htm*

CDC WONDER *wonder.cdc.gov*

General Sites

American Medical Association: *www.ama-assn.org*

MedicineNet: *www.medicinenet.com*

Medscape: *www.medscape.com*

Oncolink: *www.oncolink.upenn.edu*

ParentsPlace.com: *www.parentsplace.com*

Links Only

Hardin Meta Directory of Internet Health Sources *www.arcade.uiowa.edu/hardin-www/md.html*

CD-ROMS

The following CD-ROMs are available from IVI Publishing, 7500 Flying Cloud Drive, Eden Prairie, MN 55344.

The Virtual Body (Grades 4 and up)
A virtual exploration of the human body—a journey of exploration and discovery inside the human body that shows the body in action and explains even the most complex topics. Features include cross-sections and closeups of the human body,

answers to fifty-two of the most frequently asked questions (such as "How does a cut heal?" and "Why is blood red?"), and invaluable homework helper. Tested by students, adults, and educators. Available only in Windows.

Welcome to Bodyland (Grades K–5)
Join Ricki and Hiccup, her funny parrot friend, on an adventure through Bodyland theme park. Kids can learn about their skeletons as they stroll down Bony Boulevard. By visiting Dream Land, they'll understand why we dream at night. Teaches fundamentals of the human body. Features include fun and challenging games and activities, thirteen unique lands to explore (each with an original music theme), and a challenging quiz game reinforcing learning. Available in MacIntosh and Windows.

VIDEOS

The following videos are available from Sunburst Communications, 101 Castleton Street, P.O. Box 40, Pleasantville, NY 10570.

Looking Good, Feeling Good: (Grade 5)
Healthy You
Using catchy songs and fast-paced visual effects, this video shows students that when they eat a variety of wholesome foods; get enough exercise and rest; and take proper care of their skin, hair, and teeth, they not only improve their personal appearance, but also grow in confidence and self-respect. (17 minutes)

The New Improved Me: (Grade 5)
Understanding Body Changes
Gives young teens and preteens a supportive explanation of male and female body changes to help them accept puberty as an exciting and important event in their lives and a normal, healthy part of growing up. (23 minutes)

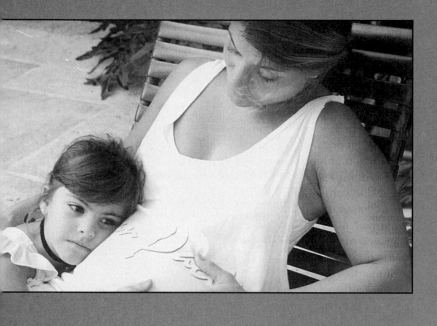

CHAPTER ELEVEN

Sexuality Education

A comprehensive sexuality education program respects the diversity of values and beliefs represented in the community and will complement and augment the sexuality education received from students' families.

—Sexuality Information and Education Council of the United States (2002a)

VALUED OUTCOMES

After reading this chapter, you should be able to:

- identify the goals of a sexuality education program
- discuss the social aspects of sexuality and family living
- discuss marriage, parenthood, and divorce
- trace the psychological development of sexuality
- describe the anatomy and physiology of the male and female reproductive systems
- explain the problems of family abuse and violence

After reading this chapter, reflect upon the type of training you believe an elementary education teacher would need to have in preparation for teaching sexuality education. Be specific in the type of content to be covered in the training. Do you think some type of certification is needed? What (if any) qualities does a teacher need to teach sexuality education? What should the emphasis be focused on at the elementary level?

Sexuality Education

Sexuality education is among the most controversial areas facing teachers. Many people view inclusion of this subject as an attempt to teach sexual technique and lower the morals of today's youth. Based on these concepts, sexuality education would involve little more than teaching the act of coitus. Sexuality education does deal with sexuality, but this is not the same thing as sex. Sexuality involves one's total being and identity. An effective sexuality education program seeks to develop an individual's sexuality, which includes an appreciation for self and the opposite sex, the ability to develop fulfilling personal and family relationships, comfort with sexual roles (mother, father, sister, brother, friend, wife, husband), recognition of bodily functions as related to reproduction, understanding how emotions play a part in sexual behavior, maturing attitudes toward the function of sex, the responsibility of being a member of a family, and, overall, a healthy attitude toward life.

The Sexuality Information and Education Council of the United States (SIECUS) says that "sexuality education is a lifelong process of acquiring information and forming attitudes, beliefs, and values about identity, relationships and intimacy" (SIECUS 2002b). The Council goes on to state that comprehensive school-based sexuality education that is appropriate to students' age, developmental level, and cultural background should be an important part of the education program at every age. The program should respect the many values and beliefs represented in a community and complement/augment the sexuality education received in the home.

The primary responsibility for teaching facts, attitudes, and values about sexuality should remain with the parents. However, there is frequently a gap between the education children receive about family life in their homes and their level of questioning, need, and interest. School is not the only source of information outside the home. Churches and other organizations can contribute significantly in this area. The school is an increasingly important contributor to education about family life. Before a family life curriculum can be taught, parental approval must be obtained. Most communities will support such a program if the school administration and community understand what is to be

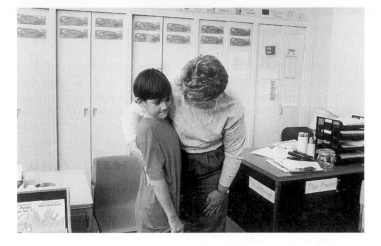

It is important that a positive self-image be developed if children are to grow to adulthood with the ability to respect others.

taught. This is the most important first step, which cannot be ignored if sexuality education is to be successful.

The appreciation for self must start early in life and be built on each year if children are to feel comfortable with their sexuality through the preadolescent, adolescent, and adult years. As should be emphasized in all aspects of health education, children must recognize that they will eventually have to accept the responsibility of their sexuality.

If society is not willing to promote comprehensive sexuality education, then that component of a student's total being will be shortchanged. Personal and social problems such as unwanted pregnancies, sexually transmitted infections (STIs), sexual unresponsiveness, and divorce will continue to plague society. A worthwhile educational effort in sexuality and family life must include social, psychological, moral, and biological components. In this chapter, these areas of concern are examined while providing the necessary overview of content for teaching sexuality education.

Implications for Sexuality Education

Few subjects in society evoke more discussion and controversy than sexuality education courses taught in our schools. It is amazing that one of the most significant aspects of our being is such a taboo topic. Humans are sexual from the moment they are born until well into old age. The adage that we are sexual beings from womb to tomb is certainly true. Although humans have learned a great deal about sexuality that can be taught in the educational process, we seek to repress and hide sex information and avoid discussing sexuality with our children. Many people believe that it is better to ignore unwanted pregnancies, the increasing rate of STIs, and the many misconceptions of the nation's youth.

There are basically two philosophical positions concerning sexuality education in our society. One group advocates comprehensive sexuality education, and the second group promotes the concept of abstinence-only education. Both positions stem not only from the desire to promote specific sexual ideologies and social visions, but also from each group's perception that the opposition represents a crucial component in an encroaching political movement. What is at stake is each group's visions of morality, family, and gender (Nelson 1996, 16).

Parents greatly influence the views their children hold concerning sexuality. Parents provide the young child with a basic orientation by the verbal and non-verbal messages they send concerning nudity, masturbation, sex values, and so on. If the message is that sex is shocking, dirty, or disgusting, this is transmitted to the child. These types of messages are likely to interfere with enjoyable healthy sexuality in the adult years. It is important to note that when children learn about sex and sexuality from their parents, the information is more likely to be accurate and positive than that learned from peers. Children are more likely to view sex as "dirty" or something to be "ashamed of" if learned from peers. Research indicates that adolescents who report good communication with parents are more likely to use contraception than those adolescents who report poor communication, and adolescents who receive sex education from their parents are more likely to behave in ways consistent with their knowledge.

The dilemma facing educators and schools is the teaching of abstinence versus responsibility. In question is whether schools should approach sexuality education from the perspective that all sexual problems can be avoided if students remain sexually abstinent, or if a more pragmatic approach should be followed, acknowledging that young people are going to be sexually active and that issues associated with such activity need to be discussed so sexual responsibility can be advocated. This latter approach fits well with the wellness approach and self-responsibility. However, since the early 1980s, a variety of abstinence education programs have been adopted by several states. In these curricula, students are taught chastity is the only answer and that premarital sex can only lead to disease, pregnancy, and emotional turmoil. Opponents of this approach point out that such views can cause extreme reactions toward sex. In addition, issues such as preventing pregnancy, HIV, and other STIs are not discussed in abstinence programs. Omitting such information from sexuality education is actually dangerous to the welfare of students. Most educators favor a middle position on teaching sexuality education: Abstinence is encouraged, but with the realization that students may have premarital intercourse and that they do need to be informed and responsible for protecting themselves from unwanted pregnancies and possible infection with HIV or some other STI.

Sexuality education must include an open learning atmosphere, improved materials, and improved training of educators. In addition, the curricular planning process, the implementation of the curriculum, training of the teachers, and multimedia materials should all be open to parents and the community for inspection and evaluation.

Health Highlight

STATE MANDATES
Sexuality Education and HIV/AIDS and STI Education

State	Mandate: Sexuality Education	Content: Abstinence	Content: Contraception	Mandate: STI Education	Mandate: HIV/AIDS Education	Content: Abstinence	Content: Prevention
AL	No	Required*	—	Yes	Yes	Required	Required
AK	No	—	—	No	No	—	—
AR	No	—	—	No	No	—	—
AZ	No	Required	—	No	No	Required	—
CA	No	Required*	Required	Yes	Yes	Required	Required
CO	No	Required	—	No	No	—	—
CT	No	—	—	No	Yes	—	—
DE	Yes	Required	Required	Yes	Yes	Required	Required
DC	Yes	—	Required	Yes	Yes	—	—
FL	No	Required*	—	Yes	Yes	Required*	Required
GA	Yes	Required*	Required	Yes	Yes	Required*	Required
HI	Yes	Required	Required	Yes	Yes	Required	Required
IA	Yes	—	—	Yes	Yes	—	Required
ID	No	—	—	No	No	—	—
IL	Yes	Required*	—	No	Yes	Required*	Required
IN	No	Required*	—	No	Yes	Required*	—
KS	Yes	—	—	Yes	Yes	—	—
KY	Yes	Required	—	Yes	Yes	Required	Required
LA	No	Required*	—	No	No	—	—
MA	No	—	—	No	No	—	—
MD[1]	Yes	—	Required	Yes	Yes	—	Required
ME	No	—	—	No	No	—	—
MI	No	Required	—	No	Yes	Required	Required
MN	Yes	—	—	Yes	Yes	Required*	Required
MO	No	Required*	Required	Yes	Yes	Required*	Required
MS	No	Required*	—	No	No	Required*	—
MT	No	—	—	No	No	— —	
NC	Yes	Required*	Required	Yes	Yes	Required*	Required
NE	No	—	—	No	No	—	—
NH	No	—	—	Yes	Yes	—	—
NJ	Yes	Required	Required	Yes	Yes	Required	Required
NM	No	—	—	No	Yes	Required	Required
NV	Yes	—	—	Yes	Yes	—	—
NY	No	—	—	No	Yes	Required*	Required
ND	No	—	—	No	Yes	—	—

State	Mandate: Sexuality Education	Content: Abstinence	Content: Contraception	Mandate: STI Education	Mandate: HIV/AIDS Education	Content: Abstinence	Content: Prevention
OH	No	—	—	Yes	No	Required*	—
OK	No	Required	—	No	Yes	Required	Required
OR	No	Required	Required	Yes	Yes	Required	Required
PA	No	—	—	No	Yes	Required	Required
RI	Yes	Required	Required	Yes	Yes	Required	Required
SC	Yes	Required*	Required	Yes	No	—	Required
SD	No	—	—	No	No	—	—
TN[2]	Yes	Required*	Required	Yes	Yes	Required*	Required
TX	No	Required*	—	No	No	Required*	—
UT	Yes	Required	—	Yes	Yes	Required*	Required
VA	No	Required*	Required	No	No	Required*	Required
VT	Yes	Required	Required	Yes	Yes	Required	Required
WA	No	—	—	No	Yes	Required*	Required
WI	No	—	—	Yes	Yes	—	—
WV	Yes	Required	Required	Yes	Yes	Required	Required
WY	Yes	—	—	Yes	Yes	—	Required

*Indicates abstinence until marriage is required specifically

1. Contraception and STI education required in elective courses

2. If the pregnancy rate in Tennessee County exceeds 19.5 pregnancies per 1,000 females aged 15–17, the county's local education agencies must provide sexuality, STI, and HIV education.

State Mandate Totals

Mandate		Sexuality Education	STI Education	HIV Education	HIV and STI
Yes	20	27	35	37	
No	31	24	16	14	

Content Total—Abstinence Until Marriage

Abstinence Until Marriage	Sexuality Education	HIV/AIDS and STI Education
Yes	15	15
No	36	36

SOURCE: Sexuality Information and Education Council of the United States (SIECUS) 2002b

Where Do Children Learn About Sexuality?

In 1999, the Henry J. Kaiser Family Foundation conducted a study that determined 59 percent of adolescents ten to twelve years old and 45 percent of adolescents thirteen to fifteen years old indicated that they personally learned the "most" concerning sexuality from their parents. The same study found that 44 percent of parents of ten- to twelve-year-olds and 70 percent of thirteen- to fifteen-year-olds said they had talked with their children concerning relationships and becoming sexually active.

Children also learn about sexuality from sources outside the home such as friends, teachers, neighbors, television, music, books, advertisements, and toys. They learn from institutions such as churches, synagogues, and other places of worship as well as from community agencies and schools. To help illustrate this concept, another study conducted by the Kaiser Foundation found that teenagers identified the sources from which they had learned "a lot" about pregnancy and birth control. Forty percent indicated teachers, school nurses, or classes at school; 36 percent named parents; and 27 percent named friends other than boyfriends or girlfriends (Henry J. Kaiser Foundation 2002).

School-Based Sexuality Education

Sexuality education taught by trained teachers can add significantly to children's ongoing learning. The content should be developmentally appropriate and should include topics on issues such as self-esteem, family relationships, values, communication techniques, dating, and decision-making skills. It is imperative that communities plan sexuality programs to respect the diversity of values in the classroom and community.

The primary goal of any sexuality education effort is to promote adult sexual health. It seeks to assist young people in understanding a positive view of sexuality and provide information that can help them protect their health and make sound decisions.

In 1990, SIECUS brought together a group of professionals representing a cross section of foundations, associations, government agencies, and the medical profession to formulate a framework to promote and facilitate the development of comprehensive sexuality education programs. This task force was to develop curricula, textbooks, and programs, as well as evaluate existing programs. It produced the document *Guidelines for Comprehensive Sexuality Education: Grades K–12* (*Guidelines*) that outlines the steps needed in establishing comprehensive sexuality education programs (SIECUS 1996). In 2002, the *Guidelines* were updated to reflect more recent societal and technological changes.

According to *Guidelines,* a comprehensive sexuality education program has four goals:

1. **To provide accurate information about human sexuality**—Topics include growth and development, human reproduction, anatomy, physiology, masturbation, family life, pregnancy, childbirth, parenthood, sexual response, sexual orientation, contraception, abortion, sexual abuse, HIV/AIDS, and other sexually transmitted infections.

2. **To provide an opportunity for young people to develop and understand their values, attitudes, and beliefs about sexuality**—Teachers should help them understand their family's values, develop their own values, increase self-esteem, develop insights concerning relationships with families and individuals of both genders, and understand their obligations and responsibilities to their families and others.

3. **To help young people develop relationships and interpersonal skills**—Education should help young people develop communication and decision-making skills, assertiveness, peer refusal skills, and the ability to engage in satisfying relationships. This includes helping to develop the capacity for caring, supportive, noncoercive, and mutually pleasurable intimate and sexual relationships.

4. **To help young people exercise responsibility regarding sexual relationships**—Topics include abstinence, pressure to become prematurely involved in sexual intercourse, the use of contraception and other sexual health measures, prevention of STIs, and sexual abuse (SIECUS 2002a).

Guidelines for Comprehensive Sexuality Education

The *Guidelines for Comprehensive Sexuality Education Grades: K–12* are organized into six key concepts (see Health Highlight box on page 288). In addition, they contain a total of 36 topics and 778 developmental messages at four levels of development:

Level 1: Middle Childhood—Ages five through eight; early elementary school

Level 2: Preadolescence—Ages nine through twelve; upper elementary school

Level 3: Early Adolescence—Ages twelve through fifteen; middle school/junior high

Level 4: Adolescence—Ages fifteen through eighteen; high school

Health Highlight

CONCEPTS AND TOPICS IN A COMPREHENSIVE

SEXUALITY EDUCATION PROGRAM

Key Concepts

1. Human Development
Reproductive anatomy and physiology
Reproduction
Puberty
Body image
Sexual identity and orientation

2. Relationships
Families
Friendship
Love
Dating
Marriage and lifetime commitments
Parenting

3. Personal Skills
Values

4. Sexual Behavior
Sexuality throughout life
Masturbation
Shared sexual behavior
Abstinence
Human sexual response
Fantasy
Sexual dysfunction

5. Sexual Health
Contraception
Abortion
STDs and HIV infection
Sexual abuse
Reproductive health

6. Society and Culture
Sexuality and society
Decision making
Communication
Assertiveness
Negotiation
Finding help
Gender roles
Sexuality and the law
Sexuality and religion
Diversity
Sexuality and the arts
Sexuality and the media

SOURCE: SIECUS 2002a

The *Guidelines* are value based, and the task force has attempted to develop specific values found in most communities in a pluralistic society. However, every community should review these values to make sure they are consistent with community norms and diversity. The values expressed in the *Guidelines* include (SIECUS 1996):

- Sexuality is a natural and healthy part of living.

- All people are sexual.

- Sexuality includes physical, ethical, social, spiritual, psychological, and emotional dimensions.

- Every person has self-worth.

- Young people should view themselves as unique and worthwhile individuals within the context of their cultural heritage.
- Individuals express their sexuality in varied ways.
- Parents should be the primary sexuality educators of their children.
- Families provide their children's first education about sexuality.
- Families share their values about sexuality with their children.
- In a pluralistic society, people should respect and accept the diversity of values and beliefs about sexuality that exist in a community.
- Sexual relationships should never be coercive or exploitative.
- All children should be cared for and loved.
- All sexual decisions have effects and consequences.
- All persons have the right and the obligation to make responsible sexual choices.
- Individuals, families, and society benefit when children are able to discuss sexuality with their parents and/or trusted adults.
- Young people develop their values about sexuality as part of becoming adults.
- Young people explore their sexuality as a natural process of achieving sexual maturity.
- Premature involvement in sexual behavior poses risks.
- Abstaining from sexual intercourse is the most effective method of preventing pregnancy and STI/HIV.
- Young people who are involved in sexual relationships need access to information about health care services.

Any community or school considering the development or evaluation of an existing sexuality education program should consider the *Guidelines* and the topics provided by the task force. The group responsible for such development should represent a cross section of the community, and the curriculum developed must meet the needs and approval of that community. The complete *Guidelines* are available from SIECUS at *www.siecus.org*.

Teaching Sexuality Education

Teaching sexuality is different from, yet has aspects in common with, teaching any other subject. Like all teaching, sexuality education requires teachers who have effective communication skills; empathize with their students; understand the needs, interests, and characteristics of the various age levels; and believe in the need to develop students' critical thinking skills. Effective sexuality educators must be comfortable with their own sexuality and be able to overcome any embarrassment or self-consciousness they may feel. Another aspect of being an effective sexuality educator is using appropriate terminology. Kilander pointed

Health Highlight
A SAMPLE LETTER TO PARENTS

Dear Parent/Guardian:

Our school is developing a program in family living, including sexuality education, following the guidelines recommended by the Steuben County Board of Education. Selected teachers have been trained in the program. The philosophy of the program stresses

- the awareness and importance of family, religious, and moral values in making personal decisions
- understanding the need for consideration, love, respect, and responsibility in family life
- recognition of responsibilities to the school, the community, and society

We recognize that you, as parents, have the major responsibility for the formation of desirable attitudes toward family living and sexuality education. The role of the school is to support your efforts. We have the professional resources to create a comprehensive, sequential, and up-to-date program that will assist your child in developing these important life attitudes. The course contents, books, and multimedia materials for this program have been carefully screened. Every effort is being made to meet the varied needs and interests of our children.

We invite you to join us in developing our school program. Our first parent workshop has been scheduled for _____ (date) at _____ (time) in room _____. You are invited to review our course of study and the instructional materials. You are also welcome at any time to discuss this program with me.

Your interest and cooperation, as evidenced by the return of the tear-off form below, is very valuable to us. The response form also allows you the option of having your child excused from the program.

Sincerely,

Principal

Please return to _____ (school name) on or before _____ (date).

_____ I would like to have my child excused from the Sexuality Education program.

_____ I can attend the parent workshop.

_____ I cannot attend the parent workshop.

I would like an appointment to speak with _____ my child's teacher _____ the principal

Parent/Guardian Signature: _____

Date: _____

out thirty-five years ago that using acceptable terminology helps children learn to respect their bodies, helps prevent negative connotations for body parts and functions, provides a common vocabulary for children, and makes children more comfortable when asking questions (Kilander 1968).

The acceptance of any program must involve the community in the planning process. People are more comfortable if they have opportunities to give input and to view the actual content, materials, and activities associated with the curriculum. Successful sexuality programs have a high degree of parental involvement, administrative efforts at teacher training, a cooperative relationship between a school and a family planning agency, and strong support from the school board (Scales 1984). However, the value system taught to each child should come from the family. The attitudes the students reflect are still the responsibility of the family to instill. The school can impact the student by providing knowledge, decision-making training, and opportunities for examining sexuality issues in a nonthreatening environment. At their best, sexuality education programs in the school can strive to help students recognize and have insight into their own values. These values should be drawn from the family and the institutions most important in their lives, such as the church or synagogue. What is important to remember concerning sexuality education is that, even though opponents have received a lot of attention, most Americans support such education in the schools. As teachers we must take a stand for sexuality education and strive to make sure what students receive in the classroom is balanced and accurate. As Susan Spalt (1996) has suggested, every school professional should repeat the Serenity Prayer of Alcoholics Anonymous: "God grant me the serenity to accept the things I cannot change, courage to change the things I can, and wisdom to know the difference."

Any teachers who teach in the sexuality education program at any level need to train in that area. Teachers also need to be objective concerning controversial issues and have the ability to appreciate the views of others. Of course, a sense of humor helps, as well as being comfortable with one's own sexuality. Finally, they need a broad base of knowledge concerning the biological, psychological, and social aspects of human sexuality (Byer and Shainberg 1994, 422).

If a school district does not have a curriculum or is considering a change in its existing sexuality education curriculum, an excellent source is *Sexuality Education Curricula—The Consumer's Guide.* This publication helps educators determine what is available in school-based sexuality education curricula, provides evaluations of each curriculum by leading sexuality educators, and provides criteria with which local curriculum developers/evaluators can evaluate the various programs under consideration (Ogletree et al. 1994).

Social Aspects of Sexuality and Family Living

Various cultural, historical, legal, religious, and other institutional factors influence families and the sexuality roles within the family. It is important to remember that many forms of the family can be found. With this in mind, some typical characteristics of the family will be examined.

Types of Families

The family fulfills a most important role in providing stability for the individual and society. The term *family* is used to describe two or more people living together who are related by blood, marriage, or adoption (Eshleman 1996). A **nuclear family** might be composed of a husband and wife, a brother and sister, one parent and a child or children, or both parents and one or more children. An **extended family** consists of a number of nuclear family groupings, often with blood ties. Extended family members can include uncles, aunts, grandparents, or cousins.

Because most people marry, they will be part of at least two different nuclear families, one in which they are born and one they start after selecting a marriage partner. The nuclear family to which we are born is the first and most basic provider of socialization. The extended family also has an influence on our socialization.

The Changing Nature of the American Family

American youth in past generations generally grew up in one city or town, married someone from the surrounding area, and lived in the immediate locality. Chances were that members of the extended family, such as aunts, uncles, and grandparents, lived in the area also. In today's society, the nuclear family may be intact, but chances are that the extended family is not. For example, parents and grandparents may live in widely separate locations. As a result, grandparents may visit only on holidays or other special occasions. Thus, the interaction between these family members is not as frequent as in the past. The mobility of today's society and frequent job changes or transfers have served to separate the nuclear family from the extended family.

The advent of two-career households has brought about several changes as well. Families tend to have fewer children, and the care of the children may be left to daycare centers or other individuals who are not family members. Consequently, children may come in contact with caretakers of various ages who influence the social/psychological and value system development of the child.

In 2002, 19.3 million adults were divorced, representing 9.9 percent of the population. Almost 28 percent of all children under eighteen (19.8 million) lived with one parent; 84.5 percent of these children lived with their mother (Single Parent Central 2002).

Divorce may also change children's perspectives and the roles and responsibilities they have to handle. Estimates indicate that 50 percent of all children under the age of eighteen will spend some time in a female-parent-only situation. Several researchers have found that the increased divorce rate in

North American society is strongly correlated with a significant increase in sexual problems, juvenile delinquency, and emotional and psychological maladjustment (Haas and Haas 1993, 320). See Chapter 6 on additional effects of divorce.

Technology has influenced the family. Easy access to transportation has enabled people to move throughout the country quite easily. Sometimes this has led to family members engaging in activities as individuals rather than as a unit. Television, video games, computers, and other media have presented a variety of social values to children. In the past, the value system an individual initially accepted was a combination of beliefs fostered by the church, family, and school. Now, young people can witness a whole spectrum of values in a relatively short period of time by viewing, listening, or reading.

Individuals become socially, morally, and psychologically influenced by all the factors just described. Understanding the world is perhaps more difficult than ever because of these transitions and because of a barrage of mixed signals. No wonder, then, that many young people are confused about their roles in, and the expectations of, society.

The family has changed. However, it seems that people will always need others to whom they are bonded through closeness, sharing, and love. Such factors as the dual-career family, where both the father and the mother share child-rearing and household responsibilities, have required adjustments to the family model of the past. And divorce, separation, and death have made single-parent families very common today. Because the stigma of divorce is not as great as it once was and more opportunities exist for women to work, couples who in the past stayed together, often unhappily, now have the option of divorcing. An interesting aspect of divorce is that the fastest growing type of single-parent family is the male-headed household. Another outgrowth of divorce is the blended family, which brings together children from previous marriages. When divorced parents remarry, blending the children may well be the largest problem they need to overcome.

Another interesting change in family structure is the return of adults to the home of their parents because of divorce and/or lack of job opportunities. These adults are referred to as *boomerang children,* because they left the household once but now return to live with their parents. Situations where children return to the parents' home can cause adjustment problems for everyone. Issues of financial responsibility, privacy, and household responsibilities are all important.

Another issue for the family is the growing elderly population. As people live longer, caregiving for the elderly often falls to the family. In two-career families, this can create financial, as well as career-related, challenges.

Even with the problems and issues facing families today, couples continue to marry, remarry, and have children. Whatever problems are faced by the family, the desire to give love, share love, and be a part of the family unit will continue to perpetuate the family.

Concepts of Love and Family

Children can discuss what they like in friends and begin to realize that choosing the person with whom they want to spend their life is a very important decision. Some concepts to discuss in relation to family life are love and intimacy, courtship and marriage, parenthood, single parenthood, and divorce.

LOVE AND INTIMACY

From the socialization process, we learn that we are supposed to form relationships and "fall in love." Attempting to define love is a difficult task. Without caring, what is thought to be love instead may be strong desire. E. Fromm (1989, 17) wrote that caring and respect for another is central to love and that people can achieve a meaningful type of love only after they are secure in their own identity. Fromm goes on to define mature love as "union under the condition of preserving one's integrity, one's individuality." Fromm suggests that a lover must feel, "I want the loved person to grow and unfold for his own sake and in his own ways, and not for the purpose of serving me" (26).

The English language is limited in that only one word is available to describe a wide variety of feelings and relationships called love. The ancient Greeks had several terms to describe more precisely the different kinds of love. *Eros* referred to passionate or erotic love. *Storge* meant affection such as the feelings parents have for their children. *Philia* indicated the type of love in friendships, and *agape* referred to a kind of love associated with the traditional Christian view of being undemanding, patient, kind, and always supportive. In our society, love has been defined in terms of romantic, rational, and mature love. Romantic love is an intense emotional experience that can totally captivate our existence. Rational love is based on acceptance of a partner's imperfections as well as affections and is more likely to lead to fulfilling, long-lasting relationships. Mature love is maintained through communication and separateness of the partners. It involves respect, admiration, and the desire to help each other. Lovers who exhibit maturity are best friends who are committed to each other and their relationship. J. Gevinger-Woititz (1993) states that there are three key ingredients of love. They are:

1. **Intimacy**—The emotional component involving feelings of closeness.
2. **Passion**—The component that reflects romantic and sexual attraction to another individual.
3. **Decision/commitment**—The cognitive component that an individual makes about being in love and committing to the relationship.

According to this model the greater the levels of intimacy, passion, and commitment, the more likely a person is involved in a positive love relationship. As relationships progress, the passionate feelings tend to become less intense and are replaced with a deep, caring, enduring type of love that is capable of sustaining a long-term commitment. This is not to say that passionate love should be

Health Highlight

HOW DO YOU KNOW IT IS LOVE?

Strong, DeVault, and Sayad (1999) have suggested several factors that indicate some common experiences of an individual in love:

- Valuing the partner's presence
- Being able to communicate concerning intimate things
- Giving emotional support to the partner
- Sharing oneself and one's possessions with the partner
- Being able to understand each other
- Being able to count on the partner in time of need
- Holding the partner in high regard
- Feeling happiness with the partner
- Tolerating the partner's idiosyncrasies, routines, or forgetfulness

- Physically expressing love by hugging, kissing, making love
- Giving material evidence such as gifts, flowers, small favors, sharing tasks
- Expressing nonverbal feelings such as feeling happy, more content, more secure when the person is present
- Giving nonmaterial evidence such as emotional and moral support in times of need and respecting the opinion of the partner
- Offering self-disclosure such as revealing intimate facts about oneself
- Verbally expressing affection such as saying "I love you"

SOURCE: Strong, DeVault, and Sayad 1999

allowed to leave relationships. In fact, couples should strive to maintain romance in their relationship. This requires a great deal of effort in learning how to communicate effectively, considering the spouses' feelings, striving to meet one another's needs, and the continuing commitment to the spouse.

To be intimate means to be vulnerable. It means risking rejection or suffocation of one's self. However, compatible partners replace those risks with trust and satisfaction. Essentially, individuals must remain responsible for themselves yet help each other with their goals, problems, and desires. Enjoying, sharing, and caring should be the outcomes of living with someone with whom love and intimacy are shared.

DATING COURTSHIP AND MARRIAGE

People marry for both personal and societal reasons. There is no single reason why people marry. Some marry because they do not want to be alone. They want someone to share confidences, and they want to give and receive affection. A happy marriage can offer intimacy, support, and stimulation for personal growth. Some people marry for economic reasons; they may wish to pool their incomes, or one spouse may provide financial security to the other while he or she runs the home and cares for the children. Most people marry because they enjoy a person and can depend on that person in times of need. Marriage theoretically provides someone to share both joy and sorrow.

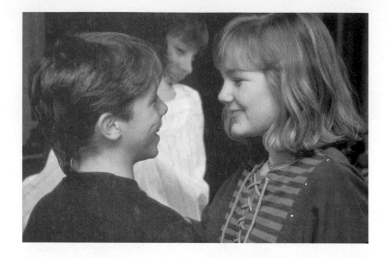

Dating helps in the processes of socialization, personality development, and learning to get along with the opposite sex.

Marriage serves many functions for individuals, including establishment of a family, companionship, economic strength, emotional security, a sexual outlet, and children. The greater the success in meeting these needs, the greater the likelihood the marriage will remain intact. Because each year more than two million marriages take place in the United States, it seems safe to say that marriages exist to fulfill basic needs associated with the husband–wife relationship. For these individual needs to be met, each partner must be committed to the marriage, develop effective communication skills, and accept the responsibility to nurture and enhance the marriage.

PARENTHOOD

When children enter a family, couples must assume new roles. The wife must become a mother and the husband a father. The exclusive attention of the partners toward each other, as well as the time demands and interests of the couple, must change. Parenthood is a difficult task, yet couples are expected to fulfill this role with little or no formal training. Parenthood is a lifetime commitment. Individuals can quit their jobs or divorce their mate, but there is no honorable way to withdraw from the role of father or mother. Many groups are now providing parenthood education programs that promote parenting skills. These courses attempt to teach ways to facilitate communication between parents and children, improve methods of discipline, and develop appropriate behavior for parents and children.

Advantages and Disadvantages of Parenthood. The obvious advantage of parenthood is the opportunity to love and nurture another human being. The psychological pleasure derived from being part of a loving family and helping to direct its development can bring a couple closer together, with the long-term benefit of pride in having done so. Besides the extreme economic cost of having and raising children, parenthood usually requires an adjustment in the career of

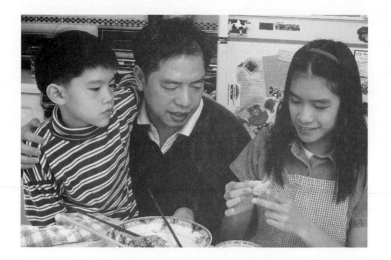

One of the greatest joys of parenthood is the opportunity to love and nurture another human being.

at least one of the partners. Further, a child takes away from the emotional sharing time of the couple. Much time is spent in guiding and showing affection to the child. Some personal activities must be changed or eliminated, and there is a constant need to transport the children to and from various activities and functions as they become older.

SINGLE PARENTHOOD

Parenthood is difficult when two partners share the nurturing and love that children require. It can become even more difficult if only one parent is present. Through death, desertion, or divorce, single-parent situations often arise. Some individuals cope quite successfully with single parenthood, whereas others struggle with the many roles and situations they face in raising their children.

A single parent may experience a variety of problems. It may be difficult to meet the emotional needs of the child. There are a variety of ways to express love for a child. Telling a child he or she is loved and demonstrating that love with quality time serve to express love; however, the demands of working and maintaining a home may be so overwhelming that a child's emotional needs may not be met adequately. It also may be hard for the single parent to provide proper supervision for the child. Making arrangements for the child's care and supervision is difficult and costly and may take a large share of the budget. In addition, because women tend to make less money than men, households headed by women can experience financial difficulties. Finally, the single parent may experience unfulfilled emotional and sexual needs. Unmet emotional needs can develop because of the lack of time to seek a relationship. Because most single parents wish to hide their sexual involvement from their child, finding a time and place can present problems. Nevertheless, being a single parent does not have to be a disaster. It is important that single parents have sufficient financial, material, and emotional support to meet their own and their child's demands.

DIVORCE

The most frequent method for dissolving a marriage is through divorce. In 1997 there were 4.3 divorces per 1,000 people. The 1997 marriage rate was 8.9 per 1,000, which means that about half of all marriages are destined to end in divorce (U. S. Bureau of the Census 2002).

Divorce is usually viewed as a failure of the family system, as well as a great personal crisis. However, it is also a way to end physical abuse and emotional tension. Personal factors most often given as reasons for divorce include financial problems, physical abuse, mental abuse, drinking, in-law problems, lack of love, adultery, and sexual incompatibility. Six social factors that seem to have contributed to the increased divorce rates are (Byer and Shainberg 1994):

1. **Changing family functions**—Outside sources may now fulfill functions that were once considered primary family responsibilities. These may include medical, religious, and recreational aspects of family life.

2. **Casual marriages**—Hasty and youthful marriages complicated by pregnancy are often unstable.

3. **Jobs for women**—With greater job/career opportunities available to a large number of women, which allows greater economic freedom, a great barrier to divorce is removed.

4. **Decline in moral and religious sanctions**—Although not all churches openly state it, most have taken a more liberal attitude toward divorce. Also, society does not attach the severe stigma to divorce that it once did.

5. **The philosophy of happiness**—If happiness does not materialize to the degree anticipated, divorce or separation is accepted as a way of dealing with the feeling.

6. **More liberal divorce laws**—The liberalization of divorce laws, including no-fault divorces, has made it easier to terminate a marriage.

The emotional impact of a divorce is most difficult. Anyone who has experienced a divorce will usually describe it as a painful, devastating experience. Problems with finances, personal adjustment, and children can create an extremely stressful situation. Children whose parents are divorcing may develop deep feelings of guilt, fear, anger, loneliness, and/or sadness. Many times children feel that they must take sides in the conflict, which only serves to enhance their feelings of guilt. Because of the emotional conflict between the marriage partners, they may fail to recognize the worry the children feel concerning their own welfare. It is important to remember that despite the family fighting, the children will continue to love both parents. It is extremely important that children have sensitive parents and understanding teachers during and after a divorce. Many children will require counseling, which places an even greater burden on the teacher and school system.

BLENDED FAMILIES

Indications are that about 80 percent of individuals who divorce will remarry. Many times children from previous marriages find themselves in a stepfamily or

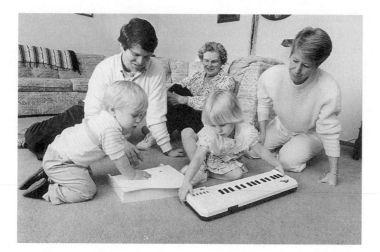

The family serves an important role by providing stability in the individual and society.

blended family situation. The transition and adjustment for both the parents and the children may be difficult. Dealing with sibling jealousy and new rules and striving for affection can put stress on the blended family.

Psychological Aspects of Sexuality and Family Living

Individuals have a wide variety of options for displaying their psychological and physiological traits. Also, in today's society there is greater flexibility in sex roles. This section deals with those psychological aspects of human sexuality and family life that help determine how people feel and react as individuals.

Gender Development

From birth, social expectations largely guide gender development. Parents consciously and unconsciously manipulate their children's gender development from infancy based on the sole criterion of sex. From dress and toys to behavior, the child learns to accept the parameters of being either a girl or a boy. By age two, children know what sex they are and understand some of their society's expectations for that sex. By the time children have reached school age, task orientation and emotional responses are based almost solely on what has been learned about gender.

The key to gender development is the creation of gender equality. Gender is socially constructed from the exercise of cultural conditioning. Making the sexes appear to be opposite and of unequal value requires the suppression of natural similarities by the use of social power. Social power can take the form of pushing boys toward what society considers the more masculine occupations while girls are expected to follow those occupational paths that women have traditionally followed. An example of stereotypical gender roles is expecting women to become elementary teachers or nurses. In reality, males and females are more like each other than they are different. Both can be reasonable, emotional, aggressive, or passive. Contemporary gender roles are evolving from traditional gender roles in which one sex is subordinate to the other to more equal roles in which both sexes are treated equally and to androgynous roles in which both sexes display the instrumental and expressive traits associated with one sex or the other. It is important for teachers not to perpetuate artificial gender differences in the classroom. Imperative to this is recognition by teachers that boys and girls do not have innate abilities or disabilities in areas (academic, social, emotional, etc.) because of their gender.

Gender identification is a most important organizer of expectations and conduct. Society places a great deal of emphasis on socializing and maintaining gender differences. In some cases this process may be beneficial; in other cases it may be detrimental to the potential of both boys and girls.

Both males and females have a right to expand their individual potential and not be held to traditional roles and stereotypes. Traditional behavioral roles are learned in the same ways as gender identity. The emphasis should be on the humanness of people, not on their gender. Through such an emphasis, factors that inhibit the complete development of the individual can be discarded. Sharing household duties, child rearing, and economic responsibilities can all contribute to the personal development of both partners. Males need not always be expected to be aggressive, nor females always passive.

Overcoming traditional gender roles is not easy because they are established early in life and are constantly reinforced throughout the years. Self-evaluation and a sense of adequacy are linked to gender role performances as defined by parents and peers in childhood.

Developing Sexuality

All aspects of human sexuality develop over a long period of time, from early childhood through the adult years. The groundwork for sexual values begins to develop in infancy, as children learn trust, initiative, and love. As they grow older, children try to achieve self-confidence in their interactions with parents, adults, and peers. Development of self-confidence is crucial to the development of the child's sexuality. If children grow up feeling at ease with themselves, they are more likely to appreciate themselves and members of the opposite sex.

Anything that affects a child's developing identity will eventually affect his or her sexuality as well. If the child learns to be defensive, unforgiving, or mistrusting in daily life, these attitudes will carry over into the sexual component of that individual's personality. Consequently, it is imperative that children learn to give and receive love and have a positive self-image if they are to be at ease with their sexuality later in life.

SEXUAL ORIENTATION

Some children in the classroom may not identify with a heterosexual orientation, that is, sexual attraction to members of the opposite sex. They may instead be sexually attracted to members of the same sex, or a homosexual orientation.

Reasons for sexual preference are not well understood. Some research suggests that it may have a biological basis in the size of certain brain structures (Allen and Gorski 2002). Other research suggests genetic, environmental, or hormonal factors may influence sexual orientation. There is probably no single reason or theory that accounts for all differences in sexual preference.

Teachers need to understand that a person's sexual orientation is not a matter of choice. An individual has no more choice about being homosexual than heterosexual. Teacher sensitivity is most important when interacting with gay and lesbian students because these students can become socially isolated, withdraw from activities and friends, have trouble concentrating, and develop low self-esteem (American Academy of Child and Adolescent Psychology 2002).

Problems generally begin in early adolescence. Some of the problems encountered by gay/lesbian adolescents may include:

- feelings different from peers
- feeling guilty about their sexual orientation
- worrying about the response from their families and loved ones
- being teased and ridiculed by their peers
- worrying about HIV infection and other STIs
- fearing discrimination when joining clubs, playing sports, seeking admission to college, and finding employment
- being rejected and harassed by others

Biological Components of Sex Education

It is essential for all teachers to have a basic knowledge of the reproductive system and how it works. Obviously all the material presented in this section will not be presented in the elementary classroom, but teachers need the information for their own understanding of the reproductive system.

Figure 11.1
*The Male Reproductive
System*

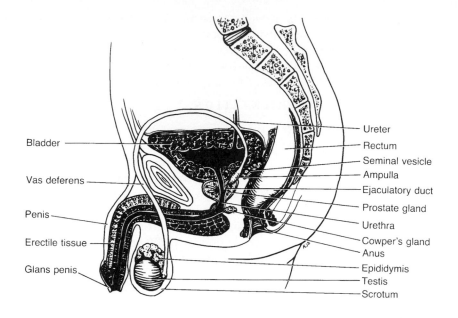

Bladder

Vas deferens

Penis

Erectile tissue

Glans penis

Ureter
Rectum
Seminal vesicle
Ampulla
Ejaculatory duct
Prostate gland
Urethra
Cowper's gland
Anus
Epididymis
Testis
Scrotum

The Male Reproductive System

The male reproductive system, shown in Figure 11.1, is not as hormonally complex as that of the female because men do not have sexual cycles. The major male sexual endocrine glands are the two *testes,* or **testicles,** which are contained and protected in a saclike structure called the **scrotum.** At puberty, the testes (singular *testis*) begin producing mature **sperm,** the male reproductive cells. Attached to the top of each testis is the **epididymis.** This structure consists of tightly coiled tubes through which the sperm pass to the *vas deferens* (also called the *ductus deferens* or *spermatic ducts*). The two vas deferens serve as storage areas for the mature sperm and are the means by which sperm move to the urethra. The two vas deferens eventually merge into one structure called the *ejaculatory duct.* This tube connects with the **urethra.** The urethra is a tube that runs the length of the *penis* and is used to transport both urine and semen (described below). The penis is the male organ for sexual intercourse and consists of spongy vascular material called erectile tissue that swells when blood fills the vascular spaces in response to psychological and/or physical stimulation. The head of the penis is called the *glans penis.* This area contains many nerve endings and is very sensitive to sexual stimulation.

The *seminal vesicles,* the *prostate gland,* and the two **bulbourethral glands (Cowper's glands)** manufacture substances important to the sperm and ejaculate. The seminal vesicles produce a simple sugar, fructose, that adds volume to the ejaculatory fluid, called semen, and activates the movement of the sperm. The prostate gland provides a highly alkaline milky fluid that helps neutralize the highly acidic vagina, and which facilitates the movement of sperm. The pea-sized bulbourethral glands also produce an alkaline fluid that lubricates and neutralizes the acidity of urine in the urethra. The bulbourethral glands secrete this substance prior to ejaculation of sperm. The combined fluid produced by the seminal vesicles, prostate, and bulbourethral glands, along with the sperm it contains, is **semen.**

It should be noted that the testes constantly manufacture mature sperm from puberty through old age. On release of interstitial cell-stimulating hormone (ICSH) into the bloodstream from the anterior lobe of the pituitary gland, the testes also secrete testosterone. Although it plays many diverse roles, testosterone is needed to trigger the male adolescent growth spurt, which is accompanied by the development of secondary sex characteristics, including appearance of facial and genital hair, deepening voice, oilier skin, and increased muscle size and mass.

The Female Reproductive System

The female reproductive system, shown in Figure 11.2, is composed of the external genitalia and the internal organs consisting of the vagina, uterus, uterine tubes (fallopian tubes or oviducts), and ovaries. The external genitalia are the *labia majora* (the outer lips or folds) and the *labia minora* (the inner lips, or folds). The *clitoris* is a small structure at the top of the labia minora that facilitates sexual stimulation. The *vagina* is an elastic canal extending from just behind the cervix to the opening of the external genitalia. It serves as the organ for sexual intercourse and as the birth canal. The *uterus* (or womb) is a pear-shaped organ

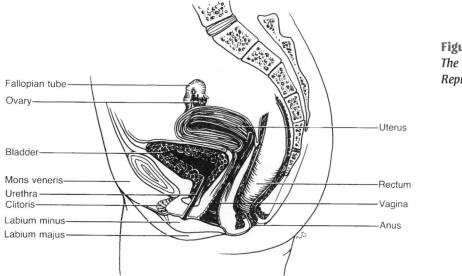

Figure 11.2
The Female Reproductive System

Fallopian tube
Ovary
Bladder
Mons veneris
Urethra
Clitoris
Labium minus
Labium majus

Uterus
Rectum
Vagina
Anus

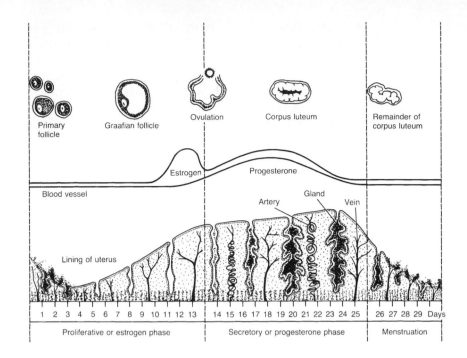

Figure 11.3
The Female Monthly Reproductive Cycle

Primary follicle

Graafian follicle

Ovulation

Corpus luteum

Remainder of corpus luteum

Estrogen

Progesterone

Blood vessel

Artery

Gland

Vein

Lining of uterus

1 2 3 4 5 6 7 8 9 10 11 12 13	14 15 16 17 18 19 20 21 22 23 24 25	26 27 28 29 Days
Proliferative or estrogen phase	Secretory or progesterone phase	Menstruation

where the fetus develops. The uterus has three layers: the *perimetrium* (outer layer), the *myometrium* (muscular middle layer), and *endometrium* (inner layer). The endometrium is sloughed off during menstruation. Two armlike projections called the *uterine tubes* branch from the top of the uterus. These tubes are three to five inches long and have *fimbria* (small fingerlike projections) at the far ends next to the ovaries. Through these tubes the eggs, or *ova,* pass. If fertilization takes place, it occurs in the upper third of one of the uterine tubes. Two *ovaries* produce ova and secrete hormones that bring about the development of the female secondary sex characteristics, such as the rounding of the female figure, breast development, and pubic hair.

Each ovary contains 200,000 to 400,000 saclike structures called *follicles* that store immature egg cells. At the onset of puberty several follicles are activated in the ovary each month by follicle-stimulating hormone (FSH) being released into the bloodstream from the anterior lobe of the pituitary gland. Only one follicle will evolve into a mature ovum and simultaneously secrete estrogen. Estrogen signals the uterus to prepare for a potential pregnancy by filling its lining with blood and nutrients for nourishment of the embryo. As the maturing follicle and its ovum move to the surface of the ovary, with the follicle continuing to secrete estrogen, lutenizing hormone (LH) is released into the bloodstream from the anterior lobe of the pituitary. The production of LH causes the follicle to rupture and release the mature ovum into the uterine tubes. This process, known as *ovulation,* usually occurs midway into the monthly reproductive cycle of twenty-eight days. This cycle is shown in Figure 11.3.

Table 11.1   *Development during Pregnancy*

First-trimester development

A small mass of cells is implanted in the uterus.

Becomes embryo until seventh/eighth week

Development into a fetus begins after seventh/eighth week.

Major organ systems are present and recognizable.

During the fourth to eighth weeks, the eyes, ears, arms, hands, fingers, legs, feet, and toes develop.

By the seventh week, the liver, lungs, pancreas, kidneys, and intestines have formed.

By the end of the first trimester, the fetus weighs two-thirds of an ounce and is about 4 inches in length.

From this time on, development consists of enlargement and differentiation of the existing structures.

Second-trimester development

By the end of the fourteenth week, movement can be detected.

By the eighteenth week, a fetal heartbeat can be detected.

By the twentieth week, the fetus will open its eyes.

Around the twenty-fourth week, the fetus is sensitive to light and can hear sounds. It will also have periods of sleep and wakefulness.

Third-trimester development

Fat deposits form under the skin.

During the seventh month, the fetus turns in the uterus to a head-down position.

By the end of the eighth month, the fetus weighs an average of 5 pounds, 4 ounces.

At birth, the average infant weighs approximately 7.5 pounds and is 20 inches long.

During ovulation, estrogen is at its highest level and causes cessation of additional secretions of FSH. At the same time, LH continues to be secreted and produces closure of the ruptured follicle. The empty follicle, now called the *corpus luteum,* and the mature ovum begin to produce another hormone, in addition to now-declining levels of estrogen, called *progesterone.* Progesterone further prepares the uterus for implantation of a fertilized egg and continues to maintain the uterus during pregnancy.

From the moment that conception occurs, the woman's body begins to change. Through pregnancy a weight gain of seventeen to twenty-four pounds is normal and looked on as desirable because this helps ensure adequate development of the fetus. The average fetus weighs approximately seven pounds at birth. Table 11.1 lists the development of the fetus through each trimester.

If the mature ovum is not fertilized within twenty-four to forty-eight hours after ovulation, it disintegrates, thus diminishing the amount of estrogen and progesterone in the bloodstream. Around the twenty-fourth day of the cycle, the corpus luteum also stops secreting progesterone and estrogen. As a result, several days later the uterus expels its blood-rich lining through the vagina in a process referred to as *menstruation.* Following menstruation, the reproductive cycle begins again in preparation for possible fertilization and pregnancy. Menstruation begins with puberty. The onset of menstruation is called *menarche.*

Conception

Conception occurs when a single sperm fertilizes an egg to produce a *zygote.* Conception usually occurs in the upper third of the uterine tube and must take place in the first or second day following ovulation. To facilitate conception the sperm go through a series of biochemical changes known as *capacitation,* which enables penetration of the egg (Denney and Quadagno 1992, 132). When a sperm enters an egg, the membrane thickens to prevent further penetration by sperm.

Genetics

The human body is made up of trillions of cells that perform various specialized functions. Each cell contains a *nucleus,* which contains genes that provide the hereditary information in smaller rod-shaped bodies called *chromosomes.* Twenty-two pairs of autosomal (non-sex-determining) chromosomes account for individual facial features, hair color, height, body build, and a myriad of other characteristics. Gender is determined by the twenty-third, or sex-determining, chromosomal pair. One member of the pair is an X chromosome inherited from the mother's ovum. The other (inherited from the father's sperm) can be either an X or Y chromosome. If a Y chromosome is present, the offspring is male; if no Y is present, the offspring is female.

Mitosis is ordinary cell division. This process results in two new cells that each contain the full complement of forty-six chromosomes. *Meiosis* is the cell division by which sperm and ovum are formed. These cells are called *gametes* and contain only twenty-three chromosomes. When a male gamete (sperm) unites with a female gamete (ovum), the twenty-three pairs unite to form the complete set required to produce a new individual from the zygote.

The Embryonic Period

Immediately after conception, the zygote begins to divide to form other cells. It travels down the uterine tube and within ten days attaches to the uterine wall. From the time it attaches to the wall until the eighth week, it is called an *embryo.* The embryo divides into three layers of cells from which the various body organs and systems develop. The innermost layer, the *endoderm,* becomes the digestive and respiratory systems; the next layer, the *mesoderm,* forms the skeletal, muscular, circulatory, and reproductive systems; and the *ectoderm,* or outermost layer, becomes the nervous system and skin. The head develops first, with the lower body developing last. After eight weeks, the embryo is called the *fetus.* (For simplicity, both the embryo and fetus will be described as the embryo in the following two paragraphs.)

The *amnion* is a thin protective membrane that is filled with a fluid called the *amniotic fluid.* This fluid serves as insulation and protection for the embryo against shocks and blows to the mother's abdomen. The fluid also permits changes in position as growth and movement occur. The *umbilical cord* connects the placenta and the developing embryo.

The *placenta* is the organ through which nutrients, vitamins, antibodies, and other substances (such as drugs, alcohol, and diseases) are moved inward. Waste products, such as nitrogen compounds and carbon dioxide, are carried outward to diffuse across the placenta to the mother's blood, which carries them to the mother's kidneys and lungs for disposal (in urine and exhaled gas). This is accomplished even though there is no mixing of the embryo's and mother's blood. The placenta is expelled shortly following the birth of the child and is referred to as the *afterbirth.*

Multiple Births

Several factors contribute to multiple births. Heredity, the increased use of fertility drugs, age of the mother, and social factors seem significant (Haas and Haas 1993). Some families are genetically more likely to have multiple births than others. Women in their thirties and forties are more likely to have multiple births than are women in their twenties.

Identical twins develop from a single fertilized ovum that divides to form two individuals. Such twins are always the same sex and look alike. *Fraternal twins* develop from two different ova fertilized at the same time. However, fraternal twins may not be of the same sex and look no more alike than any other siblings born to the same parents.

Triplets usually involve two fertilized ova, one of which separates and then develops into twins. *Quadruplets* usually involve two fertilized ova that then divide and develop into two pairs of identical twins.

Childbirth

The process of childbirth occurs in three stages and is referred to as *labor* (see Figure 11.4). This process begins when the amniotic sac that has protected the fetus ruptures and the amniotic fluid flows from the vagina. Labor pains occur at regular intervals, usually fifteen to twenty minutes apart, with the cervix dilating three to four inches to permit passage of the fetus through the vagina. This first stage of labor may last twelve to sixteen hours (or even longer) for the first birth but usually is shorter in subsequent births.

The second stage begins when the cervix has fully dilated and the baby's head enters the vagina. It ends with the birth of the baby. Contractions are quite severe and last from a minute to a minute and a half, with a two- to three-minute interval between contractions. The contractions serve to move the baby

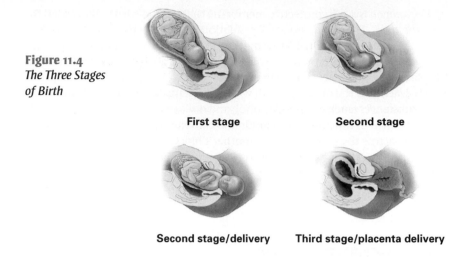

Figure 11.4
The Three Stages of Birth

First stage   Second stage

Second stage/delivery   Third stage/placenta delivery

down the birth canal. Just before the head of the child appears, it rotates to the side to pass the pelvic bone. The neck and shoulders emerge, and the rest of the body follows rather quickly.

The third and final stage lasts only a few minutes and consists of the delivery of the placenta. The placenta separates from the wall of the uterus and is expelled as afterbirth. It is examined to determine that all of the organ has been delivered.

Occasionally, complications arise during labor. For example, some conditions may require a *caesarean section.* When this procedure is used, an incision is made through the abdominal wall and another in the uterus, and the baby is removed. The reason for a caesarean section is usually a contracted pelvis through which the baby is unable to pass into the vagina. Other reasons are that the baby is in a breech (buttock or leg presenting first) position; the placenta has prematurely separated from the uterus, causing a loss of oxygen; a vaginal infection is present; or the mother is incapacitated because of injury or trauma. To help identify potential complications, a fetal monitor may be used during the birth process.

Unwanted Pregnancies

The abortion issue is far from settled. Many states have circumvented the 1973 Supreme Court ruling allowing abortions by establishing laws that make abortions difficult to obtain. The U.S. Congress has placed restrictions on federally funded abortions by prohibiting Medicaid funds from being used to pay for the procedure except when the mother's life is in danger. The issues associated with abortion continue to be hotly debated.

If the decision is made to not terminate an unwanted pregnancy, there are other options. The woman may choose to keep her child or place the infant for adoption. In general, the younger the woman, the more difficult her decision. Parenting is a demanding job, and if the woman is single, the difficulty is even greater. Many times she must rely on her parents or other relatives to aid in caring for the child. Unfortunately, too often the maturity necessary to be a good parent is lacking. The woman is faced with the difficulty of supplying a safe place for the child to grow and develop; providing adequate nutrition; developing sufficient economic resources; and having a secure, supportive environment. The options open to a single, young parent may be severely lacking from a social, educational, and economic perspective. Even if marriage occurs, the chance of a teenage marriage surviving is much less than if marriage occurs later in life.

Adoption is also a difficult decision, but many couples want to provide the love, closeness, and resources a child needs. Being an adoptive parent is not different from being a natural parent. The same love, rewards, and frustrations are experienced by both parents and children.

Problems of Child Abuse and Violence

Child abuse consists of any act of commission or omission that endangers or impairs a child's physical or emotional health and development (Childhelp USA 2000). The major forms of child abuse are:

- **Physical abuse**—any nonaccidental injury to a child. This includes hitting, kicking, slapping, shaking, burning, pinching, hair-pulling, biting, choking, throwing, shoving, whipping, and paddling.

- **Emotional abuse**—any attitude or behavior that interferes with a child's mental health or social development. This includes yelling, screaming, name-calling, shaming, negative comparisons to others, telling a child he or she is "bad," "no good," "worthless," or a "mistake."

- **Sexual abuse**—any sexual act between an adult and child. This includes fondling, penetration, intercourse, exploitation, pornography, exhibitionism, child prostitution, group sex, oral sex, or forced observation of sexual acts.

- **Physical neglect**—failure to provide for a child's needs in the form of supervision, housing, food, clothing, medical care, and hygiene.

- **Emotional neglect**—failure to provide affection and support necessary for the development of emotional, social, physical, and intellectual well-being.

Child abuse is a particularly difficult problem to combat because the abuse usually occurs in the home and because there is often a public reluctance to intervene or report what is thought to be a private matter.

Data reported in 2000 indicate that approximately 879,000 children were victims of child maltreatment. Maltreatment includes neglect, medical neglect,

Health Highlight
INDICATORS OF SEXUAL ABUSE

Psychological Signs
1. Fear of being alone with a specific person
2. Sleep disturbances, such as nightmares, fear of going to bed, and fear of sleeping alone
3. Irritability or short temper
4. Clinging to parent or parents
5. Unexplained fears
6. Changes in behavior and schoolwork or in relating to friends or siblings
7. Behaving like a younger child (regression)
8. Sexual sophistication or knowledge greater than age group
9. Running away from home or fear of going home

Physical Signs (Caused by Sexual Acts)
1. Difficulty in walking or sitting
2. Pain or itching in genital areas
3. Torn, stained, or bloody underwear
4. Bruises or bleeding in external genitals, vagina, or anal areas
5. Sexually transmitted diseases
6. Pregnancy

Source: Denney and Quadagno 1992

physical abuse, sexual abuse, and psychological maltreatment. Almost two-thirds of child victims suffered neglect: 19 percent were physically abused, 10 percent were sexually abused, and 8 percent were psychologically maltreated. The rate of child victims per 1,000 children in the population had been decreasing steadily from 15.3 victims per 1,000 in 1993 to 11.8 victims per 1,000 children in the population in 1999. Victimization rates increased slightly in the year 2000 (12.2 per 1,000 children), but researchers cannot determine if this represents a trend until additional information is collected. Data indicate that rates decline as the age of the child increases. The rates for victimization were similar for male and female victims (11.2 and 12.8 per 1,000 children, respectively) except for sexual abuse. The rate for sexual abuse was 1.7 victims per 1,000 female children compared to 0.4 victims per 1,000 male children. The perpetrators of these acts of child abuse or neglect were reported as 60 percent female and 40 percent male. A perpetrator is most often a parent or other caretaker, such as a relative, babysitter, or foster parent, who has maltreated a child. More than 80 percent of victims were abused by a parent or parents. The mother acting alone was responsible for 47 percent of neglect victims and 32 percent of physical abuse. The father acting alone was responsible for 29 percent of child neglect cases and 22 percent of abuse cases. There were approximately 1,200 child fatalities in the year 2000. Youngest children were the most vulnerable. Children younger than one year old accounted for 44 percent of child fatalities, and 85 percent of fatalities were children younger than six years of age. (Administration for Children & Families 2002).

Health Highlight

INFORMATION FOR TEACHERS ON ABUSE

1. Child sexual abuse (molestation) involves the misuse of power by an adult or older child to engage a younger child in sexual activities to gratify the perpetrator's (offender's) needs.

2. Both touching and nontouching offenses are included in the category of sexual abuse. Examples of nontouching behaviors include showing children pornography or having children pose for pornographic pictures. Touching offenses include fondling and penetration.

3. Although the actual behavior involved in child sexual abuse varies, the following characteristics are common:

    a. It usually starts at an early age before children are aware of the inappropriate nature of the acts.

    b. The adult takes advantage of the child's need for approval, trust, and lack of knowledge.

    c. The behavior is surrounded with secrecy.

    d. The adult uses authority to threaten, bribe, or trick the child into complying.

    e. The child feels responsible for the abuse.

4. The child's reaction to the situation depends on his or her perception of the offense and the reactions of those important to him or her, rather than the legally defined severity of the offense.

5. Current information suggests that at least 1 in 4 girls and 1 in 7 boys are physically molested by the age of 18. In 80 to 90 percent of the reported cases, the perpetrator is someone who is known to the child; in over 50 percent of the cases, the offender is a family member.

6. Most often, the perpetrator is someone the child knows well. The child may be emotionally tied to the individual and may even love him or her. Therefore, it should be emphasized that abuse can happen with someone we know or love; do not overemphasize danger from strangers.

7. Some children are aware of the inappropriateness of abusive behavior but are still unable to terminate it. Others are unable to recognize or respond appropriately to abusive or potentially abusive behaviors.

8. The educator should be sensitive to the manner in which material is presented and to the reactions of the students. Disclosure is often vague or indirect.

9. Define the subject according to the child's age. For young ones, explain that, although most adults are good and caring, some do not make good decisions about touching children. They may try to touch children on private parts of the body for no good reason. A broader range of offenses and behaviors can be included when defining molestation to older children. Describe examples of touching and nontouching behaviors to make sure they understand the entire concept.

10. It is equally important for children to understand the characteristics of healthy interpersonal and familial relationships. Indicate that most adults do care and want to help children. Describe examples of positive interpersonal relationships as well as negative ones in teaching the material.

11. Lessons for younger children need to stress developing the self-confidence and self-esteem needed to resist the attention and gifts often "earned" through participating in the abuse. Older children should begin to recognize characteristics of cooperative and exploitative relationships and relate these to their daily activities.

12. Touches can be categorized according to one's personal reaction to the touch. Good touches make one feel warm, secure, or happy; bad touches make one feel angry, hurt, or ashamed. Those touches that confuse are often sexual touches or touches that are delivered in a contradictory manner that perplexes the child. Teachers can refer to resource materials, the local school district, or the state department of education for additional information.

13. Lessons should include opportunities to role-play and use the skills taught. For examples of assertiveness and decision-making activities, refer to the various resource materials available through state departments of education and local school districts.

Aside from the obvious physical effects, a child's psychological development can be seriously handicapped by abusive treatment. Many abused children are emotionally affected for the rest of their lives. A child who is abused in the home is one who loses the chance to be a child. Unable to understand why they are being punished, these children come to believe that they deserve such treatment because they are "bad." They see the world as cold and hostile and have little faith in themselves or in their ability to succeed in life. They learn that using force is an acceptable way to deal with others and, tragically, often become child abusers themselves.

Parents most often become physically or emotionally abusive because of their own history of abuse, failure to understand the needs of their children, or as a response to unmanaged stress. They typically do not have the self-confidence, ingenuity, and ability to cope with crises within the family. Crisis presents a greater danger for them than for someone with better coping skills. Even a minor occurrence may be enough to lead to loss of self-control and an abusive attack on an innocent child. In many instances, abusing adults reverse roles with their children, requiring the child to love and care for them without providing the emotional support the child needs. With sexual abuse, abusers may actually convince themselves that they are doing a child a favor by showing him or her the "facts of life" in a more loving way than an outsider would do (Office of the Attorney General 1985). In 90 percent of child sexual abuse cases, the offenders are male and are often described as being unassertive, withdrawn, and emotionless. Other characteristics include a history of either physical or sexual abuse, alcohol or drug abuse, little satisfaction with sexual relationships with adults, lack of control over their emotions, and occasionally mental illness. (Prevent Child Abuse America 2002) There is hope for reeducation of the adult if the matter can be brought to the attention of the proper authorities. Successful therapy seems directly related to the perpetrator's willingness to change.

Every state has laws that make it mandatory for teachers to report suspected abuse. Not every bruise should be considered abuse, but if a pattern of injury is observed, teachers should report this concern. Proper authorities include the state's department of family and child services or a local health agency (see Health Highlight box on page 311).

Summary

- No area in health education is more controversial than that of sexuality education.
- The majority of teachers and parents support sexuality education.
- Some individuals oppose sexuality education.
- Schools can assist students in developing critical thinking skills, communication skills, self-esteem, and a solid knowledge base.
- The family should provide the value base on which students make their decisions.

- Sexuality education at the elementary level consists of many components, including biological aspects, self-esteem, relationships, personal skills, social mores, and sexual health.

- The family is the basic unit of society. Because of the increase in divorce the family is an institution in transition, leading to variations of family units such as single-parent and blended families.

- Factors that may contribute to the increased divorce rate include changing family functions, casual marriages, increased job availability for women, decline in moral and religious sanctions, the philosophy of happiness, and more liberal divorce laws.

- Human sexuality develops over an extended length of time, ranging from early childhood to the adult years.

- The various structures of the male and female reproductive system are designed to enable human reproduction.

- Unwanted pregnancies are a continuing issue; the options available for consideration are keeping the child, planning for adoption, or terminating the pregnancy. For all three options, there are consequences that must be faced by the individuals involved.

- Estimates are that about 3 million children are maltreated by their parents and other adults each year.

- Every state has laws that require teachers to report suspected abuse.

DISCUSSION QUESTIONS

1. What are some reasons for opposition to sexuality education?
2. What are some of the groups that oppose sexuality education, and what are their grounds for opposition?
3. Discuss the anatomy and physiology of female and male reproductive systems.
4. What important functions does the family fill?
5. What factors should the classroom teacher be aware of when there are children of divorce in the classroom?
6. What are the shortcomings of inflexible gender roles?
7. Differentiate among and explain the different types of abuse.
8. What are the key concepts that a comprehensive family life and sexuality education program should contain?

CRITICAL THINKING QUESTIONS

1. Does sexuality education promote premature sexual activity? On what rationale do you base your opinion?
2. Does sexuality education belong in the home, school, or both?
3. From what sources did you discover your sexual information? What effect has that had upon your perception of sexuality?

4. In today's world, is it realistic to expect to marry once and have it last a lifetime?

5. To what extent should a couple stay married for the sake of the children involved?

WEB SITE ACTIVITY

Investigate the SIECUS Web site. What is being advocated for how to approach sexuality education in the school?

WEB SITES OF INTEREST

American Social Health Association (ASHA): *www.ashastd.org*
Provides information on STIs and their harmful effects upon individuals, families, and communities. Site has hotline, sexual history glossary, surveys, and recent research.

Child Care Experts National Network: *www.childcare-experts.org*
Provides information for community-based resources and referral agencies for a wide variety of child- and family-related service and information.

Relationship Growth Online: *www.relationship.com*
Provides information on how to develop better relationships.

Sexuality Information and Education Council of the United States (SIECUS):
    www.siecus.org
Advocate for family life education. Excellent source of education policies and programs at the national and state level.

Work and Family: *www.workfamily.com*
Clearinghouse for information concerning work-, life-, and family-related issues.

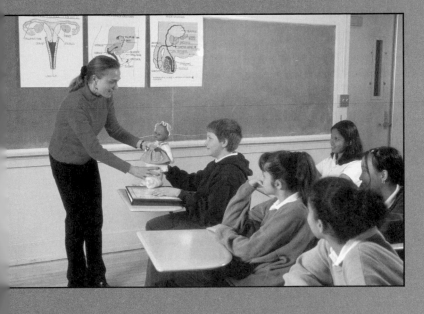

CHAPTER TWELVE

Strategies for Teaching Sexuality Education

The primary goal of sexuality education is the promotion of adult sexual health. It assists children in understanding a positive view of sexuality, provides them with information and skills about taking care of their sexual health, and helps them acquire skills to make decisions now and in the future.

—Guidelines for Comprehensive Sexuality Education Fact Sheet SEICUS (2002)

VALUED OUTCOMES

After doing the activities in this chapter, the student should be able to express and illustrate the following guidelines:

- There are many different types of families; not all families consist of a husband, wife, and children living together.

- Each member of a family is important, and each has certain privileges and responsibilities.

- Interpersonal skills are necessary for strengthening individual and family life.

- Friends help one another feel good about themselves and provide support.

- A positive self-image is necessary if we are to be at ease with ourselves.

- Understanding of self and others is a foundation for successful adulthood.
- Children have rights, and no one should be mistreated, taken advantage of, or abused by another person.
- Heredity and environment influence growth and development.
- Physical, social, and emotional growth occur over a long period of time; such growth differs in each individual.

- Procreation is a function of both males and females.
- Menstruation is a normal process that each healthy female experiences.
- Wholesome attitudes toward sexuality constitute a basic factor for happiness throughout life.
- Sexual values and sexual responsibilities are often individual decisions.

REFLECTIONS

Review the quote at the beginning of this chapter. What is your reaction to the idea that the primary goal of sexuality education is the promotion of adult sexual health? What topic taught at the elementary and middle school levels would be most difficult for you to deal with in the classroom? Discuss what information you would need to have as a teacher to be successful in teaching the topic(s)? What sensitive areas for students and parents would you be most concerned about when teaching the content?

Building Self-Esteem and Responsible Decision Making

Traditionally, providing sexuality education has been the responsibility primarily of the family. Organized religion and other social institutions have also played a significant role. For a variety of reasons, these sources are no longer completely adequate. The schools, by supplementing, not replacing, traditional sources, can provide well-designed and tested sexuality education programs that can benefit all concerned—children, parents, and society in general.

The classroom is a nonthreatening atmosphere where reliable and accurate information can be presented about sex and family matters. But sexuality education is more than just factual information. An effective program must be based on the development of self-esteem and responsible decision making. If children learn to feel good about themselves, they are less likely to need to exploit others and less likely to be open to exploitation in sexual and family functioning. Sexuality education strives to teach equality and respect between the sexes and an appreciation for self and others.

The suggestions in this chapter will help you work toward these goals. These learning opportunities will assist students in obtaining factual knowledge, developing their value systems, and growing psychologically as individuals.

Shown to the right of each activity title in this chapter is the suggested grade level(s) for which the activity might be appropriate. However, through modification, many of the suggested activities could be used at various grade levels. This modification could include the changing of questions that might be more age appropriate for the activity than those provided.

Value-Based Strategies

RIGHTS AND RESPONSIBILITIES   Grades (4–6)

Valued Outcome: The students will be able to identify the factors that help families live in happy environments.

Description of Strategy: Have the class prepare two-column lists of their rights and responsibilities as family members. Under the Rights column, they may list such things as being provided with food and shelter, having free time to play or watch television, being allowed to express their opinions on certain family matters, and spending their allowances as they wish. Under the Responsibilities column, students may list such things as keeping their rooms clean, taking out the trash, helping with housework, caring for a younger sibling, being honest in family matters, and accepting parental decisions. After the lists have been prepared, discuss the significance of the items listed. Ask questions such as the processing questions below.

Materials Needed: pencils or pens and paper

Processing Questions:

1. Do you think your rights and responsibilities are equally balanced?
2. How have your rights and responsibilities changed as you have gotten older?
3. Do boys in a family have certain rights and responsibilities that girls do not have?
4. Do girls in a family have certain rights and responsibilities that boys do not have?
5. How much input should children have about their rights and responsibilities?
6. If you made all the rules in your home, what changes might you consider? Why?
7. What do your rights and responsibilities suggest to you about your own level of maturity?
8. How would you feel if you had no responsibilities?

ATTITUDE INVENTORY—   Grades (4–6)
HOW DO I FEEL?

Valued Outcome: The students will identify feelings concerning family, friends, and themselves.

Description of Strategy: Prepare individual sheets like the one shown here, and ask the students to offer their opinion about each statement. Follow with a general class discussion.

How Do I Feel?

	Agree	Disagree	Not Sure
1. Each child is an important member of his or her family.	____	____	____
2. Families do a lot of fun things together.	____	____	____
3. Mothers should hug and kiss their children more than fathers should.	____	____	____
4. Children who have no brothers or sisters are unhappy.	____	____	____
5. Mothers and fathers should not hug and kiss each other in front of their children.	____	____	____
6. The more I learn about myself, the better I like myself.	____	____	____
7. Children who don't help with the housework should not get an allowance.	____	____	____
8. The best way to learn about sex is to ask friends.	____	____	____
9. I'd be too embarrassed to ask my parents about sex.	____	____	____
10. Sometimes I dread becoming a teenager.	____	____	____
11. I have trouble telling friends how I really feel.	____	____	____
12. My friends often pressure me to do things I don't want to do.	____	____	____
13. When a friend does something wrong, I usually tell the person how I feel.	____	____	____
14. Children should be allowed to set some of the family rules.	____	____	____
15. Adults are free to do what they want most of the time.	____	____	____

Materials Needed: attitude inventory sheet for each student, pencils

Processing Questions:

1. Were there questions that were difficult to answer?
2. Why were the answers to some of the questions difficult?
3. What three things did you learn from your responses?

GETTING TO KNOW ME

Valued Outcome: Students will be able to list their unique characteristics.

Description of Strategy: Prepare sheets or cards with the following statements or categories on them. Pass out a sheet to each student to complete, then collect and shuffle all the responses. Either as a class or small-group activity, see if students can identify each other by the responses. Have the students consider what this suggests about the unique individuality of each person.

Something that I do well: _____

Music that I like: _____

Three words that describe me: _____

If I could have a dream come true, it would be: _____

What I like to do in my spare time: _____

I'm looking forward to: _____

One thing I like about myself: _____

Who am I? _____

Materials Needed: one prepared paper or card for each student, pencils

Processing Questions:

1. Were there any questions that were difficult to answer?
2. What were you proud of in your answers?
3. What would you like to change about your answers?
4. Did anything surprise you about your answers?

THAT'S MY OPINION

Valued Outcome: The students will develop insight into what boys and girls look for and expect from individuals of the opposite sex.

Description of Strategy: This activity is designed to help boys and girls understand the many misconceptions about qualities desired by the opposite sex. Divide the class into groups of males and females and assign a recorder and spokeperson for each group. Have each group respond to the questions "I like girls (boys) who. . . ." and "I dislike girls (boys) who. . . ." The recorder keeps a record of all responses and the spokeperson reads the responses aloud (the teacher may wish to screen the responses first).

Materials Needed: pencils and paper

Processing Questions:

1. What did the boys seem to like about the girls? What did they dislike?
2. What did the girls seem to like about the boys? What did they dislike?
3. Why do you think there were differences between the two lists for both the likes and dislikes?
4. What do you think we can learn from the likes and dislikes of boys and girls?

Decision Stories

Present decision stories such as the following, using the procedures outlined in Chapter 4, pages 80–83. The content of the stories that you present should be appropriate for the developmental levels of your students. The examples here range from stories suitable for the early elementary grades to the upper grades, but remember that appropriateness must be determined in the social context of your own group.

AM I STUCK WITH ME?   Grades (K–3)

Kevin is overweight and not very good at sports. He is often chosen last in team sports and games; although this bothers him, he tries to make a joke of it. In fact, he makes a great many jokes because he wants the other kids to like him. And they do. They think Kevin is a lot of fun. But Kevin doesn't just want to be the class clown. He wants the other kids in class to respect him for what he is. He would like the girls in class to think more highly of him too.

Focus Questions:

1. What might Kevin do to feel better about himself?
2. Are there some things that he should not change? Why or why not?

THE CRUSH   Grades (4–6)

Jackie couldn't seem to stop thinking about the boy who lived down the street. He was a lot older than she was, and he thought she was "just a kid." Jackie went out of her way to be around him. She hoped that he would invite her out on a date, even though she wasn't really old enough to start dating. Then one day Jackie saw him with another girl—one closer to his own age. She felt terrible. How could he do this to her?

Focus Question: What should Jackie do next?

JOHN'S WORLD   Grades (4–6)

John's parents were divorced last year. John is living with his mother, but he sees his father regularly. One weekend, while John is staying with his father, he finds out that his father is going to get married again. "John," his father says. "This is Janet. I know that you're going to like each other." But John doesn't like his father's woman friend. He is still feeling bad about the divorce. Now this! Will this woman become his stepmother? What will happen to his real mother? What kind of a family will this be? John is confused, very angry, and deeply unhappy.

Focus Questions:

1. Should John pretend he likes this woman, or should he treat her badly so she will know how he feels?
2. What could John say to his father about this situation?

Health Highlight

WHAT'S HAPPENING?

Martin Heesacker, in *Portraits of Adjustment,* has stated, "Long-term studies indicate that many of the behavioral, psychological, and academic problems shown by children following divorce are traceable to conflict in the dysfunctional family prior to the divorce." Some of the research findings indicate that girls tend to act out less than boys; that eleven-year-old boys whose parents had divorced within the last year had 19 percent more behavioral and academic problems than eleven-year-old boys living in an intact family; and divorces tended to generate their own problems, whether in reducing economic well-being or in further disrupting relations among parents and children.

SOURCE: Heesacker 1994, 254

STORIES OR FACTS?   Grades (4–6)

One day after school, some of the girls are talking about how babies are made. Susan is listening with interest. Some of the things she hears are new to her. She has learned a little bit about sex education from her parents and in school, but she is still not sure about all the details. Now she is more confused than ever. She wishes that she knew which of these things were really true.

Focus Questions:

1. What can Susan do to get accurate information?
2. Who should she try to talk with?
3. Should she rely on her friends for information?

FOOLING AROUND   Grades (6–8)

Bob and his friend George are spending the afternoon together in George's home. It is raining, so they have to stay inside. George's parents are not at home. The two boys start to talk about sex. Then George suggests that the two of them "fool around" together and play with each other's bodies. Afterward, Bob feels that maybe he did something wrong. He feels guilty and frightened. The next day, he feels even worse. He is afraid to tell his parents what happened.

Focus Question: What should Bob do?

THE PARTY   Grades (6–8)

Tina's friend Marie is having a party and has invited her. At the party, Tina knows only a few of the other guests. Everyone seems to be having a good time. There is music, and the boys and girls are dancing. Later, Tina notices that some of the couples are kissing and making out. A boy named Carl comes over to her.

"Would you like to dance with me?" he asks. She is not sure. She doesn't really know Carl. What if he tries something? What could she do? She feels flattered that Carl is paying attention to her, but she is also unsure of herself in situations like this.

Focus Questions:

1. What should Tina do?

2. What are some possible reasons she feels uncomfortable?

3. What decisions does Tina have to make now and in the future?

BEING FRIENDLY

Grades (4–8)

Sharon was playing in her backyard one day when Mr. Smith, the man next door, asked her if she would like to come over and have some ice cream. Mr. Smith had always been nice, so Sharon quickly accepted his invitation. Once inside his house, Sharon learned that Mrs. Smith was not there. Mr. Smith started putting his arms around Sharon and brushing up against her. That made Sharon feel uncomfortable. Sharon wanted to leave, but Mr. Smith was very anxious to have her stay.

Focus Questions:

1. Is Mr. Smith acting appropriately?

2. What should Sharon do in this situation?

3. Should she worry about hurting Mr. Smith's feelings?

4. How should Sharon react if the person touching her is her stepfather or another relative?

Other Strategies for Teaching

BEING MY OWN PERFECT FRIEND

Grades (1–6)

Valued Outcome: The students will be able to assess the qualities they desire in themselves and others who are friends.

Description of Strategy: Ask the students to make a list of five qualities they would like in a perfect friend. Have them describe each of these qualities in a sentence, such as "My perfect friend gives me good advice when I am not feeling happy" or "My perfect friend accepts me for who I am." Ask students to share their ideas in class, and prepare a master list on the board, poster board, or overhead projector.

Materials Needed: index cards or sheets of paper, pencils, board, posterboard, or overhead projector and markers or pens

Processing Questions:

1. How can each of you be your own "perfect friend"?

2. If you cross out "my perfect friend" in your sentences and substitute the word "I," what do you notice about the sentence?

3. How can each of us be more of a "perfect friend" to ourselves instead of sometimes being our own "worst enemy"?

4. What are the implications for ourselves and our friends?

LOVE, LOVE, LOVE   Grades (6–8)

Valued Outcome: The students will list nonsexual ways to express love toward others.

Description of Strategy: Have a "love discussion" in which the class talks about all the different kinds of love (between them and brothers and sisters, parents and stepparents, relatives, friends, teachers). Have students list different appropriate ways of expressing love to family members by their words, the tone of their voices, body language, and actions toward each other.

Materials Needed: pencils and paper

Processing Questions:

1. How many different people do you love?

2. What are some ways in which you express your feelings to everyone you love?

3. How can you tell if someone loves you?

SOLVING PROBLEMS   Grades (4–6)

Valued Outcome: The students will develop possible choices for solving problems they may encounter.

Description of Strategy: Divide students into an even number of groups of four or five each. One student in each group will be a recorder. Have each group write three problems that require a decision. Emphasize that these problems should be typical ones that their age group faces and should be about relationships or risky behavior. When finished, pair the groups and have them exchange problems. Each group then writes possible solutions for the new problems. The recorders can report the results to the class.

Materials Needed: pencils and paper

Processing Questions:

1. Did any groups list the same problems?

2. Is it always easy to make positive decisions?

3. Does it sometimes help to get other opinions about what to do?

Valued Outcome: The students will complete sentences describing how they will respond to various situations associated with growing up.

Description of Strategy: The passage to adulthood can be an especially awkward and confusing time as young people struggle with new signals from their bodies and the maturing young men and women around them. Many will experience emotional changes, mood swings, feelings of uncertainty, and increased feelings of independence and sexuality. A positive and confident attitude can help them handle these changes better.

As students grow, fewer adults will be making decisions for them, but the pressure to be part of the peer group will increase. They will need to rely on their own values to help make the choices most appropriate for developing a positive and healthy life. Have your students read the following statements and complete each sentence.

- I want to drive my friend's car, but I don't have my license. I'm going to _____.

- I know my girlfriend has cramps because she has her period. I'm going to _____.

- My parents can use my help around the house more often. I think I'll _____.

- I haven't developed physically as fast as my friends. This makes me feel _____.

- I have acne on my face. I will _____.

- My parents are going away next weekend. I'm going to _____.

- Some of my friends like to talk about sex. This makes me feel uncomfortable. I should _____.

Materials Needed: list of statements for each student

Processing Questions:

1. Why are some of the statements more difficult to deal with than others?
2. Is a person's maturity indicated by what he or she says? does?
3. Are there certain pressures to say or do certain things? Give examples.
4. Can you identify some decisions based upon these statements that might (or might not) indicate good decision making?

THE ANSWER IS NO   Grades (4–6)

Valued Outcome: The students will gain experience in having to tell others they may not do something they want to do. The students will then report how it feels to be in the position of saying no.

Description of Strategy: Have the students divide into pairs of their own choosing. Explain that one student will play the part of a parent, and the other will play the part of that parent's child. The child will ask permission from the parent to go to a party where both boys and girls will be present. The student act-

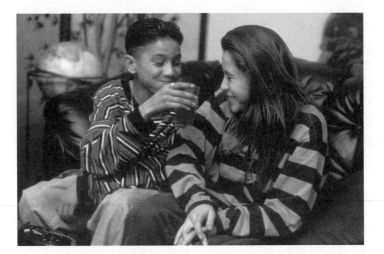

In developing relation-ships, adolescents need to rely on their values and learn to communi-cate effectively.

ing the part of the child will explain about the party—who will be there, where it will be, and so on. After listening, the student acting as parent refuses permission. The son or daughter argues for permission but is still refused. Let several pairs of students act out the situation in front of the class, but do not require anyone to do so who does not wish to participate. Discuss how the different pairs of students handle the same situation. Then, without forewarning the class that you will do so, have selected pairs of students switch roles and repeat the activity. Use discretion in choosing which pairs of students to use for this second part of the activity. Be prepared to discuss how the parents might feel when they have to say no.

Materials Needed: none

Processing Questions:

1. What differences do you note in individual roles when these roles are reversed?
2. What did you learn from this activity?
3. How do you think parents feel when they have to say no?
4. What are some potential reasons for saying no?
5. Why might saying yes be good or bad?

HOW WOULD YOU HANDLE IT?   Grades (6–8)

Valued Outcome: The students will act out commonly faced situations.

Description of Strategy: Divide the class into pairs; make sure that close friends are not paired. (There will be no role switching in this activity.) Have each pair act out situations such as the following:

  - asking for and getting a date
  - asking for and being refused a date

- introducing a friend to one's parents (a third child should play the part of the friend)
- telling a divorced parent that you don't care for the person the parent is dating
- introducing yourself to a member of the opposite sex to whom you feel attracted
- being polite to someone you don't like
- handling rejection when socially rebuffed

Materials Needed: none

Processing Questions:

1. Which of the preceding situations do you find the most difficult?
2. What is most important when attempting to convey a message to someone?
3. How many ways can you think of to handle each of the situations?

UNDERSTANDING OTHERS   Grades (7–8)

Valued Outcome: The students will imitate personal characteristics that they do not have.

Description of Strategy: Not everyone is alike; some people are bossy, and others are shy. Assign different roles to various children, such as Noisy Ned, Bossy Betty, Shy Sam, Iceberg Irene, Chatterbox Chester, Silent Sylvia, Blustery Ben, Whirlwind Wanda, Studious Stu, Laughing Larry, Somber Sarah, and Flighty Frank. Make sure that the children assigned to each role do not have the characteristics of the role they are to play. One by one, have each child act out the part for a few minutes.

Materials Needed: none

Processing Questions:

1. How can you deal with these different personality types?
2. What do you find appealing about the characteristics of each personality type?
3. Why might others be put off by some of these characteristics?
4. Why is it good that all people are not alike?

SUPERKID   Grades (5–6)

Valued Outcome: The students will verbally list ways that life is difficult for everyone, no matter what talents or gifts they have.

Description of Strategy: Have the students divide into pairs. One student plays the part of Superkid and the other will be his or her press agent. Each pair decides what abilities each Superkid will have. These abilities might include flying, speaking any language, singing or playing a musical instrument so well that the person is a superstar, possessing great athletic talent, and so on. First, the student playing the press agent introduces the Superkid and describes his or her abilities in the most glowing terms. Then, Superkid acknowledges his or her popular acclaim but notes to the class that life is not perfect even for a Superkid. Have the student explain why being a Superkid isn't as completely wonderful as the press agent has said. If the person is described as an athlete, for example, he or she might explain the anxieties about getting injured on the field, the pressure of competition, and so forth.

Materials Needed: none

Processing Questions:

1. Does anyone have all their problems taken care of?
2. Is it possible that extreme talents sometimes can create more problems?
3. If you had one incredible ability, what would you like it to be?
4. What talents do you have that make you super in some way?

ME AND MY SELF-CONFIDENCE   Grades (7–8)

Valued Outcome: The students will recognize that many people are very successful even though they may not look perfect.

Description of Strategy: Discuss characteristics that can cause people to feel self-conscious, such as being overweight or underweight, being very short or very tall, having a large nose, or having skin problems. Note that some of these characteristics are either temporary or ones that can be changed while others are permanent or difficult to change. All characteristics can actually become an asset. Discuss famous individuals noted for unique or unusual physical features. These might include Barbra Streisand and her nose, or Dudley Moore and his shortness. Emphasize that each of these individuals relied on developed talent rather than inherited physical characteristics to achieve success and that self-confidence was often the key to success.

Materials Needed: none

Processing Questions:

1. Can you name some people you really admire who may have an unusual physical characteristic?
2. What physical characteristics do you have that you feel are less than perfect?
3. What characteristics and talents do you have that make you proud?

OPPORTUNITIES FOR ALL   Grades (4–6)

Valued Outcome: The students will recognize and name professions that were once male- or female-dominated but in which both genders now have increasing opportunity to participate.

Description of Strategy: In years past, many occupations were considered as appropriate only for males or females. Today, this social attitude is changing, as are our conceptions of gender roles and gender stereotyping in general. After discussing this point with the class, divide students into small groups to talk about and research individual instances of changing professions for the sexes. Have some groups look into changing occupational opportunities and others look at changing social or familial roles. For example, many police officers in cities and towns throughout the nation are now women, and some men now stay home and care for the children. Ask each group to compile a report on how changes in their area of research have resulted in greater opportunity for both men and women.

Materials Needed: none

Processing Questions:

1. Do you think it is appropriate for females to engage in all professions? Why or why not?

2. Do you think it is appropriate for males to engage in all professions? Why or why not?

3. What profession do you think you would like to be a part of when you grow up?

INFORMATION PLEASE   Grades (4–6)

Valued Outcome: The students will rank sources of information concerning sexuality questions.

Description of Strategy: Prepare a worksheet that gives possible sources of information on sexuality such as the list below. Have each student rank the list from the source most likely to provide accurate information to the source least likely to provide accurate information. Then discuss the different rankings in class. Be sure to point out that even what might be considered the most informed source may not be able to supply information on a particular question without research. Avoid disparaging any valid source of information, but suggest that some are probably more useful than others. If appropriate, you might also note that sometimes more than one source should be consulted for more complete information.

Possible sources of sexuality information

_____ Movies and television	_____ Books from the library
_____ Health teacher	_____ Physician (doctor)
_____ Minister, priest, or rabbi	_____ Newspaper columns
_____ Friends	_____ Magazines
_____ Parents	_____ Textbooks used in schools

Materials Needed: worksheet generated from list above

Processing Questions:

1. Can any one source answer all the questions you might have?

2. Why is it wise to check several sources of information concerning questions of sexuality?

3. Should you ever consult more than one source about a question you have?

LEGAL RIGHTS   Grades (7–8)

Valued Outcome: The students will learn what sexual abuse is and what options they have if they are abused.

Description of Strategy: Unfortunately, many children in this country are sexually abused. Such abuse may come from other family members or from trusted adults or friends. Often, children are completely unaware of their legal and moral rights in such instances. After becoming informed on legal recourse available in your area, present an objective lecture on the subject to your class. It is very important that you preface your discussion by emphasizing that the child has no reason to feel guilty or ashamed for being a victim of sexual exploitation of any kind. Further, point out there are authorities who can protect against that person ever hurting them (reprisal) again. Suggest sources that children can turn to for help if such exploitation is occurring. A good first choice is the school psychologist, counselor, or physician.

Materials Needed: none

Processing Questions:

1. Is it ever a child's fault if he or she is sexually abused?
2. If you are being treated in a way that makes you think you are being abused, what should you do?
3. Who are some people you could tell if you are being abused?

FAMILIES ARE DIFFERENT   Grades (4–6)

Valued Outcome: The students will realize that any family structure can provide a loving and healthy environment for personal growth, even if that family structure is not "typical."

Description of Strategy: Invite adults of your acquaintance to come to class to discuss the different types of families in which they grew up. Include individuals from a wide variety of familial backgrounds, including traditional American nuclear families, extended family situations, single-parent families, and so forth. This is not an easy activity to do, but it can be a most valuable one. Your guests should not gloss over any difficulties they had growing up in their particular situation, but children should not get the impression that singular events are typical of any situation.

Materials Needed: guest speakers who can effectively address identified issues

Processing Questions:

1. Are all families the same?
2. Can you be a normal person if you do not live with your real mother and father?
3. Is growing up easy for anyone?

INDIVIDUAL REPORTS   Grades (7–8)

Valued Outcome: The students will learn more about human development.

Description of Strategy: As appropriate for the developmental level of your particular students, assign individual report topics on aspects of physical and emotional growth. Have the students use your health textbook and other approved informational sources to research particular areas, such as the growth spurt that occurs in adolescence, puberty, menarche, first encounters with the opposite sex in social situations, and dating behavior in the early teen years. On a separate sheet of paper, have students list questions for which they did not find answers during their research. Consult with each student on an individual basis to assist in finding appropriate solutions to these questions. In doing this activity, rely on the advisory committee to your sexuality education program for appropriate responses to individual student questions or dilemmas.

Materials Needed: paper, pencils or pens, reference materials

Processing Questions:

1. What kinds of questions do you have for which you did not find answers?
2. What did you learn that you did not know before about human development?

WHY NOT?   Grades (6–8)

Valued Outcome: Increase student awareness of possible consequences of some kinds of sexual behavior.

Description of Strategy: After discussion and approval of this activity by all members of the family life advisory committee, invite various representatives of sex education groups in your community to lecture to the class on the ramifications of certain sexual decisions that each individual must make, such as the decision to have intercourse outside of marriage. Make it clear before the activity that you as the teacher are not advocating any behavior that goes against general community norms.

Materials Needed: guest speakers who are screened carefully before talking to the group

Processing Questions:

1. Is it wise to make sexual decisions based on how you feel at a certain time?
2. What are some reasons for delaying some kinds of sexual behavior?

DICTIONARY WITH A DIFFERENCE   Grades (4–6)

Valued Outcome: The students will develop a page about themselves in a "human dictionary."

Description of Strategy: Have students make a "different dictionary" about themselves to be exhibited in the classroom. Each child has a page that is his or her dictionary entry. Included should be a picture, below which is the last name, first name, the phonetic respelling, and birth date. There should be a line telling the age and grade, a line listing identifying characteristics, a line for interests, and a qualitative statement (for example, I am good at basketball, baseball, and swimming).

Materials Needed: photos of students, paper, pencils or pens

Processing Questions:

1. What is something really special about yourself?
2. How are you different from the way you were last year?

GUPPIES   Grades (K–3)

Valued Outcome: The students will recognize that birth and reproduction are a normal part of the life cycle of all living things.

Description of Strategy: After discussing the concept that all living things can reproduce, let students observe the birth process in live-bearing fish. Obtain some young female guppies and young male guppies. Raise them in separate aquariums. Point out to the class the physical differences between the females and the males. Note that the female guppy is larger and somewhat drab in coloration in contrast to the smaller, brightly colored male. Explain that in many animal species there are obvious differences between males and females, as there are with human beings. When the fish are mature, place one or more males in the tank with the females. In a few weeks, one or more of the females will become pregnant. This will soon be obvious. With luck, birth may take place while class is in session. Have the children observe the birth process. Also point out differences in the birth process for different species, for example, many fish and all birds are egg layers. (As soon as the female guppies give birth, separate the adults from the young, as guppies are cannibalistic.)

Materials Needed: functioning aquarium apparatus, guppies, fish food

Processing Questions:

1. What are some examples of species where their babies are not born alive? How are they born?
2. Were you born alive?

BABY ANIMALS   Grades (K–3)

Valued Outcome: The students will observe mammalian birth.

Description of Strategy: If appropriate, you may wish to breed white mice or other rodents in the classroom. After the female has given birth, have the children observe the offspring.

Materials Needed: mice, cage, food, nesting materials

Processing Questions:

1. How are the adults and children alike? How are they different?

2. How does the mother take care of her young? Why does she take such good care of her children?

3. Do all animals nurture their children?

4. How are animal families like human families? How are they different?

GENETICS

Grades (4–6)

Valued Outcome: The students will observe how offspring inherit different traits from their parents.

Description of Strategy: If you decide to breed mice or other animals in the classroom, you can also use the project to demonstrate inherited traits by using a male and a female with different physical characteristics, such as fur coloration. Observe how many of the offspring have inherited coloration traits similar to those of one parent or the other. For upper elementary school children, discuss dominant and recessive traits.

Materials Needed: mice, cage, food, nesting materials

Processing Questions:

1. What traits did you inherit from your mother? What traits did you inherit from your father?

2. Can you give other examples of some traits you have observed in the offspring of pet cats or dogs?

INHERITED TRAITS

Grades (4–6)

Valued Outcome: The students will realize that some personal characteristics are inherited.

Description of Strategy: The human genetic code contains information about thousands of inherited traits. These include hair, eye, and skin color; shape of ears and nose; and general physique. Emphasize to your class that even individual rates of growth are to a large extent genetically controlled, which explains why some children grow more quickly than others. To demonstrate that some genetic traits are less obvious than others, ask the class to roll their tongues. Some students will be able to roll their tongues, but others will be unable to do so. This ability is a genetic trait.

Materials Needed: none

Processing Questions:

1. What are some other characteristics that you have that are unique?

2. Does having a certain genetic trait make you better or worse than anyone else?

Puzzles and Games

REPRODUCTION SYSTEMS CROSSWORD PUZZLE

Grades (6–8)

Valued Outcome: Students will increase their vocabulary about reproduction.

Description of Strategy: Prepare a crossword puzzle worksheets (see the Teaching in Action box below).

Materials Needed: crossword puzzle worksheet and pencils for each student

Processing Questions:

1. Can you define all the words in the crossword puzzle?

2. Can you use each word in a sentence?

TEACHING IN ACTION *Reproduction Systems Crossword Puzzle*

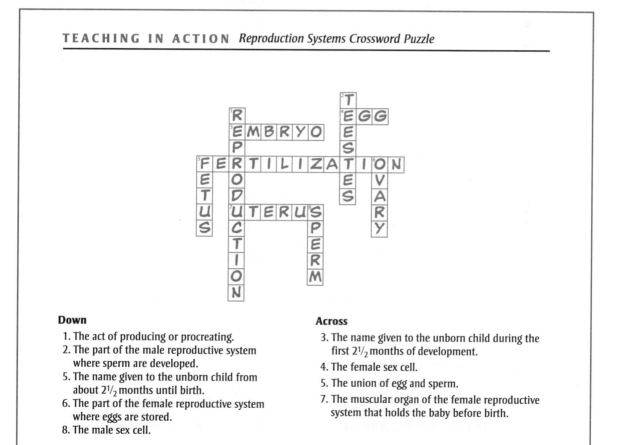

Down

1. The act of producing or procreating.
2. The part of the male reproductive system where sperm are developed.
5. The name given to the unborn child from about 2¹/₂ months until birth.
6. The part of the female reproductive system where eggs are stored.
8. The male sex cell.

Across

3. The name given to the unborn child during the first 2¹/₂ months of development.
4. The female sex cell.
5. The union of egg and sperm.
7. The muscular organ of the female reproductive system that holds the baby before birth.

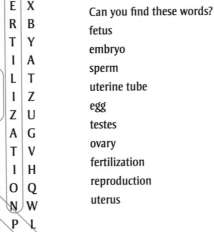

Can you find these words?

fetus

embryo

sperm

uterine tube

egg

testes

ovary

fertilization

reproduction

uterus

WORD SEARCH   Grades (4–6)

Valued Outcome: Through a word search puzzle, the students will become more familiar with words associated with reproduction.

Description of Strategy: Recreate the word search puzzle in the Teaching in Action box above—or create your own—and have the students find and circle each of the words listed. The words may read in any direction—up, down, across, or diagonally.

Materials Needed: word search worksheet and pencils for each student

Processing Questions:

1. Can you define all the words in the word search list?

2. Can you use the words in a sentence?

SCRAMBLED SENTENCES   Grades (7–8)

Valued Outcome: Students will review the reproductive system by unscrambling sentences.

Description of Strategy: Create a worksheet using the following scrambled sentences about the human reproductive systems. Have the students unscramble the sentences.

canal acts birth as the vagina a _____
  (*The vagina acts as a birth canal.*)

ova the hormones and ovaries produce _____
  (*The ovaries produce ova and hormones.*)

tubes occurs in fertilization the uterine _____
  (*Fertilization occurs in the uterine tubes.*)

begins females in at menstruation puberty _____
  (*Menstruation begins in females at puberty.*)

in the fetus uterus the develops _____
  (*The fetus develops in the uterus.*)

are cells the male sperm reproductive called _____
  (*The male reproductive cells are called sperm.*)

testes produced in the cells sperm are _____
  (*Sperm cells are produced in the testes.*)

fluids other and semen of made is up sperm _____
  (*Semen is made up of sperm and other fluids.*)

puberty begin at sperm produced to be _____
  (*Sperm begin to be produced at puberty.*)

at testosterone the triggers spurt male puberty growth _____
  (*Testosterone triggers the male growth spurt at puberty.*)

Materials Needed: worksheet for each student generated from scrambled sentences above

Processing Questions:

1. Are there any terms you did not understand?
2. Can you take each unscrambled sentence and describe the process that is occurring within each situation?

MATCHING PARTS AND FUNCTIONS   Grades (7–8)

Valued Outcome: The students will review information on the reproductive system by labeling the parts in a team competition.

Description of Strategy: Draw a large diagram of the female reproductive system on the board. Draw leader lines from each of the parts, and allow room for labeling. Prepare a similar diagram for the male reproductive system. (Refer to Figures 11.1 and 11.2 on pages 302 and 303.) Divide the class into two teams. Point to a part on either diagram and ask the first player from Team A to identify it. If the student knows the answer, he or she should come to the board and label the part. If the student does not know the correct answer, the first player from Team B gets a chance. Score one point for each correct answer. After a part has been correctly labeled, ask the next player to explain one function of that part. If the student knows the correct answer, she or he should come to the board and write the function next to the name of the part.

Materials Needed: board and markers or overhead projector and pens

Processing Questions:

1. What were the most significant things we learned?
2. What were some of the most difficult questions to answer?

TRUE OR FALSE?   Grades (7–8)

Valued Outcome: The students will review information about human sexuality through team competition.

Description of Strategy: Divide the class into two teams and ask each player to decide whether a statement that you make is true or false. Score one point for each correct answer. Then write each of the true statements on the board. Review the true statements at the end of the game. Sample statements might include the following:

> Girls should not swim during menstruation. (false)
>
> A wet dream is a sign that a boy is reaching puberty. (true)
>
> Fertilization leading to pregnancy occurs when a sperm unites with an egg. (true)
>
> The beginning of menstruation means that a girl can now become pregnant. (true)

Materials Needed: board and markers, prepared list of statements

Processing Questions:

1. What were the most difficult questions to deal with? Why?
2. Were there questions you wanted to know more about?

Other Ideas

GROWING UP   Grades (4–6)

Valued Outcome: Students will increase understanding of the growth process.

Description of Strategy: Have each student trace his or her hand on a sheet of paper. Ask the students to take their tracings home, and have one or both parents trace their hands over the child's tracing.

Materials Needed: paper, pens

Processing Questions:

1. Is your parent's hand larger than yours? Why?
2. How do body parts grow?
3. Will your whole body be larger when you are grown?

FAMILY ACTIVITIES COLLAGE   Grades (K–3)

Valued Outcome: Students will make a collage of activities they engage in with their families.

Description of Strategy: Have each student search through magazines to find pictures of family activities. These activities can include watching television together, going on trips or outings, working around the house, talking with one another, and so forth. Explain to the students that the pictures they choose need to represent a family activity. Thus, a picture of a television set by itself can represent watching television together, an airplane can represent a trip to relatives in another part of the country, and so on. Have each student prepare a colorful collage and then explain to the class the meaning of each component.

Materials Needed: poster board, magazines, scissors, glue

Processing Questions:

1. What activities do you do most often with your family?
2. What family activities are your favorite?

MY FAMILY TREE   Grades (4–6)

Valued Outcome: Students will develop a family tree and discuss characteristics they might have inherited from other family members.

Description of Strategy: Distribute copies of the Teaching in Action box on page 338. Have each student prepare his or her family tree (younger children may need the assistance of their parents to fill in the names). After the diagrams are completed, discuss the family trees. This may be an area where sensitivity will be needed since some students may be adopted or have stepparents. If approached carefully, this activity may provide an opportunity to discuss what adoption is, why people adopt, and which traits any of the adopted children in the class perceive they have that are similar to those of their adoptive parents.

Materials Needed: photocopies of the family tree for each student

Processing Questions:

1. What physical features do you have in common with siblings, parents, grandparents, stepparents, and so on?
2. Do you have any interest(s) similar to those of your ancestors?
3. Which relative do you think you most resemble?

CAUGHT IN THE ACT   Grades (4–6)

Valued Outcome: The students will observe and record classmates' behaviors.

Description of Strategy: What positive behaviors do you see your classmates use? Are they responsible, cooperative, or courteous? Read the following examples. See if you can catch your classmates in the act. Write in the names of the people who use these behaviors.

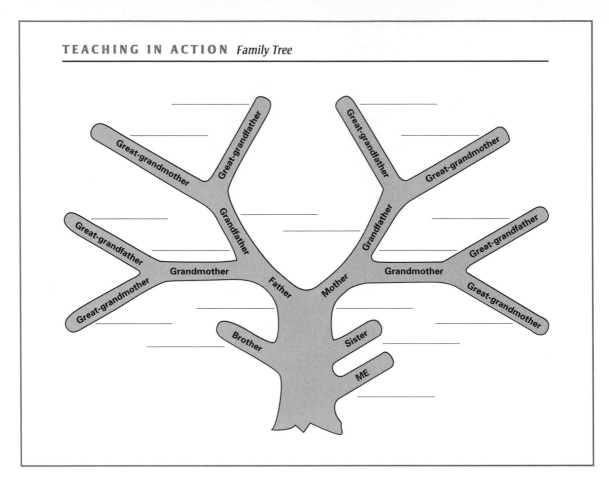

Being Responsible

Returned something that was borrowed

Admitted making a mistake

Finished all schoolwork and turned it in on time

Being Cooperative

Followed the line leader

Worked well with someone to get a job done

Tried hard in a game or in physical education

Who Did It?

_____

_____

_____

Who Did It?

_____

_____

_____

Being Courteous	Who Did It?
Helped someone who had a problem	_____
Waited for his or her turn in line	_____
Gave someone else a compliment for doing something well	_____

Materials Needed: worksheet for each student

Processing Questions:

1. Why is it important for us to be responsible, cooperative, and courteous?
2. How do you feel when someone is not responsible, cooperative, and courteous?
3. How does it make you feel when you are responsible, cooperative, and courteous?

RESPONSIBILITY   Grades (4–6)

Valued Outcome: The students will list the responsibilities of different family members.

Description of Strategy: Create a worksheet of the chart below. Have the students write their name and their family members' names in the first column. Put an X in each column that tells a responsibility each person has in the home. Add other responsibilities if needed.

Family Member	Cooking	Washing Clothes	Doing Dishes	Paying Bills	Taking Out Trash	Cleaning Bathroom	Other

Materials Needed: chart for each student, pencil or pen

Processing Questions:

1. What are the consequences of people not completing their responsibilities?
2. Do you always fulfill your responsibilities?
3. Do you have to be reminded to do your jobs around the house?

HOW MY DECISIONS AFFECT OTHERS

Valued Outcome: The students will list how they think their decisions to perform various tasks affect their family.

Description of Strategy: Use the following list as an example. Students should consider different situations they may face and think about how the decisions they make affect their family. Have students record their responses and then discuss them as a class.

If I Decided to . . .	I Think My Family Would Feel . . .
say no to a drug a friend offered me	_____
not clean my room after being told to do so	_____
try to do my best in math	_____
do my homework for a week without being reminded	_____

Materials Needed: list of situations for each student

Processing Questions:

1. Do your actions affect the people around you?

2. Can you do things that will make life easier for your family?

HELPING OTHERS

Valued Outcome: The students will develop a list of ways that they can help their friends and family.

Description of Strategy: Prepare individual worksheets of the chart below. Using this chart, have students compile a list of things they can do to help out family and friends. These acts of kindness need not be big chores or sacrifices. They can be little things that may make a difference in the day of the people they love.

Whom I Can Help	How I Can Help	How Many Times I've Helped
Parents	_____	_____
Grandparents	_____	_____
Brother or sister	_____	_____
My teacher	_____	_____
My best friend	_____	_____

Materials Needed: worksheet for each student

Processing Questions:

1. Was it difficult to think of ways to help any of the people on the list? Why?
2. Do you feel you have helped the people on the list as much as you should?
3. How does helping others make you feel?

FAMILY RULES   Grades (7–8)

Valued Outcome: The students will list various rules they are supposed to follow every day.

Description of Strategy: Create a worksheet of the following chart and give a copy to each student. Discuss with the students the different kinds of rules they may be expected to follow every day. Two rules are given. Have the students discuss rules and then complete their own daily lists, placing an X in the columns of the days they successfully followed each rule.

	M	T	W	Th	F	Sa	S
Get up on time							
Brush my teeth							

Materials Needed: worksheet for each student

Processing Questions:

1. Are some rules more difficult to follow? Why?
2. Why are there rules to follow?
3. What would happen if there were no rules? Would you really like that?

THE MENSTRUAL CYCLE   Grades (5–6)

Valued Outcome: Students will learn the different phases of the menstrual cycle.

Description of Strategy: About every twenty-eight days, a new menstrual cycle begins in the female body. The cycle begins with the shedding of the lining of the uterus. This is called menstruation and takes about four or five days. For the next several days, the lining (or endometrium) is very thin, and an egg cell in an ovary begins to ripen. The lining starts to thicken, and, by the fourteenth day, a ripened egg is released into a uterine tube. This is called ovulation. The endometrium continues to thicken as the egg moves toward the uterus. If the egg is not fertilized, it disintegrates and menstruation takes place, which signals the beginning of a new cycle.

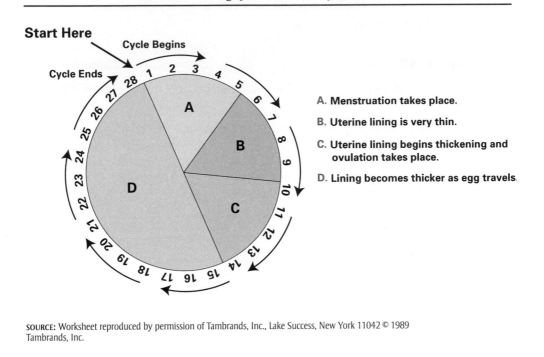

Start Here

Cycle Begins

Cycle Ends

A. **Menstruation takes place.**

B. **Uterine lining is very thin.**

C. **Uterine lining begins thickening and ovulation takes place.**

D. **Lining becomes thicker as egg travels.**

SOURCE: Worksheet reproduced by permission of Tambrands, Inc., Lake Success, New York 11042 © 1989 Tambrands, Inc.

The Teaching in Action box above shows a twenty-eight-day menstrual cycle. Have students put the letter of each phase on the blank spaces of the diagram in the correct order. Then tell them to indicate on the circle when ovulation takes place. (Answers have been included in the cycle for your reference.)

Materials Needed: worksheet for each student

Processing Questions:

1. What is menstruation?

2. Why is menstruation called a twenty-eight-day cycle?

WHY ARE THEY LIKE THAT?   Grades (5–6)

Valued Outcome: The students will have an opportunity to ask questions about the behavior of the opposite sex.

Description of Strategy: Certain aspects of the behavior of boys is often a puzzle to girls and vice versa. Have each student write one question about some aspect of the "typical" behavior of the opposite sex that is puzzling or perhaps annoying. The questions should be unsigned. Collect all the questions and read aloud those that seem most germane to a discussion of behavior among boys and girls at your class's grade level. Have volunteers attempt to explain the point of view of the opposite sex that might shed light on a particular aspect of behavior. For example, at a certain age girls may be more interested in boys than boys are interested in girls as a result of maturational differences. Therefore, girls may be attracted to older boys, thus giving boys their own age the feeling that they are not seen as sexual peers. Act as moderator in the discussion, and provide factual information as necessary.

Materials Needed: slips of paper, pencils or pens

Processing Questions:

1. Did you learn anything new about the opposite sex?
2. Do you think the behavior of the opposite sex makes any more sense than it did before?
3. Do males and females think the same way?

ADVICE COLUMN   Grades (7–8)

Valued Outcome: The students will ask questions about family and human sexuality.

Description of Strategy: With your assistance and supervision, have the class put together a newspaper advice column. First, have each student write a letter to the column asking for some advice about a sexuality or family life matter. Students may ask for simple factual information, such as "What is masturbation?" or for advice on handling a personal problem, such as "How can I ask someone for a date?" Collect all the letters, which should be unsigned or signed with something like "Puzzled" or "Wondering," and group them into categories. Restate a typical example of each category, writing this paraphrase on the board or overhead projector. Then have each student write an answer for the "column." Again using your discretion, collate the different suggestions offered and discuss them with the class. Properly handled, this activity can offer you important insights into the sexual development of students in your class. As "managing editor" of the advice column, however, you must make sure that topics covered stay within guidelines set up for your school's sexuality education program.

Materials Needed: paper, pencils or pens, board and markers or overhead projector and pens

Processing Questions:

1. What did you learn that you did not know before?
2. What do you think is the most important part of relationships with others?
3. Did you find out what you most wanted to know?

Resources

PAMPHLETS

101 ways to say no to sex. Santa Cruz, CA: ETR Associates. Suggestions on how teens can say no to sex. (Grades 6–12)

101 ways to survive puberty. Santa Cruz, CA: ETR Associates. Suggests staying away from drugs, choosing friends wisely, and not dating until ready. (Grades 5–8)

Draw the line, respect the line. Santa Cruz, CA: ETR Associates. Three different pamphlets with same name. Discusses social pressures, challenges to personal limits, communication, and how to say no. (Grades 6–8)

Female facts. Santa Cruz, CA: ETR Associates. Gives young women important facts and information on the menstrual cycle and how hormones control it. (Grades 5–8)

Five smart steps to abstinence. Santa Cruz, CA: ETR Associates. Helps students develop a decision to abstain and to maintain that decision. (Grades 5–12)

Here we go . . . watch me grow! Santa Cruz, CA: ETR Associates. A preschool curriculum containing over thirty lessons on a variety of topics including growth and development. (Preschool)

Male facts. Santa Cruz, CA: ETR Associates. Provides basic information about male reproductive anatomy and physiology. (Grade 5–8)

Touch talk. Santa Cruz, CA: ETR Associates. Teaches children what to do if someone touches them and they are uncomfortable with the touching. (Grades K–4)

When sex is the subject—Attitudes and answers for young children. Santa Cruz, CA: ETR Associates. Provides age-appropriate answers to children's questions and what parents should know about teaching sexuality at home. (Grades K–6)

WEB SITES

General Health

American Medical Association: *www.ama-assn.org*

Yahoo.com: *www.yahoo.com/health*

Sexuality Information and Education Council of the United States (SIECUS): *www.siecus.org*

CD-ROMS/COMPUTER SOFTWARE

A.D.A.M. essentials. Available for both Macintosh and PCs. Contains all body systems, including the reproductive systems of males and females. (Grades 7–9)

Human sexuality. Available for both Macintosh and PCs from NASCO, 901 Janesville Avenue, P.O. Box 901, Fort Atkinson, WI 53538-0901. Relationships, communication, and decision-making are discussed. Allows students to consider sexuality in the larger context of values, relationships, and communication. (Grades 6 and up)

VIDEOS

101 ways to make love without doing it   (Grades 6–8)
Provides the message that abstinence is the responsible choice and can be a fun choice as well.

Growing up! For girls   (Grades 4–6)
Provides the facts on becoming a young woman. Information on changes, good health and hygiene, and promoting self-confidence in girls. Takes a realistic look at the responsibilities of adulthood. Available from NASCO, 901 Janesville Avenue, P.O. Box 901, Fort Atkinson, WI 53538-0901. (15 minutes)

Growing up! For boys   (Grades 4–6)
Information on physical and psychological changes that are a part of growing up. Seeks to foster self-esteem. Available from NASCO, 901 Janesville Avenue, P.O. Box 901, Fort Atkinson, WI 53538-0901. (15 minutes)

Kids and divorce   (Grades 2–5)
Provides insights into kids and divorce through children's firsthand accounts of their feeling about parents and the breakup of their families. Available from Sunburst Communications, 101 Castleton Street, Pleasantville, NY 10570-0040. (20 minutes)

We're growing up!   (Grades 5–8)
Designed for mixed audiences and covers a review on male/female anatomy, sexual development, and provides an emphasis on responsible choices during adolescence. Available from NASCO, 901 Janesville Avenue, P.O. Box 901, Fort Atkinson, WI 53538-0901. (15 minutes)

When mom and dad break up   (Grades K–6)
Helps children work through the confusion and pain of parents' divorce. Available from the National Center for Elementary Drug and Violence Prevention, 117 HWY. 815, P.O. Box 9, Calhoun, KY 42327-0009. (32 minutes)

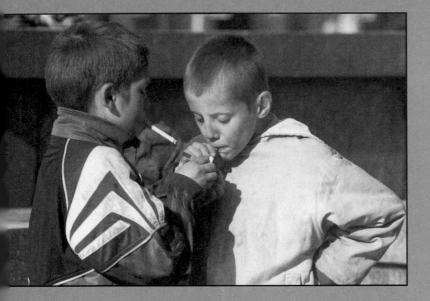

CHAPTER THIRTEEN

Substance Use and Abuse

Today, drug abuse is a more acute problem and more widespread than in any previous era.

—Hanson, Venturelli, and Fleckenstein (2001, 2)

VALUED OUTCOMES

After reading this chapter, you should be able to:

- define substance use, misuse, and abuse
- identify reasons that people abuse substances
- describe the various effects of different drugs on the body
- describe how tobacco advertising influences youth to use tobacco products
- list recommendations for schools to reduce alcohol, tobacco, and other drug abuse problems among their students
- give examples of the signs and symptoms of substance use and abuse
- describe the most effective drug abuse education and prevention programs

As you read through the chapter, note the patterns of use of the various drugs and the reasons some youth abuse drugs. As you consider these facts, think of how you could develop an effective substance abuse prevention program for your community.

Substance or Drug Abuse

Virtually anyone can abuse or become addicted to drugs. Today's rapid pace of change exerts a constant pressure to keep up that can be overwhelming. To handle this pressure and other life stressors, many people turn to using or abusing drugs. Some people do not act in accordance with what they know about the harmful effects of these drugs. Rather, they value what they feel the drugs do for them—calm them down, speed them up, and so on (Hanson, Venturelli, and Fleckenstein 2001, 4).

In this chapter, we examine those substances that are commonly abused or misused. Some of them have little or no therapeutic value but can be purchased by adults for their personal use. Over-the-counter (OTC) drugs, such as cough medicines, can have beneficial effects when used carefully. Because many people wrongly consider these drugs to be essentially harmless, however, misuse and abuse are common. Prescription drugs, such as tranquilizers, are more closely controlled, but these substances are also widely abused. Finally, we look at illegal substances, such as marijuana, heroin, hallucinogens, and cocaine.

REASONS FOR SUBSTANCE ABUSE

Individuals misuse or abuse drugs for a variety of reasons. Young people are especially likely to do so for the following reasons:

> **Curiosity**—humans intrinsically desire to experience the unknown; this desire is especially pronounced during the ages of strong peer influence, when many of a youngster's friends are experiencing drugs.

> **Low self-esteem**—many individuals have poor opinions of themselves. By using drugs, these people attempt to avoid coming to grips with their feelings of inadequacy. Drugs thus serve as a coping mechanism.

> **Peer pressure**—particularly during adolescence, individuals have a strong need to belong to "the group." If peers are abusing drugs, there is strong pressure on the part of all members of the group to do likewise.

> **Adult modeling**—young people want to feel grown up, and they view drug taking as a form of adult behavior to be emulated. Smoking tobacco or marijuana, drinking alcohol, or taking pills may all result from adult modeling.

Mood alteration—some people take drugs simply to change their psychological state. The mellow feeling or the excitement produced is the motivation for this behavior.

Boredom—many young people, especially during the teenage years, are unsure about their place in society. The activities of childhood no longer interest them, but they are not yet able to engage in adult activities. As a result, they feel bored with life.

Alienation—Some individuals feel that they have little or no power to control their own destiny. They may also feel unwanted and unloved. Often, such people have few friends and view themselves as social misfits. Drugs provide an outlet for the expression of feelings of alienation.

YOUTH AT RISK FOR SUBSTANCE ABUSE

The National Household Survey on Drug Abuse (2002) provides insights regarding trends in youth substance abuse. The Health Highlight box on page 348 has excerpts from the 2000 National Household Survey on Drug Abuse.

SYMPTOMS OF POSSIBLE SUBSTANCE ABUSE IN YOUTH

Drug use is a preventable behavior, and drug addiction is a treatable disease. As with many other diseases, the sooner it is detected and addressed, the sooner a sick person can begin to get well. How can a teacher tell if a student is abusing drugs? This is a difficult question when behavioral signs and symptoms are used as a basis for suspicion. It is difficult to separate the typical adolescent behavior from drug-induced behavior. Just because a student exhibits some of the behaviors listed below, it doesn't mean that child is using drugs.

Young people use drugs for many reasons that have to do with how they feel about themselves, how they get along with others, and how they live. No one factor determines who will use drugs and who will not, but several indicators can alert adults that a young person might be involved in substance abuse:

- low grades or poor school performance
- aggressive, rebellious behavior
- excessive influence by peers
- lack of parental support and guidance
- behavior problems at an early age
- withdrawn, depressed, and tired
- hostile and uncooperative
- relationships with other family members have deteriorated
- dropped his or her old friends
- lost interest in his or her appearance; personal hygiene has deteriorated
- lost interest in hobbies, sports, and other favorite activities
- eating or sleeping patterns changed

Health Highlight

2000 NATIONAL HOUSEHOLD SURVEY ON DRUG ABUSE

In the year 2000, an estimated 14 million Americans were using illicit drugs (defined as having used an illicit substance during the previous 30 days). This estimate represents 6.3 percent of the population over the age of 12. Unfortunately, this figure indicates no statistically significant change from the numbers found in the previous year's illicit drug use survey.

With 76 percent of the population indicating use, marijuana is the most commonly used illicit drug. Of the 5.7 million users of other illicit drugs, 3.8 million (1.7 percent of the population aged 12 and older) were using psychotherapeutics nonmedically; this included pain relievers, tranquilizers, stimulants, and sedatives.

The drug Ecstasy was used at least once by an estimated 6.4 million people, an increase of 1.3 million over the previous year. An estimated 1.2 million Americans (0.5 percent) have used cocaine, 1 million (0.4 percent) have used hallucinogens, about 265,000 indicated they had tried crack, and 130,000 (0.1 percent) have used heroin.

Almost seven million people (3.1 percent of the population aged 12 and older) reported having driven under the influence of an illicit drug at some time in the past year. This is a significant decrease from 1999 estimates of 3.4 percent.

SOURCE: National Household Survey on Drug Abuse 2002

Effects of Drugs on the Body

A *drug* is any substance that has mind-altering properties or in other ways interacts with and modifies the structure and function of the body. Drugs include OTC and prescription medicines, caffeinated beverages, alcohol, tobacco, illegal substances, herbs, and volatile chemicals such as airplane glue, correction fluid, and paint.

Drug misuse includes the unintentional or inappropriate use of prescribed or nonprescribed medicine resulting in the impaired physical, mental, emotional or social well-being of the user. Some individuals take more than the recommended dosages, or they reduce the standard time interval between doses (Carroll 2000, 8).

Drug abuse generally refers to chronic, excessive use of a drug. Drug abuse may also refer to a person's intent. If a person drinks to excess for the purpose of getting drunk, that could be considered abuse. If a person uses an illegal drug for any reason, that is considered abuse. This includes anyone under the age of twenty-one drinking alcohol, if their state considers this action illegal (underage drinking).

ROUTE OF ADMINISTRATION

Drugs can be taken orally in the form of pills, capsules, or liquids. They may be injected intravenously (directly into the bloodstream through a vein), intramuscularly (into a muscle), or subcutaneously (under the skin). Certain substances may be inhaled. Others may be administered topically, that is, by the external application of the substance to the skin or mucous membranes.

The amount of time required for a drug to take effect largely depends on the technique employed to administer it. The method of administration yielding the strongest and most rapid effect is intravenous (IV) injection. This procedure is considered the most dangerous because the risk of infection, vein collapse, or overdose is extremely high. Overdose is a significant problem with IV injection because chemicals enter the circulatory system rapidly, bypassing the body's first line of defenses. Smaller amounts of a drug are needed than for any other form of application.

Intramuscular injection works most rapidly in the deltoid muscle and least rapidly in the buttocks (because the blood supply found in the buttocks is poor). Subcutaneous injection can be extremely irritating to the tissue. Topical administration is usually short acting and may damage the skin or mucous membranes because the chemical being administered often serves as an irritant.

Even oral ingestion creates problems. This technique requires the drug to enter the bloodstream by passing through the stomach, where it may be destroyed or altered to an inactive form. Then the substance must be lipid (fat) soluble in order to cross cell membranes and reach its target. Lipid-soluble products tend to be retained by the body and show cumulative effects; if water soluble, the substance is rapidly excreted by the body. Substances absorbed in the digestive tract then go to the liver before being absorbed into general circulation. The function of the liver is to break down chemicals for excretion, so at least some of the substance may be inactivated there. Ultimately, oral ingestion creates difficulty in controlling the actual dosage absorbed by the body.

DISTRIBUTION

Drugs are carried to body parts through the bloodstream. Some drugs are absorbed and then excreted quickly. Aspirin is an example of a drug that is excreted within a few hours. Other drugs are cumulative and are excreted very slowly. It may take several days to build up the level of the drug in the body to produce the desired therapeutic effect. Once drug levels are built up, only maintenance doses are needed to maintain the drug's level. Certain heart medications are of this type.

DOSAGE

Dosage is the amount of a drug that is administered. The dosage determines the effect of the substance on the body, or the dose-response relationship. The larger the amount taken, the greater the probability of several different effects. The *threshold dose* is the minimum amount required to produce a therapeutic effect. The dose in which maximum effect is obtained is called the *maximum dose.* The *effective dose* is the dose needed to produce a desired effect. A *lethal dose* is the amount that will produce death. The ratio between the effective dose and the lethal dose is the *therapeutic index.* This is obtained by dividing the amount of a lethal dose by the amount required for an effective dose. The higher the index, the lower the chance of a given dosage being lethal.

Another important concept concerning dosage is the potency, or the difference in effective doses between drugs that are used for the same purpose. For example, substance A may require twice the dosage to achieve the same effect as substance B. Therefore, substance B is a more potent drug. The time required for the substance to produce an effect after the body receives it is called the *time response.* As a general rule, the more quickly an effect appears, the shorter its effectiveness.

The presence of more than one drug can produce what is called *synergism,* in which the combined action of the drugs is greater than the sum of the effects of any one of the drugs taken alone. For example, some drugs *potentiate,* or increase the effect of, another drug. The effect of one substance may be enhanced because of specific enzymes or formation of more potent metabolites or for unknown reasons. Pesticides, traces of hormones in meat and poultry, traces of metals in fish, nitrites, nitrates, herbs, and a wide range of chemicals used as food additives have been shown to interact with and potentiate some drugs. The classic example of synergism causing a dangerous potentiation is that a safe dose of alcohol mixed with a safe dose of a barbiturate can become lethal by depressing respiration. Conversely, a drug that acts as an *antagonist* blocks or interferes with the function of another drug when used in combination with it, or it may inhibit a normal biological compound, such as a hormone.

EXPECTATIONS OF THE USER

The mood of the user and the setting in which the drug is taken may also affect the reaction to the drug. If the person expects the substance will help a problem or produce a particular effect, then the probability of that effect actually occurring increases. The effect may occur even when the substance administered is only a placebo, or inert substance. The *placebo effect* is quite common. Friends, soft lights, and music may help create an environmental setting for particular drug effects.

Placebos are substances that produce an apparent cure or perceived health improvement based on the expectations of the user. Many patients report improvements after taking simple sugar pills that they believed were powerful drugs. About 10 percent of the population is believed to be exceptionally susceptible to the power of suggestion and may be easy targets for advertisers of these "drugs." People who use placebos unintentionally when medical treatment is urgently needed increase their risk for health problems (Donatelle 2002, 584–585).

FREQUENCY OF USE

When some drugs are used frequently, larger dosages are required to maintain the effect. This is called *tolerance.* There are several forms of tolerance: disposition tolerance, cross-tolerance, pharmacodynamic tolerance, and reverse tolerance. *Disposition tolerance* concerns the rate at which the body disposes of a drug. Certain drugs tend to increase the rate of action of enzymes in the liver and, consequently, the deactivating of the drug. For example, alcohol and barbiturates cause the liver to increase production of metabolic enzymes that deactivate certain drugs. Alcohol and barbiturates are examples of drugs that cause the liver to produce the metabolic enzymes. Another important point is that these enzymes are not very discriminating; therefore, tolerance to one substance may lead to tolerance of other drugs that are pharmacologically similar. This effect is called *cross-tolerance.* Usually a heavy drinker will exhibit tolerance to barbiturates, tranquilizers, and anesthetics.

Evidence indicates that a considerable degree of central nervous system tolerance to certain drugs may develop independent of changes in the rate of absorption, metabolism, or excretion. This is called *pharmacodynamic tolerance* and occurs when the nervous tissue or other target tissues adapt to the substance so that the effect of the same concentration of a chemical decreases. In the case of *reverse tolerance,* users will have the same response to a lower dose of a drug that they had with initial higher doses. Reverse tolerance is believed to be primarily a learning process and does not result from a physiological response. However, it is possible for some drugs, such as marijuana, to be stored in the fat cells and released later as the fat cells are broken down. The fact that drug products remain in the body for extended periods of time may account for some of the reverse tolerance effect (Ray and Ksir 2002, 417). Usually, tolerance to a substance that requires increasing amounts of a chemical to maintain normal body functioning will lead to a physical dependence.

Some drugs, such as aspirin, cause neither tolerance nor dependence. *Psychological dependence,* or habituation, occurs when a person has a strong desire to repeat the use of a drug either occasionally or continually for emotional reasons. With psychological dependence, there is a feeling of satisfaction or psychic drive that requires repeated administration of the substance to produce an effect or avoid discomfort (Carroll 2000, 58).

Substance dependence, either physiological or psychological, appears to be synonymous with substance abuse. The model of addiction-producing drugs is based on the opiates, which require the development of tolerance, along with physical and psychological dependence. Opiates, alcohol, and barbiturates are examples that fit the traditional addiction model.

Over-the-Counter Drugs

Over-the-counter (OTC) is a term that is interchangeable with nonprescription drugs (Pinger et al. 1998, 391). In 1951, an amendment to the Food, Drug, and Cosmetic Act of 1938 marked the official recognition of medicines that could be purchased for self-treatment as being OTC drugs (Pinger et al. 1998; 167). OTC drugs were identified as non habit forming, having no harmful side effects, and not requiring professional supervision for use. Many OTC drugs are on the shelves in grocery, convenience, or drug stores and are accessible for purchase without regulation. According to the National Clearinghouse for Alcohol and Drug Information (NCADI), over $78 billion in prescription and OTC drugs are produced each year in the United States (NCADI 1998, 1).

Most OTC drugs are somewhat effective in relieving the symptoms of the mild illnesses and disorders for which they were developed, as long as they are used according to directions. However, despite regulation by the Federal Trade Commission and other government agencies, advertising claims for many OTC products are often misleadingly optimistic. As a result, when the product fails to produce instant relief, some individuals may be tempted to exceed the recommended dosage in hopes of additional or faster aid. This sort of misuse can create health hazards. Additional health hazards are created when those with a predilection to addictive behavior, such as alcoholics, become dependent on and thus abuse such OTCs as cough syrup.

Individuals should also recognize that there is some risk involved in using any medication, including aspirin, even when the directions are carefully followed. First, there is a possibility of allergic reaction. In rare cases, such reactions can be fatal. Second, relief provided by an OTC drug may mask symptoms of another illness or underlying disorder. For this reason, self-medication should only be attempted when the problem is minor and obvious, as in the case of a mild cold.

Another risk in using OTC drugs comes from *synergism*. As mentioned earlier, if two or more drugs or medications are taken at the same time, one substance can cause an increase or decrease in the potency of another. This synergistic reaction can have harmful and even fatal results.

As with any drugs, OTC drugs can have a stronger effect on children than on adults. Recently, for example, children's aspirin, formerly thought to be safe, has been identified as a cause of a severe reaction that can lead to death under certain conditions. Epidemiological research has shown an association between the development of Reye's syndrome and the use of aspirin (a salicylate compound) for treating the symptoms of influenza-like illnesses such as chicken pox and colds. The U.S. Surgeon General, the Food and Drug Administration, the Centers for Disease Control and Prevention (CDC), and the American Academy of Pediatrics recommend that aspirin and combination products containing aspirin not be given to children under nineteen years of age during episodes of fever-causing illnesses (National Reye's Syndrome Foundation 2000).

Depressants

Drugs that slow down, inhibit, or depress the nervous system are classified as depressants. The most commonly used depressant drug is alcohol. There are dozens of other depressants, most of which are prescription drugs. Whether obtained legally or illegally, however, depressants are among the most common of misused and abused drugs.

Depressants can have a calming effect, and strong depressants can produce sleep. They have been used to treat insomnia, but their most important use is the treatment of epileptic seizures (Levinthal 1999, 296). The use of depressants has an extremely high risk of both physical and psychological addiction. Prolonged use builds up a tolerance, which may eventually lead to a coma and

Health Highlight

ABUSE-RESISTANT OXYCONTIN?

OxyContin is a very powerful painkiller that has a recent history of increasing abuse. When used medically, OxyContin is swallowed in pill form and can produce up to 12 hours of pain relief; however, if it is chewed, inhaled, or injected, it produces a quick, and potentially lethal, heroin-like high.

There have been recent attempts to create an abuse-resistant form of OxyContin by adding drugs that would block the "high" if OxyContin is taken at too high a dose. One method under consideration is to use the narcotic blocker naloxone hydrochloride in OxyContin tablets. If the tablets are crushed and injected, naloxone hydrochloride would enter the bloodstream to block OxyContin's effects. The problem is that in some research studies naloxone hydrochloride also blocked pain relief for patients who used the drug correctly.

Creating abuse-resistant painkillers is very difficult and complex. There are no formulas to date that are 100 percent effective in preventing abuse. Some critics have called for OxyContin to be banned until an abuse-resistant version is developed; however the Food and Drug Administration is not yet considering this option.

SOURCE: Neergaard 2002

death. The withdrawal process from depressants can be life threatening and should be carried out under medical supervision. Because of the high risk of addiction and tolerance, many doctors are reluctant to prescribe these drugs as sleep aids.

Depressant drugs have four main effects on the body. As *sedatives,* they can produce relaxation. As *tranquilizers,* they can reduce anxiety and act as muscle relaxants. As *hypnotics,* they can promote sleep. As *anesthetics,* they can create a loss of sensation. Various depressant drugs differ in their potencies, but in sufficient amounts they can all produce these four effects.

The sedative-hypnotics include barbiturates and tranquilizers. Examples of barbiturates by trade name include Amytal, Nembutal, and Seconal. Commonly prescribed tranquilizers include Valium, Librium, and Miltown. Both of these types of drugs are usually taken orally, although some can be given intravenously as a general anesthetic.

Alcohol

The use of alcohol by youth still remains a problem, despite declining levels of use and increased awareness of the inherent dangers. Fifty-three percent of eighth-graders, 72 percent of tenth-graders, 77 percent of twelfth-graders, and 89 percent of college students have tried alcoholic beverages (Hanson, Venturelli, and Fleckenstein 2001, 203). Further, alcohol use among young people appears to stimulate a progression to other drug use. The use of alcohol and tobacco among youth is correlated with other health problems, including adolescent suicide, homicide, school dropout, delinquency, early sexual activity, sexually transmitted infections (STIs), unwanted pregnancy, and motor vehicle crashes. Alcohol-related traffic crashes are the leading cause of death and spinal cord injury for young Americans. Young adults are unlikely to develop alcohol problems if the age of first use is delayed beyond childhood and adolescence.

Ethyl alcohol is the active ingredient in beer, wine, and distilled beverages such as whiskey. Ethyl alcohol is not as toxic as are some other forms of the chemical, such as isopropyl alcohol, which is used as rubbing alcohol. In this discussion, we use the term *alcohol* to refer to ethyl alcohol. Alcohol is a colorless, flammable liquid formed by the fermentation of fruits, juices, or cereal grains. Alcoholic beverages contain varying amounts of alcohol, depending on the type of beverage. Beer usually contains from 5 to 7 percent alcohol. Wines may vary from 11 to 20 percent. Distilled beverages have the highest alcohol content. This content is measured by the proof of the beverage, which is a number that is twice the alcohol content. For example, a 100-proof whiskey contains 50 percent alcohol, whereas a 90-proof whiskey contains 45 percent.

Effects of Alcohol. Alcohol is a central nervous system depressant. In small doses, the substance has a mellowing or tranquilizing effect. The individual may feel relaxed and free from tension. As a result, behavior may become less inhibited, leading to the misconception held by some that alcohol is a stimulant. Actually, what appears to be stimulated, or at least animated, behavior results from the anesthetic, depressant effect that alcohol has on the cerebral cortex area of the brain.

The effects of alcohol on the body correspond with the amount of alcohol in the system. The amount of alcohol can be measured by the percentage of the blood that is composed of alcohol. In large amounts, alcohol impairs brain activity, muscular control, coordination, memory, reaction time, and judgment. Heavy intake over a short period can bring about a dulling of the senses. Continued heavy drinking can result in coma and death.

Consumption of alcohol over a long period can result in damage to the brain and liver. The brain may be damaged to the extent that memory, judgment, and learning deteriorate. Cirrhosis of the liver is a potentially fatal condition caused by alcohol damage. Cirrhosis of the liver does occur in nonalcoholic drinkers, but this is rare. Recently, the harmful effects of even moderate amounts of alcohol consumed by pregnant women have become known. Alcohol can have a deleterious effect on the developing fetus, resulting in a condition known as *fetal alcohol syndrome.* A child born with this condition may suffer permanent impairment. Characteristics of the condition include low birth weight, smaller head circumference, abnormal formation of the nose, small fingernails, smaller stature, poor joint movement, ear abnormalities, and mental retardation.

In moderation, alcohol does not seem to harm the adult body permanently. However, an adult who decides to partake of alcoholic beverages should exercise care. Alcohol should be consumed slowly, with adequate food in the stomach. Individuals should also recognize that tolerance to alcohol is cumulative. More of the substance may be required to produce the pleasant, mellow effect associated with its use. Drinking without recognizing the potential dangers of alcohol can lead to tragedy.

Why Do Youth Begin Abusing Alcohol? Why do underage youth drink? Decisions to drink are influenced by an array of interacting individual and environmental factors. Two main reasons are reported: to see what it is like and to be sociable. Youth drinking is usually group behavior with rituals of sharing and turn-taking, free from adult control. Teens also report drinking to feel good, to feel grown-up, to relax, to get away from problems, and to relieve boredom. Parents and other family members play a crucial role in the development of their children's drinking patterns and establishment of future goals, and peers play an important role in present lifestyle issues and activities. For teens who go on to develop problems with alcohol abuse, risk factors such as genetic predisposition or conduct disorder may be evident. However, no one factor can play a role without being influenced by other factors. Psychosocial, biomedical, and psychological problems are associated with the consumption of alcohol in adolescents—a population experiencing rapid change due to physical, psychological, social, and cognitive development. Accident statistics are a prime indicator of this.

Alcohol drinking is also associated with sexual risk-taking, which creates risk for teenage pregnancy, STIs, and HIV/AIDS. Although a direct causal relationship between the two has not been empirically shown and may not be generally applicable to all adolescents, alcohol is perceived by adolescents and some adults as a sexual disinhibitor.

Alcohol and other drug abuse may also contribute to the higher rates of low birth weight and mortality among infants born to adolescent mothers. Alcohol use is associated with psychiatric conditions such as depression, conduct problems, and antisocial behavior. Prolonged use can result in psychological problems such as escapism, poor self-image, and alienation. Alcohol can affect mood, judgment, and self-control, resulting in such outcomes as suicidal behavior.

Finally, alcohol dependence in itself can be a consequence of alcohol abuse, a health problem affecting both mental and physical health. Youth represents a risky population of alcohol users and abusers, one in which the consequences of use tend to be more severe than with adults. Prevention, intervention, and treatment are required to effectively reduce present and future harm.

The key to dealing with adolescent alcohol and other substance use is prevention, which should begin in early childhood and continue throughout adolescence. Prevention programs can be school, family, or community based. The information-only and "scare tactic" approaches of the past are now considered ineffective. The mass media approach, although information oriented, is useful in increasing public awareness and putting an issue on the social agenda. Current programs tend to be more psychosocial in approach, addressing social, cognitive, biological, attitudinal, and developmental factors aimed at building skills within a supportive group context.

School-based programs have the advantage of being able to use age-specific strategies in a learning environment. Highly structured programs are appropriate for younger ages. Community approaches depend on a coordinated effort on behalf of the public and private agencies and other groups within the community. Possible community strategies include recreational alternatives for youth and community.

Drinking and Accidents. Alcohol remains the primary cause of automobile accidents among drivers. Alcohol is involved in 50 percent or more of all fatal traffic accidents. Without question, drinking and driving don't mix. Two of the many groups who are keeping the drunk driving issue alive by increasing awareness of the problem are MADD (Mothers Against Drunk Driving) and SADD (Students Against Drunk Driving). MADD also serves to mobilize the public to help individuals modify their drinking habits and protests the judicial system when an individual with a history of drunk driving is allowed to continue to drive. MADD has been successful in reducing the legal blood-alcohol concentration in various states and has initiated several effective programs to limit drinking and driving.

The purposes of SADD include helping students save their own lives and the lives of others, educating students on the problem of drinking and driving, developing peer counseling among students about alcohol use, and increasing public awareness and prevention of alcohol abuse. An important feature of the SADD program is the "Contract for Life," a teenager–parent contract in which the teenager agrees to call the parent for advice and/or transportation at any time from any place if the teenager or his or her driver has had too much to drink. The parent in return agrees to transport the teenager and also agrees to seek sober transportation for him- or herself in a similar situation.

Alcoholism and Alcohol-Related Problems. Perhaps the area of greatest concern among substance abuse professionals is alcoholism among young people. According to the National Council on Alcoholism, alcoholism is the number one drug problem among the nation's youth. Forty percent of children have tasted alcohol by age ten. The average age for a first drink is just under thirteen. Nearly 30 percent of teenagers have experienced negative results from abuse of alcohol. These range from auto accidents to arrests to detrimental effects on schoolwork and others mentioned earlier in this chapter. Ironically, 42 percent of fourth-graders failed to recognize alcohol as a drug. Only 72 percent of children in the upper grades realize it is a drug and, therefore, dangerous.

Definitions of the term *alcoholism* vary from source to source. In general, the disease alcoholism can be described as when a person is unable to choose whether he or she will drink and is unable to stop drinking. Alcoholics use the substance in such a way that their personal, social, and occupational behavior is interfered with or totally disrupted. The problem is common among people from all walks of life, including the clergy, homemakers, politicians, factory workers, musicians, police officers, and retired people. Both rich and poor, young and old, are susceptible. As many as 10 million Americans have a serious drinking problem.

The disease model of alcoholism has received support from many medical practitioners and has been endorsed by the American Medical Association and other professional groups. However, there are many scientific critics of the disease concept. There is considerable evidence that indicates some degree of vulnerability to alcoholism may be inherited. Alcoholism does tend to run in families, but this may be due to similar expectancies developed through common cultural influences and children learning from their parents. These studies imply that inheritance plays a strong role but is far from a complete determinant of alcoholism (Ray and Ksir 2002, 251–253). Ethnicity as well as heredity may also play a role in alcoholism. Many Asians, for example, have a genetic variant of aldehyde dehydrogenase that is slower than the allele found in non-Asians. This is typically blamed for the accumulation of acetaldehyde that is associated with the marked facial flushing and increased heart rate that many Asians experience when drinking alcoholic beverages.

Regardless of how important the heredity factor is, social and psychological factors also influence the development of alcoholism. Because alcohol is generally accepted in our society, many individuals feel free to use it. Too often, however, use leads to misuse, and alcoholism is the result. The drug becomes a crutch for dealing with everyday problems until the individual can no longer get along without it.

Alcohol-related problems are all too well known in our society. Aside from the thousands of traffic deaths and injuries that occur each year because of alcohol abuse, alcohol is also related to the high divorce rate, job absenteeism, crimes of violence, suicide, and social disorder.

Alcoholics and their families can receive help from many sources, including such nonprofit groups as Alcoholics Anonymous (AA). AA is a support group of fellow alcoholics designed to help each other remain sober. There are also many commercial alcoholic treatment programs. These can be expensive, but many insurance companies now pay for such treatment. Al-Anon, Alateen, and Alatot are groups specifically established to assist the families of alcoholics. Al-Anon is a group for spouses, relatives, and friends of alcoholics. Alateen and Alatot are groups that are designed for children of alcoholics. These groups are designed to help friends and relatives understand the alcoholic and thereby better cope with the alcoholic's lifestyle. These groups also help the family members understand the roles they play as codependents—that is, the behavior of family members that sometimes enables the alcoholic to continue his or her lifestyle. For example, if a spouse calls her alcoholic husband's employer and tells the employer that her husband will not be at work because he is sick, this action enables the alcoholic to continue his behavior.

BARBITURATES

Barbiturates have historically represented one of the nation's biggest drug abuse problems. Generally known as downers, barbiturates are often taken as a way of escaping from the problems of daily living. Since the 1970s, the use and abuse of barbiturates have declined because a safer group of sedative-hypnotics called benzodiazepines are being prescribed instead (Barry 2002, 2). Today, less than 10 percent of all depressant prescriptions in the United States are for barbiturates (U.S. Drug Enforcement Administration 2002). Because of its decline in use, the addiction to barbiturates is fairly uncommon today.

The effects of barbiturates depend on the dosage ingested. In small doses, a person feels drowsy, uninhibited, and intoxicated. In moderate amounts, depressants produce a state of intoxication that is remarkably similar to alcohol intoxication. In high doses, the user staggers as if drunk, develops slurred speech, and is confused. At higher doses, the person is unconscious (coma), and death from cardiac or respiratory arrest is very possible (Barry 2002, 3). Some people use depressants in order to obtain a "high" or to counteract the effects of stimulant drugs. The margin of safety between a safe and a lethal dose is very narrow; therefore, barbiturates are considered dangerous and are less likely to be prescribed than safer alternatives.

Withdrawal symptoms associated with the discontinued use of barbiturates indicate a strong physical dependence of the body on the drug. Some of these symptoms may include a combination of tremors, vomiting, general confusion, nausea, intense perspiring, convulsions, and increased heart rate (Levinthal 1999, 296). Withdrawal from barbiturates and tranquilizers should be supervised by a physician.

TRANQUILIZERS

Tranquilizers are classified as major and minor. The major tranquilizers, such as Thorazine, are used to treat psychosis. Minor tranquilizers, such as Valium and Librium, are prescribed for stress and anxiety and are also useful as muscle relaxants. However, partly because they are so widely prescribed, such tranquilizers are often abused. Physical and psychological dependency can result. Symptoms of physical dependency include drowsiness and slurred speech. Psychological dependency may be characterized by increased irritability and irrational fear. As is the case with barbiturates, withdrawal from tranquilizers can be highly traumatic.

CROSS-TOLERANCE AND THE DEPRESSANT DRUGS

Tolerance to depressant drugs can be developed fairly quickly. Then higher and higher doses of the drug must be taken to produce the desired relaxing effect. Tolerance to one kind of depressant drug also produces tolerance to other types of depressant substances that are not even being taken. This phenomenon is known as *cross-tolerance*. The danger of cross-tolerance may not be as obvious to drug abusers as it should be. Once tolerance to one depressant drug has developed, the individual may decide to switch to another depressant in hopes of achieving the same desired effect. However, because of cross-tolerance, the outcome is not as hoped. A higher dose may then be taken. If the new drug is more potent, a fatal overdose may result.

Narcotics

Narcotic drugs are produced for the most part from opium and its derivatives, although some are synthesized substances. Such drugs act on the central nervous system and gastrointestinal tract. They are excellent painkillers, but they can be highly addictive, both physically and psychologically. Opium, morphine, codeine, and heroin are derived from the opium poppy. Morphine is a potent painkiller used primarily to relieve severe pain such as that caused by acute sickle cell crisis and heart attack. Codeine is often used in conjunction with acetaminophen to relieve moderate pain; codeine is also effective in suppressing the cough reflex.

Heroin is not used for medical purposes and is one of the most dangerous drugs abused. Much heroin is produced illegally in Asia and smuggled into the United States. The drug can be smoked, swallowed, injected under the skin, or injected directly into a vein. The latter method is used most often by heroin addicts because the drug reaches the brain most quickly this way. The desired effect is a sudden rush of euphoria, followed by a dreamy state of complete relaxation. This period may last up to several hours, depending on a variety of factors, including the strength of the dosage.

Although considered physiologically "clean" in the sense that it does not damage organs, heroin is extremely addictive, and a user soon may live for no other reason than to inject more heroin. Tolerance also quickly develops, leading to a need for higher and higher or more frequent doses of the drug. The result is too often a fatal overdose, which results in death from cardiorespiratory failure.

Withdrawal from heroin is agonizing. It is characterized by chills, fever, diarrhea, and vomiting. However, painful as it is, heroin withdrawal is seldom life threatening. Still, most heroin addicts, even when they would like to quit, find it almost impossible to do so because of the craving they have developed for the drug.

The dangers from heroin use are manifold. Aside from weight loss, lethargy, sexual inadequacy, and the constant problems of withdrawal that require regular doses of the drug, injection of heroin can lead to other health problems, including hepatitis and HIV/AIDS because of dirty needles and anemia caused by disregard for proper nutrition. "Street heroin" is always sold in an adulterated state (such as being mixed with baking soda or milk sugar) so that the actual percentage of heroin is small. Toxic adulterants in heroin sold on the street can also kill.

After the Harrison Act of 1914, there was a decline in the number of addicts using opiates, including heroin. In the early years after World War II, heroin use slowly increased in the lower class, partially because it was inexpensive. During the 1950s and 1960s, heroin use spread rapidly. Because of laws, eradication programs in Turkey and Mexico, and diminished supplies, heroin use in the United States fell slightly in the 1970s and 1980s. However, surveys show that heroin use was on the rise in the 1990s, paricularly among high school students (Ray and Ksir 2002, 344–348).

Stimulants

Stimulants are drugs that stimulate, or speed up, the nervous system. Physiologically, the stimulant drugs increase heart rate, blood pressure, and amount of circulating blood sugar. They also constrict the blood vessels and dilate bronchial tubes and the pupils of the eyes. Some can produce a temporary euphoria.

CAFFEINE

The most common stimulant is caffeine, which is contained in coffee, tea, cola drinks, and even chocolate. Caffeine is a mild stimulant that is often abused. Nonetheless, it is a drug and should be recognized as one that can lead to health problems.

Caffeine is absorbed rather quickly into the bloodstream and reaches a peak blood level in about thirty to sixty minutes. It increases mental alertness and provides a feeling of energy. However, high doses of caffeine can overstimulate and cause nervousness and increased heart rate. Caffeine can also cause sleeplessness, excitement, and irritability. In some cases, high doses of caffeine can induce convulsions.

Coffee or cola drinking, let alone chocolate eating, cannot be considered drug abuse by most commonly accepted standards. But some individuals seek out caffeine for its own sake, in OTC products and in illegal substances to produce a caffeine "high." Because it is not considered a dangerous drug, the opportunities for caffeine abuse are often overlooked.

AMPHETAMINES

Amphetamines, or "uppers," represent a more serious stimulant drug abuse problem than caffeine. These drugs have limited legitimate and useful medical applications, but because of their wide availability, they are often abused.

Amphetamines are related in structure to the neurotransmitters norepinephrine and dopamine, which produce stimulatory effects on the nervous system (Hahn and Payne 1998, 386). They can be helpful if taken correctly, or they can be detrimental to a person's health if taken incorrectly or illegally. Amphetamines are used in many medical treatments. Ritalin is a prescription drug that aids in attention deficit hyperactivity disorder (ADHD), and Sudafed is an OTC drug that is a powerful nasal decongestant. Adderall, an amphetamine that was once used to treat exogenous obesity, has been outlawed in some states due to abuse. Adderall has also been used to treat cases of ADHD and narcolepsy. Many states in the United States restrict the use of Adderall as an anorectic agent (i.e., for the treatment of anorexia); the long-term effects of Adderall are not known.

The FDA has approved short-term use of amphetamines for weight-loss programs but has warned against their potential for abuse. The U.S. medical associations have asked all physicians to be more careful about prescribing amphetamines. Only 1 percent of amphetamine prescriptions are now written for weight loss, compared with 8 percent in 1970. In fact, amphetamine use is currently recommended only for narcolepsy and some cases of hyperactivity in children.

Use of traditional amphetamines declined among students from the late 1980s to the early 1990s, and this was accompanied by an increase in the trend in cocaine abuse. However, in 1993, there was an alarming rise in the number of adolescents who abused amphetamines. By 1999, approximately 4.5 percent of high school seniors used amphetamines at least once a month (Hanson, Venturelli, and Fleckenstein 2001, 267).

A potent and commonly abused form of amphetamine is "speed," a white, odorless, and bitter-tasting powder. Speed is an illegal, highly addictive methamphetamine that is cheaper and has longer-lasting effects than cocaine. Methamphetamine is a relatively easy and inexpensive stimulant to make, so the Comprehensive Methamphetamine Control Act was passed in 1996 to discourage its illicit manufacture.

Abusers of amphetamines pass into an extremely excited state and may feel omnipotent until the drug begins to wear off. A depressed period, called a "crash" by abusers, then follows, leading to a craving for more amphetamines. Taking a large amount of amphetamines on a regular basis leads to dependence. Tolerance develops rapidly, necessitating increased dosage levels to obtain the desired effects. When the regular use of amphetamines is stopped, one can experience severe mental depression, fatigue, irritability, long periods of sleep, and extreme hunger. These withdrawal symptoms are considered by medical authorities as evidence of physical dependency (Carroll 2000, 202).

COCAINE

Known on the street as "snow" or "coke," cocaine is an illegal drug that continues to rise in popularity. Currently, cocaine trafficking and consumption represent the most significant drug problem in the United States. The groups most vulnerable to cocaine use include adolescents and young adults who demonstrate higher than average levels of tobacco, alcohol, and especially marijuana use. The risk of becoming a cocaine user does not decrease after the teen years. Initiation to cocaine use occurs anytime from adolescence to adulthood.

In 1998, an estimated 1.8 million Americans were current cocaine users. This represents 0.8 percent of the population age twelve and older. The number of cocaine users declined from 5.7 million in 1985 (3 percent of the population) to 1.4 million (0.7 percent of the population) in 1992 and has not changed significantly since then (NCADI 1998).

Cocaine is legal and useful for limited medical purposes. Because of its vasoconstrictive and anesthetic properties, cocaine is used as a local ingredient in Brompton's cocktail, a preparation for treating severe pain in individuals with a terminal illness. Cocaine is taken to produce a feeling of intense euphoria and boundless energy. As this fades, depression—sometimes severe—follows, along with the strong desire for another dose, or "hit." Although physical dependence is not strong with cocaine, psychological dependence is common and can be very potent. Paranoid thinking, hallucinations, and psychosis can occur with heavy, extended use. Withdrawal symptoms from cocaine are limited to mild depression and anxiety with limited use.

Cocaine is most often found in the form of a white powder, which is usually sniffed or "snorted" up the nostrils or smoked. The drug enters the bloodstream through the nasal membranes when sniffed or snorted. The cocaine concentration in the blood rapidly increases for about thirty to forty minutes, then gradually declines for three or more hours after use (Hanson, Venturelli, and Fleckenstein 2001, 267–279).

Following intravenous administration, the total amount of cocaine enters the bloodstream in a few minutes. Within seconds after injection, cocaine users experience an incredible state of euphoria. The high is intense but short lived; within fifteen to twenty minutes, this high is followed by a depression that may last ten to forty minutes (Hanson, Venturelli, and Fleckenstein 2001, 280). Oral use is not common in the United States, but the resulting high is comparable to other forms of use.

A process used for purifying or refining cocaine is called *freebasing.* This method produces a more potent form with an accelerated and intense high. The drug is heated to a high temperature and mixed with other substances, some highly volatile, resulting in explosion on occasion. The final mixture is then smoked in a water pipe.

Another form of cocaine, "crack" or "rock," gets its name from the sound made by the crystals when heated or from the rocklike appearance. Crack may be 90 percent pure, compared to 15 to 25 percent purity in regular cocaine. The drug is smoked in a water pipe and reaches the brain in less than ten seconds, with the high lasting from five to seven minutes. Following this intense rush, crashing depression may occur and may last two to three times longer than the high.

Many people perceive smoking to be less dangerous, but this route provides direct absorption via the lungs, into the blood, and to the brain in less than ten seconds. The speed with which crack acts and the purity it displays make it very dangerous. Crack is widely available for about five to ten dollars a hit, which erases the notion that cocaine is an upper-class drug (Abadinsky 2001, 111).

Cocaine's action on the body most directly affects the cardiovascular system. Heart rate increases and small blood vessels constrict, thus raising blood pressure. This sudden increase in cardiac activity, coupled with vasoconstriction, leads to an elevated risk of cardiac ischemia, resulting in heart attack or rhythm disturbances. These risks can occur when using small amounts, either by sniffing, snorting, smoking, or IV use. The absence of an underlying heart condition *does not* make an individual immune from cardiac consequences.

Treatment of cocaine dependence varies for different programs and has improved over time. From 30 percent to 90 percent of the patients who persist in outpatient treatment programs are considered successful, but these figures may be misleading since they do not take into account the patients who drop out of programs (Ray and Ksir 2002, 283).

TOBACCO

Tobacco has been used for hundreds of years. It can be sniffed in the form of snuff, chewed (placed between the gum and lips), or smoked. Smoking is the most popular use of tobacco. Cigarettes became popular in the early 1900s; previously, tobacco was usually chewed or smoked in a pipe.

The Surgeon General of the United States has stated that a combination of education and public policy approaches is the most effective way to prevent the onset of smoking (CDC 2001). Since the U.S. Surgeon General's first warning about smoking and cancer, heart disease, and other health problems, the nation's smoking rate has fallen dramatically. In the mid-1960s, an estimated 40 percent of the adult population smoked. Currently, the rate of cigarette smoking is the lowest ever reported, with just 25 percent of Americans smoking.

Approximately 43 million people have quit, with the greatest decline in smoking rates occurring among males.

Cigarette smoking remains the single, most preventable cause of death in our society (Ray and Ksir 2002, 274). Smoking is directly responsible for about 390,000 deaths each year in the United States; thus, we can fairly blame smoking for more than one of every six deaths in our country.

About 90 percent of adult smokers began their addiction as children or adolescents, and these young smokers will account for many health problems in the future. The younger a person is when he or she starts to smoke, the more likely he or she is to become a long-term smoker and to develop smoking-related diseases. Preventing youngsters from taking up smoking is far more cost-effective than treating the addiction and resulting diseases later in life.

The Healthy Youth 2010 Initiative states that a carefully planned, comprehensive school health education program can make a big difference in preventing the onset of smoking. The United States has launched an initiative to reduce and/or prevent tobacco use among children by improving the enforcement of state laws against smoking by minors (CDC 2001). According to a study by the U.S. Department of Health and Human Services (DHHS), children in this country can easily buy cigarettes virtually any time they want to, in violation of the law. However, DHHS also found that where state and local officials take their responsibilities seriously and devise enforcement tools that are workable and effective, these laws can be successfully enforced. Preventing the use of tobacco products will do more to enhance the length and quality of life in the United States than any other step that could be taken.

Effects of Tobacco Smoking. According to the U.S. Surgeon General, cigarette smoking is the primary avoidable cause of death in our society and the most important health issue of our time. Cancer is the second leading cause of death in this country, and smoking accounts for nearly one-third of all cancer deaths. Prevention of smoking in young people is a critical goal, particularly in view of the mixed success that many smokers have in quitting (Ray and Ksir 2002, 287). Unfortunately, more than 64 percent of American high school seniors have used cigarettes, and more than 12 percent smoke a half a pack or more daily. White adolescents have higher smoking rates than Hispanics, with African-American adolescents being the least likely to smoke. The CDC states that roughly 29 percent of U.S. high school students are currently smoking. However, this number is down from 36 percent in 1997 (Davis and Jain 2001, 1469). The decline is due to a 70 percent jump in the price of cigarettes from the end of 1997 to May 2001, along with expanded school, state, and national smoking prevention efforts. Schools played a part in this prevention effort and by 2000, 92 percent of U.S. school districts required tobacco-prevention education, and nearly half of middle and senior high schools had no-smoking policies. The CDC believes that if these trends continue and smoking among teenagers continues to decline, their national goal to reduce teen smoking rates to 16 percent or lower by 2010 is achievable (Davis and Jain 2001, 1469).

The primary drug in tobacco is nicotine. A typical filter cigarette contains between 1 and 2 mg of nicotine, with about 90 percent of this amount being absorbed when inhaled. Nicotine acts as a stimulant on the heart and nervous system, causing an increased heartbeat and elevated blood pressure, and the constricted blood vessels also decrease skin temperature. Blood loses some of its ability to carry oxygen because of the carbon monoxide in tobacco smoke, which is more easily picked up by hemoglobin.

Cigarette smoke also contains chemicals known collectively as *tars*. These substances have been identified as carcinogens, or cancer-causing agents. Smoking is a major cause of lung cancer and may contribute to other forms of malignancies as well. Smokers not only run an increased risk of developing cancer, they also have much higher rates of coronary heart disease. Emphysema, a breathing disorder that results from deterioration of lung tissue, is also associated with cigarette smoking, as are many other respiratory diseases.

The relationship between a mother's smoking and harmful effects on a developing fetus has been established. Some of the most important findings related to smoking and pregnancy are that cigarette smoking during pregnancy causes a reduction in infant birth weight, is related to significantly higher fetal and neonatal mortality, and is associated with an increase in sudden infant death syndrome (Donatelle 2002, 364).

Both male and female current cigarette smokers experience more workdays lost, days of bed disability, and long-term limitation of activity due to chronic diseases than do people who never smoked. In addition, current and former smokers report more hospitalization than nonsmokers in the year before being interviewed in research studies. Even though most studies show a reduction in the risk of mortality among former smokers, data on disability and illness often show continued high risk among former smokers. All measures of smoking disability are dose related—that is, the more smoking there is (or was), the greater the likelihood of developing a disability or disablement (Carroll 2000, 172).

Although cigarette smokers run the highest risk of developing health problems, use of tobacco in other forms can also lead to serious problems. For example, pipe smoking is related to cancer of the lip; both pipe and cigar smokers run a higher risk of developing cancer of the mouth, larynx, and esophagus. Snuff dippers, or people who use smokeless tobacco, have a higher incidence of oral cancer than do nonusers.

Because of these deleterious health effects, several states have sued the tobacco companies for compensation to help pay for health costs due to smoking. At least four tobacco companies—RJR Nabisco, Philip Morris, Brown & Williamson, and Lorillard—reached a decision with attorneys general in nearly forty states to have the tobacco companies pay out $368.5 billion over the next twenty-five years for compensation to states for health care costs of smokers in treatment, financing health research, and promoting education programs targeted to youth. All fifty states now restrict the purchase of tobacco by minors (Hanson, Venturelli, and Fleckenstein 2001, 330).

Secondhand and Sidestream Smoke. Although an individual may choose not to smoke, being in an enclosed area with smoking forces him or her to smoke involuntarily. Sidestream smoke is the smoke that comes from a burning cigarette. Secondhand smoke is exhaled from the smoker. This smoke has much higher concentrations of some irritating and hazardous substances than mainstream, or inhaled, smoke. Carbon monoxide is especially significant with secondhand smoke. With several people smoking in an enclosed area, the Environmental Protection Agency's safe limit recommendation can be exceeded. Most standard air-filtration systems do not remove carbon monoxide gas from the air. Only dilution with fresh air can lower carbon monoxide levels.

Nicotine from sidestream smoke generally settles out of the air, with only small amounts being absorbed from heavily polluted air. Other carcinogens are absorbed in small amounts, but the carcinogenic effect is not known. Other substances from sidestream smoke probably are not hazardous, just irritating to nonsmokers. People with cardiovascular disease or bronchopulmonary disease can be adversely affected. Children of parents who smoke are more likely to have bronchitis, pneumonia, and reactive airway diseases during the first year of life and as youth.

Why People Smoke. People begin smoking for some of the same reasons that apply to drinking. Adult modeling and peer pressure are certainly factors. The appeal produced by cigarette advertising also plays a part. Some people abuse tobacco to be more alert, and others use it to relax. (The mood of the smoker plays a role in the perception of the abuser.) Many smokers find smoking extremely pleasurable. Some claim that cigarettes curb anxiety, sadness, and boredom. Some smoke because of habit, with various cues (immediately after a meal, with coffee, or being around other smokers) triggering the habit of tobacco abuse. Of course, the chemicals in the tobacco, including nicotine, produce a physiological dependence (Abadinsky 2001, 126).

A very forceful motivation for smoking is advertising. Cigarette manufacturers spend approximately $4 billion each year promoting cigarettes and the acceptance of smoking. Cigarette advertising reveals very few facts about cigarettes, but rather appeals to individual needs, a memory of good feeling, the universal need for companionship, and a desire for escape and adventure. Cigarette ads also are designed to reduce one's anxieties about growing old, being alone, and losing one's health and sex drive. And they are designed to result in the trial and/or purchase of tobacco products. Free samples may encourage initiation of tobacco use among children and adolescents, especially when distributed at youth-oriented events, such as concerts. Cigarette sponsorship of sporting events allows cigarette brand names to be shown or mentioned on television (even though cigarette commercials are prohibited in the broadcast media), and cigarette sponsorship of televised sporting events is reported to increase cigarette brand recognition among children.

The impact of such advertising on potential smokers (primarily young people) is substantial. A sample of children, aged three through six, was shown various advertising logos, including the Disney channel's mouse ears, the Chevrolet and Ford symbols, the Nike athletic shoe symbol, and Camel cigarettes' Joe Camel. They were then asked to match the logos with product symbols. The Joe Camel character was found to be as recognizable to the children as any of the other symbols. Thirty percent of the three-year-olds and 91 percent of the six-year-olds correctly matched Joe Camel with a cigarette. This evidence led to federal regulations prohibiting the association of tobacco products with cartoonlike characters and limiting other forms of advertising such as children's caps and T-shirts with cigarette logos (Ray and Ksir 1999, 286).

Advertising of tobacco products targeted toward girls and women has been successful. Over 25 percent of females smoke tobacco. Among youths ages twelve to seventeen, the rates for males and females are similar (18.7 percent for males, 17.7 percent for females). The explanation is not only that more girls than boys have taken up the habit in the past decade, but also that fewer girls quit. The targeting of girls and women in advertising tobacco products is made easier by the fact that smoking temporarily holds down body weight, and societal pressure for girls and women to be slender is intense. Weight control is one of the most important reasons girls start smoking and one of the biggest barriers preventing them from quitting. The effects of the resulting tobacco use among girls and women have been devastating. Lung cancer has overtaken breast cancer as the number one cause of cancer death among women, and lung cancer death rates among women continue to increase at an unrelenting pace. Other smoking-related diseases, such as heart disease and emphysema, also are exacting a terrible toll on women. For example, women who smoke are significantly more likely to have a heart attack than are women who have never smoked (Donatelle 2002, 364).

A study by the CDC shows that antismoking strategies are needed in childhood to counteract the effects of advertising. Findings from the CDC's latest Youth Risk Behavior Survey indicate that students who smoke their first cigarette at less than twelve years of age are more likely to become regular and heavy smokers than students who begin smoking at a later age. Students who participate in sports activities smoke less than students who do not participate. These findings suggest that antismoking education should be available during childhood before smoking becomes a problem. Also, since another study showed that few youth who smoke receive counseling about nicotine addiction, smoking cessation education should be available to youngsters who do smoke (CDC 1999).

Reducing the Hazards of Smoking. The best way to avoid the hazards of smoking is simply not to smoke. This means not beginning in the first place or giving up the habit if smoking has already begun. People who smoke should also recognize the possible harmful effects of secondhand smoke on others. Inhaling smoke produced by a smoker can aggravate respiratory conditions and may even be the cause of such conditions in a nonsmoker. Those who refuse to stop smoking can lower the risk they run by choosing a brand of cigarettes with low tar and nicotine, by smoking fewer cigarettes, by taking fewer puffs and not inhaling deeply, and by not smoking the cigarette all the way down to the end.

Smokeless Tobacco. Advertising claims have made it appear that smokeless tobacco is a safe alternative to smoking tobacco. Evidently this effort has been successful, because smokeless tobacco is the only type of tobacco product whose use has increased in recent years. Advertisements for this product feature athletes and run in adventure and sports magazines, thereby appealing to young people, and adolescents have gotten the message. Many young people consider smokeless tobacco less physically damaging than other tobacco products, and the prevalence of smokeless tobacco use is increasing, especially among male adolescents and young adults (Hanson, Venturelli, and Fleckenstein 2001, 320).

Marijuana

After alcohol and nicotine, marijuana is the third most popular recreational drug in the United States—in other words, it is the dominant illicit drug.

Some statistics regarding use of marijuana (Hanson, Venturelli, and Fleckenstein 2001, 368–9) include the following:

- First-time use of marijuana is highest among 12- to 17-year-olds.
- Seventeen percent of students ages 12 to 17 have used marijuana in their lifetimes, and 8.3 percent have used it in the last month.
- The most frequent users are between 18 and 34 years old.
- Annual marijuana use peaked among high school students in 1979 then declined steadily for thirteen years.
- In the 1990s, there was a resurgence in use of this drug. Some decline occurred during 1999.

Marijuana is a prepared mixture of the crushed leaves, flowers, small branches, stems, and seed of the hemp plant, *Cannabis sativa*. Hashish is a more potent resin derived from this plant. Marijuana is a hard drug to classify. Depending on various factors, including the amount of drug taken, the type of drug, the setting, and the mood of the user, cannabis intoxication may resemble the effects of alcohol, a sedative, a stimulant, or a hallucinogen. Marijuana in low to moderate doses causes a sedative effect. However, at higher doses, marijuana produces effects quite similar to the mind-expanding psychedelics. Like the powerful psychedelics, there is little cross-tolerance for marijuana and, for example, lysergic acid diethylamide (LSD). In average doses, it acts much like alcohol. In addition, there is distortion of time, increased heart rate, increased appetite and thirst, dilation of the blood vessels in the eyes, and perhaps muscular weakness. Some individuals may act emotionally unstable or anxious or experience sensory distortions. The ability to think, in terms of short-term memory, seems to be reduced. The ability to drive a car effectively is hindered by reduced perception and motor coordination.

The health effects from long-term marijuana use are still under investigation. Several major problems can result from intense marijuana abuse. It is assumed from current research that chronic bronchitis, cancer, and emphysema will result from long-term marijuana smoking—in fact, the risks of these diseases is greater from marijuana than from tobacco because marijuana smoke goes into the body unfiltered. There have also been reports suggesting that marijuana smoking adversely affects the body's ability to fight off disease.

Marijuana affects the reproductive system in various ways. It affects the sympathetic nervous system, increasing vasodilation in the genitals and thus delaying ejaculation. Chronic marijuana use has been shown in some studies to reduce testosterone (male hormone) levels and lower sperm counts, but results are inconclusive (Donatelle 2002).

Although marijuana tolerance can develop, the frequent user may actually require less to gain the effects of the drug over time. Physical dependence seems to be rare. There is a danger of psychological dependence, however.

For some time, marijuana has been under investigation for possible medical use. In fact, marijuana has been used for numerous medical purposes since the ancient Chinese first employed the cannabis plant as a therapy. It is possible that some patients not helped by conventional therapies could be treated successfully with marijuana, and that cannabis might be combined effectively and safely with other drugs to produce a treatment goal.

Marijuana has been used medically in the following ways (Carroll 2000, 245–246).

- **Glaucoma**—marijuana smoking is effective in reducing the fluid pressure of the eye in a glaucoma patient.

- **Chemotherapy-caused nausea and vomiting**—a 1982 report from the National Academy of Sciences stated that medication containing tetrahydrocannabind (THC), the active ingredient in marijuana, was the only kind that was effective in reducing the severe nausea caused by certain drugs used to treat cancer.

- **Appetite stimulant**—there may well be a stimulating influence on food intake in advanced cancer patients who use marijuana in conjunction with chemotherapy.

- **Antiasthmatic effect**—short-term smoking has produced a bronchodilation effect in patients with bronchial asthma.

- **Seizures, spasticity, and other nervous system disorders**—according to the 1982 report from the National Academy of Sciences, marijuana has been found useful in treating some of these disorders (epilepsy, for example).

- **Muscle-relaxant action**—limited studies suggest that marijuana is effective in relieving muscle spasms common in patients with multiple sclerosis.

On the other hand, for each of these uses, there are other modern drugs with equal effectiveness (Ray and Ksir 2002, 414–416).

Should marijuana become an accepted drug? Marijuana is an unstable substance that has a poor shelf life. It will probably be found to contain over 1,000 chemicals, of which only about 400 are currently known. It contains dozens of things that may not be useful in treating a specific problem. At best, marijuana is a controversial drug. Although it may not be as harmful as some researchers report, it certainly is not harmless. Any use of THC for medical purposes does not stand as an endorsement for the recreational aspects of the drug.

Inhalants

Substances that are inhaled to produce altered states are called *inhalants*. These substances are classified as volatile solvents and aerosols. Common chemicals inhaled are fingernail polish remover, lacquer thinners, glue, gasoline, and liquid paper. Inhalation is a rapid means of ingesting substances, equivalent to IV injection in the time required to reach the brain. Altered consciousness can be achieved within one to two minutes of inhaling a large concentration and five to ten minutes with low doses. Inhalants can also be ingested through the mouth. This method is called *huffing,* and it is not as prevalent as inhaling.

Most volatile substances are classified as depressants, although some may exhibit hallucinogenic characteristics. The effects of inhaled chemicals include initial nausea with some irritation of airways causing coughing and sneezing. With low doses there is often a brief feeling of light-headedness and mild stimulation followed by a loss of control, lack of coordination, and disorientation accompanied by dizziness. Chronic use can result in permanent brain damage; impairment of motor behavior; severe psychological problems; and damage to lungs, kidneys, and liver. There has been a recent disturbing increase of inhalant abuse by younger children. Approximately 20 percent of eighth-graders abused inhalants in 1999 (Hanson, Venturelli, and Fleckenstein 2001, 396–398).

Designer Drugs

Designer drugs are substances produced synthetically by underground chemists and sold under the false assumption that they are some other drug (Hanson, Venturelli, and Fleckenstein 2001, 9). Compounds are altered to give the appearance of the original drug, and to some extent, the effects, but they contain only legal substances. They are often called *look-alikes.* The most familiar designer drugs were amphetamine look-alikes that contained caffeine, ephedrine, and phenylpropanolamine hydrochloride—the same ingredients as in many OTC diet and cold compounds. Designer cocaine may consist of powdered sugar and a topical anesthetic such as benzocaine. The user experiences sinus numbing, but the cocaine rush is absent. Naive users may be fooled, but experienced coke snorters quickly recognize the imposter.

In addition to differing in chemical makeup, some designer drugs are more dangerous than the drugs they imitate. They may contain very dangerous drugs that can be lethal in very small amounts, so when the user injects his or her usual dose, it may be fatal. Other effects such as brain damage and paralysis have occurred. Designer drugs are banned in the United States by a bill passed in 1986.

Hallucinogens

Hallucinogens are substances that occur naturally or are produced synthetically and which distort the user's perception of reality. Such drugs cause sensory illusions that make it difficult to distinguish fact from fantasy. Perhaps the most widely known hallucinogen is LSD, which was first synthesized in 1938. Although still occasionally used in medical research, the drug has no commonly used therapeutic applications. Even a tiny amount is enough to cause hallucinations, which manifest themselves in intensified colors, individualized sound perceptions, and bizarre visions that may be pleasant or extremely frightening. In mentally unstable individuals, LSD can produce psychotic reactions. There is also a danger of so-called flashbacks in which an individual will suddenly have hallucinations even weeks after having last ingested the drug. LSD does not cause physical dependency or seem to result in brain damage or birth defects, as once supposed. However, a "bad trip," or unpleasant experience while under the influence of the drug, can have long-lasting psychological effects.

Other hallucinogens are either derived from peyote, a kind of cactus that grows in Mexico and the American Southwest, or made synthetically. Most have effects similar to those produced by LSD, but some are particularly dangerous because of unpredictable side effects. One of the more common of these illegal drugs is phencyclidine hydrochloride (PCP), known as "angel dust." Originally synthesized as an animal tranquilizer, PCP is a relatively easy chemical to manufacture illegally. The drug is usually mixed with tobacco or marijuana and ingested by smoking.

PCP produces perceptual distortions, feelings of depersonalization, and changes in body image. Apathy, sweating, and auditory hallucinations may also result. High doses produce a stupor and overdose coma that can last for several weeks. This period can be followed by weeks of a confused mental state. In some individuals PCP also has been reported to precipitate extremely violent behavior, including murder.

Drug Education

Evaluation research on drug education prevention programs done over the last thirty years indicates that these programs have not been effective. In fact, the findings state that these programs essentially had no effect on the drug problem. Although studies of the more recently developed programs are more optimistic, the findings still do not provide strong evidence of highly effective programs. The goals of these programs have been to affect three basic areas: knowledge, attitudes, and behavior. The programs have had some success in increasing knowledge and, to a lesser extent, attitudes toward drugs; however, increases in knowledge and changed attitudes do not mean much if the actual drug behavior is not affected. In fact, those programs that only increase knowledge tend to reduce anxiety and fear of drugs and may actually increase the likelihood of drug use. For example, one approach in the past was to provide students with complete information about all the possibilities of drug abuse, from the names of every street drug, to how the drugs are usually ingested, to detailed descriptions of possible effects of the drugs and possible consequences of an overdose. Given the inquiring nature of children, such an approach could well amount to a primer on how to take drugs, not how to avoid them.

The only effective approach to drug education is one in which children come to see that drug abuse constitutes unnecessary and self-abusive consequences.

Health Highlight

STRATEGIES USED IN EFFECTIVE DRUG ABUSE
EDUCATION AND PREVENTION PROGRAMS

Effective drug abuse education and prevention programs begin in elementary schools and promote a clear "no use" message. Strategies that can be effective are:

- freeing students from the common perception, or normative belief, that they must abuse drugs to be popular or socially acceptable

- employing the "personal commitment" strategy to encourage students to voluntarily make public or private pledges not to use or abuse drugs

- using various values clarification exercises to challenge students to find conflicts between existing personal values and abuse of drugs

- fostering the development of resistance skills, where students learn how to identify and resist peer and media pressure to abuse drugs

- teaching students a system of setting and achieving goals

- teaching students a decision-making system in which they learn how to organize information and make wise choices among alternatives

- teaching students to increase feelings of self-worth and personal identity

- teaching students a variety of ways to relax under stress and cope with pressure in order to resolve problems

- teaching students life skills, like assertiveness, and how to communicate more effectively with others; with these life skills, students improve their ability to maintain social relations without the abuse of drugs.

SOURCE: Carroll 2000, 360–361

Teachers must provide realistic alternatives. Too often, the real appeal of such drugs as marijuana or alcohol is dismissed by asking children to take up a sport or go bike riding or learn to play a musical instrument. Such suggestions are fine as far as they go, but they often fail to take into account the personal problems that may tempt children into drug abuse.

Education programs that address social influence show the most promise in reducing or delaying onset of drug use. Psychological approaches in which social influences and skills are stressed are more effective than other approaches. The most effective programs in influencing both attitudes and behavior are peer programs that included either refusal skills—with more direct emphasis on behavior—or social and life skills, or both.

In order for drug abuse prevention programs to be effective, they should involve all locations and situations the student encounters. Also, the student needs to be receiving the same message from each part of his or her environment. Such community-wide comprehensive approaches to drug abuse prevention education are essential, because research indicates that school-based drug abuse prevention programs are not as effective in preventing or reducing drug problems when used independently from more comprehensive programs (Carroll 2000, 355).

A drug abuse education program is not an easy undertaking. For every strategy that has been proposed, there have been critics with good and plausible arguments as to why that strategy is the worst one possible. There are even those, including many parents, who feel that the best approach is no approach at all. This is the concept that if adults don't mention drugs, then the problem doesn't really exist. This latter view seems out of touch with reality, and yet it is understandable considering how so many drug education programs have led to unfortunate results.

The use of scare tactics in any health education program, including drug abuse education programs, is counterproductive. Children soon learn to recognize the difference between fact and possible fiction. Attempts to equate the dangers of marijuana with those of heroin, suggestions that any drug can kill or permanently impair an individual, and other dire warnings, no matter how true, are often disregarded as propaganda.

Teachers must never lie about the dangers of drugs or play down the problems that children are facing that may make drugs seem to be an appealing way to cope. Effective drug education walks a fine line, one that requires teachers' sensitivity to the environment in which children must live and function. It is always important to point out that, no matter what the circumstances, each individual has a choice and must make a choice about substance use or abuse. Drug education must be a part of a comprehensive mental health education program. Only when children realize that drugs are not the answer to a problem, but part of the problem, can instruction be considered successful.

Summary

- A drug is any substance that alters bodily functions.
- Drugs can be misused or abused.
- Reasons for substance abuse include:

low self-esteem	mood alteration	curiosity
peer pressure	boredom	alienation
adult modeling		

- Drugs act on the body by stimulating or depressing cellular activity.
- Even when drugs are prescribed for medical purposes, there is a possibility that substance abuse can result.
- Over-the-counter drugs are usually safe when taken as directed, but ingestion of any drug, no matter how mild, can cause health hazards.
- Advertisements for OTC drugs can often lead people to believe that they are safer and more effective than they actually are.
- Central nervous system depressants are some of the most widely used and abused drugs in the United States because they produce a "quality high." In addition, they relieve stress and anxiety, and induce sleep. These effects appeal to many people. Unfortunately, these depressants can cause numerous serious side effects, including a strong dependence.

- Alcohol is one of the most commonly used and abused drugs.
- Alcohol can easily lead to psychological and physical dependency, sometimes resulting in alcoholism, a disease that can wreck lives.
- The disease of alcoholism can and does occur in youth.
- Alcoholics and their families can receive help from many sources, such as AA.
- Particularly dangerous drugs include barbiturates and amphetamines, known commonly as "downers" and "uppers."
- Barbiturates are depressants, and amphetamines are stimulants. If abused, these drugs can cause serious health problems or death.
- Marijuana, for various reasons, is in a classification by itself.
- Ongoing research is determining the possible medicinal effects of marijuana.
- Narcotics are in some ways much more dangerous than barbiturates.
- The narcotics class of drugs includes opium, morphine, and heroin.
- Heroin is extremely addictive and can lead to psychological breakdowns and irrational acts.
- As with any street drug, the user can never be sure of just what chemicals are contained in the dose sold.
- A stimulant drug that is currently one of the most dangerous we have in our society is cocaine, known as "snow," or "coke," or "crack."
- Crack is cheap and readily available and is smoked and absorbed into the bloodstream in less than ten seconds.
- Most crack-related deaths result from brain hemorrhage, blocking of the heart's electrical system, lung failure, or associated heart and vessel complications.
- Smoking tobacco is a serious health problem.
- Smokers often become psychologically and physically dependent on tobacco.
- Tobacco companies' advertising and promotional activities have led many children to start smoking and to use smokeless tobacco.
- Smoking is a difficult habit to break, but failure to do so can lead to a variety of serious diseases, including cancer and emphysema.
- Sidestream and secondhand smoke can cause similar problems to nonsmokers who live and/or work with smokers.
- Smokeless tobacco can lead to similar problems as smoking tobacco.
- Hallucinogenic drugs include LSD and PCP.
- Although not physically addictive, hallucinogens can lead to psychological breakdowns and irrational acts.
- Substance education is a difficult topic, one in which there are no easy answers regarding the correct course of action.
- Factual information must be provided, and yet substance education must not be allowed to become a primer on how to take drugs.
- Effective drug abuse education programs are needed to change not only knowledge and attitudes, but behavior as well.

- Community mores and lifestyles must be considered so that information and advice given are realistic and practical.
- The best course is to build self-esteem in students so that drugs are not seen as a viable alternative for coping with personal problems.

DISCUSSION QUESTIONS

1. What is the definition of a drug? Give examples of substances that qualify as drugs under this definition.
2. List six common reasons for substance abuse, especially as these reasons apply to young people.
3. What factors contribute to the misuse and abuse of OTC drugs?
4. Describe the effects of alcohol on the body at various blood alcohol concentration levels.
5. List six reasons that contribute to the habit of smoking tobacco.
6. Discuss the adverse effects of smokeless tobacco.
7. Discuss cocaine and the various forms of the drug.
8. Why is marijuana considered to be a harmful substance? How can it effectively be used medicinally?
9. What approach to substance education is the most effective, and why?
10. What are the characteristics of a good substance abuse prevention program in the schools?

CRITICAL THINKING QUESTIONS

1. There appears to be a thin line between use, abuse, and misuse. Do you think an underage person (for example, someone who is under twenty-one and drinking alcohol) can use alcohol responsibly? Explain your answer relative to the law prohibiting the use of alcohol by those under the age of twenty-one.
2. There are a variety of reasons why some people begin to abuse drugs, and they appear to be unique for each individual. Can you synthesize the factors into the most common reasons for beginning abuse of substances?
3. Explain why some people continue to abuse substances even when they know about the harmful effects of the drugs on their body.
4. Explain your side of the debate regarding whether or not marijuana should be legalized.
5. How do you feel that the tobacco settlement monies should be used by the states?

WEB SITE ACTIVITY

Access the Youth Risk Behavior Survey Web site by the National Center for Chronic Disease Prevention and Health Promotion. Compare the various age groups among students with regard to marijuana use.

WEB SITES OF INTEREST

Centers for Disease Control and Prevention (CDC): *www.cdc.gov*
Provides information about preventing and controlling disease, injury, and disability.

Emedicine.com, Incorporated: *www.emedicine.com*
Provides informational articles on a variety of medicines and issues related to specific drugs.

Join Together: *www.jointogether.org*
Provides current information regarding substance abuse and related issues, such as safety and violence prevention.

National Center for Chronic Disease Prevention and Health Promotion:
  www.cdc.gov/nccdphp/dash/yrbs/natsum97/su97.htm
Provides summaries of the latest national Youth Risk Behavior Survey.

National Clearinghouse for Alcohol and Drug Information
  www.health.org/links/AlcDrug.htm
Provides numerous related links for Alcohol and Drug Information and Resources.

National Organization on Fetal Alcohol Syndrome
  www.nofas.org/main/ index2.htm
A very in-depth Web site that provides a large volume of information about fetal alcohol syndrome (FAS). It includes ideas for prevention, help for parents of children with FAS, and links to related Web sites.

Partnership for a Drug-Free America (PDFA): *www.drugfreeamerica.org*
PDFA is a private nonprofit, nonpartisan coalition of professionals from the communications industry. Its mission is to reduce demand for illicit drugs in America through media communication.

Substance Abuse and Mental Health Services Administration
  www.samhsa.gov/oas/NHSDA/2kNHSDA/chapter2.htm
Provides indicators of drug abuse and results of national surveys, such as the National Household Survey of Drug Abuse.

U.S. Department of Labor: *www.dol.gov/asp/programs/drugs/workingpartners*
Presents the disturbing statistics of employee drug use in the United States and what employers are doing to stop it.

Web MD: *www.my.webmd.com/encyclopedia*
Includes articles and medical advice regarding the nature and use of several licit and illicit drugs and medicines.

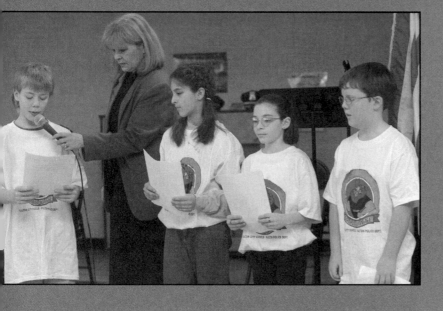

CHAPTER FOURTEEN

Strategies for Teaching about Substance Use and Abuse

It is important for teachers to realize that there are almost as many reasons for drifting into substance abuse as there are different kinds of drugs.

VALUED OUTCOMES

After doing the activities in this chapter, the student should be able to express and illustrate the following guidelines:

- dealing effectively with personal problems is important in preventing substance abuse
- poor self-image increases the potential for substance abuse
- drugs should be taken only when a doctor prescribes them and only in the amount prescribed
- people use and abuse drugs for physical, emotional, and social reasons
- certain drugs can be legally purchased only with a doctor's prescription
- some drugs, called over-the-counter drugs, can be purchased without a doctor's prescription

- smoking is dangerous to health
- tobacco smoke can be harmful to those who do not smoke, as well as to smokers themselves
- alcohol is a drug
- misuse of alcohol can cause physical, emotional, and social problems
- alcoholism is a disease
- alcoholism can lead to many health problems

- barbiturates can cause both physical and psychological dependency
- cocaine and crack are very dangerous drugs and should not be used under any circumstances
- amphetamines, like barbiturates, can be dangerous if abused
- illegal drugs, including narcotics and hallucinogens, can have unpredictable and serious health consequences

REFLECTIONS

Consider the possibility that you have a student who is abusing an illegal drug, and he or she has confided in you. What are the realistic steps that you would take as a teacher in this situation? What other pieces of information would you need? Consider the personal, ethical, and legal ramifications. Which of the strategies in this chapter would be useful to help teach students to take responsibility for their actions?

The Challenge of Substance Abuse Education

Elementary school children need to be provided with learning experiences that will help them develop attitudes and values that build self-esteem and respect for the body so that drug taking is not seen as a way of coping with life. They must be taught to accept responsibility for their own behavior so that they will know how to deal with the problem of drugs in society.

The challenge of drug education is not to make every child a drug expert, nor to frighten children with scare tactics. Instead, it is to help children recognize that there is no need for them to misuse or abuse any drug, regardless of what reason they may have for being tempted to do so.

It is important for teachers to realize that there are almost as many reasons for drifting into substance abuse as there are different kinds of drugs. A youngster may wish to start smoking for an entirely different reason from the reason a youngster might begin amphetamine abuse. The temptation to take a particular drug may not stem from any self-destructive impulse, although sometimes it does. The problem is that the resultant behavior is always self-destructive, in varying degrees, regardless of the motivation. If children recognize this fact, and if they are on their way to building a strong self-image, then substance abuse is far less likely to occur in later years.

Shown to the right of each activity is the suggested grade level(s) for which the activity might be appropriate. However, many of the suggested activities could be modified for use at various grade levels.

Value-Based Activities

SMOKING AND THE LAW   Grades (4–5)

Valued Outcome: The students will be able to describe the variables involved in making a decision about smoking.

Description of Strategy: After you have discussed the definition of a drug, point out that tobacco qualifies under the definition. Note that although smoking is known to be hazardous to health, tobacco products can be purchased legally by adults. Ask students to consider the implications of this fact. Point out that each individual must make a decision about smoking. Then have the students consider the following question: Should laws be passed that prevent people from smoking in certain public places?

Materials Needed: none

Processing Questions:

1. Should cigarettes be made illegal? Why or why not?
2. What legal rights should smokers have?
3. What legal rights should nonsmokers have?
4. What are some reasons to be considered in making such laws?
5. How do you feel about laws regulating smoking?

SMOKING AND YOU   Grades (4–5)

Valued Outcome: The students will be able to list reasons why a person might decide not to start smoking.

Description of Strategy: Have each student prepare a list with two columns. In the first column, ask the students to write reasons why they think a person might want to start smoking. In the second column, have them list reasons why a person might decide not to start smoking. Talk over the various reasons that the students list in a general discussion. Which reasons in each column are rational ones? Which are irrational ones?

Materials Needed: pencils and paper

Processing Question: What are the emotional and social reasons a person might start smoking?

LIVING WITHOUT DRUGS
Grades (4–5)

Valued Outcome: The students will be able to describe alternative ways to alleviate various health problems.

Description of Strategy: Have the students bring in advertisements for health-related products from magazines and newspapers. Look especially for ads that deal with stress ailments, such as headaches, backaches, insomnia, and diarrhea. After comparing and discussing the ads, have the students brainstorm alternative ways to deal with these problems. Alternatives to medication may include taking time to talk to a friend or loved one, listening to soft music, eating properly, exercising, drinking plenty of water, or doing something special.

Materials Needed: newspapers and magazines

Processing Question: Why is our society so drug dependent?

LIVING WITH DRUGS
Grades (4–5)

Valued Outcome: The students will be able to explain the connection between societal problems and substance abuse.

Description of Strategy: Have the students collect and bring in magazine articles and newspaper clippings about accidents, domestic problems, violence, suicide, and crime. Discuss the clippings and the role drug or alcohol use may have played. Have the class members consider reasons why these things might have occurred and what kinds of actions can be taken to avoid them in their own lives (alternatives to destructive behavior).

Materials Needed: newspapers and magazines

Processing Question: Why is there such a positive correlation between substance abuse and violence/crime?

WHERE DO YOU STAND?
Grades (K–5)

Valued Outcome: The students will be able to clarify their values regarding substance abuse.

Description of Strategy: Draw a chalk line on the floor. Explain to your students that the line is a continuum on how they feel about various decisions. One end of the line represents complete disagreement with a position, and the other end represents complete agreement. Or the line could represent degrees of willingness or unwillingness.

Then ask for volunteers to demonstrate where they stand on a variety of questions that you put forward. Try to keep the questions nonthreatening and nonincriminating. Questions that you might ask include: Where do you stand on smoking cigarettes? Where do you stand on drinking alcohol? How willing would you be to tell a friend who takes drugs that you do not approve of that behavior? How dangerous do you think it is to take a drug that you yourself don't know anything about?

Materials Needed: chalk

Processing Question: none

SENTENCE COMPLETION   Grades (3–5)

Valued Outcome: The students will be able to complete statements with their own values-related answers.

Description of Strategy: Ask the students to complete statements such as the following with values-related answers:

> For me, smoking is . . .
>
> If I saw another student using drugs, I would . . .
>
> Some people start drinking alcohol because . . .
>
> Drugs are . . .
>
> To me, substance abuse means . . .
>
> The best reason for not taking any drugs is . . .
>
> One thing I don't believe about drugs is . . .
>
> If I made the laws about drugs, I would . . .
>
> I was surprised to learn that drugs . . .
>
> People who take drugs . . .

Materials Needed: handout for each student, pencils

Processing Question: What factors in your background influence your values regarding substance abuse?

DRUG RATING SCALE   Grades (4–5)

Valued Outcome: The students will express their opinions about drugs.

Description of Strategy: Have the students complete the following rating scale on their beliefs about drugs. Then have a classroom discussion about why they feel the way they do. The rating scale is:

1 strongly agree   2 agree   3 don't know/neutral
4 disagree   5 strongly disagree

_____ It is okay to smoke marijuana every once in a while.

_____ Crack cocaine is the worst drug a person can take.

_____ Nicotine in cigarettes is a drug.

_____ Smoking cigarettes is not good for your health.

_____ Tripping on acid only affects you once, and then you never feel the effects of the drug again.

_____ The best thing I can do when asked to take drugs by someone is to say no and walk away.

_____ Drinking alcohol is not the same as taking a drug.

_____ Alcohol won't hurt you.

_____ I can smoke now and then quit when I get older, and it won't hurt me.

_____ The only kind of people who take drugs are bad students who are always getting in trouble.

Materials Needed: handout for each student, pencils

Processing Questions:

1. Why should we say no to drugs?

2. What happens when people take drugs?

3. If a person takes drugs, will it affect him or her for the rest of his or her life?

Decision Stories

Present decision stories such as the following, using the procedures outlined in Chapter 4, pages 80–83.

WANT A SMOKE? Grades (4–5)

Mark always walks home from school with a group of friends. One day, two of his friends light up cigarettes. Mark is surprised because he didn't know that they had started smoking. "Want a smoke?" his friend Jim asks. "They're real mild," his other friend George says. "Try one." Mark can see that Jim and George are trying to look grown up. He wants to look grown up, too. The other two boys in the group are not smoking. Mark wonders what he should do.

Focus Question: What should Mark say to his friends?

PROBLEMS AT HOME Grades (7–8)

Michael's problems at home are getting worse, and he feels he has nowhere to turn. He is very lonely and frightened about what is happening in his life. His parents are always fighting. They don't seem to have any time for him anymore. He wants so much to have someone show him love and concern. He also wishes that he could just leave his problems behind him.

Focus Questions:

1. What are some methods of coping that Michael might try?

2. What might be the consequences of each of these methods?

SLUMBER PARTY   Grades (3–5)

Sally is throwing a slumber party at her home. Her parents respect Sally's judgment and ask her to make sure that the party does not get out of hand. Sally doesn't think it will. But after her parents have gone to bed, some of Sally's friends start passing some pills around. They tell her that these pills are fun to take and are not dangerous. They also say that Sally doesn't have to try the pills if she doesn't want to. But they ask her not to spoil the party for them.

Focus Question: What should Sally do?

DRUGS IN THE NEIGHBORHOOD   Grades (3–5)

Darlene knows that some of the older kids in her neighborhood are using and selling drugs. They don't seem to care that Darlene sees what they are doing. "It's none of your business," one of them told her. But Darlene is not so sure. A couple of her friends bought some of these drugs and have started using them. Darlene doesn't know what will happen in the neighborhood next.

Focus Question: What can Darlene do about the drug problem in her neighborhood?

MOM DRINKS TOO MUCH   Grades (3–5)

Often, when David arrives home from school in the afternoon, his mother is sitting in the living room with a glass or a bottle beside her. Sometimes she is very loving, and other times she seems very angry at him. Sometimes she is asleep on the couch, and he has trouble waking her up. Sometimes Mom can't fix supper for David and his younger sister. David knows that his mom uses alcohol more than she should. She is frequently depressed and upset. David is afraid of how his mom will act when he comes in every day, and he is afraid that she will get hurt. He also worries about who is taking care of his sister when he is not there. David constantly worries about what will happen to his family if his mom does not stop drinking.

Focus Questions:

1. What actions should David take?
2. Who does he need to talk to about his problems?
3. Who might be able to help David, his sister, and his mom?

SLEEPOVER   Grades (4–5)

Leah had been looking forward to tonight. It was her tenth birthday, and she was having a sleepover party in her backyard. Her parents were letting Leah and her two friends, Casey and her sister, Allison, sleep in her tent. The girls had eaten sandwiches and were about to play cards when Casey pulled out a pack of cigarettes from her coat pocket. "Hey, let's light up," she said. Casey and Allison both took out a cigarette. Casey offered the pack to Leah. "No, I don't want to," she said. "What's the matter, big baby? Are you scared?" asked Casey. "We didn't know we were sleeping over with such a baby. Maybe we'd better go home." Leah had been having lots of fun, but she did not know that her friends smoked.

Focus Question: What should Leah do?

Dramatizations

DRUG COURT   Grades (3–5)

Valued Outcome: The students will be able to dramatize various drug-related court actions.

Description of Strategy: Have the students role-play various drug-related court actions. In this court, the class acts collectively as judge and jury. Various students come before the court acting the part of the arresting officer. They explain to the court that they have arrested an individual on a drug charge and then describe the offense. In each case, the defendant has already pleaded guilty to the charge. It is up to the court to decide what sentence or decision to make. The class must come up with a consensus on each offense. Follow each decision with general discussion. Also note to the students what the penalty might have been in an actual court.

Materials Needed: none

Processing Questions:

1. Why is it illegal to use/abuse certain drugs?
2. What penalties are given to those who illegally use/abuse drugs?

PUBLIC SERVICE MESSAGES   Grades (4–6)

Valued Outcome: The students will be able to devise a sixty-second message on substance education.

Description of Strategy: Divide the class into small groups. Have each group prepare a sixty-second public service message for television broadcast about substance education. Encourage imagination. Some students may wish to write and sing a song bearing their message. Others may wish to act out a skit. Still others may opt for a panel format. Have each group give its "televised" presentation in front of the class. Each presentation must be sixty seconds long. After the presentations, have the class discuss each one. You may wish to have the students vote for the most effective presentation.

Materials Needed: optional videotaping equipment to aid discussion

Processing Questions:

1. How can antidrug messages best be given to the public?
2. What should these messages include?

WHAT WOULD HAPPEN IF . . . ?   Grades (3–5)

Valued Outcome: The students will be able to simulate various activities while pretending to be under the influence of certain kinds of drugs.

Description of Strategy: After discussing the effects that various kinds of drugs can have on the body and brain, have students role-play situations in which a person attempts an activity while under the influence of a certain kind of drug. For example, what would happen if an airline pilot tried to land a plane while under the influence of alcohol? What would happen if a surgeon tried to operate while under the influence of a hallucinogen? Have one student play the affected person. Another student, at the last minute, steps in and saves the day. After the activity, emphasize to the class that sometimes no one can keep a tragedy from happening. Bring this point home by discussing drunk-driving statistics or other examples from the news.

Materials Needed: none

Processing Questions:

1. What effects do drugs have on the body?

2. How can the effects of drugs affect one's job performance?

TO SMOKE OR NOT TO SMOKE   Grades (4–5)

Valued Outcome: The students will describe the harmful effects of smoking, and demonstrate the ability to make healthful decisions about smoking when pressured by their peers.

Description of Strategy: Provide the students with the following scenario. Lately, your friends have been talking about how "cool" it is to smoke. Then, at your friend's house, while her parents are out of town, she pulls out a cigarette and lights up. She offers a cigarette to you and your other friend. You know that you do not want to smoke, but you are worried that your friends will think you are "not cool" if you don't. Your friend is also reluctant about taking a cigarette; but, after a few minutes and some teasing from the girl who is smoking, he goes ahead and takes one. Then she offers a cigarette to you. What will you do?

Have the students individually write down ideas about how to handle the situation, then divide them into groups of three for some role-playing. Give each student in the group a "part." Have one of the students be the friend who starts smoking, have one be the reluctant taker, and have the third be the one to refuse the cigarette. Have the students role-play the introductory scenario, then have the groups discuss the actions of the non-taker. Then as a whole class, discuss the different actions that could be taken to avoid taking a cigarette.

Materials Needed: pretend cigarettes (such as stick candy or short straws), paper, pencils

Processing Questions:

1. What are ways to combat peer pressure about smoking?

2. What are the effects of smoking?

SOURCE: Foster 2003

DANGERS OF HUFFING

Valued Outcome: The students will discuss the difficulties of peer pressure and ways of overcoming and reversing peer pressure. The students will be able to name some of the dangers of inhaling chemicals.

Description of Strategy: Divide the class into small groups of four or five students each. Give the groups pretend bottles of glue. Have a couple of students play the role of the persuader and the other students in the group play the role of the reluctant ones. Have the students discuss how it felt to be pressured and the possible effects of inhaling chemical products. Then have the students brainstorm ways to handle these situations and ways they might actually reverse peer pressure by preventing the other members of the group from participating.

Materials Needed: pretend bottles of glue

Processing Questions:

1. What are the dangers of inhaling chemicals?
2. What are some ways you could avoid situations like these?

PAST, PRESENT, AND FUTURE DRUGS USERS AND ABUSERS

Valued Outcome: The student will be able to explain and discuss the effects, consequences, and solutions of substance use and abuse.

Description of Strategy: Have four to five students role-play the effects and consequences of substance use and abuse. The selected students should have background knowledge on their substance and its effects and consequences. Provide appropriate information for the various drugs to ensure that students disseminate the correct information. Have the other students ask questions about the selected students' "experiences" with substance use and abuse. As a class, have students discuss different outcomes and solutions that would prevent future use and abuse of substances.

Materials Needed: note cards with appropriate information

Processing Questions:

1. What are some of the effects and consequences of substance use/abuse?
2. What are some reasons people use and abuse substances?

MOST PEOPLE DON'T USE DRUGS— DEBATE

Valued Outcome: The students will debate the differences between stereotypes and reality and make decisions about substance use and abuse.

Description of Strategy: Divide the class into two groups. Ask the class a series of questions about the different stereotypes of drug use and abuse. Have one side of the room agree and the other side disagree with the statements. Students must give reasons why they agree and disagree. Give the students time to discuss their answers with their group members. Then have a student report to the class what the groups have said. This could be discussed using a debate format or by having the students on one side make statements and the other side give counterpoints. After asking a few questions, have the students reverse the roles.

Materials Needed: pencils and paper

Processing Questions:

1. Will smoking make you popular?
2. Is it okay to drink at social functions?
3. Will smoking make your breath stink?
4. Are people who don't smoke and drink happier than people who do?

SOURCE: Hawley 1997

SUBSTANCE ABUSE INFLUENCES   Grades (3–5)

Valued Outcome: The students will be able to identify external and internal influences that affect one's choice of behavior; discuss that external influences include influences outside ourselves (environment, family, and friends); explain that internal influences include determinants within ourselves and that they are based on our values and beliefs; and describe the impact of a variety of influences that exert themselves on a daily basis.

Description of Strategy: Ask for five volunteers. Without the class hearing, explain role-play to them. Have them sit around a table on which is a plate of "wellness" cookies. Distribute previously prepared instruction sheets to the five students; tell them not to show the instructions to anyone else. Three of the volunteers (1, 2, and 3) will get instructions that read, "Take one wellness cookie, eat it slowly, and try to persuade everyone else at the table to eat a cookie." The fourth volunteer (4) will get instructions that say "Wait two minutes, then take a cookie." The fifth volunteer's (5) instructions will read, "Do not take a cookie, no matter what." After five minutes, ask the processing questions given below.

Materials Needed: plate of real cookies, instruction cards

Processing Questions:

1. Ask person 5: How did you feel being pressured to do something you were told not to do?
2. Ask person 4: How did you feel about giving in?
3. Ask person 5: How did you feel when person 4 gave in?
4. Ask persons 1, 2, 3: How did you feel persuading others?
5. Ask entire class: Who makes your decisions?
6. Ask entire class: What are some ways you can say no to someone trying to persuade you to do something you do not want to do?

SOURCE: Furtado 1994

I'M NO DUMMY   Grades (K–2)

Valued Outcome: The students will be able to demonstrate refusal skills.

Description of Strategy: Have the students make and use hand puppets to act out skits about drug use and abuse. One puppet, for example, might be offered drugs by other puppets. "I'm no dummy," the first puppet replies and then gives reasons for refusing.

Materials Needed: paper lunch bags or cloth for making puppets, markers

Processing Question: What is the best way to refuse the offer of drugs?

PEERS HELPING OTHER PEERS   Grades (3–5)

Valued Outcome: The students will be able to persuade a peer to prevent drug abuse.

Description of Strategy: Have the students role-play a drug-related incident. Pick four students who are willing to participate in the role-playing. Without the class hearing, explain to the four students that they are at the mall and see a couple of friends. They watch their friends walk around to the back of the mall. Deciding they want to see what their friends are up to, they follow them. Little did they know their two friends were doing drugs. Once approached, they started acting really funny. The good students are to tell their friends the effects of the drugs on their body and to help them understand that what they are doing is wrong. Explain to the students they are to use their prior knowledge from the unit on substance abuse to persuade the students to quit. After this is accomplished, ask the rest of the class to tell the four students what they did wrong or what they did right. Follow this with discussion on what they could have done to prevent the drug use.

Materials Needed: none

Processing Questions:

1. What can you do as a student to keep your friends off drugs?

2. What would you do if approached with a harmful substance?

3. What can you do for the community to cut down substance abuse?

CAFFEINE: THE COMMON DRUG   Grades (1–3)

Valued Outcome: The students will describe the dangers of caffeine and consume soft drinks containing it in moderation.

Description of Strategy: Discuss with the students what caffeine does to the body, such as making the heart beat faster, inhibiting sleep, and causing headaches. On a table, display a number of food items, some with caffeine and others without. Items that might be included are caffeinated and noncaffeinated soft drinks, milk, chocolate milk, juice, coffee, tea, a chocolate bar, and water. Ask the students to identify those items that contain caffeine and those that do not. Discuss with students why they should consume food items containing caffeine in moderation. Explain the importance of calcium in their diet, and the food and beverages that will provide them with calcium. Encourage the students to select a juice, milk , or water for lunch instead of a soft drink.

Materials Needed: caffeinated and noncaffeinated food items, a table

1. What drinks and other products contain caffeine?
2. What drinks can you substitute for caffeine products that would make you healthy?

Discussion and Report Techniques

PRESENTATION BY HEALTH PROFESSIONALS   Grades (K–5)

Valued Outcome: The students will learn numerous facts about substance use and abuse from health professional.

Description of Strategy: With permission from your school administration, invite an official from a substance abuse program to speak to your class about substance use and abuse. Talk with your guest alone before the presentation and emphasize that no scare tactics should be used. The presentation should be factual and objective. Allow time for a question-and-answer session afterward.

Materials Needed: none

Processing Questions:

1. What types of treatment are given in substance abuse programs?
2. How effective are these programs?

THE QUESTION BOX   Grades (3–5)

Valued Outcome: The students will be able to identify personal problems and write them on an index card.

Description of Strategy: Have each student write on an index card a personal problem he or she is concerned about. Students may fill out as many cards as they like but they are to write only one question per card. No names or other means of identification should be included. Have the students place their cards in a large ballot box. Allow them to place additional questions in the box for a week. After class, open the box and screen out any cards that inadvertently reveal any problems that would lead to identification of the student involved. Compile a numbered list of concerns from the remaining cards, hand out copies of the list, and randomly assign each student a number from the list. Each student should explain to the class how he or she would deal with the problem. Allow other students with different opinions to add comments.

Materials Needed: index cards, pencils, ballot box, handout for each student of compiled list of concerns

Processing Question: What type of problems in relationships or school could lead to a substance abuse problem?

ASSESSING THE MEDIA'S INFLUENCE TOWARD DRUGS

Grades (5–8)

Valued Outcome: The student will be able to describe how the media influences people's opinions and shapes the way society views some types of drugs.

Description of Strategy: Have each student give a five-minute oral presentation about a particular drug. Then show a movie or play a song that involves that drug. Use the following information for the oral presentation:

- What the medium is (movie title, song title), what the drug is, who is being targeted, and your view whether this media selection is acting positively or negatively regarding the drug.
- What target group is the media trying to influence (young or old, personality, nationality).
- What the media selection (news clip, movie, song) is trying to say about the drug. This can be positive or negative.
- How the media selection presents the information: Where is the drug used and how? Does the song or movie tell or show how it is used?
- Who used the drug, and why? How does it make the person feel?

Materials Needed: videocassette recorder (VCR) and videotapes, tape player and audio tapes, CD player and CDs

Processing Question: How does the media influence your opinion about drugs?

SOURCE: PE Central 2000b

DO YOU WISH YOU NEVER HAD STARTED SMOKING?

Grades (4–5)

Valued Outcome: The students will be able to explain why most smokers wish they had never started smoking.

Description of the Strategy: Assign students to ask a smoker who has been smoking for at least ten years if he or she wishes he or she never had started smoking. Tally the results on the board—write the number of people who wish they never had started in one column and the number of people who said they are glad they started smoking in another column. The likelihood is that the majority of long-term smokers will say they wish they never had started smoking.

Materials Needed: board and markers or overhead projector and pen

Processing Question: How does this activity help with your decision-making process regarding beginning to smoke cigarettes?

SOURCE: Wright 2000a

SMOKING MARIJUANA   Grades (4–5)

Valued Outcome: The students will be able to demonstrate an understanding of the physical effects and legal consequences of smoking marijuana and methods to avoid the temptation.

Description of Strategy: Invite a juvenile court representative to class to speak about the legal consequences of using drugs. The activity before the lesson will include discussion of students' experiences with jail or criminal activity. The follow-up activity will consist of asking the speaker a series of questions. Each student should be handcuffed for a few seconds.

Materials Needed: paper, pens, markers, handcuffs (provided by juvenile court representative)

Processing Questions:

1. Why is it important not to smoke marijuana?
2. What did the juvenile court representative cite as a legal consequence of using marijuana?

JUST SAYING NO IS   Grades (5–6)
OUR FINAL ANSWER!

Valued Outcome: The student will be able to use his or her prior knowledge of substance abuse/use to organize a drug-free school environment.

Description of Strategy: Divide the class into small groups. Assign each group different roles in making their school a drug-free school. For example, have the class decide on different strategies that would get the drug-free message out to the students and to the community. Different strategies might include posters, videos, or specials programs with different activities informing the students of the harmful effects of substance abuse. Have each group give at least a one- to two-minute presentation of the strategy that they would use to make their school a drug-free environment. After the presentations, discuss with the class the positive and negative aspects of each presentation.

Materials Needed: none

Processing Questions:

1. What are other ways to promote a drug-free school environment?
2. What can you do as a student to promote a drug-free community?

PREVENTING DRINKING AND DRIVING   Grades (4–5)

Valued Outcome: The students will demonstrate the ability to use decision-making steps to make healthful decisions about alcohol use.

Description of Strategy: Provide students with this scenario: Your older sister arrives to pick you up from the movies but has had too much to drink, and you know it. You both have to get home soon, and your sister is determined to get behind the wheel. What can you do to prevent this from happening? Have the students individually jot down their ideas, then break them up into small groups to compare notes, and have each group pick and present one of their preventive measures to the rest of the groups.

Materials Needed: pencils and paper

Processing Question: What would you do to prevent someone from drinking and driving?

SOURCE: U.S. Department of Education 2001

SMOKING   Grades (3–5)

Valued Outcome: The student will be able to recall the detrimental effects of smoking by writing a short paragraph on the topic.

Description of Strategy: Ask students to sit in a circle and talk about what smoking does to the body. Hold up a smoking advertisement and ask the students what the advertisement tells them about smoking. For example, does it make you look cool? Have the students respond as a group. Then have students draw pictures of how they think healthy lungs look compared to the lungs of a smoker. Tell students to list other detriments of smoking on a sheet of paper.

Materials Needed: smoking/cigarette advertisement

Processing Question: How do advertisements try to influence young people to smoke?

STIMULANTS   Grades (5–8)

Valued Outcome: To analyze the effects of tobacco, alcohol, and other drug use on crime rates and the economy.

Description of Strategy: Explain that drug use costs the United States billions of dollars every year. Much of this money is spent on law enforcement, rehabilitation, and prevention education. Point out that a portion of taxes that students' parents pay supports institutions involved in fighting the drug war (military, police, prisons, and hospitals) and in preventing drug use (schools, social services, research institutions, and others). As a class, have the students discuss the following:

- How do students feel about their families having to pay for the effects of drug use?
- How else could this money be used?
- How else could the United States get money to deal with the drug problem?
- How would the student(s) solve the drug problem?

Materials Needed: none

Processing Question: How are tax monies used to prevent drug use?

DANGERS OF SMOKING   Grades (4–5)

Valued Outcome: The students will be able to explain and discuss the dangers of smoking.

Description of Strategy: Give the students information about the dangers of cigarette smoking. Working individually, have the students create slogans or posters for a class anti-smoking campaign. Ask the principal to judge the students' work; present small prizes for originality and creativity.

Materials Needed: construction paper, markers, crayons, colored pencils, scissors, glue

Processing Questions:

1. Why do you think people smoke?
2. Why do you think it is so hard for people to quit smoking?

SOURCE: American Lung Association 2002, 2003

PRICE OF SMOKING   Grades (4–5)

Valued Outcome: The students will be able to discuss the cost of cigarettes and the paraphernalia associated with smoking.

Description of Strategy: Give students the assignment of going to a grocery or convenience store. An adult should accompany the student while in the store to explain to the clerk that the student is working on an assignment. While there, have them record the prices per package of three different brands of cigarettes and other smoking paraphernalia. During class, have the students calculate the costs of smoking for a year, assuming a smoker consumes one pack of cigarettes a day. Then have the students make a list of the things they could buy with the money spent on cigarettes.

Materials Needed: prices for cigarettes and smoking paraphernalia, pencils, paper

Processing Questions:

1. Do you think smokers realize how much money they spend each year on smoking?
2. Do you think money is the only thing smokers are wasting by smoking?

SOURCE: The Nemours Foundation 1995–2003c

DANGERS OF INHALANTS   Grades (4–5)

Valued Outcome: The students will identify the effects of inhalants on body systems.

Description of Strategy: After a class lesson on the dangers of inhalants, divide students into six small groups. Help the students complete Part 1 of the worksheet in the Teaching in Action box "To Air Is Human." Have the students fill out the rest of the worksheet in their groups. Then have each group discuss and

DANGER OF INHALANTS

Directions: For Part I, fill in the information about the dangers of inhalants as your teacher discusses them. Then make a list of your favorite activities in Part II. Tell how these activities would be affected by use of inhalants.

Part I—Dangers

1. Hepatitis _____

_____

2. Muscle weakness _____

_____

3. Weakened immune system _____

_____

4. Coordination affected _____

_____

5. Thinking ability _____

_____

6. Death _____

_____

Part II—Favorite Activities

1. _____
2. _____
3. _____
4. _____
5. _____

How would these activities be affected by inhalants?

Now	Later
1. _____	_____
2. _____	_____
3. _____	_____
4. _____	_____
5. _____	_____

choose one of the dangers listed in the worksheet and what type of activities might be impaired by the use of inhalants. After completion of this task, have a spokesperson from each group present one idea discussed by the group in a class discussion.

Materials Needed: pencils, worksheet for each student

Processing Questions:

1. Do you think a person could die if he or she only used an inhalant once or twice?

2. Why are inhalants so harmful?

3. How old do you think most kids are who use inhalants?

SOURCE: HealthTeacher 2001

SHARING Grades (K–5)

Valued Outcome: The students will be able to relate personal positive experiences to each other in the class.

Description of Strategy: Have the students sit in a circle on the floor. Ask each student to share one positive experience that happened to him or her in the last month. Sharing may relate to home, school, athletics, play, and so on. No one is to interrupt or ask any questions until every student has had an opportunity to share. Follow the activity with a discussion, asking questions such as: Was it hard to find something to share? What were the similarities among the things shared? Did people share more as the activity progressed? What does this indicate?

Materials Needed: none

Processing Question: What types of positive activities can serve as effective alternatives to substance abuse?

DEALING WITH PROBLEMS Grades (K–5)

Valued Outcome: The students will be able to identify personal problems and then share solutions with each other in class.

Description of Strategy: Divide the class into small groups and have them complete these four sentences:

> I have a problem . . .
>
> This is what happened . . .
>
> My feelings were (or are) . . .
>
> I need your help to . . .

Have each group discuss or role-play for the rest of the class a real problem for them personally. Then let the group present their ideas for positive solutions and get the class response.

Materials Needed: pencils and paper

Processing Question: If you find effective solutions to problems, can that keep you from using/abusing drugs?

WHO INFLUENCES YOUR DECISIONS? Grades (K–5)

Valued Outcome: The students will learn about decision making and whom they can talk to when making difficult decisions.

Description of Strategy: Talk with students about how all people make decisions every day. Some decisions affect our lives more drastically than others. There are easy decisions to make—such as which shoes to wear to school—and there are much more difficult decisions—such as what to do if a friend wants to copy your test answers. It is important to know where to go for advice or help when making important decisions. Have students brainstorm a list of people, places, and institutions that are important to consider when making a decision. This list might include family, television, friends, church, teachers. Have each student decide who or what he or she considers to have the greatest influence on his or her own life. Then have students create collages about the many different influences that affect their thinking and decisions every day.

Materials Needed: paper, magazines, scissors, markers, crayons, glue

Processing Questions:

1. What is the most effective way to make a wise decision?
2. How can effective decision making help prevent a substance abuse problem?

WHAT WOULD HAPPEN IF . . . ? Grades (3–5)

Valued Outcome: The students will be able to identify consequences that follow certain actions.

Description of Strategy: Consequences are the results of our actions. All actions have some kind of consequences. Although it is impossible to always know what all the consequences of a particular action will be, it is important to attempt to figure out logical consequences of important decisions. Have students title a paper "What would happen if . . . ?" and provide them with some situations such as you helped a friend with a chore; you cheated on your homework; you cleaned the house for your mother before she got home from work; a friend asked you to do something you felt uncomfortable doing, such as stealing from a store; or you become angry and hit a friend. Students may want to contribute their own ideas for actions they confront every day. In the paper, have students write about possible consequences for the situation they chose.

Materials Needed: pencils and paper

Processing Questions:

1. Why is it important to consider the consequences of all our actions?
2. How can this type of consideration prevent a substance abuse problem?

THE SPACE COLONY

Valued Outcome: The students will be able to originate a drug policy and drug laws for a new planetary settlement.

Description of Strategy: Tell the class that they are about to travel to a new planet by spaceship. On this planet there are as yet no governments or laws. As a group, the class must decide on the drug policy and drug laws for the new planetary settlement. The class, acting as a committee, must decide what drugs, if any, are to be taken to the new planet and how such drugs will be distributed or made available. Have the class keep in mind that drugs include useful medications, but that such medications can be abused. Laws relating to the misuse of drugs on the new planet must also be discussed. After thorough discussion, have the class come to a consensus about a drug policy on the new planet. Write their conclusions on the board. Then have each student prepare an individual report, including any dissenting opinions. Students must support their opinions.

Materials Needed: markers, board

Processing Questions:

1. Why are drug laws needed?
2. Are current laws effective in preventing substance abuse? Why or why not?

INDIVIDUAL REPORTS

Valued Outcome: The students will be able to initiate research and prepare a report on a drug-related problem.

Description of Strategy: Ask students to do research on a drug-related problem and prepare individual reports on what they find. Topics can include smoking and health, alcohol abuse and accidents, drugs and the law, and dangers of substance abuse.

Materials Needed: none

Processing Questions:

1. What is the relationship between smoking and health?
2. What are the dangers of substance abuse?

SAYING NO TO DRUGS

Valued Outcome: The students will demonstrate drug awareness.

Description of Strategy: Discuss with the students what drugs are. Explain to them that drugs can hurt them badly, and it is not good to use them. Tell the students it is all right to say no to using drugs and that people who want them to try drugs are not their friends. Allow the students to talk about drug abuse. Advise them on the right and wrong thing to do. Tell them about famous people who have died from drug abuse. Following the discussion, give each student a piece of drawing paper and some crayons or markers. Give them suggestions for drawing campaign signs against using drugs (e.g., "Just Say No"). Have them make the signs as colorful and noticeable as possible. Hang the signs throughout the school as a reminder to the rest of the students that drug abuse is not welcome.

Materials Needed: crayons or markers, paper

Processing Questions:

1. What should you do if someone offers you drugs?
2. What is drug abuse?
3. Are drugs good for your body?

RESEARCHING SUBSTANCE ABUSE   Grades (5–8)

Valued Outcome: The students will learn more about different drugs and know the effects that drugs have on the human body.

Description of Strategy: Discuss different types of drugs with the students. Allow the students to share anything (within reason) they know about the different drugs and the effects they have on the human body. Tell the students that they will be writing a research paper on drugs and the effect they have on the body. Make materials such as encyclopedias, written information on drugs or drug abuse, and Internet access, if possible, accessible to the students throughout the entire time they are working on the project. Have the students pick a drug or type of drug, and describe it and the effects it has on the human body. First, have them research their topic; this can be started on the first day of the assignment. Make sure they document their information. The second step is a rough draft, which should be approximately six pages and handwritten on every other line. Finally, have students correct his or her rough draft and turn in the final copy, which should be three pages handwritten or one and one-half pages typed and double spaced. Have each student make an oral presentation of his or her research paper.

Materials Needed: paper and pencils, research materials such as encyclopedias, drug abuse manuals, computer(s) with Internet access

Processing Question: What types of drugs are there?

EFFECTS OF DRUG USE   Grades (3–5)

Valued Outcome: The students will become aware of the effects of drugs on the body.

Description of Strategy: To begin this activity, define the word *drug*. Explain how some drugs can be helpful and others harmful. Then, discuss how some drugs that are helpful can be harmful if used wrongly. Divide the students into groups of four. Give each group on index card with a drug use situation on it. Have each group discuss a particular situation and decide if the drug being used is helpful or harmful and why. Then, write *harmful* and *helpful* on the board. Have each group share the siuation they discussed and say whether the drug is helpful or harmful. Write the situation down. To close this activity, summarize why it is important to know how and what drugs are used for. Also discuss a few helpful things that drugs do and a few harmful things they do.

Materials Needed: index cards, board, markers

Processing Questions:

1. Why is it important to know about the effects of drugs?
2. How can people abuse helpful drugs and make them harmful?

DEBATING DRUG ABUSE   Grades (5–8)

Valued Outcome: The students will be able to explain the pros and cons of taking drugs.

Description of Strategy: Divide the class into two groups. Half the class should be on one side of the room (side A), and the other half should be facing them (side B). Tell the students on side A that they are against taking drugs and cannot stand to be around those who do. Tell side B that they all take drugs, and they think drugs should be legal. These two sides are both given this question: "Should drugs be legalized?" Give the students the rest of the class period to do research. On the next day, hold a debate between Side A and Side B. Side A should detail the facts of the effects of drugs, and side B should give excuses about those facts and excuses that people taking drugs would make. Then discuss the harm that drugs do cause with the exceptions of the drugs that are legal for medicinal purposes only.

Materials Needed: none

Processing Questions:

1. Should all drugs be legalized?
2. Is it dangerous to take illegal drugs without a prescription?

DEFENDING YOURSELF FROM PRESSURE   Grades (4–6)

Valued Outcomes: The students will see that the media do not always portray life accurately, especially regarding substance abuse, and will learn techniques that can help them resist false advertising.

Description of Strategy: Explain the effects alcohol, smoking, and illegal substances may have on the body. Ask for examples they know of in which drugs have had an ill effect on someone. Then have the class discuss why people become involved in such things. Lead the class in discussing peer pressure, what is considered "cool," and the effects of the media. Have the class discuss how the media influences our way of thinking and how they can defend themselves from such pressures. At the end of the discussion, have the students make a substance-abuse collage from magazine advertisements. Have them develop a theme such as "just say no to false advertisement" for their collage. Students should be able to explain their slogans and collage clippings and tell how the pictures apply to the slogan. Grade them on (1) doing the project and doing it well, (2) originality, (3) time and effort put into it, and (4) explanation of collage. When the collages are done, display them around the school (such as in the cafeteria) to remind other students of false advertising.

Materials Needed: poster board, magazines for clippings, construction paper or markers, glue, scissors

Processing Questions:

1. How does the media misrepresent information?
2. What are some ways you can resist false advertising?

EFFECTS OF SMOKING   Grades (3–5)

Valued Outcome: Students will discuss the negative components of smoking cigarettes and the effects smoking has on the lungs.

Description of Strategy: Discuss with the students the effects of cigarette smoke on the human lungs. Have students find statistics on smoking related to the health of the human body. Show the students pictures of a human lung affected by cigarette smoke and a healthy lung. Divide the students into small groups and have them make a list of positive and negative effects of smoking. Then have the groups discuss and compare their lists with the rest of the class.

Materials Needed: paper, pencils, resource material and statistics on smoking, pictures comparing healthy and diseased lungs

Processing Questions:

1. What is the job of our lungs?
2. What are the effects of smoking cigarettes?
3. What do statistics show is the proper thing to do regarding smoking?

EFFECTS OF DRUGS   Grades (4–5)

Valued Outcome: The students will be able to accurately complete sentences about the effects of drugs.

Description of Strategy: Give students a handout with a list of sentences to complete regarding the effects of drugs. Some ideas for sentences are:

1. Fetal alcohol syndrome is the leading cause of _____.
2. Pregnant women should check with a doctor before taking any _____.
3. AIDS can be transmitted to the baby through _____.
4. Marijuana use during pregnancy may produce defects similar to _____.

Materials Needed: handout with questions for each student

Processing Question: How can the preceding information help you make a wise decision about substance abuse?

SOURCE: Gerne and Gerne 1991

Experiments and Demonstrations

SAYING NO!   **Grades (3–5)**

Valued Outcome: The students will recognize the power in asserting themselves when confronted with possible substance abuse.

Description of Strategy: This lesson in assertiveness is accompanied by a physical demonstration of how assertiveness strengthens itself with repetition. Students are encouraged to develop an arsenal of assertive responses telling why they won't indulge in a harmful substance. The more they practice their responses, the more powerful their will becomes. Sample responses might include "No! That is harmful, and I won't become involved with it." Or "I've seen (heard) what can happen by using that. It's not for me." Or "I respect my body too much to do that to it." Assertive behavior includes more than just a set of words. Encourage students to be firm and quick with their rejections of the substance. Help students realize that anyone who would tempt them to harm themselves in such a way is definitely not a friend, no matter how long he or she may have known them.

To illustrate the importance of will power, hold one dowel out in front of you with both hands (thumbs extended toward the middle of the rod). Explain to the class that the dowel represents willpower and the ability to say "No!" to using harmful substances such as cigarettes, drugs, or alcohol. Tell the students if they are tempted by someone to try such a harmful substance for the first time (slowly and firmly place pressure on the center of the dowel by pulling the ends in toward you), their will is being tested just as the strength of the dowel is being tested. Ask the students, if a person has never said "No!" to this substance before, do they think that person's will could withstand the temptation? (Allow students to offer responses. Their answers may vary.) Continue the even pressure until the dowel breaks in the middle. Explain to the students that since some people never learn to say "No!," their will could break easily the first time. Now take four dowels and stack two on top of the other two. Secure the grouping of dowels at either end with rubber bands. Hold them out in front of you as you did earlier. Explain that these four dowels represent someone who has said "No!" several times before. Ask the students if they think it will be easier or harder for their will to be broken. (Allow for student responses.) Again, with the thumbs extended toward the middle of the bundle of four dowels, attempt to pull back on the ends (holding the dowels away from students). More than likely, it will be rather difficult to break this bundle. Explain to the class that putting the four dowels together is as if someone had been able to say "No!" four times to the offer of a dangerous substance.

Materials Needed: five wooden dowels, each approximately eighteen inches long

Processing Questions:

1. What are some good responses when confronted with drugs?
2. What is likely to happen to someone who has never said no before?
3. Is it easier to say no after you have said it once before?

HOW TO SAY NO TO SMOKING   Grades (5–8)

Valued Outcome: The students will describe the dangers of smoking and learn assertive techniques for saying no to smoking.

Description of Strategy: Describe assertiveness, how to say no, and nonverbal behavior that accompanies saying no assertively. Provide a sponge to represent the lung and dark poster paint to apply to a sponge to represent the effects of tar and nicotine on the lungs and have students describe what they see. Discuss how to make the decision to want to say "no" by making a pros and cons list. After discussing how harmful smoking is and how to not give in to peer pressure, reinforce it by having the students act out a role play. For example, one student could be offering a friend a cigarette while another student would decide what to say to him or her.

Materials Needed: sponge, dark poster paint

Processing Questions:

1. What does cigarettes smoking do to your lungs?
2. What would you say to a peer who offers you a cigarette to smoke?

SMOKING MACHINE   Grades (K–5)

Valued Outcome: The students will become aware of what cigarette smoking does to the body.

Description of Strategy: The purpose of this demonstration is to show the effect of cigarette tars on the human body by way of analogy. Check with school and state policies regarding experiments in the classroom before engaging in this demonstration. If there are no policies prohibiting the experiment, send a letter home to the parent or guardian that informs them in advance of this demonstration. Be sure to perform this experiment in a well ventilated room.

You will need a large glass bottle, a two-hole rubber stopper, glass delivery tubes, a cigarette holder, cigarettes, and a small hand pump. Most of this equipment can be found in a school chemistry lab or can be obtained from a scientific supply house. Set up the apparatus as shown in Figure 14.1 on page 402. Fill the bottle halfway with water. Place a cigarette in the holder and light it. Operate the pump to draw smoke from the cigarette into the bottle and water. Continue to pump until the cigarette is burned completely. Burn additional cigarettes as necessary until tars can be seen in the water. Have the students examine the

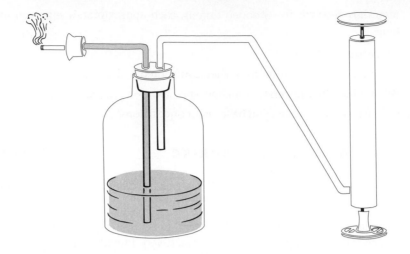

Figure 14.1
Smoking Machine Apparatus

water and note the distinct smell. Tars may also collect in the glass tubing. Ask students how this demonstration illustrates what happens when a person smokes a cigarette.

Materials Needed: water, a large glass bottle, a two-hole rubber stopper, glass delivery tubes, a cigarette holder, cigarettes, a small hand pump

Processing Questions:

1. What happens to cigarette smoke when it enters the body?
2. What are the short-term and long-term health effects of cigarette smoking?

GOLDFISH DEMONSTRATION   Grades (K–5)

Valued Outcome: The students will learn about the toxic qualities contained in cigarette smoke.

Description of Strategy: Check with school and state policies regarding experiments in the classroom before engaging in this demonstration. If there are no policies prohibiting the experiment, send a letter home to the parent or guardian that informs them in advance of this demonstration. Be sure to perform this experiment in a well ventilated room.

Before you begin, explain to the class that there are more than 300 chemical substances in cigarette smoke including nicotine, cyanide, formaldehyde, lead, arsenic, and carbon monoxide, which are all poisons. Set up a smoking machine apparatus like the one shown in Figure 14.1. This time, first add two or three goldfish to the water in the bottle. Then process three or more cigarettes by using the pump. The fish will begin to lose their equilibrium as they are affected by the chemicals in the cigarette smoke. *As soon as this begins to happen,* remove the fish by pouring the water into a net. Place the fish into a bowl of clean water. *Do not pour the contaminated water into the clean water as you do this, or the fish will die from continued exposure to the contaminants.*

Materials Needed: water, a large glass bottle, a two-hole rubber stopper, glass delivery tubes, a cigarette holder, cigarettes, a small hand pump, two or three goldfish, fish net

Processing Questions:

1. What are some of the chemicals in cigarette smoke?
2. How does the body react to these chemicals when they enter the body?

BREATHALYZER DEMONSTRATION   Grades (K–5)

Valued Outcome: The students will learn the dangers of drinking and driving.

Description of Strategy: Invite a local police officer to demonstrate how a Breathalyzer works. This device is used to test the amount of alcohol in a person's bloodstream. Have the officer explain the dangers of drinking and driving. The officer should note that even a small amount of alcohol has a deleterious effect on driving ability.

Materials Needed: none

Processing Questions:

1. What are the effects of alcohol on the body?
2. Why do police officers have to test drivers' blood alcohol concentration?

IMPAIRED   Grades (4–5)

Valued Outcome: The students will be able to describe how drug and alcohol use diminishes the ability to perform tasks that require manual dexterity.

Description of Strategy: Divide the class into teams of equal size (five or six students per team). Explain that each person must thread a nut all the way onto a screw and off again; when each student has finished, he or she passes the screw and nut to the next teammate and repeats the process until the entire team has completed the task. Time this process and record each team's time. Repeat this process with students wearing gloves or mittens and again record each team's times. Repeat the process with students wearing the sunglasses smeared with Vaseline or hand lotion and record the time again.

Materials Needed: for each team: one pair of gloves or mittens, one screw and corresponding nut, one pair of sunglasses that have been covered with Vaseline or lotion, a stopwatch, paper

Processing Questions:

1. How is the use of the gloves and the sunglasses comparable to the way drugs and alcohol can impair you?
2. Compare the time each team took to complete the three different tasks. How can this relate to the impact of drugs and alcohol on reaction time?
3. Can you list some daily tasks (even some jobs) that would be influenced by alcohol and other drug use?

SOURCE: Wolfanger 2001

Valued Outcome: The students will be able to identify each of the different sobriety tests and how they are used to detect the amount of alcohol consumed by a person. Students will also understand the physical effects of drinking alcohol.

Description of Strategy: Before class, set up the four stations described below. At each station, have directions written out on index cards. At the beginning of the class, show a fifteen-minute video about the consequences of DUIs (driving under the influence) and DWIs (driving while intoxicated) and the different field sobriety tests used to determine alcohol consumption. After the video, pair students up and have them visit each stations and do the activities described.

> **Station 1: Breathalyzers**—The first station will have two Breathalyzers. Have students try using the Breathalyzers.
>
> **Station 2: Vision Impairment**—This station has two pairs of "fogged" sunglasses (use Vaseline or lotion on the lenses) to show the students how vision is affected after consuming alcohol. While wearing the sunglasses, have students walk up to the board and write down a sentence that is read to them from the index card at that station.
>
> **Station 3: Visual Tracking**—This station has five small pen lights. Use the lights to dilate the pupils of the eyes. Have students:
>
> 1. Shine the light into your partner's eyes with his or her permission, and watch how the person's pupils change shape. If the person had been drinking, his or her pupils would stay dilated.
> 2. Move the light around in several directions and have your partner follow it with the eyes only (not moving his or her head). If the person had been drinking, he or she would not be able to smoothly follow the path of the light or of any object.
>
> **Station 4: Walking a Line**—Attach a three-inch-by-ten-feet piece of tape to the floor. Have one partner put palms together and, while standing, raise the hands straight up above the head. While looking directly up, and with the help of the other partner, have the student spin around five or six time to until disoriented. Immediately, have the person who was spinning try to walk in a straight line along the tape.

Then, assemble students into five groups. Have each group write down and perform a skit that relates to the things they did in the four stations or to what they learned from the stations and the fifteen-minute video. These skits will be used to check for understanding.

Materials Needed: index card of instructions for each station, two Breathalyzers, two pairs of fogged sunglasses, five small pen lights, video about consequences of DUIs and DWIs and the field sobriety tests that are used to determine how much alcohol a person has consumed, roll of wide masking tape, additional blank index cards. (Note: your local police departments or sheriff's office may also lend you some Breathalyzer tests for educational purposes and may have officers who present alcohol awareness programs with additional specialized equipment.)

Processing Question: What did you learn from the stations about the physical effects of alcohol?

MARSHMALLOW READINGS   Grades (K–5)

Valued Outcome: The students will be able to explain how too much alcohol can affect speech and body.

Description of Strategy: Select one or more students to read aloud a section of text using a normal speaking voice and clear speech. Then have the student place a marshmallow in the center of his or her mouth and—without pushing it to the side or squashing it down—re-read the same text. The students' speech should be slurred and muffled, mimicking the effects of alcohol on a person's speech. More marshmallows can be added to simulate the effect of additional drinks of alcohol being consumed.

Materials Needed: bag of large marshmallows, reading material

Processing Question: Why is a person's speech slurred after they have abused alcohol?

SOURCE: PE Central 2000a

SMOKING AEROBICS   Grades (4–5)

Valued Outcome: The students will be able to show how smoking tobacco affects a person's everyday physical activity.

Description of Strategy: Have each student check his or her heart rate using a stethoscope or by placing their fingers along the side of their necks. Do a ten-minute aerobic routine with the students to raise their heart rates. After exercising, have them check their heart rate again and compare it with their first reading. Then have them do the following:

- Write any two facts you know about smoking.
- Write down your two favorite physical activities.

Now give each student a straw. While they are breathing through the straw, lead students through the same aerobic routine as before. The straws represent the restricted air passages through which a smoker breathes when doing physical activity. At the end of the exercise, have the students check their heart rates again to see if there is a difference compared to the first heart rate taken. Then have students do the following and discuss their answers as a class.

- Write two words expressing feelings you experienced when doing aerobics while breathing through the straw.
- How can smoking affect the two favorite physical activities that you wrote down?

Materials Needed: stethoscopes, straws

Processing Question: How can smoking affect your fitness?

SOURCE: PE Central 2000c

Match the drug with its commonly used street names. (There will be at least two names for each drug.)

A. *cocaine*

B. *crack*

C. *methamphetamine*

D. *marijuana*

E. *alcohol*

_____ Mary Jane	_____ brew
_____ juice	_____ pot
_____ roaches	_____ freebase rocks
_____ rock	_____ crank
_____ coke	_____ joints
_____ snow	_____ meth
_____ grass	_____ flake
_____ vino	_____ booze
_____ blow	_____ dust
_____ girl	_____ weed
_____ reefer	_____ crystal

Answers to Match Game

D Mary Jane	D grass	D pot	A flake
E juice	E vino	B freebase rocks	E booze
D roaches	A blow	C crank	A dust
B rock	A girl	D joints	D weed
A coke	D reefer	C meth	C crystal
A snow	E brew		

STREET NAMES

Grades (4–5)

Valued Outcome: The students will identify street names of various substances that are abused.

Description of Strategy: Using the Internet, have the students research various substances that are abused. During their research, they are to locate and identify street names of the various substances. After a class discussion about the information found, divide the class into groups of three or four. Give each group a copy of the "Match Game" worksheet to complete (see the Teaching in Action box above). Allow fifteen minutes to complete the worksheet. The members of the group with the most correct answers during the allotted time limit will be given one No Homework pass or other prize.

Materials Needed: Internet access, pencils, Match Game sheet for each group

Processing Question: Why do you think people use so many different names for the same drugs?

SOURCE: National Clearinghouse for Drug and Alcohol Information 2002

RISK OF STEROID USE   Grades (3–5)

Valued Outcome: The students will be able to explain how using steroids can create problems for tendons in your body.

Description of Strategy: As a demonstration in front of the class, stretch a good rubber band. Then stretch a partially cut rubber band. The partially cut rubber ban should snap. Follow this demonstration with a discussion about how steroids cause muscles to grow while simultaneously causing tendons to deteriorate in elasticity and strength. Tendons attach muscles to bones so their deterioration reduces the tendons' ability to support the larger muscles. The result is that the tendons snap like the partially damaged rubber band.

Have students draw muscles and tendons that are properly proportioned. Then have them do the same for muscles and tendons that are not properly proportioned.

Materials Needed: a good rubber band, a partially cut rubber band, paper, pencils or markers

Processing Question: How do steroids affect the bones and muscles?

SOURCE: Geiger and Reynolds 2000

DRUGS ABSTINENCE SKILLS   Grades (3–5)

Valued Outcome: The students will be able to state refusal skills to promote abstinence from tobacco, drugs, and alcohol.

Description of Strategy: Prior to class, arrange a set of cones, jugs, or boxes in the gymnasium or playground. Each cone, jug, or box should be posted with signs or other illustrations of tobacco, drug, and alcohol products (a pack of cigarettes, a can of beer, and so on). Create a challenging obstacle course wide enough for the scooters to navigate. Place bicycle helmets, blindfolds, and scooters near the beginning of the obstacle course.

At the beginning of class, ask students to generate a list of practical refusal skills that promote abstinence from tobacco, drugs, and alcohol. Sample refusal skills include: assertive communication (saying "No!"); walking away from a tempting situation; telling a responsible adult; finding new friends; talking to a friend or relative who is practicing abstinence; and finding something else to do (hobby, sports, or other physical activity).

Divide students into small teams of three or four. Have students select a team color or name—blue or Dream Team, for example. Then have them select a race driver who is blindfolded and must remain silent while negotiating the obstacle course. The other team members act as a pit crew of peer supporters. The aim of the activity is to successfully complete the obstacle course without running into cones, jugs, or boxes. The pit crew may shout out directional cues to the race driver to avoid obstacles. During the race, members of the pit crew may each remove a cone, jug, or box once they recite aloud a refusal skill. This aids the race driver in avoiding the obstacles of tobacco, drugs, and alcohol. At the conclusion of the race, discuss with students the most difficult parts of the activity. Review again the refusal skills selected by students.

Materials Needed: gymnasium, paved parking lot, or playground surface; one scooter per group; set of playground cones, plastic half-gallon milk jugs, or cardboard boxes; signs or other illustrations of tobacco, drug, and alcohol products; bicycle helmets; scarves for blindfolds

Processing Question: How can refusal skills help you abstain from abusing drugs?

SOURCE: Wright 2000b

Puzzles and Games

DRUGS SPELL TROUBLE   Grades (3–5)

Valued Outcome: The students will be able to match the names of drugs with clues about those drugs.

Description of Strategy: Prepare individual puzzle pages as shown in the Teaching in Action box "Drugs Spell Trouble" below. Have students write the name of the drug that answers each clue given in the letter spaces provided. The completed puzzle spells out vertically a message about substance abuse.

TEACHING IN ACTION *Drugs Spell Trouble Puzzle*

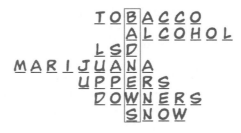

1. What cigarettes are made of
2. The drug in beer, wine, and whiskey
3. Three letters for a substance that causes hallucinations
4. Substance made from the cannabis plant
5. Street name for amphetamines
6. Street name for barbituates
7. Street name for cocaine

Materials Needed: puzzles for each student, pens or pencils

Processing Question: What clues about drugs can identify those drugs?

WHY ARE DRUGS BAD FOR YOU?   Grades (4–5)

Valued Outcome: The students will be able to explain and discuss the definitions of substance abuse, and other key words associated with substance abuse.

Description of Strategy: Hand out to each student a copy of the *KidsHealth* article, "What You Need to Know About Drugs" (The Nemours Foundation 1995–2003c, d) for silent reading during the class period. Then, divide the class into small groups of three or four. Have students discuss what they have learned from the article in their small groups. After each group has completed this activity, have a whole class discussion about the words and their definitions. Give each student a word search puzzle with a hidden message about substance abuse to be completed for homework and returned the next school day. (See the Teaching in Action box "Why Are Drugs Bad for You? Word Search" on page 410.) An alternate puzzle without a hidden message is provided in the Teaching in Action box on page 411.

Materials Needed: *KidsHealth* article "What You Need to Know About Drugs," pencils, word search puzzle

Processing Questions:

1. Is alcohol a drug?

2. Is cigarette smoking substance abuse?

3. If a person only smokes marijuana occasionally, is that considered substance abuse?

SOURCE: The Nemours Foundation 1995–2003c, d

SMOKING CROSSWORD PUZZLE   Grades (3–5)

Valued Outcome: The students will be able to use their knowledge of the detrimental health effects of smoking to complete puzzles.

Description of Strategy: Prepare individual puzzle sheets as shown in Teaching in Action box on page 412. After you have discussed smoking in class, distribute the worksheet and have the students complete the puzzle. In this example, the correct answers have been provided.

Materials Needed: puzzle worksheet for each student, pens or pencils

Processing Question: What are the detrimental effects of smoking?

Find each of the words listed below and circle them. The words may read in any direction—up, down, across, or diagonally. The words may even intersect.

```
B  D  R  U  G  S  A  C  T  R  E  D  A  N  G  E  R  O  U  S
S  R  O  M  E  T  I  M  I  N  E  S  D  D  E  A  D  L  Y  B
F  G  A  Z  Z  L  T  H  A  G  A  U  A  E  R  S  U  T  H  Y
S  H  Z  I  Z  L  T  X  U  H  A  S  R  L  A  Z  I  Y  A  J
Z  X  T  I  N  T  W  G  F  K  I  R  S  M  H  D  X  D  Z  D
Q  A  D  D  I  C  T  I  O  N  G  G  E  E  C  C  L  B  V  A
S  N  B  Y  L  H  E  R  O  I  N  T  H  T  R  K  G  Y  O  F
S  M  V  Y  C  I  Y  L  S  I  I  C  L  Y  T  P  Q  F  W  G
O  E  R  D  W  Y  N  T  L  M  U  T  I  D  K  E  E  D  A  E
M  S  F  H  V  V  H  V  E  S  Z  I  G  X  N  Y  S  D  N  Q
E  P  M  Y  O  A  K  S  Z  E  Y  H  J  C  K  W  H  R  A  O
T  N  A  L  A  H  N  I  X  Y  A  P  N  S  K  E  N  V  U  P
I  N  C  C  O  C  A  I  N  E  R  B  W  G  S  B  D  T  J  S
M  A  A  K  U  P  A  Z  L  Y  E  K  F  U  U  H  O  B  I  S
E  D  T  L  L  E  V  Y  G  N  R  T  U  R  F  L  V  Z  R  L
S  J  H  Z  U  X  S  H  K  R  G  G  F  D  G  O  U  I  A  C
P  Y  F  O  H  M  B  N  V  Y  B  B  N  B  E  U  S  R  M  W
O  E  Y  B  X  N  I  B  M  O  O  D  Y  A  N  N  E  B  B  O
C  H  P  H  G  F  B  T  P  I  Z  V  H  S  X  F  C  P  N  K
I  P  P  L  S  F  S  P  S  G  A  A  L  C  O  H  O  L  M  X
```

addiction
alcohol
angry
are
braincells
cigarettes
cocaine
depressant
heroin
high
inhalant
marijuana
moody
sad
sometimes
stimulant

Moving horizontally across the top of the word search, circle all the letters that are not used in the word search and write them below in the order in which they occur in the word search. This will give you a message about drug abuse.

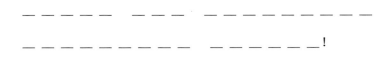

— — — — — __ — — — · — — — — — — — — — —

— — — — — — — — — — — — — —!

Find each of the words listed below and circle them. The words may read in any direction—up, down, across, or diagonally. The words may even intersect.

Can you find these words?

emphysema
cigarette
cancer
smoke
chemicals
incurable
hashish
counselor
stimulants
pharmacy
dosage
dependence
withdrawal
tolerance
hangover
tar
caffeine
hallucinogens
narcotics
depressant
overdose
marijuana
alcoholic
cirrhosis

```
          E J D K D            I D F I N
          R O T V W X Z        A C O P B N R
        Z P V A Q H M O      A L C O H O L I C
        T O L E R A N C E  I E N J D S J K L D K D J
      B L P V R N Q P H A R M A C Y I R J F M O D S M
      W I T H D R A W A L S J K I M Q P C N E L E K D
      S L I D O S A G E E E I N C U R A B L E I P F B
      C O F K S T I M U L A N T S D K S M W M J R W L
      A D E P E N D E N C E M S O E M F P K P A E J S
      C I R R H O S I S M S L K T N D H A S H I S H N
      N S J S M S J E U L L S O N O F S N P Y C S D F
      B E A U T F U K L S K C H E M I C A L S T A X S
      F O R H A L E I N D P O T S Y G O R I E I N N D
      F E C H K W V A J D U U Q T O A L C O M T T S L
      H A L L U C I N O G E N S C U E L O Z A X N D A
        A K T U C H E D V H S M S T U O T E N E U N
        N K N S J L O S N E O A W S X I D B A A
          G M S J S L O L L K N F G R C V L U
          O N E J S E C O E H H G J S Q J
          V C C I G A R E T T E E F I
          E C A F F E I N E E N R
          R O C A N C E R G A
          A Q F E R N B M
          G K J N S D
          D O O S
          N Y
```

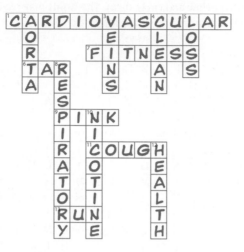

Across

1. The _____ system contains the heart and blood vessels.
6. The cancer-causing substance in tobacco smoke is _____.
7. Cigarette smoking can lower your physical _____.
9. Normally, the lungs are a _____ color.
11. Many smokers awake every morning with a _____.
13. Cigarette smoking may cause you to lose your breath quicker when you _____.

Down

2. The blood vessel that carries blood from the heart to the rest of the body is the _____.
3. The blood vessels that carry blood back to the heart are _____.
4. Nonsmokers have a right to breath _____ air.
5. When a person develops emphysema, there is a definite _____ of lung function.
8. Smoking is also bad for your _____ system.
10. A substance in tobacco that causes blood vessels to get smaller is _____.
12. Warning: The Surgeon General has determined that cigarette smoking is dangerous to your _____.

LET'S PLAY TIC-TAC-TOE

Grades (3–5)

Valued Outcome: The students will be able to distinguish facts from misconceptions with regard to several substance abuse–related statements.

Description of Strategy: Using the tic-tac-toe frame provided in the Teaching in Action box below, tell the students to write "T" in the squares with true statements and write "F" in the squares with false statements. Each square corresponds with the question having the same number.

1. The family does not cause the drug-dependent person to take drugs.
2. Drug dependency does not occur in "good" families.
3. Talking to someone you trust about a drug problem is helpful.
4. Family members of drug-dependent people never need help.
5. Drug-dependent people may be unable to stop taking drugs unless they get special help.
6. Family members can make drug-dependent people stop taking drugs by being good and by doing nice things.
7. A drug-dependent person has an illness.
8. "Bad" children cause their parents to drink.
9. Drug-dependent people do not love their families.

How many students scored tic-tac-toe? Have students change some of the false statements to true so they can be winners.

TEACHING IN ACTION *Tic-Tac-Toe*

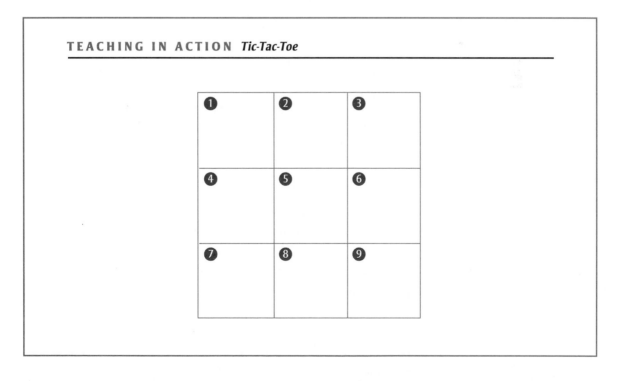

Materials Needed: tic-tac-toe worsheet for each student, pens or pencils

Processing Questions:

1. Why are there so many misconceptions about substance abuse?

2. How can we reduce the number of misconceptions in the public about substance abuse?

SAFE USE OF MEDICINES   Grades (3–5)

Valued Outcome: The students will learn to identify the safe use of several common over-the-counter (OTC) medicines.

Description of Strategy: In advance, make an enlarged transparency of the front side of a flattened box or wrapper for several OTC items for use on an overhead projector. Cut a piece of construction paper to cover the transparency. Then cut this paper into four or five interlocking shapes, creating a sort of jigsaw puzzle. Number each piece according to its difficulty, from 1 to however many total pieces are used to cover the image; the most obvious puzzle piece clues would have the higher numbers on them. Place number 1 over the directions for the medication's use. Use a little bit of tape to hold each cover piece to the transparency.

Divide students into groups. Explain to the class that on the overhead is the image of an OTC medicine with which they may be familiar. It is presently covered by several pieces of a jigsaw puzzle. Each group in rotation will be asked a true/false question about the safe use of OTC medicine. If the group answers the question correctly, the students ask to have a specifically numbered piece of the puzzle removed. They then have ten seconds to see if they can identify the mystery medication. If no one correctly guesses the product, the puzzle piece is replaced on the overhead, and the second team is offered a true/false question with the possibility of removing a puzzle piece and correctly identifying the hidden product. When a correct identification of the hidden product is given, that team obtains a point value equal to the sum of the numbered puzzle pieces left on the transparency. If the puzzle originally had four pieces and only pieces number 1, number 2, and number 4 were left on the transparency, that team would score 7 points. Continue the game until either all the true/false questions have been covered or all the images have been identified. The highest score wins.

Materials Needed: the outer boxes or wrappers of several well-known OTC medicines—aspirin, nasal spray, acetaminophen, eye drops, and so on; transparency sheets (one for each product); overhead projector; several sheets of construction paper (one for each product); true/false questions; clear tape

Processing Questions:

1. Can an OTC drug be bought without a doctor's prescription?

2. What should you do before taking an OTC drug?

Other Strategies for Learning

DEALING WITH PEER PRESSURE   Grades (K–5)

Valued Outcome: The students will be able to describe how peer pressure can be a positive and/or negative influence with regard to substance abuse.

Description of Strategy: Divide the class into groups of six to eight. Have each group form a circle and place pieces of candy in the center of each group. Give five members of each group a slip of paper stating that they are to eat the candy and attempt to get anyone not eating it to do so. Give the remaining students in each group a slip of paper stating that they should not eat the candy and should resist all attempts to get them to do so. Let this interaction go on for about five minutes. Then ask the students to take their regular seats. Ask the following questions:

What were you feeling when you were doing this exercise?

What do you think the purpose of this exercise was?

What is peer pressure?

Why is it important to know about peer pressure?

Materials Needed: written instructions for each student, pieces of candy

Processing Questions:

1. What is peer pressure?

2. How can peer pressure be a positive factor in your life?

3. How does negative peer pressure lead to substance abuse?

SLOGANS   Grades (3–5)

Valued Outcome: The students will be able to develop a list of slogans against drug use.

Description of Strategy: Have the students develop a list of slogans used by tobacco, alcohol, and OTC drug manufacturers. Discuss what the slogans are attempting to convince the consumer to do. Discuss the irrational appeal often used in this advertising approach. Then have the students come up with counterslogans that seek to convince the consumer to do the opposite.

Materials Needed: none

Processing Question: How can antidrug messages convince the public not to abuse drugs?

AFFIRMATIONS   Grades (K–5)

Valued Outcome: The students will be able to describe how support from friends can prevent substance abuse problems.

Description of Strategy: Have each student come to the front of the class and say, "Sometimes I don't feel so good about myself." Then have the student turn his or her back to the class. Have other students then volunteer to affirm one fine quality about that individual. Every student should get three affirmations from the class. These may refer to being a loyal friend, being kind, being a good student, being fair, being friendly, and so on.

Materials Needed: none

Processing Questions:

1. How can young people offer moral support to their friends through praise?

2. How can such praise prevent substance abuse problems?

BE A FRIEND TO YOURSELF!   Grades (K–5)

Valued Outcome: The students will be able to discuss the importance of having hig self-esteem.

Description of Strategy: Pose the following questions to your students:

- If you had a best friend who was very special to you, how would you act toward that person?
- Would you say nice things to him or her?
- What kind of nice things would you say?
- Would you let your friend know that you liked him or her?

After class members have shared their ideas, follow up with these points: You do have a best friend. You are your own best friend. The most important person for you to be a friend to is yourself. Being a friend to yourself means saying nice things about yourself and doing nice things for yourself.

Materials Needed: none

Processing Questions:

1. What are some nice things about you that you like about yourself?

2. What are some special things you can do for yourself?

MY CHOICE, YOUR CHOICE . . .   Grades (K–2)
CONSEQUENCES!

Valued Outcome: The students will be able to explain to a friend or peer why he or she does not use or abuse substances.

Description of Strategy: Have the students make hand puppets using a sock or paper sack. Decorate faces on the puppets using markers or colored buttons. After the puppets are completed, have the students decide whether or not his or her puppet will have a positive name, such as Sober Joe, or negative name such

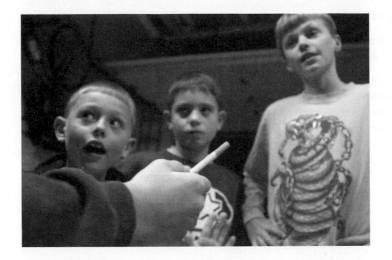

Peer pressure can be a positive or negative influence in a person's life.

as Bobby Booze. Pair students up so that each pair has a positive and negative puppet. Working in pairs, have the students tell why he or she does not use or abuse substances. For example, one puppet—Bobby Booze—may tell Sober Joe how he sneaked into his dad's cabinet and had a sip of alcohol. The other puppet—Sober Joe—should tell Bobby Booze his reasons for not drinking.

Materials Needed: socks or paper bags, buttons (different colors) or other materials to use to decorate the puppets, glue, markers

Processing Questions:

1. What is your best refusal line to the peer pressure to use substances?
2. How can you be a positive influence on your friend(s) when they begin to use/abuse substances?

DRUGS COMIC BOOK   Grades (3–5)

Valued Outcome: The students will create a comic book about a child who abuses alcohol or some other substance.

Description of Strategy: Have the students create a short comic book about a child who is a substance abuser. Have them illustrate and write the text for the comic strip as well as create an illustrated cover for their comic book. Give students the opportunity to read his or her comic book to the class during a substance abuse lesson.

Materials Needed: paper; markers, crayons, or colored pencils

Processing Question: Do you think you could show your comic book to some of your friends who either are, or have considered, using or abusing a substance such as alcohol?

SOURCE: The Nemours Foundation 1995–2003a

WHY SHOULDN'T I DRINK?   Grades (4–5)

Valued Outcome: The students will be able to describe the harmful effects of drinking alcohol.

Description of Strategy: Divide students into groups of three or four. Using the Internet, have each group research the harmful effects of drinking alcohol. Then, use their research to create a "televised" public service announcement to present to the class. Each member of each group must participate in the research and creation of the presentation. Give students one minute for their presentation. Have a class discussion about the Internet sites the students found and interesting bits of information they discovered on each site.

Materials Needed: computer, paper, printer, Internet access

Processing Questions:

1. Do you think occasional drinking is okay for kids?
2. Why do you think some kids feel the need to drink?

SOURCE: The Nemours Foundation 1995–2003b

DRUG POSTER   Grades (4–5)

Valued Outcome: The students will be able to list things a person could do instead of using drugs.

Description of Strategy: Have each student make a poster that creatively lists ten things a person could do instead of using drugs. After they have all finished, ask each student to name just one item from his or her list. Engage the students in a discussion about why he or she chose that particular item. Display the posters in the hallway for public viewing.

Materials Needed: pencils, markers, crayons, colored pencils, construction paper, poster board

Processing Questions:

1. Do you think a person may use drugs because he or she is bored?
2. Do you think a person may use drugs just to fit in?
3. Why do you think a person may use drugs?

SOURCE: Utah Lesson Plans 1996

DRUG COLLAGE   Grades (3–5)

Valued Outcome: The students will be able to describe the harmful effects of tobacco use.

Description of Strategy: Have the students create a collage showing in detail the effects of tobacco use, and state reasons that they believe people start using tobacco. They can find information by searching magazines they have brought to class and finding tobacco ads. They can also use articles from the newspaper about drug-related incidents that have happened recently that they can cut out and paste to the backboard for their collage.

Materials Needed: magazine advertisements, newspapers that have a youth editorial section, paper, markers, glue

Processing Question: What are some harmful effects that tobacco products bring to a person's health and overall lifestyle?

Resources

BOOKS

Carroll, C. R. 1996. *Drugs in modern society.* 4th ed. Madison, WI: Brown & Benchmark.

Hahn, D. B., and W. A. Payne. 1997. *Focus on health.* St. Louis: Mosby.

Hanson, G., and P. J. Venturelli. 1995. *Drugs and society.* 4th ed. Boston: Jones & Bartlett.

Ray, O., and C. Ksir. 1996. *Drugs, society, and human behavior.* 7th ed. St. Louis: Mosby.

Witters, W., P. Venturelli, and G. Hanson. 1992. *Drugs and society.* 3d ed. Boston: Jones & Bartlett.

WEB SITES

Drugs/Drug Addiction

Food and Drug Administration (FDA) *www.fda.gov*

Join Together Online: *www.jointogether.org*

National Clearinghouse for Alcohol and Drug Information: *www.health.org*

National Institute on Alcohol Abuse and Alcoholism: *www.niaaa.nih.gov*

National Institute on Drug Abuse *www.nida.nih.gov*

Substance Abuse and Mental Health Services Administration: *www.samhsa.gov*

Food and Drug Safety

American Academy of Family Physicians *www.aafp.org*

FDA Center for Drug Evaluation and Research *www.fda.gov/cder*

FDA Center for Food Safety and Applied Nutrition *www.vm.cfsan.fda.gov/list.html*

Food and Drug Administration (FDA): *www.fda.gov*

Institute of Medicine, Food and Nutrition Board *www2.nas.edu/Fnb/2102.html*

USDA Food Safety and Inspection Service *www.usda.gov/agency/fsis/homepage.htm*

General Health

About Health: *www.abouthealth.com*

Adolescent Health On-line *www.ama-assn.org/ama/pub/category*

American Cancer Society: *www.cancer.org*

CDC Prevention Guidelines Database *www.wonder.cdc.gov/wonder/prevguid/prevguid.htm*

Healthy People 2000 *www.dphp.osophs.dhhs.gov/pubs/hp2000/default.htm*

National Health & Education Consortium (NHEC) *www.nhec.org*

Physical Activity and Health: A Report of the Surgeon General: *www.cdc.gov/nccdphp/sgr/sgr.htm*

Resources for School Health Educators *www.indiana.edu/~aphs/hlthk-12.html*

General Sites

American Medical Association: *www.ama-assn.org*

MedicineNet *www.medicinenet.com*

Medscape *www.medscape.com*

Oncolink *www.oncolink.upenn.edu*

Surveillance and Data Systems

Agency for Health Care Policy and Research Data and Methods: *www.ahcpr.gov:80/data*

CDC National Center for Health Statistics *www.cdc.gov/nchswww/nchshome.htm*

continued

CDC Scientific, Surveillance, and Health Statistics, and Laboratory Information
www.cdc.gov/scientific.htm

Health Care Financing Administration, 1996 Statistics at a Glance: *www.hcfa.gov/stats/stathili.htm*

Tobacco/Smoking Cessation

American Cancer Society: *www.cancer.org*

American Dental Association Online: *www.ada.org*

American Heart Association: *www.amhrt.org*

American Lung Association: *www.lungusa.org*

CDC Office on Smoking and Health, Tobacco Information & Prevention Sourcepage
www.cdc.gov/nccdphp/osh/tobacco.htm

Food and Drug Administration (FDA): *www.fda.gov*

SAMHSA National Clearinghouse for Alcohol and Drug Information: *www.health.org*

Substance Abuse and Mental Health Services Administration: *www.samhsa.gov*

Tobacco BBS: *www.tobacco.org*

VIDEOS

General

The following videos are available from Sunburst Communications, 101 Castleton Street, Suite 201, Pleasantville, NY 10570.

Addiction: The problems,   (Grades 7–12)
the solutions
Through a series of interviews with young people, a medical expert, and a clinical psychologist, this video explores what addiction is, who is vulnerable, and what can be done. (31 minutes, Item 2351)

Drugs, your friends, and you: (Grades 5–9)
An update
Their powerful need for peer acceptance leaves young teens particularly vulnerable to pressure to use drugs or alcohol. In an update to the Sunburst bestseller, the *Drugs, Your Friends, and You* program re-emphasizes that students can respect their own best interests and say no. This video makes it clear that they do have choices, then teaches specific techniques for dealing assertively with pro-drug or alcohol pressures. (24 minutes, Item 0678)

The truth about inhalants   (Grades 5–9)
This video gives the facts about inhalants—the fumes or vapors found in common household products—and shows how breathing them in,

purposely or accidentally, can quickly damage body organs and may even cause death. Interweaves real-life vignettes and graphics about the dangers of and inhalants and offers tips on their safe use; a powerful indictment of inhalant abuse. (15 minutes, Item 2397)

Tobacco and you   (Grades 5–9)
This program interweaves a TV talk show on tobacco's health dangers and interviews with young teen smokers to show that smoking is neither cool, sexy, nor grown-up, but is instead a nonglamorous and socially offensive habit that is very hard to break. (22 minutes, Item 2341)

The truth about alcohol   (Grades 5–9)
Alerts students to the facts they need to know about alcohol—what it is, how it acts on the body, and why young people are so vulnerable to its dangers. (20 minutes, Item 2362)

Why I won't do drugs   (Grades 3–5)
Designed for earliest drug education, this video helps young viewers make the connection between understanding and respecting your body and how drug use can harm it. (10 minutes, Item 2378)

Professional Education

Alcohol withdrawal syndrome. (1986; health professionals)
Provides step-by-step training in an effective method of assessment and management of alcohol withdrawal syndrome. The method, developed in the Clinical Institute of the Addiction Research Foundation, helps ensure adequate and prompt treatment of the alcoholic patient and prevent serious complications of alcohol withdrawal syndrome. The program includes three modules: (1) *Introduction:* Alcohol withdrawal syndrome is defined, causes and clinical manifestations are examined, and characteristics of withdrawal reactions are summarized. (2) *Assessment:* In order to determine the most effective treatment procedure, severity of withdrawal must be assessed. This module demonstrates the actual process of assessment, using simulations of a patient in minor and major withdrawal. (3) *Treatment:* A variety of treatment approaches, both with and without drug therapy, are demonstrated. Available from Addiction Research Foundation, 33 Russell Street, Toronto, Ontario, Canada M5S 2S1 1 (800) 661-1111 or (416) 595-6059. (48 minutes, Item 2002)

Double trouble I: Mood and anxiety disorders.
(1992; health professionals, EAP, addiction specialists)
Leo, a recovering alcoholic, feels paralyzed by depression. Neither his wife, Mary, nor his boss can find a way to lift his spirits. Mary suffers from panic attacks and uses alcohol and tranquilizers to quell her symptoms, while her worried family tries to cope. The video dramatizes their symptoms and follows both through diagnosis and treatment. Leo is prescribed antidepressants (which don't violate his sobriety, his psychiatrist says), and psychotherapy helps him resolve long-standing feelings of grief and anger toward his father. Following detoxification, Mary follows a comprehensive program of therapy, relaxation, and other coping skills.

Evaluation: Good. The subject of dual disorders is emerging as a key issue in the health field. Professionals in the mental health field need to know more about drug use and its effects, and addiction professionals must learn more about some of the mood and personality disorders that may coexist with—or even prompt—alcohol or drug abuse. This video covers some of the basics but seems geared more to the mental health professional than the addiction specialist. Viewers may find the attitudes of Mary's husband and therapist rather paternalistic. Available from Kinetic Communications Inc., 408 Dundas St. E., Toronto, Ontario, Canada, M5A 2A5 (416) 963-5979. (30 minutes, Item 1005)

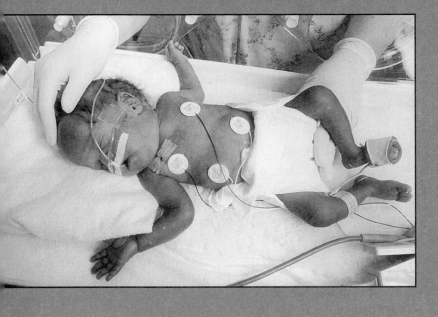

CHAPTER FIFTEEN

Infectious and Noninfectious Conditions

You can do more for your own health and well-being than any doctor, or any exotic medical service.

—Joseph Califano, former Secretary of Health, Education, and Welfare

VALUED OUTCOMES

After reading this chapter, you should be able to:

- describe the disease agents for infectious and noninfectious conditions
- describe the typical stages through which a disease progresses
- describe how the body is protected from disease
- discuss the major childhood communicable diseases
- discuss the human immunodeficiency virus
- discuss the types of cardiovascular disease and cancer
- identify the risk factors associated with the major noninfectious diseases
- discuss the recent trends in the diagnosis and treatment of diseases

Helping children understand how diseases are prevented is important to their long-term quality of life. Check your state's requirements for vaccinations and immunizations. Are there risks associated with any of the suggested or required vaccinations? What are your feelings concerning the potential risks?

Diseases—Then and Now

Many conditions affect the quality of life. Over the past centuries, the types of diseases that have killed and debilitated humans have changed. At one time infectious diseases were the biggest killers, but now chronic diseases are the leading causes of death. Some say that the infectious diseases may again become our biggest enemy, primarily in the form of the acquired immunodeficiency syndrome (AIDS) epidemic.

Communicable Diseases

At various times throughout history, communicable diseases such as the bubonic plague, smallpox, syphilis, and polio have been common throughout the world. Occasionally a disease such as Legionnaires' disease also causes an epidemic. Currently the AIDS epidemic threatens the welfare of our citizens. The common cold, influenza, and the persistence of the many childhood diseases also are constant problems. (See Table 15.1.)

The Stages of Diseases

When a pathogen invades a human host, the body's reaction to the invasion proceeds through several broad phases—incubation, prodromal, clinical, convalescence, and recovery. Figure 15.1 illustrates these typical stages.

The **incubation stage** is the time between initial infection and the appearance of symptoms. The incubation period can be as short as a few hours (for the common cold) or as long as a few years (as in the case of AIDS). The **prodromal stage** is the short period in which the body begins to react to the pathogens. Fever, headache, nasal discharge, and irritability are common but the actual characteristics of the disease are not yet apparent, and diagnosis may be difficult. The disease is usually highly communicable during this period. The **clinical stage** is the time when the disease is at its worst. The characteristics of the disease are readily identified. The **convalescence stage** is that period in which

Table 15.1 *The Pathogens*

Type	Characteristics	Examples of Disease Caused
Viruses	The smallest pathogens. Composed of nucleic acid and protein. Made up of DNA or RNA but not both. Known as *obligate intracellular parasites* because they must live in living host. Penetrate cells and use cells' nucleic acids to replicate viruses. May burst out of cell, destroying it, or the cell degenerates and viruses are released as cell dies.	Warts; hepatitis A, B, C, D, E; measles; polio; mumps; oral and genital herpes
Bacteria	Single-cell microorganisms. Abundant in our environment, but very few are pathogenic to humans. Three common forms: rod shaped or bacilli, round or cocci, and spiral or spirilla. Cause harm by releasing toxins (poisons) and need not invade cells to cause disease.	Tuberculosis, strep throat, tetanus, gonorrhea, Legionnaires' disease
Rickettsias	Now considered to be small bacteria. Resemble both viruses and bacteria. Like viruses, they are intracellular parasites. Transported by insects and other arthropod vectors.	Rocky Mountain spotted fever, typhus, Q fever
Fungi	Single-celled or multicelled plantlike organisms. Release enzymes that digest cells. Seek a favorable climate for reproduction on food or anywhere there is high humidity, warmth, and oxygen supply.	Candidiasis, ringworm
Protozoa	Single-celled microscopic parasitic animals. Release toxin and enzymes that destroy cells or interface with their functions.	Trichomoniasis, malaria, amoebic dysentery, African sleeping sickness
Helminths	Multicellular parasitic animals. Vary in size from relatively small (pinworms) to a length of several feet; may lodge in various parts of the body and block the digestive tract, blood, and lymph vessels.	Pinworms, tapeworms, trichinosis

Figure 15.1
Typical Periods of Illness

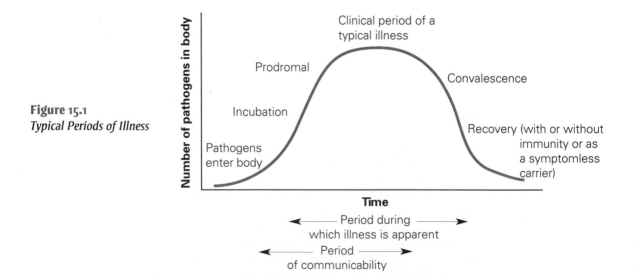

the host feels better but may or may not feel like returning to normal activities. The **recovery stage** is the time in which recovery seems complete. However, the disease may still be communicable. The host may relapse, recover with immunity to the disease, recover but not have immunity, or recover from the disease but be a source (carrier) for the disease.

Protection against Diseases

For an infectious disease to invade a human host, some change must take place in either the host or the environment. The mere presence of a pathogen does not necessarily lead to infection; the host must be susceptible to the disease. Factors such as age, sex, stress level, nutrition, and genetic makeup influence susceptibility. For a pathogen to gain entry to a human host, it must overcome several effective barriers (Table 15.2). These barriers are diagrammed in Figure 15.2.

THE IMMUNE SYSTEM

If the defenses listed in Table 15.2 do not prevent development of a disease, the host body turns to another powerful line of defense. **Immunity** is the state of being protected against diseases or through the activities of the immune system.

Table 15.2   *The Body's Defenses against Disease*

Barrier	Defense against Pathogens: Viruses, Bacteria, Fungi, Protozoa, Rickettsia, Helminths (parasitic worms)
The Skin	Skin must break for invader to penetrate
Body Secretions	Sweat and oil glands kill or repel invaders
	Secretions at body entrances such as earwax, tears, nasal secretions
	Secretions contain enzymes that destroy invaders
Mucous Membranes	Trap and engulf invaders
	Cilia function to sweep invaders toward body openings
	Contain enzymes that destroy or slow pathogen reproduction
Enzymes and Compounds in Blood	Kill invader by causing it to burst, destroying its cell membrane, preventing/slowing reproductive cycle
Immune System	Antigen/antibody response
	White blood cell action
	Attempts to reject unrecognized enemies or develop antibodies against them
Interferon and Natural Substances	When virus invades, protein is produced that protects healthy cells making subsequent infections difficult
	Properdin: large protein that destroys gram-negative bacteria
	Polypeptides: same action as properdin
	Lysozyme: enzyme that kills bacteria; found in saliva, tears, and breast milk

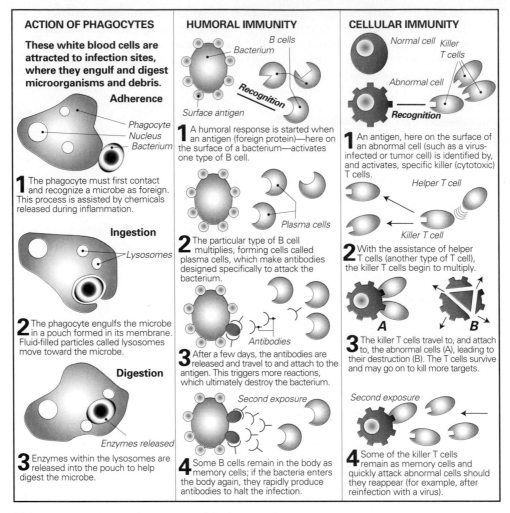

ACTION OF PHAGOCYTES

These white blood cells are attracted to infection sites, where they engulf and digest microorganisms and debris.

Adherence

Phagocyte
Nucleus
Bacterium

1 The phagocyte must first contact and recognize a microbe as foreign. This process is assisted by chemicals released during inflammation.

Ingestion

Lysosomes

2 The phagocyte engulfs the microbe in a pouch formed in its membrane. Fluid-filled particles called lysosomes move toward the microbe.

Digestion

Enzymes released

3 Enzymes within the lysosomes are released into the pouch to help digest the microbe.

HUMORAL IMMUNITY

B cells
Bacterium
Recognition
Surface antigen

1 A humoral response is started when an antigen (foreign protein)—here on the surface of a bacterium—activates one type of B cell.

Plasma cells

2 The particular type of B cell multiplies, forming cells called plasma cells, which make antibodies designed specifically to attack the bacterium.

Antibodies

3 After a few days, the antibodies are released and travel to and attach to the antigen. This triggers more reactions, which ultimately destroy the bacterium.

Second exposure

4 Some B cells remain in the body as memory cells; if the bacteria enters the body again, they rapidly produce antibodies to halt the infection.

CELLULAR IMMUNITY

Normal cell   Killer T cells
Abnormal cell
Recognition

1 An antigen, here on the surface of an abnormal cell (such as a virus-infected or tumor cell) is identified by, and activates, specific killer (cytotoxic) T cells.

Helper T cell
Killer T cell

2 With the assistance of helper T cells (another type of T cell), the killer T cells begin to multiply.

A   B

3 The killer T cells travel to, and attach to, the abnormal cells (A), leading to their destruction (B). The T cells survive and may go on to kill more targets.

Second exposure

4 Some of the killer T cells remain as memory cells and quickly attack abnormal cells should they reappear (for example, after reinfection with a virus).

Figure 15.2 *Actions and Responses of the Immune System*

When the host is invaded by a pathogen, the immune system swings into action to destroy the infectious agent. Anything that invades the body and causes the immune system to react is called an **antigen** (foreign body). The body develops **antibodies** that destroy or lessen the effects of the invading antigen. Each type of antibody is specific for each type of antigen. For example, antibodies for measles have no effect on the common cold antigens.

The immune system works in several ways to protect against diseases and infections. The first is through the action of **phagocytosis,** which is the ingestion and destruction of pathogens by several different types of white blood cells (Thibodeau and Patton 1993). **Humoral immunity** is the protection provided by antibodies derived from B cells. In **cellular immunity** T cells are activated and attack microbes or abnormal cells such as viral or tumor cells. Figure 15.2 illustrates these three mechanisms.

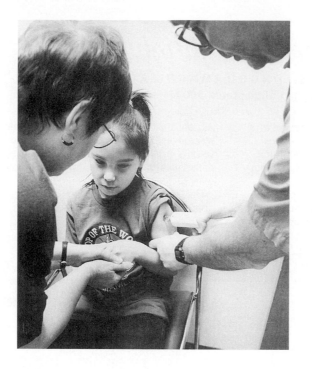

Artificial immunity is acquired by vaccination.

Lymphocytes are the type of white blood cells most responsible for the preceding actions. Two forms of lymphocytes are **T cells** and **B cells.** T cells circulate through lymphatic tissue and the bloodstream, neutralizing antigens. **T helpers** or **T suppressor cells,** respectively, increase or release the response of other lymphocytes. When stimulated by an antigen, B cells produce antibodies that destroy the antigens.

Immunity can be developed through having a disease (**natural immunity**) or through **artificial immunity.** Artificial immunity is acquired by vaccination when killed or attenuated (weakened) organisms or **toxins** (poisons) are injected into the body to stimulate antibody formation. Antibodies for a particular antigen can be injected that will provide short-term protection against a disease.

Selected Infectious Diseases

Common childhood diseases include the common cold, chicken pox, rubella (German measles), influenza, rubeola (measles), strep throat, meningitis, tuberculosis, mumps, and pertussis (whooping cough). Of these, the diseases most commonly found in schools are the common cold; influenza; strep throat; and the childhood diseases of chicken pox, mumps, and rubella. To a lesser extent, diseases such as infectious mononucleosis, hepatitis, and human immunodeficiency virus (HIV) are now affecting the classroom. In schools, childhood

Health Highlight

RECOMMENDED CHILDHOOD IMMUNIZATION SCHEDULE
United States, 2002

This schedule indicates the recommended ages for routine administration of currently licensed childhood vaccines, as of December 1, 2001, for children through age 18 years. Any dose not given at the recommended age should be given at any subsequent visit when indicated and feasible.
■ Indicates age groups that warrant special effort to administer those vaccines not previously given.

Additional vaccines may be licensed and recommended during the year. Licensed combination vaccines may be used whenever any components of the combination are indicated and the vaccine's other components are not contraindicated. Providers should consult the manufacturers' package inserts for detailed recommendations.

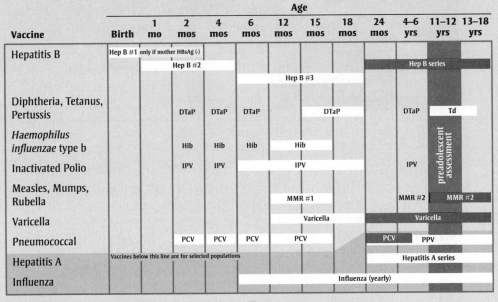

Vaccine	Birth	1 mo	2 mos	4 mos	6 mos	12 mos	15 mos	18 mos	24 mos	4–6 yrs	11–12 yrs	13–18 yrs
Hepatitis B	Hep B #1 only if mother HBsAg (-)		Hep B #2			Hep B #3					Hep B series	
Diphtheria, Tetanus, Pertussis			DTaP	DTaP	DTaP		DTaP			DTaP	Td	
Haemophilus influenzae type b			Hib	Hib	Hib	Hib					preadolescent assessment	
Inactivated Polio			IPV	IPV		IPV				IPV		
Measles, Mumps, Rubella						MMR #1				MMR #2	MMR #2	
Varicella						Varicella					Varicella	
Pneumococcal			PCV	PCV	PCV	PCV			PCV	PPV		
Hepatitis A	Vaccines below this line are for selected populations									Hepatitis A series		
Influenza						Influenza (yearly)						

KEY: ☐ = range of recommended ages, ■ = catch-up vaccination, ■ = preadolescent assessment

SOURCE: National Immunization Program 2002

diseases constitute the greatest problem. Students face days of restricted activity and school absenteeism because of these diseases.

THE COMMON COLD

The cold is the most common of all infectious diseases found in schools. A cold alone is not considered serious, but secondary infections resulting from improper care can be a problem. There are more than 200 different viruses or rhinoviruses that can cause the common cold. Symptoms usually develop within twenty-four hours after exposure and include teary eyes, obstructed breathing, and a runny nose. When a fever is present, it indicates a secondary infection. Once a cold develops, it typically will run its course in seven to fourteen days.

There is no cure for a cold; antibiotics are of no benefit. Once a cold has developed, bed rest, good nutrition, and plenty of fluids are the best treatment. Over-the-counter cold remedies may help treat the symptoms of the cold but cannot treat the virus itself. A cold is most contagious in the first twenty-four hours.

STREP THROAT

Strep throat is commonly found in the school setting. The causative agent is the streptococcal bacterium. The infection is passed primarily through sneezing, coughing, or the use of soiled objects, such as handkerchiefs, that reach the mouth. Incubation time for strep throat is three to five days. Symptoms may include sore throat, fever, nausea, and vomiting. In some cases, people may develop a rash on the neck and chest area. Strep throat is treated with antibiotics. Students should be excluded from school until the fever and sore throat are gone for twenty-four to forty-eight hours.

INFLUENZA

Influenza, or flu, is a commonly experienced virus. Three forms of the virus are currently isolated, with a multitude of strains within each variety. Forms of the virus include types A (the most pathenogenic), B, and C. Short-term immunity may be acquired from any particular form, but this does not transfer to a different variety. Today, fortunately, the flu is not extremely hazardous to normally healthy people. However, deaths can occur in adults over sixty-five, children under five, and people experiencing chronic diseases.

The symptoms of influenza include aches and pains, nausea, diarrhea, fever, and coldlike ailments. The best treatment for flu is bed rest, ingesting plenty of fluids, eating nutritious foods, and taking medicine, if prescribed. Although obvious symptoms last only a few days, a feeling of weakness may persist for some time, so extra rest may be needed. It is important to take extra care following the flu, so that complications do not develop. Because influenza is caused by a virus, Reye's syndrome can develop as a secondary disease. Children should not be given aspirin to relieve discomfort as it may contribute to the development of Reye's syndrome. This syndrome can involve the pancreas, heart, kidneys, spleen, and lymph nodes. Symptoms may include an upper respiratory infection, nausea, vomiting, disorientation, coma, and seizures. Although rare, this is a serious and often life-threatening disorder.

INFECTIOUS MONONUCLEOSIS

Infectious mononucleosis is initiated by the Epstein-Barr virus and is transmitted through saliva, hence its more common name, the kissing disease. In reality, mononucleosis does not seem to be highly contagious. Initial symptoms may include moderate fever, discomfort, lack of appetite, fatigue, headache, and sore throat. Lymph nodes usually become enlarged, as does the spleen about one-third of the time. Occasionally mild liver damage may occur, leading to jaundice for a few days. Diagnosis is made using a blood test. A positive test indicates extremely high levels of mononucleocytes, a type of white blood cell. Treatment consists of possibly prolonged bed rest, sound nutrition, and medicine for secondary problems, as indicated. For two to three months after recovery, the person may feel depressed, lack energy, and feel sleepy during the day. Symptoms may exist up to a year after infection.

HEPATITIS

Seven types of hepatitis have been isolated: hepatitis A, B, C, D, E, F, and G. Hepatitis A is often the result of poor sanitary conditions and is a common infection in the United States, with almost half the adult population carrying antibodies against the virus. Hepatitis A vaccine (Harvix) is highly effective in preventing the illness. If a susceptible person is exposed to hepatitis A, gamma globulin administered within ten days provides protection. Hepatitis A is transmitted through person-to-person, fecal-oral contact, sexual contact with infected persons, and contaminated blood (rare). Persons traveling internationally should receive the hepatitis A vaccine (Centers for Disease Control and Prevention [CDC] 2002).

Hepatitis B is currently transmitted primarily by drug addicts sharing contaminated needles and through body secretions such as sweat, breast milk, and semen. Hepatitis B is more serious than hepatitis A, with a higher potential for liver damage. Since 1982, there has been a vaccine that will prevent hepatitis B.

Health Highlight

PROTECTING AGAINST BLOOD-BORNE PATHOGENS

The Occupational Safety and Health Administration (OSHA) has issued regulations concerning job exposure to blood-borne pathogens. Teachers and other school personnel must be aware of the hazards and protect themselves from harm when there is potential contact with body fluids from a child infected with HIV or hepatitis. Obviously the consideration is for more than just casual contact. The beginning point for a teacher's personal safety is to make sure all immunizations are up to date. OSHA standards require that an employer make the hepatitis B vaccination series available to all employees who are exposed to blood or other body fluids on the job. OSHA also requires postexposure evaluation and follow-up to all employees who are exposed.

The Centers for Disease Control and Prevention (CDC) has identified what it calls Universal Precautions for protection or preventing the risk of exposure from any type of bodily substance. These precautions include personal hygiene (washing hands, face, etc.) after potential exposure, wearing personal protective equipment (having a face mask, apron, and rubber gloves), having work practice controls for protocol and procedures for disposing of potentially contaminated materials, and procedures/protocol for cleaning and disinfecting areas of contamination.

It is imperative that every school district have guidelines and protocol for dealing with blood- and fluid-borne pathogens. The school should provide every teacher with a kit containing the above listed items. Training should be provided each year on the guidelines/protocol for dealing with blood/fluids in the school setting.

The vaccination consists of three injections spaced over a period of several months. Routine vaccination is recommended for anyone under 18 years of age.

Hepatitis C is caused by the hepatitis C virus, which is found in the blood of an infected person, and the infection is spread by contact with that blood. The sharing of items such as toothbrushes, razors, personal care items, or intravenous syringes can spread this virus. The disease is rarely spread through sexual contact. Further protection consists of getting the A and B vaccinations, not getting a tattoo or body piercing, not having sex with more than one partner, and using latex condoms when having sex (CDC 2002).

Hepatitis D can only be contracted by a person suffering from hepatitis B. The C virus seems to intersect with hepatitis B to create a chronic and more severe form of the disease. Hepatitis D is spread in the same fashion as hepatitis B.

Hepatitis E is similar to hepatitis A but is acute rather than chronic in nature. This type is rare in the United States but has resulted in large outbreaks in other parts of the world. Direct or indirect contact with an infected person's feces, contamination of food or water supply, raw shellfish, unwashed hands, and cooking utensils may have enough of the virus to cause an outbreak.

At the present time characterizations of the epidemiology and clinical features of hepatitis F and G are not listed until diagnostic procedures can be developed. Hepatitis F appears to produce a type of hepatitis similar to C, but experts are unsure if it is a separate hepatitis virus. Hepatitis G is a newly identified virus that is in all likelihood transmitted in a similar fashion to hepatitis C. It has not been determined if it produces chronic symptoms (CDC 2002).

HUMAN IMMUNODEFICIENCY VIRUS AND ACQUIRED IMMUNODEFICIENCY SYNDROME

The human immunodeficiency virus (HIV) can lead to a complex array of diseases resulting in AIDS. The CDC lists a variety of clinical conditions to be used in diagnosing AIDS, along with an HIV-positive seroconversion and a T cell count below 200 (CDC 1997).

Conditions used in diagnosing AIDS include the following:

Opportunistic Infections (infections that take advantage of a weakened immune system)

- *Pneumocystis carinii* pneumonia (PCP)—a type of lung disease caused by a protozoan fungus, which is usually not harmful to humans
- Tuberculosis—either *Mycobacterium avium-intracellulare* complex (MAI) or *Mycobacterium tuberculosis* (TB); MAI is most common among AIDS patients
- Bacterial pneumonia—caused by several common bacteria
- Toxoplasmosis—disease of the brain and central nervous system

Cancers

- Kaposi's sarcoma—a cancer causing red or purple blotches on the skin
- Lymphomas—cancers of the lymphatic system
- Invasive cervical cancer—more common in women who are HIV positive

Other Conditions

- Wasting syndrome—involves persistent diarrhea, severe weight loss, and weakness

- AIDS dementia—impairment of mental functions, mood changes, impaired movement as a result of HIV infection of the brain

Other Infections

- Candidiasis (also called *thrush*)—a fungal infection that affects the vagina, mouth, throat, and lungs

- Herpes—a common viral sexually transmitted infection (STI)

- Cytomegalovirus—a virus that, in AIDS patients, can lead to brain infection, infection of the retina, pneumonia, or hepatitis

AIDS remains a devastating disease. It took eight and one-half years for the first 100,000 cases of AIDS to be reported. In only two and one-half years the second 100,000 cases were reported. More than 50 percent of individuals whose cases have been reported since 1981 have since died. In 1993, AIDS became the leading cause of death for Americans between the ages of twenty-five and forty-four. The best protection young people have is education and practicing safe sex if they become sexually active. The Health Highlight box on page 433 provides information on preventing the spread of HIV/AIDS and lists sources of information on the nature of HIV treatment and prevention.

Individuals infected with HIV may experience a variety of symptoms or may appear to be quite healthy. However, even people with no obvious symptoms can transmit HIV to others. The indicators of possible HIV infection include persistent diarrhea, dry cough, shortness of breath, fatigue, skin rash, swollen lymph glands (neck, armpits, groin), candidiasis, unexplained fever or chills, night sweats (over several weeks), and unexplained weight loss of 10 percent of body weight in less than two months. Women may also experience abnormal Pap smears, persistent vaginal candidiasis (a yeastlike fungal infection characterized by an itchy white discharge), and abdominal cramping as a result of pelvic inflammatory disease (PID). These infections are a result of HIV infection and are caused by immunodeficiency, but they are not yet considered AIDS.

It was previously thought that HIV did little in the body immediately after infection and simply stayed within a few immune system T cells for seven to ten years. It is now known that the real battle starts immediately within the lymph nodes, where day after day, year after year, the body is in mortal combat with the virus before finally exhausting its immune response reserves (Cray and Park 1996, 64).

HIV-1 is the HIV subtype found in the vast majority of infected individuals in the United States. Two tests are currently being used to detect HIV. The enzyme-linked immunoabsorbent assays (ELISA) test is the antibody test initially used. If the ELISA results indicate that the patient has HIV, another test—the Western blot—is administered for confirmation. Since the ELISA is an antibodies test and it may take from two to thirty-six months for antibodies to develop, there is a possibility of a false negative test for HIV antibodies. Usually the Western blot, a more precise antibodies test, shows clearly either HIV positive or negative. If there is an inconclusive Western blot test, a person should be retested in six months. Anyone who tests positive for HIV can transmit the virus. Enzyme

Health Highlight

PREVENTING THE SPREAD OF HIV/AIDS AND SOURCES OF INFORMATION

Recommendations to reduce the possibility of becoming infected:

- Practice abstinence or mutual monogamy.

- Always use protection (that is, latex condoms and spermicide, such as nonoxynol-9) if having sex with multiple partners or with persons who have multiple partners.

- Do not have unprotected sex with individuals with AIDS, those who engage in high-risk behavior, or those who have had a positive test for the AIDS virus.

- Avoid sexual activities that might cut or tear the rectum, vagina, or penis, such as anal intercourse.

- Do not have sex with prostitutes.

- Do not use IV drugs or share needles. Refrain from having sex with IV drug users.

Information on AIDS and HIV

CDC National AIDS Hotline
(800) 342-2437

Information on HIV and AIDS, free information available in several languages.

CDC National AIDS Clearinghouse
(800) 458-5231

Information on education services. Copies of Public Health Service publications available.

Lina National de SIDA (Spanish)
(800) 344-7432

24-hour hotline that provides information and referrals for HIV and AIDS.

Local health departments also have valuable information concerning HIV and AIDS.

SOURCE: CDC 2002

immunoassays are used to detect the presence of HIV-1 in clinical samples. ELISA tests are used as the primary screening test for HIV-1 infection, and the Western blot tests are used to double-check and confirm positive ELISA results. Both these variations of agglutination tests use antigen-specific antibodies labeled with specific enzymes to detect the presence of HIV-1 antigens. Additional tests using other techniques may also be performed to detect the presence of HIV and to monitor the status of an HIV-infected patient (Brooks, Butel, and Morse 2001). In addition to the above-mentioned tests, a home-testing kit for HIV is now available. However, any results of home testing should be confirmed by a proper medical authority.

HIV is transmitted primarily through sexual contact. Secondary transmission occurs among intravenous drug users. Screening techniques have reduced the chances of receiving HIV in blood transfusions to approximately one in one million. The heterosexual transmission of HIV has become a significant problem. The CDC has reported that heterosexual transmission makes up 33 percent of new infections. Men having sex with men still account for the largest percentage of new infections (42 percent). Intravenous drug users and sharing of needles account for 25 percent of new infections (CDC 2003). In fact, the potential for an AIDS epidemic through heterosexual transmission of HIV is staggering. Estimates are that one million Americans are already infected with

Infectious and Noninfectious Conditions   **433**

Health Highlight

SUPPORT FOR CHILDREN WITH HIV INFECTION IN SCHOOL: BEST PRACTICES GUIDELINES

I. Preparation of the School Setting

1. An **advisory committee on HIV-related issues** shall be established for the school district and commissioned by the superintendent. Membership shall be composed of health professionals (community physicians, school nurses, and other child and adolescent health workers), parents, teachers, students, persons with HIV infection, attorneys, advocates, and persons representing diversity in the community. At regular meetings, matters shall be discussed concerning HIV that relate to administrative practices, legal and policy questions, educational programs, universal infection control standards, and student welfare. Consultants shall be used as appropriate.

2. The school district shall adopt **policy statements of relevance to students with HIV infection** in collaboration with the advisory committee. These shall conform with state and federal laws and regulations, and draw on state-of-the-art medical and scientific information from appropriate government sources, documents from national organizations, research studies, and expert consultation. It may be helpful to use public hearings to gain input into these matters. The policy statements shall then be disseminated to all administrative levels; made available to staff, students, parents, and community leaders; and included in student and parent handbooks. They shall be reviewed at yearly intervals.

3. **Staff education and in-service training** concerning the issues of HIV infection, including transmission, prevention, civil rights, mental health, and death and bereavement, shall be carried out at least annually for all school personnel, including the school board. The program content shall be determined by a multidisciplinary team of appropriate individuals that shall include families of children with HIV infection and also persons with HIV infection. It shall aim to affect staff members' knowledge, feelings, attitudes, behavior, and acceptance of people who are HIV positive. For new employees, this education shall be built into the orientation program and offered within three months of hire. Teachers responsible for instruction of students regarding HIV infection shall receive specific in-service training.

4. **Universal precautions relating to blood-borne infections,** as adapted for schools, shall be in effect. School clinics and nursing offices shall follow OSHA guidelines for health care facilities. It is the responsibility of the school district to ensure adequate gloves, bleach, sinks, and disposal containers. There shall be systems of quality assurance or monitoring to document compliance with universal precautions in all school settings. These matters shall be featured in the staff education program.

5. The school district shall provide **education relating to the prevention of HIV infection for students in grades K–12,** within the context of a quality comprehensive school health program. Delivered by trained teachers, health educators, and nurses, it shall be developmentally, culturally, and linguistically appropriate. It shall actively promote abstinence as the best protection and shall also offer explicit information about the use and availability of condoms. Acknowledgment shall be given to the special needs of adolescents regarding emerging sexual orientation. An additional effect of this effort should be to enhance understanding of the needs of students, staff, and others who are infected with HIV.

II. The Enrollment Process

6. The parent, guardian, or student shall decide **whether or not to inform the school system** about HIV status or other health conditions.

He or she may support the transfer of this information by another professional or person, including a personal physician or a case manager, but only in the context of strict informed consent procedures. It shall be recognized that disclosure of HIV status often involves revealing related facts, such as medication, parent condition, transmission, and other matters. Under no circumstances shall parents, guardians, or students be required by school personnel to obtain HIV testing or to release information about HIV test results on the student or other family members.

7. Few, if any, personnel in the school or school district shall **receive information about the HIV status** of a student. Determination of those who are to be informed is the prerogative of the parents, guardian, or student, and shall be made in the setting of consideration about special health care or social services that are needed while the student is in school. The terms *need to know* and *right to know* are usually not applicable for school staff and are best eliminated. Specific release of information by the family as they wish it is obviously acceptable, but such material should then be treated confidentially regarding further dissemination.

8. **Information about a student's HIV status** shall not be included in the educational record, usual school health records, or any other records that are accessible to school staff beyond those the parents, guardian, or student has determined should know. Documentation about specific health care given by school nurses, counselors, clinicians, or other personnel to students with HIV infection shall be put in special health records kept in locked files. If the student changes schools, a plan for the transfer of these records shall be developed with the family and student.

III. Assurance of Appropriate Services

9. The **design of an individual student's program** shall be based on educational needs and not the status regarding HIV infection. The curriculum and other activities of a student with HIV shall be modified only as required per developmental and/or personal health needs. Exclusion or segregation of students solely on the basis of HIV infection is never appropriate.

10. **In-school health services** shall be provided as needed, including special regimens required because of HIV infection, but the origin of these programs shall not be identified at the classroom level. Specific health care plans may be formulated by school health personnel for students with symptomatic HIV infection. Notification for families about the presence of other communicable diseases at school (e.g., chicken pox) that place students at risk shall be forwarded universally.

    Particular notification will be given to families who have informed key school personnel about HIV infection. School nurses, and others with appropriate training, shall participate in counseling for students regarding HIV matters, including the availability of testing. They shall establish quality linkages with youth-serving HIV programs in the community that can provide culturally sensitive, age-appropriate medical, mental health, social, and drug treatment services.

IV. Other Elements

11. School administrators shall provide culturally sensitive information, technical assistance/consultation, and access to resources on HIV issues to the **school's parents and families** through PTAs and other parent organizations. Appropriate issues for discussion include prevention, confidentiality, classroom educational services and related supports, and community resources.

12. Relevant to existing federal and state statutes, teachers, school health professionals, and other qualified employees shall have the **right to employment and confidentiality** regardless of their own HIV status or other health conditions. If they choose to disclose their HIV status to students or other staff, this shall not have ramifications regarding employment.

SOURCE: Crocker et al. 1994. Used with permission.

Health Highlight

DECIDING WHAT TO SAY TO ELEMENTARY AND MIDDLE SCHOOL STUDENTS CONCERNING HIV AND AIDS

Since most students in this age group are not sexually active or trying drugs, you may decide that the young people you speak with do not need to know the details of how HIV is transmitted through unprotected sexual intercourse and injecting drug use. However, if you think they may be considering or may be doing things that put them at risk of infection, you will need to be sure they know the risk regardless of their age.

Students this age probably have heard about AIDS and may be scared by it. Much of what they have heard may have been incorrect. To reassure them, make sure they know that they cannot become infected through everyday contact, such as going to school with someone who is infected with HIV.

Students also may have heard myths and prejudicial comments about HIV infection and AIDS. Correct any notions that people can be infected by touching a doorknob or being bitten by a mosquito. Urge students to treat people who are infected with HIV or who are infected with HIV or who have AIDS with compassion and understanding, not cruelty and anger. Correcting myths and prejudices early will help students protect themselves and others from HIV infection and AIDS in the future.

Consider including the following points in a conversation about HIV infection and AIDS with students in the late elementary and middle school levels:

- AIDS is a disease caused by a tiny germ called a virus.
- Many different types of people have AIDS today—male and female, rich and poor, Caucasian, African American, Hispanic, Asian, and Native American.
- Because a person can be infected with HIV for as long as ten or more years before the signs of AIDS appear, a significant number of young people may have been infected when they were teenagers.
- Correct the many myths concerning AIDS.
- You can become infected with HIV either by having unprotected sexual intercourse with an infected person or by sharing drug needles or syringes with an infected person. Also, women infected with HIV can pass the virus to their babies during pregnancy or during birth. If not treated during pregnancy there is increased likelihood that the disease will be passed to the baby.
- A person who is infected can infect others in the ways described, even if no symptoms are present. You cannot tell by looking at someone whether he or she is infected.
- People who have AIDS should be treated with compassion.

SOURCE: CDC 1999

HIV. Considering that the incubation period can be as long as ten years and that the HIV-infected person is unaware of the disease, transmission has the potential to grow exponentially. In 1986, a second type of HIV virus, HIV-2, was discovered. Studies of HIV-2 are rather limited; while there seem to be many similarities to HIV-1, differences are noted. Both types of HIV have similar means of transmission, and both lead to the opportunistic infections listed on page 431. However, persons infected with HIV-2 are less infectious early in the course of infection. Most cases of HIV in the United States are HIV-1, whereas HIV-2 is more predominant in West Africa (CDC 2002).

HIV infection is not contracted through contact with food, eating utensils, clothing, furniture, swimming pools, or insects. Such contact as shaking hands, coughing, sneezing, or even living with an HIV-positive person will not transmit the disease. HIV has been found in tears, saliva, and urine, but transmission through contact with these substances has not been found to be directly implicated (Peterman 1986).

At present, no cure is available for HIV/AIDS, and the disease must still be considered fatal. The type of treatment that seems most effective in the treatment of HIV/AIDS is a triple-drug therapy consisting of a protease inhibitor, which blocks an enzyme (protease) that aids the virus in development at a later stage in its cycle. Two drugs from another group of antiviral drugs called nucleoside analogs—AZT (zidovudine) and ddI (didanosine)—work by blocking reverse transcriptase, the enzyme used by HIV to replicate itself inside a host cell. Early and very aggressive treatment with these drugs has cut the death rate by 70 percent and inhibited opportunistic infections by 73 percent. This mode of treatment is not without serious side effects, however, including diabetes, abnormally high cholesterol and triglycerides levels, shrinking limbs, and bizarre appearance of fat deposits on different parts of the body (Palella et al. 1998).

Chronic and Noninfectious Diseases

Americans are commonly afflicted by chronic and noninfectious diseases. Diseases of this type are not "caught" but are developed over time, often are progressive in effect, and may be due to genetic predisposition. Under normal circumstances, these conditions do not usually lead to death, but they are uncomfortable and, in more severe cases, can cause suffering. Although medicine is used in treatment, development of a wellness lifestyle may decrease both the incidence and the effects of these diseases.

The Cardiovascular System

Chronic diseases affecting the cardiovascular system are now among the leading causes of death. The cardiovascular system is complex and is subject to a range of diseases.

ANATOMY AND PHYSIOLOGY

The heart is composed of specialized muscle tissue called *cardiac muscle.* This muscle is extremely thick and strong and has amazing endurance capacity. Although the heart is only the size of a fist and weighs a mere eight to ten ounces, it contracts an average 70 to 80 times per minute, 100,000 times per day, and nearly one billion times in an average life of seventy years, and pumps thirty million to forty million gallons of blood. The heart is divided into two pumps by a wall called the septum. Each half is divided into an upper chamber called the atrium and a lower chamber called the ventricle. The right side of the heart

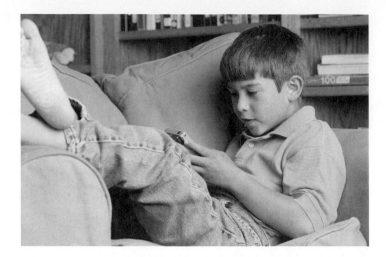

Inactivity at any age contributes to heart disease.

receives deoxygenated blood from the body and pumps it to the lungs so that carbon dioxide can be exchanged for a new supply of oxygen. This oxygen-rich blood is then sent to the left side of the heart so that the oxygenated blood can be pumped throughout the body.

On leaving the heart, blood travels throughout the body as part of the circulatory system. Blood containing oxygen and nutrients travels away from the heart, first in arteries, then in arterioles, and then in capillaries. It is through the very thin walls of the capillaries that oxygen, carbon dioxide, nutrients, and waste products are exchanged. Even the heart receives its nourishment in this manner. The waste products and carbon dioxide that are picked up by the blood in its deoxygenated state are returned to the heart through venules (small veins) and then veins, before reentering the venae cavae to the right atrium.

The heart has its own system for controlling its rhythmic pace. This mechanism begins with a group of specialized cells called the **sinoatrial node** (SA node) or *pacemaker*. The heartbeat begins when the SA node emits electrical impulses that signal the atria to contract and simultaneously travel toward the atrioventricular node (AV node). There is a momentary pause before the electrical impulse is distributed through the **bundle of His,** or AV bundle, and then throughout the Purkinje fibers, thereby causing the ventricles to contract. This conduction of electrical charge occurs slightly later in the ventricles and accounts for the characteristic "lub-dub" heart sound heard through a stethoscope (Thibodeau and Patton 1995).

TYPES OF CARDIOVASCULAR DISEASE

The most common cardiovascular diseases do not originate in the heart, but in the arteries. **Arteriosclerosis** is the generic term for a collection of diseases characterized by hardening of the arteries. The most common form of arteriosclerosis is known as **atherosclerosis.** Atherosclerosis is a degenerative disease that begins early in life, perhaps as early as two years of age. Atherosclerosis is the result

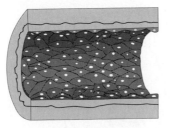

Cross section of a
normal artery

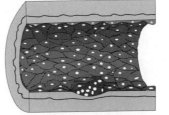

Fatty deposits form
on the inner lining

Figure 15.3
*Progress of
Atherosclerosis*

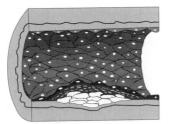

Channel narrows as
fat deposits increase

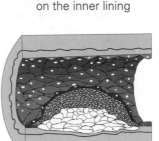

Blood clot blocks
narrowed channel

of a buildup of plaque, fat, and other materials that aggregate at sites of damaged cells inside arterial walls (Figure 15.3). The earliest formations are composed of fatty streaks in the inner lining of the arteries. As atherosclerosis progresses, the arteries harden and thicken. With this hardening, the arteries begin to lose their ability to dilate and constrict, an ability needed to meet all the body's requirements for oxygen in the various parts.

Over time, more and more plaque accumulates, gradually narrowing the flow of blood through the arteries. This narrowing can result in **ischemia,** or diminished blood flow. Also, as channels narrow, the chances for developing a **thrombus,** or stationary blood clot, increase. If the channels become sufficiently narrow, a free-floating clot (air or gas bubble or clump of bacteria, tissue, tumor, or thrombus), known as an **embolus,** can become stuck and block blood flow, resulting in a **heart attack** (or **myocardial infarction**) or a stroke (if the blood vessel is in the brain). A heart attack may be severe enough to result in death or may be sufficiently mild so that heart function can return to normal. In either event, a certain amount of heart tissue dies, and heart tissue does not regenerate. In time, scar tissue can form, and if it is located in strategic areas (such as along the electrical conducting pathways), full recovery from a heart attack may not be possible. If atherosclerosis affects arteries going to the brain (the carotid and cerebral arteries), a **stroke** (or shortage of blood to the brain) may result. Between 70 and 80 percent of all strokes are due to either a thrombus or embolus. Figure 15.4 shows the possible effects of atherosclerosis in the arteries.

Coronary heart disease (disease of the coronary vessels, rather than of the heart itself) is the leading cause of death in the United States today. Coronary atherosclerosis is the leading form of coronary heart disease. Current research

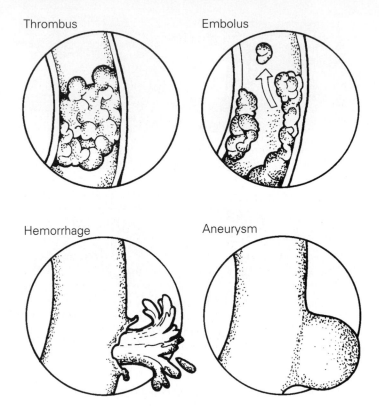

Figure 15.4
Possible Effects of Atherosclerosis on Arteries

Thrombus

Embolus

Hemorrhage

Aneurysm

has indicated that some heart attacks may be caused by spasms (cramping) in the coronary arteries. The origin of these spasms is at present unknown, although there is the possibility of a relationship between stress, tension, and heart spasms. Other experts believe that spasms are due to overabundance of calcium in cells that are being deprived of oxygen, or that the release of chemical substances at diseased sites causes the artery to close down. When these spasms occur in cases where sufficient atherosclerosis is present, the chances of having a heart attack increase. An aneurysm, a ballooning in an artery or vein due to weakened or damaged arterial walls (see Figure 15.4), is another source of coronary heart disease. An aneurysm in arteries in the brain may hemorrhage and cause a stroke.

Other forms of heart disease include **congenital heart defects** that originate during the development of the fetus. These difficulties usually affect the septum or valves of the heart so that they do not function properly. In congestive heart failure, the heart has lost strength and cannot pump all the blood out of the chambers. Circulation is negatively affected. The primary reason for congestive heart failure is high blood pressure or **hypertension** that is uncontrolled, although it may also be due to a previous heart attack, atherosclerosis, or a birth defect. Hypertension usually has no symptoms and may affect people of all ages, including children. Men are more susceptible than women to high blood pressure, and blacks are more susceptible than whites.

Table 15.3   Risk Factors for Cardiovascular Disease

Major Risk Factors That Cannot Be Changed

1. Age	According to the American Heart Association, 55 percent of all heart attacks occur in people over 65; this age group accounts for more than 80 percent of all fatal attacks.
2. Gender	Women have less heart disease than men, particularly before menopause. After menopause the heart attack rate among women increases significantly until the mid-60s, when women's risk is equal to that of men the same age.
3. Heredity	Father, grandfather, and brothers who die of coronary heart disease before the age of 55 or female relatives (mother, grandmother, and sisters) who died of coronary heart disease before the age of 65 indicate a strong familial tendency.

Major Risk Factors That Can Be Changed

1. Cholesterol	There are several types of cholesterol. Very low-density lipoproteins (VLDL) and low-density lipoproteins (LDL) cholesterol have been referred to as the bad cholesterol or type that enhances the depositing of plaque in the lining of the arteries. High-density lipoproteins (HDL) cholesterol in contrast picks up fat from the cells and linings of the arteries and delivers it to the liver, where it is degraded and eliminated or used to form other tissue.
2. Cigarette smoking	Tars, carbon monoxide, and nicotine adversely affect the body. The effects of these products increase heart rate, raise blood pressure, increase arterial spasms, reduce the ability of the blood to carry oxygen, and elevate cholesterol levels. Smoke destroys the alveoli in the lungs and paralyzes the cilia.
3. Hypertension	Systolic blood pressure is the force exerted against the arteries when the heart is contracting. Diastolic pressure is the force against the arteries when the heart is relaxed. These pressures are measured in millimeters of mercury (mmHg). As a result of hypertension, the heart receives inadequate rest between beats that produces muscle fibers that are overstretched and lose the ability to contract. This increases pressure, damages the kidneys and arteries, and accelerates atherosclerosis.
4. Inactivity	Research has shown that the impact of physical inactivity on heart disease is similar in magnitude to that of cigarette smoking, high serum cholesterol levels, and hypertension; 78 percent of Americans exercise too infrequently. In addition, exercise has a modifying effect on many of the risks for cardiovascular disease.
5. Obesity	There is a strong positive association between obesity and abnormal cholesterol and triglycerides, hypertension, and excessive production of insulin. These factors lead to increased likelihood of coronary artery disease and type II diabetes.
6. Diabetes mellitus	Long-range complications lead to degenerative disorders of the blood vessels and nerves. Diabetics often are victims of cardiovascular lesions and accelerated atherosclerosis. The incidence of heart attacks and strokes is higher among diabetics than nondiabetics. Diabetes increases the risk of coronary artery disease by 2 to 3 times the normal rate in men and 3 to 7 times in women.
7. Stress	Experts agree that chronic stress produces a complex array of physiological changes in the body. Some of these physiological responses can constrict the arteries and increase the workload of the heart.
8. Homo cysteine	When building blocks of protein (amino acids) are found in high levels in the blood, the probability of having a heart attack increases to 3 times that of normal level subjects.

The common childhood illness of strep throat is the source of an infection that can cause **rheumatic heart disease.** Undiagnosed strep can result in rheumatic fever; in a portion of these cases, rheumatic heart disease results, causing damage to one or more of the heart's valves. Abnormal heart sounds, known as **heart murmurs,** may be indicative of turbulence in the blood flow resulting from such problems as narrowed or leaky heart valves or an incomplete closure of a congenital hole in the heart's septum (prior to birth, there is a hole, the foramen ovale, between the two atria to allow the blood to bypass the nonfunctional lungs). *Functional heart murmurs,* on the other hand, are considered normal and may be the result of changes in blood turbulence due to increased exercise; this type of murmur is especially common in young people (Spence and Mason 1992).

Angina pectoris is defined as chest pains. Angina is not a heart attack, nor is it a disease. It is a frequent symptom of coronary heart disease, however. An angina attack usually lasts less than five minutes, often after unaccustomed exercise or stress. A primary symptom is a squeezing sensation in the chest, as if a weight had been placed there. For some, it is pain elsewhere in the upper body, frequently the left arm, or a pain that feels similar to indigestion or heartburn. Angina usually subsides with rest and medication. The positive aspect of angina is that it is an early warning of progressive heart disease. For one-third of all victims, the actual heart attack is the first symptom. Recognized and properly treated, angina can lead to prevention of more serious heart disease or even a heart attack. The risk factors for cardiovascular disease are shown in Table 15.3. See Table 15.4 for information about cholesterol levels and hypertension in children.

Table 15.4 *Blood Cholesterol and Hypertension in Children*

Total Blood Cholesterol and LCL-Cholesterol Levels for Children Ages 2 to 19

Cholesterol Type	Cholesterol Levels (in mg per deciliter)		
	Normal	Moderately High	High
Total cholesterol	Below 170	170–185	Above 185
LDL cholesterol	Below 110	110–125	Above 125

Hypertension in Children

Age Group	Hypertension		
	Normal	Significant	Severe
1 mo–2 yrs	105/69	112/74	118/72
3–5	107/69	116/76	124/84
6–9	114/72	122/78	130/86
10–12	120/76	126/82	134/90
13–15	126/79	136/86	144/92
16–18	126/79	142/92	150/98

SOURCE: Elster and Kuznets 1994, 102; Task Force on Blood Pressure Control in Children 1987

Once a heart attack has occurred the most common forms of surgical treatment are coronary bypass, angioplasty, coronary atherectomy, or coronary stents. **Coronary bypass** is designed to shunt blood around the blocked segment of a heart artery or arteries. A vein from the leg is removed and one end sewed into the aorta and the other into the coronary artery below the blockage—thus restoring blood flow. **Angioplasty** (also known as balloon angioplasty) uses a catheter with a balloon at the tip. The catheter is positioned at the narrow point in the artery end, and the balloon inflated, compressing the blockage against the vessel wall and thus returning blood flow to the blocked area. **Coronary atherectomy** uses a specially tipped catheter with a high-speed rotary cutting blade to shave off plaque in the blocked area of the heart artery. Another type of catheterization is used to implant a **coronary stent** in a diseased artery. The stent is a flexible, metallic tube that maintains an open passage for blood flow through a diseased artery. This procedure is much like the angioplasty, but the supporting stent is left in place to help insure the artery will remain open. When the stent is placed in an artery, blood-thinning medications must be taken for two to three months. Thereafter the patient must take aspirin every day to maintain the blood thinning.

Cancer

The term **cancer** does not refer to one disease, but rather to a large group of diseases. Cancer is characterized by uncontrolled growth and spread of abnormal cells or **neoplasms.** These neoplasms often form a mass of tissue called a **tumor.** These masses or tumors can be **malignant** (cancerous) or benign. **Benign** tumors usually cause no harm. However, if they are located in an area where they obstruct or crowd out normal tissues or organs, benign tumors can be life threatening; for example, a benign tumor in the brain could restrict the flow of blood. Benign tumors are enclosed in a fibrous capsule that prevents their spreading to other areas of the body. To determine if a tumor is malignant or benign, a **biopsy** (microscopic examination of tissue) must be done.

TYPES OF CANCER

There are four major categories of tumors: carcinoma, sarcoma, lymphoma, and leukemia. **Carcinoma** is the most common form of cancer. Cancers of the skin, breast, uterus, prostate, lung, stomach, colon, and rectum are examples of carcinoma. **Sarcomas** are cancers of the connective tissue and include muscle, bone, and cartilage cancers. These cancers occur less often than carcinomas but usually spread more quickly. **Lymphomas** are cancers that affect the lymph nodes. **Leukemia** is cancer of the blood-forming cells, causing an overproduction of immature white blood cells. Data on the incidence of cancer appear in Figure 15.5.

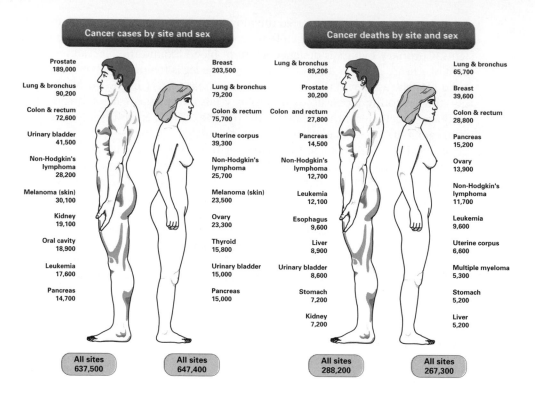

Figure 15.5 *Leading Sites of New Cancer Cases and Deaths—1999 Estimates*
SOURCE: American Cancer Society 2002

HOW CANCER SPREADS

Malignant tumors are not contained in a fibrous capsule. Consequently, the malignant cells can spread from one part of the body to another, a process known as **metastasis.** Cancers metastasize by invading adjacent tissues or dislodging and moving through the blood and lymphatic vessels to other parts of the body. Early diagnosis is vital for any type of cancer. If the cancer metastasizes, treatment becomes much more difficult. As the malignant cells spread, they begin to disrupt the chemical functioning of the normal cells in the area they invade. The cancerous cells disrupt the ribonucleic acid (RNA) and deoxyribonucleic acid (DNA) within the normal cells. When this disruption occurs, **mutant** cells that differ in form, quality, and function are developed.

CAUSES OF CANCER

Cancer is a problem of cell regulation. In simplistic terms, cells fail to perform in a prescribed fashion. To control what is an orderly replacement of cells in the body there are **regulatory genes.** A failure of these genes to regulate the specialization and replication will result in the abnormal production of cells and the development of cancer. Cells also have genes that repair any mistakes in the copying of genetic material found in each cell. Normally, if genes fail to work

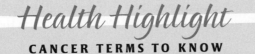

CANCER TERMS TO KNOW

The following terms are commonly used in the language of cancer treatment:

antibody: a substance made by specialized cells in the body that defends against infections due to viruses, bacteria, and other foreign substances

benign: a noncancerous growth

biopsy: removal and microscopic examination of tissue from a living body for diagnosis

cancer: a general term for more than 100 diseases involving abnormal and uncontrolled growth of cells

grading: a method physicians use to identify the severity of cancer

malignant: a growth of cancerous cells

metastasis: the spread of cancer from part of the body to another; cells in the new site are like those in the original growth

remission: a lessening or stopping of symptoms of a disease when the disease is under control

staging: a numerical method indicating the extent to which the cancer has spread; helps determine best form of treatment and prognosis

tumor: a palpable mass; may be malignant or benign

properly and result in the development of abnormal cells, the immune system will destroy the abnormalities before cancer can develop.

The genes responsible for specialization, replication, repair, and suppression can become **oncogenes,** or cancer-causing genes. Prior to becoming onccogenes they are referred to as proto-oncogenes (Lichtenstein et al. 2000). The mechanisms that cause proto-oncogenes to become oncogenes have received much attention. Many different factors may cause cancer, but three seem to be especially important: genetic mutations, viral infections, and carcinogens. Carcinogens are environmental agents that have been associated with causing cancer. Examples include tobacco smoke, environmental pollutants (water, air, toxic wastes), food preservatives, and even high-fat foods.

In humans it appears that the same proto-oncogenes (noncancerous; normally found in the DNA) can be converted to oncogenes (cancer-inducing genes) either by undergoing some form of mutation that is not associated with a virus or by passage through a retrovirus. A **retrovirus**—such as Rous sarcoma virus (RSV)—enters a cell and converts its own genetic information from RNA to DNA (RNA and DNA contain the genetic information necessary for the body to develop and function). Then the RSV adds its own DNA to that of the host cell so that it is replicated along with the normal DNA every time the host cell divides. A single change to the proto-oncogene is probably not enough to cause the cell to become cancerous—it is accumulated changes that are the likely cause, with each successive change triggering the occurrence of additional abnormalities associated with cancer (Mange and Mange 1990). (Abnormalities include cell proliferation, invasion of adjacent tissue, and metastasis.) Some genes, such as the BRCA-1 breast cancer gene, have been clearly tied to an increased tendency to develop certain kinds of cancer. Individuals in families with a high incidence of breast cancer, for example, may be tested for the presence of such proto-oncogenes and given special counseling on ways to modify their habits (i.e., environmental influences) to reduce their chances of having the oncogenes develop (Mange and Mange 1990).

Although the evidence is still under investigation, there are indications that viruses enhance the probability for the development of cancer. There is evidence that the herpes viruses may contribute to the development of some forms of leukemia, Burkitt's lymphoma, Hodgkin's disease, cervical cancer, and some forms of leukemia (Donatelle, Davis, and Hoover 1991).

Cancer, Nutrition, and Physical Activity. Although useful as preservatives, many chemical food additives and preservatives such as cyclamate saccharin and the nitrosamines have been linked with cancer. It has been estimated that 40 to 50 percent of cancers derive from environmental chemicals such as pesticides, herbicides, preservatives, and other chemicals. The Food and Drug Administration (FDA) has developed a list of over 14,000 chemicals suspected of causing cancer. Instead of concerning itself with all the ill effects of these chemicals, the American Cancer Society (ACS) (2002) has developed the following nutritional guidelines for preventing cancer:

- **Eat a variety of foods.** No one food provides all the nutrients your body needs. Eat a variety of foods such as fruit and vegetables, whole cereals, lean meats, fish, poultry without skin, beans, and low-fat dairy products.

- **Maintain desirable weight.** Obesity increases the risks for colon, breast, gallbladder, and uterine cancer.

- **Avoid too much fat, saturated fat, and cholesterol.** A low-fat diet may reduce the risks for cancers of the breast, prostate, colon, and rectum. A low-fat diet will help control weight and reduce the risk of heart disease.

- **Eat foods with adequate starch and fiber.** Starch and fiber can be increased by eating more fruit, vegetables, potatoes, and whole-grain breads and cereals. A high-fiber diet helps reduce the risk of colon and rectal cancer.

- **Include foods rich in vitamins A and C.** Foods such as carrots, spinach, oranges, strawberries, and green peppers are high in vitamin C. Vitamin A can be found in dark green and deep yellow fresh vegetables. These foods may help reduce the risk for cancers of the larynx, esophagus, and lungs.

- **Include cruciferous vegetables.** Cabbage, broccoli, brussel sprouts, and cauliflower are high in fiber and may help prevent cancer.

- **Eat salt-cured, smoked, and nitrate-cured foods in moderation.** Consuming these foods in large amounts is associated with higher incidence of cancer of the esophagus and stomach.

- **If you drink alcohol, do so in moderation.** Moderation is considered to be no more than two drinks a day for men and one drink a day for women (ACS 2002). Heavy drinking is associated with cancer of the mouth, throat, esophagus, and liver.

Finally, the ACS recommends that all children and adults adopt a physically active lifestyle. The recommendation for adults is to engage in moderate activity for thirty minutes or more at least five times per week. A more refined schedule requires vigorous activity on five or more days per week for forty-five minutes. This schedule may reduce the risk of breast and colon cancers. Children and adolescents are advised to engage in moderate to vigorous activity for sixty minutes at least five days a week.

WARNING SIGNS OF CANCER

The ACS states that the following warning signs should be carefully monitored. The chances of survival are significantly better if early detection and diagnosis take place. None of the risk factors are sure indicators of cancer, but they should be checked by a physician. The warning signs are:

- a change in bowel or bladder habits
- a sore that does not heal
- unusual bleeding or discharge
- thickening or lump in the breasts or elsewhere
- indigestion or difficulty in swallowing
- obvious change in a wart or mole
- nagging cough or hoarseness

TREATMENT OF CANCER

Surgery offers the greatest chance for cure for many types of cancer. Almost 60 percent of people with cancer will have some type of surgery. The malignant tissue and some additional noncancerous tissue is removed to attempt to ensure that all the cancerous cells are removed. Surgery is combined with chemotherapy and/or radiation. Surgery is used most often with breast, female reproductive organ, prostate, and testicular cancers. Other treatment options for cancer include:

Radiation—uses high-energy X rays or gamma rays to destroy or damage cancer cells so that they cannot replicate. Radiation causes side effects such as diarrhea, itching, and difficulty swallowing. Over the last few years, because of the ability to be more precise in focus and length of exposure, the damage to noncancerous cells has lessened and the potential side effects have decreased.

Chemotherapy—the use of drugs to treat cancer. Some of the most important advances in the treatment of cancer have been in this area. These advances include new drugs, as well as more effective combinations of new drugs and drugs already used in treatment. The drugs are usually given by mouth or intravenously. They enter the bloodstream and reach all areas of the body, which makes them useful in reaching cancers that have spread. Most chemotherapeutic agents work

PREVENTING CANCER:
GUIDELINES FROM THE AMERICAN CANCER SOCIETY

Primary prevention refers to steps that might be taken to avoid those factors that might lead to the development of cancer.

Smoking Cigarette smoking is responsible for 85 percent of lung cancer cases among men and 75 percent among women—about 83 percent overall. Smoking accounts for about 30 percent of all cancer deaths. Those who smoke 2 or more packs of cigarettes a day have lung cancer mortality rates 15 to 25 times greater than nonsmokers.

Sunlight Almost all of the more than 500,000 cases of nonmelanoma skin cancer developed each year in the United States are considered to be sun related. Recent epidemiological evidence shows that sun exposure is a major factor in the development of melanoma and that the incidence increases for those living near the equator.

Alcohol Oral cancer and cancers of the larynx, throat, esophagus, and liver occur more frequently among heavy drinkers of alcohol.

Smokeless Tobacco Increased risk factor for cancers of the mouth, larynx, throat, and esophagus. Highly habit forming.

Estrogen For mature women, certain risks associated with estrogen treatment to control menopausal symptoms, including an increased risk of endometrial cancer. Use of estrogen by menopausal women needs careful discussion by the woman and her physician.

Radiation Excessive exposure to radiation can increase cancer risk. Most medical X rays are adjusted to deliver the lowest dose possible without sacrificing image quality. The American Cancer Society (ACS) believes there is a potential problem of radon in the home. If levels are found to be too high, remedial actions should be taken.

Occupational Hazards Exposure to a number of industrial agents—for example, nickel, chromate, asbestos, vinyl chloride—increases risk. Risk factors are greatly increased when combined with smoking.

Nutrition Risk for colon, breast, and uterine cancers increases for obese people. High-fat diet may be a factor in the development of certain cancers such as breast, colon, and prostate. High-fiber foods may help reduce risk of colon cancer, and can be a wholesome substitute for high-fat diets. Foods rich in vitamins A and C may help lower risk for cancers of larynx, esophagus, stomach, and lung. Eating cruciferous vegetables may help protect against certain cancers. Salt-cured, smoked, and nitrite-cured foods have been linked

by destroying the cancer cells' ability to replicate. There are side effects, such as suppression of the immune system, diarrhea, and hair loss.

Hormone therapy—treatment with hormones that interfere with hormone production or their action. This modality is sometimes classified as chemotherapy.

Immunotherapy—the use of a variety of substances to trigger an individual's own immune system to the cancer. The substances are made through genetic engineering techniques and work by attacking malignant cells or keeping them from becoming active. Among these technologies are interferon, interleukin-2, tumor necrosis factor, and bone marrow growth regulators.

Other technologies have enhanced the diagnosis and treatment of cancer. Such technologies as magnetic resonance imaging (MRI) and computerized to esophageal and stomach cancer. The heavy use of alcohol, especially when accompanied by cigarette smoking or chewing tobacco, increases risk of cancers of the mouth, larynx, throat, esophagus, and liver.

Summary of American Cancer Society Recommendations for the Early Detection of Cancer in Asymptomatic People

Cancer-related checkup A cancer-related checkup is recommended every 3 years for people ages 20 to 40 and every year for people age 40 and older. This exam should include health counseling and, depending on a person's age, possibly examinations for cancers of the thyroid, oral cavity, skin, lymph nodes, testes, and ovaries as well as for some nonmalignant diseases.

Breast Women 40 and older should have an annual mammogram and annual clinical breast exam (CBE) performed by a health care professional and should perform monthly breast self-examinations. The CBE should be conducted close to the scheduled mammogram. Women ages 20 to 39 should have a clinical breast exam performed by a health care professional every 3 years and should perform monthly breast self-examinations.

Colon and rectum Men and women over 50 should follow one of the following examination schedules:

■ A fecal occult blood test every year and a flexible sigmoidoscopy every 5 years

■ A colonoscopy every 10 years
■ A double-contrast barium enema every 5 to 10 years
■ A digital rectal exam at the same time as the sigmoidoscopy, colonoscopy, or double-contrast barium enema (people at moderate or high risk for colorectal cancer should talk with a doctor about a different testing schedule)

Prostate The ACS recommends that both the prostate-specific antigen (PSA) blood test and the digital rectal examination be offered annually, beginning at age 50, to men who have a life expectancy of at least 10 years and to younger men who are at high risk.

Men in high-risk groups, such as those with strong familial predispositions (i.e., 2 or more affected first-degree relatives) or African Americans, may begin at a younger age (that is, 45 years).

Uterus

Cervix: All women who are or have been sexually active or who are 18 and older should have an annual Pap test and pelvic examination. After 3 or more consecutive satisfactory examinations with normal findings, the Pap test may be performed less frequently. Discuss the matter with your physician.

Endometrium: Women at high risk for cancer of the uterus should have a sample of endometrial tissue examined when menopause begins.

SOURCE: American Cancer Society 2002

tomography (CT) scanning help to detect and map tumors that once were hidden.

Respiratory Disorders

The term **allergy** can be used synonymously with the term **hypersensitivity.** Both terms refer to an exaggerated response to an antibody-forming substance **(antigen).** Many people with the most common allergic disorders have an inherited tendency to develop this hypersensitivity. Although it may seem to those who suffer from allergies that the vast majority of people do experience hypersensitivity, each specific reaction is theoretically harmless to 80 percent of the population. Table 15.5 on page 450 lists the more common allergic reactions.

Table 15.5   *Common Allergic or Sensitivity Reactions*

Reaction	Causes	Symptoms	Relief
Hay fever	Pollen from trees, grasses, or weeds; molds; dust mites; furry animals	Stuffy nose, sneezing, runny nose, itching eyes and nose, watering eyes	Avoidance of allergens; medications
Eczema (atopic dermatitis)	Food allergies; contact with pollen, dust mites, furry animals, makeup, soaps, detergents	Patchy, dry, red itchy rash—often in creases of arms, legs, and neck	Avoidance of allergens; medication
Food allergies and/or sensitivities	Any food, but most common are eggs, peanuts, milk, fish, soy, wheat, peas, and shellfish	Vomiting, hives, diarrhea, or breathing/circulation problem	Avoidance of products

ASTHMA

Because of their small airways, children are prone to asthma. Childhood asthma tends to improve as the lung airways become larger. Older children tend to become relatively free of symptoms, yet may experience problems throughout their lives. If a child's asthma is more than mild, a proper treatment plan should be undertaken. This plan should be shared with the child's teachers so that the child can fully participate in school activities.

Asthma is characterized by spastic contractions of the air passageways, resulting in difficulty breathing. The typical cause is a hypersensitivity of the air passageways to foreign substances found in the air; for about 70 percent of people under the age of thirty, this sensitivity is the cause of their asthma, pollen being the most common culprit (Guyton and Hall 1997). Such *extrinsic asthma* is episodic or seasonal, and attacks may be provoked psychologically if the air passages have already been sensitized by antigens. Hyposensitization treatments (a form of immunotherapy in which increasingly graduated doses of an allergen are given in order to develop immunity) may be helpful for some types of antigens that trigger extrinsic asthma; medications may relieve some symptoms. For people over thirty, asthma is almost always due to hypersensitivity to such nonallergenic types of irritants as those found in smog, strong cooking odors, and paint fumes. This form of asthma, known as *intrinsic asthma,* is chronic and persistent, and it may also be triggered by sudden inhalation of cold dry air, physical exercise, or violent coughing or laughing (Anderson, Anderson, and Glanze 1998).

Other Conditions

There are several other significant conditions of which a teacher needs to be aware. Teachers need to understand not only the nature of these disorders, but also the signs and symptoms so they can help identify problems students might be experiencing. These conditions include diabetes, sickle cell anemia, and epilepsy.

DIABETES MELLITUS

Diabetes can result from the secretion of too little insulin from the pancreas, insufficient numbers of insulin receptors on target cells, or defective receptors that do not respond normally to insulin (Tate, Seeley, and Stephens 1994, 175). **Hyperglycemia** (high blood sugar) is the hallmark symptom of diabetes. Obesity is a contributing factor to lack of receptor sites in older people. Insufficient amounts of insulin are available to metabolize sugar, the primary source of fuel. When fat is metabolized without sugar, a residue called a **ketone body** develops, increasing acid in the bloodstream. Sufficient amounts of ketone bodies produce a diabetic coma and can cause death. The earliest symptom of characteristically elevated blood glucose levels is excessive urination. Other common warning signs of diabetes include unusual thirst, irritability, blurred vision, frequent infections, extreme hunger, and sudden weight loss.

There are three types of diabetes mellitus. **Type I diabetes,** or insulin-dependent diabetes mellitus (IDDM), is usually caused by a lack of insulin secretion. Viral infection of the pancreatic islets or an autoimmune response that destroys the insulin-making beta cells of the pancreas may be responsible for the development of the condition. Type I usually appears in people under the age of thirty-five, most commonly between the ages of ten and sixteen years. Type I diabetics must be aware of their sugar levels at all times and take daily insulin injections. **Type II diabetes,** or non-insulin-dependent diabetes (NDDM), is considered a metabolic disease in that the beta cells of the pancreas secrete too little insulin, there are insufficient numbers of insulin receptors on target cells, or defective receptors that do not respond normally to insulin (Tate, Seeley, and Stephens 1994, 175). The onset is gradual and usually occurs in people over the age of forty; however, over the last few years there has been a significant increase in the number of adolescents developing type II diabetes. This increase has been attributed to an increase in the numbers of adolescents who are overweight or obese and who lead sedentary lifestyles. **Gestational diabetes** is the third type. This can develop in a woman during pregnancy. The condition usually disappears after childbirth, but it does put the woman at greater risk for diabetes later in her life.

Approximately 17 million people (6.2 percent of the population in the United States) have diabetes; an estimated 11.1 million have been diagnosed while one-third or 5.9 million people are unaware they have the disease (American Diabetes Association 2002). Breakthroughs in the ability to implant insulin monitors and insulin infusion pumps that regulate/dispense insulin as needed by the body have greatly changed the lives of diabetics. Now being tested is an insulin inhaler that would allow the diabetic to inhale rather than inject insulin when needed. These devices help to eliminate many of the potential side effects associated with treatment and allow more normal lives for diabetics; however, they are very expensive and thus not available to all diabetics. A new type of insulin called

Humalog supposedly is capable of acting more than twice as fast as other versions (Cray and Park 1996, 64).

Insulin shock can develop when too much insulin is present. This occurs when a diabetic is either injected with too much insulin or has not eaten after an insulin injection. Disorientation, convulsions, and loss of consciousness may result.

Extra care with personal hygiene is part of treatment. Diabetics are very prone to infections, so it is important for them to maintain sterile conditions for shaving and to treat cuts and abrasions carefully. The feet and legs are particularly susceptible to infection. Long-term complications include heart disease, stroke, hypertension, blindness, kidney disease, nerve damage, dental disease, and amputations. Some new classes of drugs work in the small intestine to inhibit the absorption of carbohydrates (which raise blood sugar levels), while others stop the liver from producing excess amounts of sugar.

SICKLE CELL ANEMIA

Sickle cell anemia is an inherited blood disease that can cause pain, damage to vital organs, and, for some, early death. The effects of the disease vary greatly from person to person, but most people with the condition enjoy good health much of the time. Most cases of sickle cell anemia in the United States occur among African Americans and Hispanics of Caribbean ancestry. Approximately 1 in every 400 to 600 African Americans and 1 in every 1,000 to 1,500 Hispanics inherit sickle cell anemia. The physical growth of children with the disease is often slower than normal.

Normally, red blood cells are round and flexible. However, the red blood cells of a person with sickle cell anemia may change into a sickle shape within their blood vessels. The sickle cells tend to become trapped in the spleen and elsewhere and are destroyed. This results in a shortage of red blood cells, which causes the person to be pale, short of breath, easily tired, and prone to infections. Viral infection and vitamin deficiency can worsen the condition.

When the cells become stuck in the blood vessels, they lose oxygen. This loss of oxygen causes severe pain in the abdomen, chest, and joints; fever; chronic anemia; lethargy; and weakness. If the condition is long lasting, damage to the brain, lungs, or kidneys can even lead to death.

Sickle cell anemia is not contagious, but it is inherited. Individuals may carry one gene for the disease (sickle cell trait) but have no signs of the disease. When two persons who have the trait have a child, that child may inherit two sickle cell genes and develop the disease. A test can identify people who either have the disease or carry the trait. Unfortunately there is no medication or therapy that will correct the effects of the disease-causing gene.

EPILEPSY

The word *epilepsy* comes from the Greek word for seizures. **Epilepsy** is a disorder of the central nervous system characterized by sudden seizures, which usually last only a few minutes. Seizures are not always convulsive, and, even when they

A STUDENT WITH SICKLE CELL ANEMIA IN THE CLASSROOM

There may be a student in your class with the severe chronic disease sickle cell anemia. Your understanding of this handicap will help him or her on the road to learning.

Such a student is often thin and small for his or her age. When not experiencing physical discomfort, the student is usually as active as any student in the class. Intelligence is not affected. As noted in earlier chapters, the majority of those affected are African Americans, but the disease also occurs in people from Mediterranean countries, South and Central America, Caribbean countries, and southern India.

There are periods when the disease is more active (crises). These episodes often occur with colds and other infections and are more frequent in early childhood. At such times, the child becomes listless and complains of pain, usually in the back, extremities, or abdomen. The whites of his or her eyes may be slightly yellow. Most of these attacks will necessitate a week or two of absence from school. Sometimes, hospitalization and special procedures, such as blood transfusion, will be required.

The disease is due to a hereditary defect in the red blood cells, causing them to assume the crescent shape that gives the disease its name. The pains are due to aggregations of sickled cells causing a temporary blockage of the small blood vessels. These cells are subject to early destruction in the circulation, causing a chronic anemia.

Sickle cell anemia is inherited as a recessive trait affecting both males and females. If both parents carry a recessive sickle cell gene, the affected child receives one such gene from each parent. When both parents have sickle cell trait, their offspring has a 25 percent chance of being normal, a 25 percent chance of having sickle cell anemia, or a 50 percent chance of having sickle cell trait.

An examination of the blood by laboratory tests will show whether a person has sickle cell anemia or sickle cell trait. Individuals with the trait have a very small percentage of sickled cells in their circulation. They never develop sickle cell anemia per se, and as a rule, they are free of symptoms that could be attributed to the presence of an abnormal hemoglobin in their red blood cells.

Points for the Teacher to Keep in Mind

1. Sickle cell anemia is a chronic hereditary handicapping illness.
2. Crises cause frequent absence from school, especially in younger students.
3. Colds and other infections may precipitate crises.
4. Between crises, a student with sickle cell anemia may carry on the usual activities of his or her peer group, with the exception of strenuous sports.
5. The disease does not affect intelligence.
6. Education should be encouraged because this handicap will necessitate a sedentary occupation as an adult.
7. When long hospitalizations are required, students should be able to continue schoolwork in the hospital with the help of a visiting teacher.
8. Psychological problems may arise from adjustment to the handicap and the environment.
9. It is important that there be some activity in which the student can excel to gain acceptance with the peer group. This could be music, art, handicrafts, games, and so forth.
10. The disease tends to become milder as an individual grows into adulthood. Crises become less frequent and less severe after adolescence.

SOURCE: Scott and Kessler 1988, 1–4

are, they are not as dangerous as they look. Epilepsy is not contagious, and, between seizures, epileptic children function normally. Seizures occur when there are excessive electrical discharges in some nerve cells of the brain. When this happens, the brain loses conscious control over certain body functions and consciousness may be lost or altered.

There are more than twenty different kinds of seizures. Only three will be described here.

General Tonic Clonic Seizures (Grand Mal). These are the most disruptive in the classroom. The child becomes stiff and slumps to the floor unconscious. Rigid muscles give way to jerking, breathing is suspended, and saliva may escape from the lips. The seizure may last for several minutes, and the child will regain consciousness in a confused or drowsy state but is otherwise unaffected.

For tonic clonic seizures:

- Keep calm. Ease the child to the floor, and loosen his or her collar. You cannot stop the seizure. Let it run its course, and do not try to revive the child.

- Remove hard, sharp, or hot objects that may injure the child, but do not interfere with his or her movements.

- Do not force anything between his or her teeth.

- Turn the child on one side to release saliva. Place something soft and flat under his or her head.

- When the child regains consciousness, let him or her rest.

- If the seizure lasts beyond a few minutes or the child seems to pass from one seizure to another without gaining consciousness, call for medical assistance and notify his or her parents. This rarely happens but should be treated immediately.

Generalized Absence (Petit Mal) Seizures. The most common in children, generalized absence seizures usually last for only five to twenty seconds. They may be accompanied by staring or twitching of the eyelids and are frequently mistaken for "daydreaming." The child is seldom aware he or she has had a seizure, although he or she may be aware that his or her mind "has gone blank" for a few seconds.

Complex Partial (Psychomotor or Temporal Lobe) Seizures. The most complex behavior patterns occur with these seizures and may include constant chewing or lip smacking, purposeless walking or repetitive hand and arm movements, confusion, and dizziness. The seizure may last from a minute to several hours. The person should not be restrained, but also should not be allowed to harm himself or herself. Medical assistance is required if the seizure lasts more than a few minutes or if it is the first time such a seizure has occurred.

Summary

- Microorganisms (microbes) are living agents. Microbes that cause disease in humans are called *pathogens.*

- There are six general types of pathogenic microbes: viruses, bacteria, rickettsiae, fungi, protozoa, and helminths.

- Every illness follows a pattern from the time the pathogen enters the body to the incubation period, prodromal period, typical illness, convalescence, and recovery.
- The immune system protects against disease.
- Body defenses include the skin, body secretions, mucous membranes, enzymes, blood compounds, and interferon.
- Common diseases that can impact children include the common cold, streptococcal throat infection, influenza, infectious mononucleosis, and the various types of hepatitis.
- HIV is the virus responsible for AIDS. It cannot be contracted through casual contact.
- There are no cures for AIDS, but a combination of drug therapy seems promising.
- Teachers must be aware of the emotional, social, and legal support an HIV-positive child needs.
- The risk factors for cardiovascular disease include heredity, sex, age, tobacco use, high cholesterol, hypertension, inactivity, obesity, diabetes, and stress.
- Conditions of the heart and cardiovascular system include congenital heart defects, congestive heart failure, myocardial infarction, angina pectoris, hypertension, and rheumatic heart.
- The term *cancer* is used to describe conditions characterized by uncontrolled cell growth.
- Neoplasms (tumors) can be benign (noncancerous) or malignant (cancerous).
- Types of cancer include carcinomas, sarcomas, lymphomas, and leukemia.
- Cancer spreads through a process called *metastasis*.
- Sickle cell anemia is an inherited blood disease that can cause extreme pain, damage to vital organs, and possible early death.
- Epilepsy is one of more than twenty types of disorders of the central nervous system.
- The three most common types of epilepsy are general tonic clonic (grand mal); generalized absence (petit mal); and complex partial (psychomotor).

DISCUSSION QUESTIONS

1. List and describe the pathogens.
2. Discuss immunity and the various protective mechanisms the body has to protect itself against disease.
3. Trace the stages through which a communicable disease typically progresses.
4. Describe the antigen-antibody response.
5. Trace the possible physiological effects experienced by an HIV-positive person.
6. Trace the blood through the heart and circulatory system.
7. Distinguish between angina pectoris, heart attack, and stroke.
8. Describe the major risk factors for cardiovascular diseases.

9. What are the four types of cancer?
10. Describe how IDDM differs from NIDDM.
11. What considerations are necessary for a child with sickle cell anemia?

CRITICAL THINKING QUESTIONS

1. Reflect on the HIV/AIDS epidemic in the United States. Select a grade level, and outline the types of content that should be covered.
2. What types of guidelines and protocols do your state and local school district have regarding protecting teacher and school personnel against blood-borne pathogens?
3. What guidelines would you establish in your classroom for the prevention of diseases?

WEB SITE ACTIVITIES

Using the Reuters Health Information Services Web site, have the students investigate the site for daily stories on health and disease. The articles can be used for discussion purposes or used as resources for developing an investigation on a particular disease.

Select either the American Heart Association or the American Cancer Society Web site, and ask the students to investigate the type of information found at these sites. Have them select (or you can assign) a topic and report on the top ten facts they found concerning the assigned topic.

WEB SITES OF INTEREST

American Academy of Allergy & Immunology: *www.aaaai.org*
Information on asthma and other allergies.

American Cancer Society: *www.cancer.org*
Information on the various types of cancer, research, and treatments.

American Diabetes Association: *www.diabetes.org/default.asp*
Comprehensive source for information on all forms of diabetes and groups affected by the condition. Treatments, research, and publications are available.

American Heart Association: *www.amhrt.org*
Comprehensive site on heart disease and stroke.

Body Health Resources Corporation: *www.thebody.com/cgi-bin/body.cgi*
A multimedia AIDS and HIV information resource for learning about treatments and information concerning HIV/AIDS.

Centers for Disease Control and Prevention: *www.cdc.gov*
All types of health information can be found at this site, including information for various diseases and conditions, data and statistics related to diseases, and prevention.

National Institutes of Health: *www.nih.gov*
Web site to all other National Institutes and the health information for the various conditions and diseases each institute investigates and researches.

National Multiple Sclerosis Society: *www.nmss.org*
Information on multiple sclerosis.

Reuters Health Information Services: *www.reutershealth.com*
Latest information on medical and healthcare news.

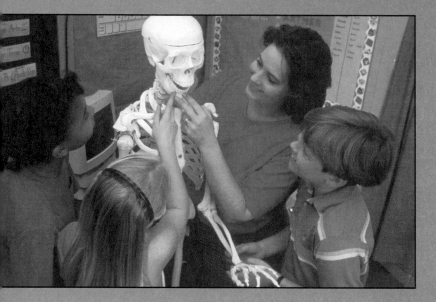

CHAPTER SIXTEEN

Strategies for Teaching about Infectious and Noninfectious Conditions

There is no shortage of good days, it is good lives that are hard to come by.

—Annie Dillard

VALUED OUTCOMES

After doing the activities in this chapter, the student should be able to express and illustrate the following guidelines:

- The diseases that are the leading causes of death in this century are the chronic diseases.

- Infectious diseases originate from pathogens.

- Protection against diseases is the work of the immune system.

- The function of the heart is to pump blood systematically and regularly through the body in order to regulate its chemical and thermal balance.

- Noninfectious diseases often develop over time, are frequently progressive, and can be positively affected by a wellness lifestyle.

Utilizing the content information for infectious and noninfectious diseases, select one disease or condition and develop the concepts that should be taught at a selected grade level. If you feel more emphasis should be placed on a particular content area, justify your feelings and outline the conceptual framework for that grade level.

Many of the values that protect and direct us as we grow are fostered during the elementary years. Learning at an early age about pathogens, the stages through which diseases progress, and lifestyles that are detrimental to high-level wellness can establish positive health values and habits. In addition, many chronic conditions detract from the quality of life for children. Awareness on the part of every teacher and child that children with chronic conditions can function effectively in the school setting improves the quality of life for the affected child.

As with other strategy chapters, the suggested grade level(s) for which the activity might be appropriate is shown to the right of each activity title. However, through modification, many of the suggested activities could be used at various grade levels. This modification could include changing the questions to be more age appropriate for the activity than those provided.

Value-Based Activities

HOW DID I GET IT?   Grades (4–6)

Valued Outcome: The students will be able to identify the risk factors associated with contracting an infectious disease.

Description of Strategy: Ask the students to think of someone who is seriously ill. Then ask them to identify some factors that may have been associated with the sick person's illness. Write the responses on the board. Make two lists, one for uncontrollable factors and one for factors that could have been better controlled if the person had followed a wellness lifestyle. Have students identify in which column each of their responses belongs. Do this for several different illnesses. You may also assign students to further research some of the conditions identified and how the illness can be prevented.

Materials Needed: board and markers

Processing Questions:

1. How many of the illnesses/conditions are related to lifestyle?
2. What lifestyle factors may have put the individual at greater risk for developing the condition?

3. Are there factors that cannot be controlled? (Point out that a wellness lifestyle can delay or prevent some of the genetic predispositions we have for certain diseases.)

4. Name some things you can do to prevent diseases.

5. What type of diseases/conditions would fall under the category of uncontrollable (hemophilia, for example)?

THE HELP I GET   Grades (5–8)

Valued Outcome: The students will appreciate the many defenses the body uses to protect them from disease.

Description of Strategy: Provide the students with a copy of the Teaching in Action box below, "The Help I Get." Have students write a brief description of how each defense listed on the handout helps protect their bodies. Then draw a line from each number in the figure to the corresponding body part. (*Example:* 3. Sweat helps our body maintain a constant temperature.) The various body

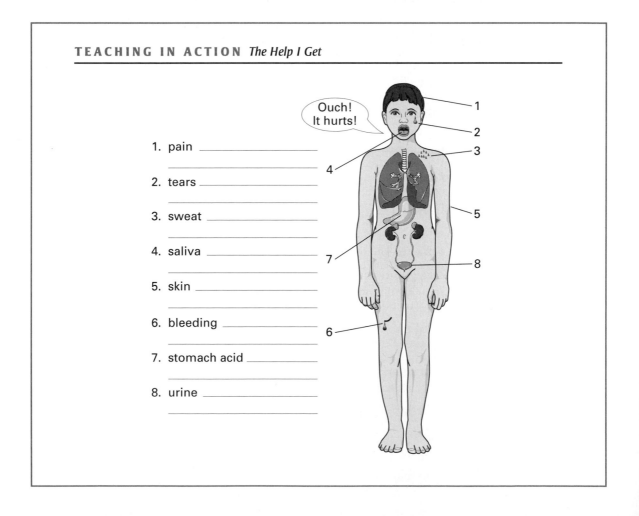

TEACHING IN ACTION *The Help I Get*

Ouch!
It hurts!

1. pain _____
   _____
2. tears _____
   _____
3. sweat _____
   _____
4. saliva _____
   _____
5. skin _____
   _____
6. bleeding _____
   _____
7. stomach acid _____
   _____
8. urine _____
   _____

defenses can be discussed in class or assigned as a group or individual activity for reporting findings back to the class.

Materials Needed: one copy of "The Help I Get" worksheet for each student, pens or pencils

Processing Questions:

1. What happens to our body defenses if we do not take care of our bodies?
2. Can you name all the body defense mechanisms?
3. How can we make sure our body defenses are operating at the highest level possible?
4. What are some lifestyle habits that inhibit our body defenses from operating at peak performance?

VALUES STATEMENTS   Grades (4–8)

Valued Outcome: The students will examine issues and lifestyle factors associated with various conditions.

Description of Strategy: The following list contains several unfinished sentences that can help initiate discussion. Use the list below or design your own questions to meet the individual needs of the students.

My heart is _____.

Smoking is _____.

Having someone sneeze on me _____.

I go to the doctor when _____.

A good diet _____.

People with diabetes should _____.

Cancer is _____.

If a friend had cancer, I _____.

Preventing heart disease _____.

AIDS is _____.

If I had a friend with AIDS, I _____.

Someone who is not feeling well should _____.

Materials Needed: none

Processing Question: none

FACTS AND MYTHS   Grades (2–5)

Valued Outcome: The students will determine what is true and false concerning various diseases and conditions.

Description of Strategy: The following are questions that students can be asked to vote on concerning heart disease, cancer, or infectious diseases. Other questions can be formulated for other topics. Have the students put their thumbs up

Health Highlight

A MOST PREVENTABLE SITUATION

Chronic disease has replaced infectious or commu-nicable disease as the leading cause of death in the United States. At the same time, however, some communicable diseases have been appearing more often. One such disease is measles, which has made a dramatic comeback. The major reason for

the increase in the incidence of measles is the fail-ure to immunize children at the recommended age intervals. This particular disease should be totally preventable if parents have access to the health care system in the United States.

if they agree and thumbs down if they disagree. Students can fold their hands if they have no opinion.

- Do you think exercise is good for your heart?
- Do you think your diet affects your heart?
- Do you think exercise is good for your health?
- How many think that there is no cure for cancer?
- Can you get cancer from another person?
- Can you get cancer from overexposure to the sun?
- Can infectious diseases be spread by sneezing?
- Do you think you should be around someone who is ill?
- Does washing your hands help prevent disease?

Materials Needed: none

Processing Question: none

Decision Stories

Follow the procedures outline on pages 80 to 83 for Decision Stories.

YOUR HEART'S EATING HABITS   Grades (4–6)

Jenny's grandmother recently had a myocardial infarction, or heart attack. The grandmother was only fifty-four years old. The heart attack was precipitated by the presence of atherosclerosis. Jenny's great-aunt, her grandmother's sister, died of heart disease when she was only sixty-one. Jenny's family eats a lot of food high in fat, and they all tend to be overweight. Jenny's mom and dad are concerned about the grandmother, and they are worried about Jenny's mom, who is thirty-four, and even Jenny, who is only eleven. The doctor has indicated that Jenny's family needs to change their eating habits, but they all really enjoy eating. Diets have never been successful in this family.

Focus Question: What are some options that Jenny and her family have in dealing with this problem?

MOLES CAN CHANGE   Grades (3–6)

Juan's dad has a mole on his foot that has been changing in appearance. It is growing and is an unusual black color. The mole has been on his dad's foot for as long as he can remember, but it has only recently changed in looks. Juan's dad insists that it is only because of the way his shoes have been rubbing his foot. Juan's mom has expressed some concern due to the changes. Juan knows that an obvious change in a wart or mole is one of the warning signals of cancer.

Focus Question: What should Juan's dad do?

PLAY BALL   Grades (2–5)

Sam has allergies in the spring. This year he is ten years old and wants to try out for the school baseball team, but tryouts occur when his allergies bother him the most. His parents told him he should just stay inside during the spring and wait until his allergies clear up. Sam says that playing baseball is really important to him. All his friends play on teams, and they have a really great time. Besides, Sam doesn't have anyone to play with because all his friends are involved in sports.

Focus Question: Should Sam try out for the baseball team or stay inside as his parents suggest?

Dramatizations

Two examples of dramatization are provided. These can be modified according to need and grade level.

BETTY BACTERIA   Grades (3–5)

Valued Outcome: The students will be able to describe how communicable diseases are spread through lack of sanitary habits.

Description of Strategy: Younger students can act out a skit stressing the importance of cleansing wounds. Discussion can include topics such as the importance of washing all wounds, cuts, and scrapes, as well as preventive care and washing hands at appropriate times. Ask the students to identify how germs are spread. Question the students on how they felt when they were becoming ill— list the symptoms on the board. Ask the students if they know how they "caught" their disease. Introduce the skit by telling the students they are going to see one way diseases can be contracted. The characters for the skit include Betty Bacteria; Zach, the little boy; Mother; and the Narrator.

Narrator:	*It is Saturday afternoon. Mother is outside washing the car when Zach comes running up.*
Zach:	Mom! Mom! (*Zach is crying.*) I hurt my leg, and it's bleeding very badly! Mom, make it stop hurting! (*Zach sits down and shows his mother his knee. Betty Bacteria is standing beside Zach's knee. She starts laughing.*)
Betty:	Now is my chance! I am going to get inside Zach's cut and infect it! I love to make people hurt! (*Betty moves closer and closer to Zach's cut.*)
Mom:	I know just what to do, Zach. First, we are going to wash it so that no germs will get inside of it and make you sick. Wait here while I get the soap and some medicine and a bandage.
Betty:	No! No! Don't use soap and water on me! I don't like soap and water! I can't live if soap and water are around and a cut is all clean. I better start making Zach's cut sick as quickly as I can. (*Betty touches Zach's knee with her hand as Zach's mom returns. Mom picks up the hose and washes off Zach's knee. Betty jerks her hand back.*)
Betty:	Stop! Stop! I don't like water. Water will make me go away, and I want to hurt Zach! (*Mom rubs the soap over Zach's knee and then rinses it off. Using a towel, she dries it and proceeds to put an antibiotic on the cut. Betty is crying and starts to shrivel up and go away.*)
Betty:	This is no fun. I can't live with soap and water. Soap and water are the end of me. (*Betty disappears offstage.*)
Mom:	Now your cut is nice and clean, and the medicine will keep any new germs from trying to hurt you. Do you feel better?
Zach:	I feel much better now, Mom. Thanks for taking care of my cut.

Materials Needed: a copy of the script for each actor, props for the skit (medicine container, Band-Aid, piece of hose, and soap)

Processing Questions:

1. What did you learn from today's lesson?
2. Can someone explain how disease germs are spread?
3. How can we prevent the spread of disease germs?

"CATCHING" COLD

Grades (4–6)

Valued Outcome: The students will describe how sneezing can spread disease.

Description of Strategy: The students role-play the following situation. Bill and Jay are eating lunch together. Bill has a cold. Bill sneezes (sprays a short squirt of water from a spray bottle) and doesn't cover his nose and mouth while sitting beside Jay. Jay is wiping himself off when Aimee comes up and sits down beside them. She asks Jay why he is so upset.

Materials Needed: one spray bottle of water that can be used as the "sneeze"

Processing Questions:

1. Why do you think Jay is upset?
2. What should Bill have done when he had to sneeze?
3. Do you think Jay can catch a cold from Bill? Why?
4. Can Aimee catch the cold from Bill, since he just sneezed?

Discussion and Report Techniques

DISEASE SEARCH

Grades (6–8)

Valued Outcome: The students will be able to identify the most common diseases and discuss how they might have been prevented.

Description of Strategy: Have the students ask their parents which chronic and communicable diseases have been experienced within the immediate family (parents, grandparents, aunts, and uncles). These diseases probably would include heart disease, cancer, arthritis, allergies, measles, chicken pox, mumps, and so on. Students can then bring in lists of these diseases and turn them in to be placed on the board. Going down the list, have students raise their hands if someone in their family has had the disease and record the totals for each disease on the board. When finished, note the diseases that have been experienced the most, ranking from least to most common.

Materials Needed: board, overhead projector, or butcher paper; markers

Processing Questions:

1. What are the diseases experienced most often by our group?
2. How many of the diseases listed have you personally had?
3. How could some of these diseases have been avoided?

NAME THAT DISEASE

Valued Outcome: Each student will be able to discuss the important signs and symptoms of various diseases.

Description of Strategy: Students working in groups can select a disease (infectious or chronic) and research the causes, signs or symptoms, and methods of treatment for the disease. The information should be placed on large sheets of paper and posted on the walls for each student to read. Oral reports may be given, using the large sheets as teaching aids.

Materials Needed: markers, butcher paper, and references for students to research the various diseases

Processing Questions:

1. What were some important points we learned about diseases in general?

2. For the diseases each of you read about, what were some facts that surprised you?

3. How are diseases treated?

WHAT SHOULD BE DONE?

Grades (6–8)

Valued Outcome: The students will be able to discuss the school policy concerning illness.

Description of Strategy: Allow the students to investigate the school policy on illness. Hold a discussion on appropriate actions to take when someone becomes ill. What should the teacher do? What should the students do? What is the responsibility of the school? How can the school nurse help (if one is available)? A variation of this strategy is to have the students write the policy and present it to the principal.

Materials Needed: copy of the school policy on illness for each student

Processing Questions:

1. Do you think the policies cover everything needed?

2. What would you do if a friend became ill?

3. What should be done if the school nurse is not at school when someone becomes ill?

Experiments and Demonstrations

PHYSICAL FITNESS TEST

Grades (6–8)

Valued Outcome: After participating in the various fitness tests, the students will be able to discuss how being fit enhances their health.

Description of Strategy: Physical fitness can contribute significantly to the prevention of cardiovascular diseases. Several groups have developed fitness tests for school-age children. One of the newest is published by the American Alliance for Health, Physical Education, Recreation, and Dance (AAHPERD). Physical Best is a comprehensive fitness education and assessment program that has three components. They are (1) a health-related fitness assessment, (2) an education component, and (3) a set of awards to reinforce positive health changes and recognize personal achievement. The fitness assessment contains norms for girls and boys, ages five to eighteen.

Materials Needed: materials from AAHPERD or other professional groups

Processing Questions:

1. What did you learn about your physical fitness level?
2. How does being physically fit make you a healthier person?
3. Does being physically fit protect you from diseases?

THE ANATOMY OF THE HEART   Grades (4–8)

Valued Outcome: The children will be able to identify the various structures of the human heart and explain the function of each.

Description of Strategy: Ask the meat department at the local grocery to donate a beef heart for dissecting purposes. (You should wear protective gloves while performing the dissection and handling the heart.) The class can observe as various structures and functions of the structures of the heart are noted. The atria, ventricles, aortas, and various valves can be pointed out.

Materials Needed: rubber gloves, scalpel, paper towels, chart of the structures of the human heart

Processing Questions:

1. How many pumping stations does the heart have?
2. What function does each part of the heart fulfill?
3. How does the blood get to the heart muscle?

WASH THOSE HANDS   Grades (K–4)

Valued Outcomes: The students will be able to discuss how germs are spread from person to person.

Description of Strategy: The purpose of this activity is to teach the students the importance of washing their hands. Stress that hands must be washed before eating or touching food, before setting the table, and after using the restroom. Have the students spray water on a piece of dark colored paper. Explain that sneezes and coughs spray germs the same way water sprays on paper. Consequently the mouth must be covered each time a person sneezes or coughs, and hands must be washed each time the person sneezes. Explain that hands may look clean, but germs are still present. Demonstrate for the class the proper way to wash hands. Emphasize that germs hide on the front and back of their hands as well as between the fingers and under the nails. To thoroughly wash hands, tell students to use soap and water and scrub all parts of their hands while singing at least the first two verses of "Yankee Doodle."

Materials Needed: spray bottle of water, dark-colored paper, soap, paper towels

Processing Questions:

1. Why does sneezing and coughing spread germs?
2. Why is it important to wash your hands?
3. How should we wash our hands?

ANALYZING CIGARETTE SMOKE   Grades (6–8)

Valued Outcome:

The students will be able to list the many harmful materials found in cigarettes.

Description of Strategy: This activity was developed by Dr. David White and Linda Rudisill. Due to the danger inherent in the chemicals involved, actual ingredients are not used. All ingredients represent by-products of cigarette use. The students are not informed about what the ingredients represent. They are to guess, based on their knowledge. The entire script is provided for the activity.

> **Lesson Focus:** How many of you have ever received products in the mail to sample, such as soap, shampoo, or toothpaste? The makers provide a small amount for us to try, and then we decide if we want to purchase the product. Suppose we could sample one of these products by breaking it down and trying the main ingredients, or analyzing it. (Teacher may want to discuss the meaning of analyze.) We might know much more about a product if we could analyze it, rather than simply trying a sample. The purpose of this lesson is to help you analyze a product that is used by millions of people in the United States. Its popularity, however, has been declining for several years. (Emphasize here that it is important not to comment on what the product is until instruction is complete. Have students write the name of the product on a sheet of paper when they think they have guessed correctly.)

> **Teacher Input:** I will NOT ask you to sample these items as I describe them. When I have completed the discussion, you can then decide if you want to try them. Remember, if you do not want to try it, your grade will NOT be affected.

> **Point to [two] balloons:** The product that we are analyzing is associated with over 500 gases and several thousand chemicals. Since I would have to go to a lot of trouble to bring you over 500 gases, I just brought two of them in balloons. This balloon contains some *carbon monoxide*. Joe, after I describe the other chemicals, would you please inhale the gas in this balloon? This gas is odorless, colorless, and although this amount should not hurt you, this gas is deadly. When you use this product, your blood transports five to ten times more carbon monoxide than normal [and carries the carbon monoxide instead of oxygen]. This is because carbon monoxide binds to hemoglobin about 240 times more strongly than oxygen.

> Now, Joe, I know what you are thinking. Why should only a guy try this? Sue, I would like you to choose a balloon and try it, too. Remember, if you use the average amount of this product daily, you will lose 6 to 8 percent of your body's oxygen-carrying capacity.

Point to [next two] other balloons: I have put another of the gases from this product in these balloons. This gas is *hydrogen cyanide.* Hydrogen cyanide is a gas that has been used in the gas chamber. When you use the product we are analyzing, the hydrogen cyanide paralyzes your cilia for 20 to 30 seconds. (Teacher may need to explain the functions of the cilia here.) Now, Carl, would you and Judy sample this ingredient by breathing the gas in these balloons? I'm fairly sure that the amount I have in here will not hurt you; however, remember that this gas paralyzes, or freezes, your cilia for 20 to 30 seconds each time you use this product.

Hold up the jar of flour (arsenic): In this jar I have a little arsenic. Kathy, would you sample this for us later? I have clean spoons for both you and Tom. Arsenic is a silvery-white, tasteless, poisonous chemical used in making insecticides. It looks like flour, and that is what it is mixed with in this jar. Arsenic is associated with the product we are analyzing.

Hold up a glass jar (about one cup) of chocolate syrup (tar): In this jar I have a brown sticky substance. If you use the average amount of the product we are analyzing, your body will collect about a cup of this brown, sticky substance a year. Tom, would you put your finger in this jar and then lick your finger?

Refer students to jar of clear syrup (nicotine): This substance is a poison. It can kill instantly in its pure form, but I have mixed it so that it will not kill you. It looks like clear syrup, so that is what it is mixed with. This poison is habit forming. It speeds the heart rate an extra 15 to 25 beats per minute, or as many as 10,000 extra beats a day. Also, it constricts the blood vessels and quickens breathing. George, would you sample this for us? Remember, a one-drop injection of this substance would cause death! Jean, you are so cooperative in class, would you mind doing this with George so he won't feel so uneasy? Also, when you use this product, this poison reaches your brain in only seven seconds. If it were not for this ingredient, people would probably not be interested in long-term use of the product we are analyzing.

Now, are you all ready to sample a few of the ingredients in this product? Before you answer, I want to give you some facts about this product. (Teacher can discuss or delete from this list, as is desirable.)

- If you start using this product now and continue, you can expect to lose six and one-half years of your life.

- If you use it a lot, your chances of dying between the ages of 26 and 65 are about twice as great as for those who do not use this product.

- Over 100,000 physicians have quit using this product.

- Before this day is over, approximately 4,500 young people will have tried or started using this product. By the time they graduate from high school, half the nation's teenagers will have used this product, 18 percent on a daily basis.

- About 1.5 billion of these products are used by 54 million Americans for an average of about 27 each day. The substances in this product are the primary cause of 360,000 known deaths a year, an average of 1,000 deaths a day.

- Using this product is one of the largest self-inflicted risks a person can take. It is responsible for more premature deaths and disability than any other known agent.

- More people die from using this product than seven times our annual death toll from highway accidents.

- A pregnant woman who uses this product may be affecting the health of her unborn child. Comparing users with nonusers, users have a higher percentage of stillbirths, a greater number of spontaneous abortions and premature births, and more of the infants die a few weeks after birth. The child's long-term physical and intellectual development may be adversely affected.

- This product will stain your teeth, and users often have bad breath.

   You might say, "Surely a person can stop using this product whenever he or she wants to." My reply is "not necessarily." Remember the habit-forming substance we mentioned. Withdrawal symptoms for using this drug often include tension, irritability, restlessness, depression, anxiety, difficulty in concentrating, overeating, constipation, diarrhea, insomnia, and an intense craving for the product.

   A few of the things I have not mentioned are:

- If you use this product, you are 1,000 percent more likely to die from lung cancer than those who do not use it.

- You are 500 percent more likely to die of chronic bronchitis and emphysema if you use it.

- Average users of this product are 70 percent more likely to die of coronary artery disease. They also tend to suffer from more respiratory infections, such as colds, than nonusers.

- Finally, this product is so dangerous that four rotating warning labels are required by law to be on the package.

   If you were sent this product in the mail to sample, would you be likely to try it? If you received a box in the mail and, on the outside, these facts were printed, would you try it?

Ask students to tell you what they think the product is. End the lesson with a statement about the importance of making wise decisions that influence your life in positive ways. For example, you might say, "You have the power to influence your future in vital ways. The choice is up to you. No one can keep you from smoking, and it definitely will affect your entire life, however short or long it may be. Why start and get hooked? If you want to smoke, it is your life. But it is the only one you will ever get. The only safe cigarette is an unlit cigarette."

Materials Needed: four balloons (two representing carbon monoxide and two representing hydrogen cyanide), one small glass jar of flour (representing arsenic), two spoons, one cup of chocolate syrup (tars), and one cup of clear syrup (nicotine)

Processing Questions:

1. Who is responsible for your using or not using cigarettes?

2. What are some of the bad things found in cigarettes?

3. What are some of the scariest things about cigarettes?

SOURCE: White and Rudisill 1987. Used with permission.

MINIDOCUMENTARY FOR CANCER
AND INFECTIOUS DISEASES

Grades (6–8)

Valued Outcome: The students will be able to discuss cancer and the many forms it can take.

Description of Strategy: The concept is for each child to be a "star" of his or her own television show. Set the activity up like the *Sixty Minutes* or *20/20* television programs. Videotaping the show allows everyone to see the production again. The videotape would be good for showing at Parent-Teacher Association functions.

Each student chooses a notecard on a particular area of cancer. On this card are several questions that the student will research and discuss. They are also given a title for themselves and may choose their own names. As an example, a student chooses "cancerous tumors." Her card will read:

Dr. _____, a leading oncologist from Harvard.

1. What are tumors?
2. What are two different types of tumors?
3. Are there any special tests to detect tumors?
4. Do tumors exhibit any special symptoms?

The rest is left up to the student. The student must find the correct answers and be able to report her findings on "television." The following is a list that could be consulted for the remaining cancer topics.

physiology of cancer cells	cancer of the prostate gland
cancerous tumors	cancer of the testes
most common causes of cancer	cancer of the larynx
carcinogens	oral cancer
warning signals of cancer	skin cancer
tests for cancer	cancer of the esophagus
treatments for cancer	cancer of the stomach
most common cancers in women	colorectal cancer
breast cancer	thyroid cancer
cancer of the uterus	Hodgkin's disease
most common cancers in males	leukemia
lung cancer	cancer in children
	the American Cancer Society

Two students must be chosen to fill the spots of commentator and interviewer. (The students who have the most enthusiasm and originality seem to be best suited for these roles.) The commentator's job is to introduce the show and make some concluding statements at the end, whereas the interviewer is responsible for accepting the notecards from the specialists, introducing them, and asking the questions. A small "set" consisting of chairs, a table, and a lamp could be constructed so that the camera operator can focus on both of the "stars" at once. To avoid confusion and allow continuity of the show while videotaping, a list should be posted so that everyone knows when her interview is coming up. The specialist takes her seat on the "set," gives her notecard to the interviewer, and when all is quiet, the camera operator says "ready . . . action!"

As soon as the interview is finished, the next specialist comes up and gets ready to go. The interviewee may also wear a lab coat and a stethoscope to add to the total effect. If each interview lasts one to two minutes, the whole show can be completed in a single class period. The students may be evaluated on their degree of research and their ability to answer the questions correctly. With a little enthusiasm, originality, and even humor, a fairly monotonous topic can be developed into an exciting and refreshing educational tool.

Even though cancer is a prime example of the topics that could be used, the minidocumentary does not need to be limited to cancer only. The same activity can be done using a variety of topics. The following is a list of possible topics for infectious diseases.

viruses	diphtheria	chicken pox
bacteria	whooping cough	common cold
fungi	tetanus	influenza
protozoa	poliomyelitis	tuberculosis
pathogens	measles	infectious
incubation period	German measles	mononucleosis
active immunity	mumps	infectious hepatitis
passive immunity		

Materials Needed: videotaping equipment, books and pamphlets for students to research the various topics, small set for videotaping (students can make this)

Processing Questions:

1. What new information did you discover from the television program?

2. What do all the various conditions discussed seem to have in common?

3. What are some things we might do to protect ourselves against such diseases?

DRAW A BUG   Grades (K–4)

Valued Outcome: The students will be able to identify what pathogens cause various diseases.

Description of Strategy: Show pictures of the various pathogens (viruses, bacteria, fungi, and so on; see Table 15.2 on page 425). Have the students draw and color one of the pathogens. On the board or overhead projector, list the names of various diseases. On their paper, have the students list the diseases caused by the pathogen they drew.

Materials Needed: pictures or drawings of the various pathogens, list of diseases, board or overhead projector and markers

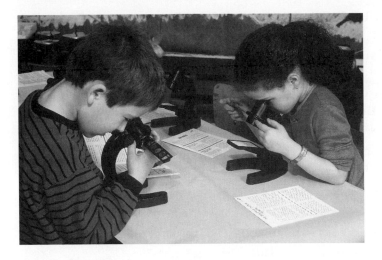

A microscope is an invaluable learning tool for students studying pathogens.

Processing Questions:

1. How many of the listed diseases did the pathogen you drew cause?

2. Are some of them more serious than others?

3. How can a certain pathogen cause so many illnesses?

THINGS I KNOW, THINGS I'D LIKE TO KNOW   Grades (4–6)

Valued Outcome: The students will identify and answer areas of concern for various diseases.

Description of Strategy: Select several diseases or conditions for students to investigate. The students must write down what they think is true concerning each disease. Students can then list some questions (establish a minimum number) they have concerning each disease. During investigation, they can determine the accuracy of their ideas on their specific disease and learn the answers to the questions they have written. Use the following form:

Disease or Condition:

Things I know	True	False	Things I'd like to know	Answers
1. _____	T	F	1. _____	_____
2. _____	T	F	2. _____	_____
3. _____	T	F	3. _____	_____
4. _____	T	F	4. _____	_____
5. _____	T	F	5. _____	_____

Materials Needed: one copy of the above form for each student

Processing Questions:

1. Was any of the information you thought you knew incorrect?

2. What was one new thing you learned from the activity?

THE "BERT BIRD KNOWS" MOBILE   Grades (K–4)

Valued Outcome: The students will be able to list the risk factors associated with various diseases and conditions.

Description of Strategy: Have the students construct a mobile as shown in the Teaching in Action box below. Each suspended card would be a risk factor for cardiovascular disease or some other disease. The bird can be reused as the students make cards for various other conditions or diseases.

Materials Needed: cardboard, paper, string or yarn, lists of factors for whatever condition is to be placed on the mobile

Processing Questions:

1. What can we do to protect ourselves against the factors listed on our Bert Bird?
2. Are any of the risk factors we have identified the same as for other conditions?
3. Of the factors listed, what seems to be the most serious?

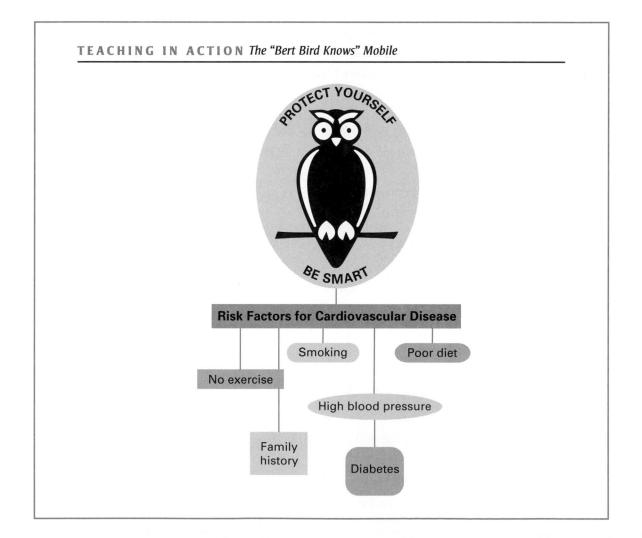

TEACHING IN ACTION *The "Bert Bird Knows" Mobile*

Puzzles and Games

Listed here are several suggestions for supplementing or building a lesson. Obviously you must design and develop these activities to fit your students' abilities. They are great fun and provide excellent learning tools.

HEART WORD SEARCH   Grades (4–6)

Instruct students to find and circle the terms listed in the word search shown in the Teaching in Action box below.

Materials Needed: copy of word search and pencils for each student

Processing Questions: none

TEACHING IN ACTION *Heart Word Search*

```
A C C Q E J D W S D M F Q H L N J E E
P F R I N S U E V F H T X G H I M L K
U I Y R S Y I Y V N Z R E X D X C V A
R Z V W H R V O S W Y W D S M S N P J
U D G T E W B E Z Z L Z O K U V S H A
W G P T O N N R I T Z T E M B O L U S
V B R W H T E I R N M L C S N M H O P
E A N O X Y H M G K S A Q M F G Z V Q
N W A T I V P H G B I M T M S X G S C
A D M M N P R E W D W A E E I M L S G
C F Z C Y K P I R N A N G I N A S Y W
A U R X W O A A N T D O A P A S Z T R
V E N T R I C L E S E R R X X P W C Q
A S T R O K E A P T G N X T W J F B N
K R T A H U M V R S V W S A A B S H A
C F S S Q O A A X D A T R I U M A E F
F S F A U T K Y G V I D X S O O I B N
I O L S F I E O N R O U W R N Z J T
B P I V H D R X L T N P M L G D O U Y
```

Can you find these words?

cardiac muscle	plaque	pacemaker	aorta	atrium
vetricles	veins	embolus	myocardium	stroke
vena cava	hypertension	angina	arteries	

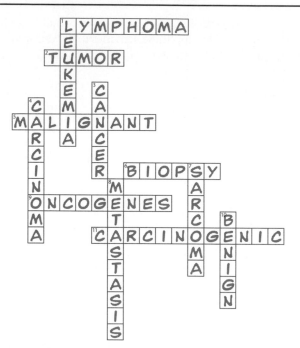

Across

1. Cancer affecting the lymph nodes
2. Abnormal growth
5. A term used to indicate a cancerous growth
6. Taking a small section of tissue to determine if it is cancerous is called a _____.
9. Genes thought to cause cancer
11. Any substance that may cause cancer is a _____ agent.

Down

1. A type of cancer affecting the white blood cells
3. Uncontrolled cell growth
4. Cancer of the soft tissue
7. Cancer of the connective tissue
8. When cancer cells move from one location in the body to another location
10. Noncancerous growth is a _____ tumor.

CANCER CROSSWORD PUZZLE   Grades (4–6)

Distribute copies of the crossword puzzle shown in the Teaching in Action box above, and have each student complete one.

Materials Needed: worsheets of crossword puzzle and pencils for each student

Processing Questions: none

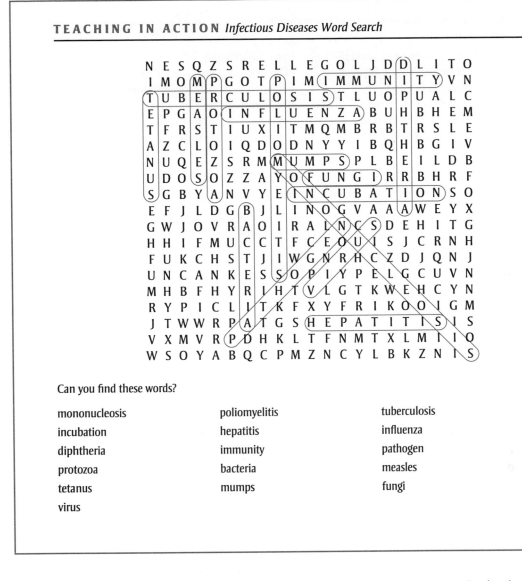

```
N E S Q Z S R E L L E G O L J D D L I T O
I M O M P G O T P I M I M M U N I T Y V N
T U B E R C U L O S I S T L U O P U A L C
E P G A O I N F L U E N Z A B U H B H E M
T F R S T I U X I T M Q M B R B T R S L E
A Z C L O I Q D O D N Y Y I B Q H B G I V
N U Q E Z S R M M U M P S P L B E I L D B
U D O S O Z Z A Y O F U N G I R R B H R F
S G B Y A N V Y E I N C U B A T I O N S O
E F J L D G B J L I N O G V A A A W E Y X
G W J O V R A O I R A L N C S D E H I T G
H H I F M U C C T F C E O U I S J C R N H
F U K C H S T J I W G N R H C Z D J Q N J
U N C A N K E S S O P I Y P E L G C U V N
M H B F H Y R I H T V L G T K W E H C Y N
R Y P I C L I T K F X Y F R I K O O I G M
J T W W R P A T G S H E P A T I T I S I S
V X M V R P D H K L T F N M T X L M I I Q
W S O Y A B Q C P M Z N C Y L B K Z N I S
```

Can you find these words?

mononucleosis	poliomyelitis	tuberculosis
incubation	hepatitis	influenza
diphtheria	immunity	pathogen
protozoa	bacteria	measles
tetanus	mumps	fungi
virus		

INFECTIOUS DISEASES WORD SEARCH   Grades (4–6)

For the word search in the Teaching in Action box above, ask each student to find and circle the designated words.

Materials Needed: copy of word search and pencils for each student

Processing Questions: none

WORD SCRAMBLE   Grades (5–8)

Have your students unscramble the following words (correct words appear in parentheses):

gahtposne (pathogens)   snxito (toxins)
brmeisco (microbes)   trovesc (vectors)
suvries (viruses)   tacinoibun gaste (incubation stage)
carebiat (bacteria)   odalmropr tagse (prodromal stage)
stekracisit (rickettsias)   yercover setag (recovery stage)
niguf (fungi)   ityummin (immunity)
orazotpo (protozoa)   gatinen (antigen)
nslehtmhi (helminths)

Materials Needed: list of words to unscramble and pencils for each student

Processing Questions: none

HIDDEN MESSAGE TO
HELP PREVENT HEART DISEASE   Grades (5–7)

Prepare a worksheet from the material below. Have each student complete the worksheet based on the following directions: Using the word list below, fill in the blanks in the sentences. Then place each answer in the corresponding spaces in the list at the top of the next page. The letters in the box reveal a hidden message.

pacemaker   hypertension   embolus
tobacco   cardiac   arteriosclerosis
aneurysm   veins   stroke

1. The heart is called the _____ muscle.

2. Cigarettes are made from _____.

3. Blood returns to the heart through the _____.

4. When a clot or vessel breakage occurs in the brain, that event is called a(n) _____.

5. High blood pressure is known as _____.

6. A free-floating blood clot is called a(n) _____.

7. _____ is the term for the collection of diseases characterized by hardening of the arteries.

8. The specialized group of cells called the sinoatrial node is also called the _____ of the heart.

9. Ballooning that occurs in weakened or damaged arterial walls is a(n) _____.

Place your answers here for the secret message.

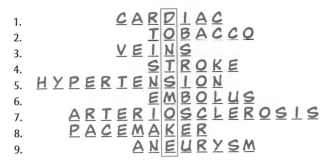

1. CARDIAC
2. TOBACCO
3. VEINS
4. STROKE
5. HYPERTENSION
6. EMBOLUS
7. ARTERIOSCLEROSIS
8. PACEMAKER
9. ANEURYSM

Materials Needed: copy of word search and pencils for each student

Processing Questions: none

Resources

BOOKS

Lammers, J. W. 1996. *I don't feel good—A guide to childhood complaints and diseases.* Santa Cruz, CA: ETR Associates. (Grades K–5)

Quackenbush, M., and Villarreal, S. 1995. *Does AIDS hurt? Educating young children about AIDS.* Santa Cruz, CA: ETR Associates. (Grades K–3)

Scheer, J. K. 1995. *Teaching kids about how AIDS works.* Santa Cruz, CA: ETR Associates. (Grades K–6 curriculum guides)

———. 1996. *Germ smart: Children's activities in disease prevention.* Santa Cruz, CA: ETR Associates. (Grades K–3)

Stang, L., and K. R. Miner. 1999. *Disease—Health facts.* Santa Cruz, CA: ETR Associates. (Grades 4–6)

Tillman, K. G., and P. R. Toner. 1990. *How to survive teaching health—Games, activities, and worksheets for Grades 4–12.* West Nyack, NY: Parker.

Vickery, D. M., and J. F. Fries. *Take care of yourself: A consumer's guide to medical care.* 1993. Reading, MA: Addison-Wesley. (Grades 4–8)

———. 2003. *How AIDS works—A curriculum for grades K–6.* Santa Cruz, CA: ETR Associates.

PAMPHLETS

HIV ABC's. Santa Cruz, CA: ETR Associates. Comprehensive information on HIV. (Grades 6 and up)

HIV fast facts—The basics. Santa Cruz, CA: ETR Associates. Explains the difference between HIV and AIDS, how you get it, and prevention strategies. (Grades 6–9)

WEB SITES

American Heart Association: *www.amhrt.org*

American Lung Association: *www.lungusa.org*

Center for AIDS Prevention Studies *www.caps.ucsf.edu/capsweb*

Centers for Disease Control and Prevention *www.cdc.gov*

Joint Committee on Smoking and Health *www.chestnet.org/smoking.html*

National Cancer Institute: *www.NCI.nih.gov*

Resource center focusing on tobacco and smoking issues: *www.tobacco.org*

University of Pennsylvania Medical Center *www.cancer.med.upenn.edu*

continued

CD-ROMS/COMPUTER SOFTWARE

Health education & (Grades 6–12)
prevention CD-ROMS
One of the CD-ROMs deals with smoking, encouraging students never to start and if having started, how to quit. Available from Sunburst Communications, 101 Castleton Street, Pleasantville, NY 10570-0040.

Human Health CD-ROM (Grades 7–12)
Looks at various health concerns including heart disease, cancer, and the auotimmune diseases. Available from NIMCO at *www.nimcoinc.com*.

Mosby's medical (Teacher; Grades 5–12)
encyclopedia for health consumers
A teacher resource that includes nearly 20,000 medical terms; audio pronunciations for over 4,000 terms; more than 1,200 full-color illustrations, video clips, and animations. Available from C.V. Mosby, 11830 Westline Industrial Drive, St. Louis, MO 63146.

VIDEOS

AIDS: The double connection (Grades 5–8)
Uses animated clay characters to explain how crack cocaine and other drugs can lead to unsafe sexual practices and to HIV infection. Explains how HIV is and is not transmitted. Available from The National Center for Elementary Drug and Violence Prevention, 117 Highway 815, P. O. Box 9, Calhoun, KY 42327-0009. (8 minutes)

Come see how we fight infections (Grades 3–6)
A series consisting of five informative and fun-filled videos. Titles include: *Come see what first aid can do; Come see about medicines; Come see about nutrition and exercise.* Available from Sunburst Communications, 101 Castleton Street, Pleasantville, NY 10570-0040. (Each video approximately 25 minutes)

Come see what the doctor sees (Grades 3–6)
Students get to see and listen through a doctor's instruments and learn various body functions. They also discover the "why" of blood and urine tests. Available from Sunburst Communications, 101 Castleton Street, Pleasantville, NY 10570-0040. (25 minutes)

Common childhood illnesses (Grades 5–8)
Addresses the common childhood illnesses, the symptoms, and possible home and professional care. Illnesses covered include ear infections, common colds, mumps, tonsillitis, measles, and abnormal bowel movements. Available from Films for the Humanities and Sciences, P.O. Box 2053, Princeton, NJ 08543-2053. (45 minutes)

Coping with childhood cancer (Grades 5–8)
Program presents five open and honest interviews with family members of childhood cancer patients. Available from Films for the Humanities and Sciences, P.O. Box 2053, Princeton, NJ 08543-2053. (28 minutes)

Kids and doctors (Grades 1–6)
Highlights the case of a ten-year-old boy with asthma and juvenile rheumatoid arthritis. Available from Films for the Humanities and Sciences, P.O. Box 2053, Princeton, NJ 08543-2053. (19 minutes)

Zardip's search for healthy wellness (Grades 1–5)
A twenty-part series of animation, live action, and songs to promote an understanding of how the body works. Disease-oriented videos include *Germs, More germs, The doctor, Hospital visit,* and *Laurie's operation.* Available from Films for the Humanities and Sciences, P.O. Box 2053, Princeton, NJ 08543-2053. (Each video 15 minutes)

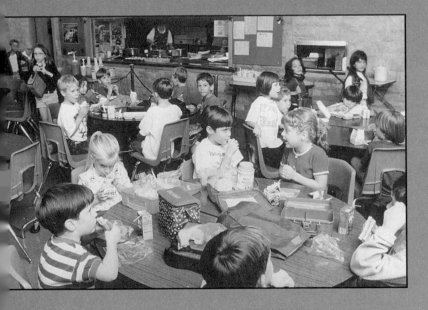

CHAPTER SEVENTEEN

Nutrition

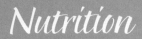

Eating well can reduce risk of
various health problems and
increase quality of life.

—Corbin et al. (2002, 311)

VALUED OUTCOMES

After reading this chapter, you should be able to:

- discuss the factors that determine food choices
- describe cultural differences in eating patterns and
preparation of foods
- discuss the U.S. Department of Agriculture's
Food Guide Pyramid
- list the basic function of the different food categories
- describe the Daily Values
- discuss the functions of vitamins and minerals in
the body
- explain the benefits of antioxidants
- list healthy ways to snack

- describe the effect of hunger and malnutrition on a student's physical and intellectual development
- describe the characteristics of an individual with anorexia and/or bulimia

- list several hints to help a student reduce or add weight
- determine the nutrient value of a food by reading the food label

REFLECTIONS

As you read this chapter, keep in mind the myriad factors (physical, social, emotional, and cultural) that affect nutritional health and fitness. Use this information to compose a complete plan for your fitness and wellness, including diet, exercise plan, change of any negative habits, stress reduction, and so on.

Knowledge and Nutrition

Human beings must eat to survive. Today, more is known about nutrition than at any other time in history, yet this knowledge has not translated into proper nutritional and/or lifestyle behavior for many people. The United States is a food-affluent society, yet many living here—and not just the poor—are malnourished (i.e., they have imbalanced nutrition from poor diet, overeating, or improper absorption). An unwillingness to alter one's lifestyle to meet sound nutritional standards and concessions to convenience are often at the heart of the problem. In our fast-paced society, people frequently skip meals, especially breakfast, or opt to eat a poorly balanced meal at a fast-food restaurant. Despite the fact that a well-nourished student is more apt to reach his or her full potential—physically, mentally, and intellectually—many parents and teachers fail to provide good examples for their students concerning nutritional habits.

Nutrition education has been included as a priority by the U.S. Department of Health and Human Services in the Year 2010 Health Objectives for the Nation, as listed by the U.S. Surgeon General (2003). The need for nutrition education is crucial. For example, U.S. elementary school students have higher cholesterol levels than students from other countries. According to the Food, Nutrition, and Consumer Services (FNCS), studies indicate that sound school nutrition programs can produce positive outcomes (USDA 2002b). Helping students develop sound nutritional habits should be a major goal in elementary health instruction. To accomplish this, teachers must do more than simply provide information; they must counter the impact of television commercials and other sources. Also, they must help students recognize that although the food they eat is strongly influenced by their culture and their lifestyle, they can learn to control these influences. Teachers must also dispel misconceptions associated with food and nutrition, help students become informed consumers, and help them develop a sense of the importance of nutrition.

THE THIRD REVIEW OF PROGRESS ON HEALTHY PEOPLE 2000

OBJECTIVES FOR NUTRITION

- Increasing body mass index (BMI) carries increased risks of heart disease, diabetes, and other chronic diseases in all populations, although there is some variation in absolute risk among different populations.

- The increase since 1980 in the prevalence of obesity in young children and youth is most probably associated with declining rates of participation in sports and other forms of physical activity. Only one state, Illinois, requires daily physical education in kindergarten through grade 12.

- A comprehensive school health program in Denver, CO, has had notable success in improving health and fitness levels of Hispanic children from families of lower socioeconomic status. The key is an integrated approach to enhancing both sound nutritional behavior and physical activity levels.

- Research on the mechanisms that control food intake and energy balance is increasing the understanding of the roles that genetic, behavioral, and physiological factors play in the development of obesity.

- Research on identifying the genetic susceptibility to obesity is advancing and should make possible the future identification of individuals who are particularly susceptible to becoming overweight.

- The Five-A-Day for Better Health Program is a multilevel (national, state, and local) nutrition education program and public–private partnership that encourages the daily intake of at least 5 servings of healthful fruits and vegetables. Data from California suggest that nutrition education must be continued over time to achieve lasting success; when suspended, consumption of fruits and vegetables drops.

- Not all vegetable products consumed are low in fat. The Continuing Survey of Food Intakes by Individuals conducted by the U.S. Department of Agriculture (USDA) found that one-third of vegetable servings consumed by persons 2 to 19 years of age in 1994–1996 were fried potatoes.

- Fruit and vegetable consumption varies by meal and day of the week. It is higher on Mondays and Tuesdays, lower on Fridays and Saturdays. Eating away from home also influences consumption.

SOURCE: Satcher 1998

Food Habits and Customs

Every culture has its own food habits and customs. Approaches to nutrition are based in part on the food resources available. Food habits and customs in the United States reflect the multicultural nature of our society. At one time, there were significant regional differences in cooking and food preferences. Seafood was a major part of the diet on the East Coast. Wild game provided much of the meat eaten in the rural South. Mexican and Indian cultures influenced the cuisine of the Southwest. Today, these regional differences have faded, largely as a result of refrigeration and modern transportation. It is now almost as easy to get fresh seafood in Kansas as it is in Massachusetts. Cultural intermixing has also diminished regional differences, while at the same time expanding the range of dishes commonly eaten. Pasta, for instance, is no longer eaten only by

Health Highlight
CHILDREN'S EATING PATTERNS

U.S. children are eating away from home more often now than 20 years ago. They are also consuming more beverages, grain-based snack foods, and combination foods (such as pizza) and are eating less fat and drinking less milk, according to data from the first year of the current 3-year USDA nationwide food consumption survey, *What We Eat In America*.

On any given day in 1994, nearly half of 3- to 5-year-olds consumed some food or drink provided outside the home, compared to one-third in the 1977–1978 survey. Food eaten away from home now contributes an average 20 percent of total calories for this age group.

Roughly two-thirds of school-age youths ages 6 through 19 consumed food and drink provided away from home in 1994, up from 55 percent in 1977–1978; on average, such food contributes about one-quarter of total calories for 6- to 11-year-olds, increasing to one-third of total calories for 12- to 19-year-olds. One in 3 school-age children get more than 40 percent of total calories from outside food.

Where are our kids eating out? The 3- to 5-year-olds most often ate at someone else's house, fol-lowed by fast-food restaurants and then daycare. Grade school–age children most often ate at the school cafeteria, followed by someone else's house and fast-food restaurants. By the teenage years, fast-food restaurants were the most frequent source of outside food for boys and a close second to the school cafeteria for girls.

Another upward trend is in consumption of beverages other than milk. The biggest increase has been in the consumption of noncitrus juices, including apple juice, grape juice, and juice blends; 2 to 3 times more children and teens drank noncitrus fruit juices on any given day in 1994 than in 1977–1978, and preschoolers consumed four times more of it. Soft drinks also had a dramatic increase in consumption among all groups, especially among teenage boys (whose intake nearly tripled between 1977–1978 and 1994). Nearly three-fourths of teenage boys drank an average of 34 ounces—almost three 12-oz. cans' worth—per day in 1994, and two-thirds of teenage girls averaged 23 ounces—about 2 cans' worth.

Milk consumption, on the other hand, has dropped markedly across all age and gender groups since the late 1970s. A little more than half

Americans of Italian heritage. Chinese, French, German, Mexican, and Middle Eastern dishes have also become popular.

ECONOMIC, PERSONAL, AND LIFESTYLE FACTORS

As an affluent, multiethnic nation, we have a greater variety of foods and dishes to choose from than almost any other people on earth. This does not mean, however, that Americans can afford to eat anything they like. Inflation has influenced the eating habits of all Americans, rich and poor alike—but especially the poor. Those living near or below the poverty level often must subsist on cheap starchy foods, which are filling but not particularly nutritious.

Although economics influences the U.S. diet, as it does the diet of every nation, most Americans cannot blame lack of money for poor nutritional habits. Instead, we must look for the reasons in personal preferences and lifestyles. Personal preference for a food often is formed by reasons that have little or nothing to do with the nourishment that will be provided by that food. For example, parents typically pass their food preferences on to their children. People develop dislikes for foods because of bad experiences, such as an allergic response or of teens drank milk in 1994, compared to some three-fourths in the late 1970s. Low-fat and skim milk are now consumed more frequently than whole milk among all but the 5-and-under group. The proportion of school-age youths drinking low- or no-fat milk has doubled since the late 1970s.

Other trends:

- U.S. youth reflected the national trend in consumption of crackers, popcorn, pretzels, and corn chips. The proportion of children and teens consuming these grain-based snack foods doubled between 1977–1978 and 1994, and they are slightly more popular among girls. Thirty-five percent of school-age girls ate at least one of these snack foods a day in 1994.

- Grain-based combinations, such as pasta with sauce, rice dishes, and pizza, also were more popular in 1994. About 45 percent of children and teens ate at least one of these combinations on a given day versus about 25 percent in the late 1970s. Pizza, tacos, and burritos are the most frequently reported grain combination foods among school-age children.

- Fruit consumption declines as children get older. Seven out of 10 children under age 5 consumed some fruit or fruit juice on any one day, dropping to less than half among teens. This decline is not seen for vegetables. At least three-fourths of all children, regardless of age, reported eating at least one vegetable on a given day. White potatoes like french fries and potato chips were most popular, followed by tomato products such as spaghetti-type sauces and salsa.

- Low on the vegetable hit parade are green beans, corn, green peas, and lima beans, with less than 16 percent of children or teens reporting having eaten them on a given day, and the percentage was even lower for the nutrient-packed dark greens or deep yellow vegetables.

- Today's youth are consuming less fat as a percentage of total calories, reflecting the trend for the population as a whole. In 1994, fat intake ranged from an average of 32 percent for teenage girls to 34 percent for preschoolers, as compared to the 37–40 percent range in the late 1970s.

- Children and teenage boys are meeting the Daily Values for most nutrients, but teenage girls averaged 85 percent or less of the RDA for calcium, magnesium, zinc, and vitamin E.

SOURCE: USDA 1996

gastrointestinal upset. The most popular foods eaten by one's subculture and peer group also influence food choices. Finally, a food might be chosen because of the way it looks, smells, and tastes.

The national lifestyle also influences our nutritional habits. When the United States was mostly a rural, agrarian society, breakfast was a major meal, and the main meal of the day was served at noon. These two meals provided the necessary energy for performing farm labor and chores. Evening dinner was typically a lighter meal. Today, the reverse is true. Most Americans eat a light breakfast, and some skip breakfast entirely. Lunch is also a light meal, often eaten in haste. The largest meal of the day is consumed in the evening, because there is more time to prepare and eat it. Unfortunately, this meal is usually followed by general physical inactivity and sleep. This is one reason why so many Americans are overweight. In addition, many overspice their foods, especially with salt and sugar. Others rush through their meals, which reduces the nourishment received from the food.

Breakfast seems to be the most frequently missed meal of the day, even though research has suggested that missing breakfast can affect concentration, ability to learn, and overall health. Recent studies have confirmed that eating

Health Highlight

DIETARY GUIDELINES FOR AMERICANS

Aim . . . Build . . . Choose . . . for Good Health

The fifth edition of *Nutrition and Your Health: Dietary Guidelines for Americans,* a joint publication of the U.S. Department of Health and Human Services and the Department of Agriculture (USDA), was released on May 30, 2000. This document serves as a guide to improve the quality of Americans' diets.

Aim for Fitness

Aim for a healthy weight.

Be physically active each day.

Build a Healthy Base

Let the USDA 's Food Guide Pyramid guide your food choices.

Choose a variety of grains daily, especially whole grains.

Choose a variety of fruits and vegetables daily.

Keep food safe to eat.

Choose Sensibly

Choose a diet that is low in saturated fat and cholesterol and moderate in total fat.

Choose beverages and foods to moderate your intake of sugars.

Choose and prepare foods with less salt.

If you drink alcoholic beverages, do so in moderation.

SOURCE: Garza et al. 2000

breakfast helps children learn better. Children who eat better perform better on standardized achievement tests and have fewer behavior problems. Other positive results from eating breakfast are improved math grades, reduced hyperactivity, decreased absence and tardy rates, and improved psychosocial behaviors compared with children who rarely ate school breakfast (Glickman 2002).

Teachers should emphasize the value of a balanced, nutritious lunch and a reasonable evening meal. This is not to suggest that teachers should criticize the eating patterns of any student's family or any religious dietary restrictions a family might have, but they can be a source of information about sound nutritional practices and encourage students to consider changes in their diet that could lead to improved nutrition. Teachers can also stimulate students' curiosity about trying new dishes that could add needed variety to their diets.

Further, teachers should emphasize that snacking on junk food, such as candy, may spoil a student's appetite for a regular meal as well as contribute to tooth decay. Although children can benefit from snacking, they often fall into the habit of constantly eating the same foods. Snacks sometimes even substitute for, rather than supplement, children's regular meals, and these snacks may not provide the variety of nutrients these youngsters need. Thus, while snacking is regarded as a potential asset to the child's diet, it can become a liability if it results in more calories than are needed. Most commercial snacks are high in fat, sugar, or salt and have few healthful nutrients.

According to the U.S. Department of Agriculture (USDA) approximately seven million children eat a school breakfast, and about twenty-five million children eat a school lunch on a daily basis. About 69,000 schools nationwide offer breakfast at school, and over 94,000 schools offer school lunch. Over the last ten years, participation in the school breakfast program has nearly doubled (USDA 2003).

Food is one of the delights of every civilization. In many cultures, preparation of some dishes is an art. Eating a fine meal is an aesthetic experience, not just fulfillment of nutritional requirements, and even the simplest dish can provide great pleasure. Teachers can use this positive approach in presenting nutritional concepts. Too often nutrition is taught as a grim and dry subject, divorced from the human perspective. No wonder students often emerge from health education with scorn for nutritional principles; they associate nutrition with the imagined somber atmosphere of a health food store!

Nutrients

The most basic function of food is to provide nutrients to the body. **Nutrients** are the substances in food needed to support life functions. One vital role of nutrients is to provide energy that the body needs. This energy, produced as a byproduct of food consumption, is measured in calories. A **calorie** is the amount of heat energy required to raise the temperature of one kilogram of water one degree Celsius. All foods have specific caloric values, and a given amount of food will produce a certain number of calories when broken down by the body.

The number of calories needed daily by the body depends on two factors: (1) the individual's basal metabolism and (2) the amount of energy expended in daily activities. **Basal metabolism** is the minimum amount of energy required by the body to maintain essential body functions (e.g., to maintain a normal body temperature, muscle tone, respiration) when at rest. The amount of energy expended by an individual varies, depending on his or her activities. Thus, someone who engages in heavy physical labor each day needs more calories than someone who works in an office. Young students need fewer calories per day than active adults because of the difference in body sizes.

During periods of rapid growth, children also need more calories. For example, a ten-year-old boy requires an average daily intake of about 2,200 calories, with this amount rising to 2,900 calories by age thirteen. A girl requires an average daily intake of 2,200 calories at age ten and 2,400 calories at age thirteen. Three categories of nutrients provide caloric energy: carbohydrates, lipids, and proteins. Together, they comprise most of the foods we eat.

CARBOHYDRATES

Foods rich in carbohydrates form about half of the typical American diet. Carbohydrates are either simple sugars, derived from such foods as sugar and honey, or more complex compounds, derived from such foods as cereals and potatoes. For example, the sweet taste of corn and peas is due to the presence of carbohydrate compounds.

Carbohydrates are found in foods as monosaccharides, disaccharides, and polysaccharides. The monosaccharides are glucose, galactose (found in human breast milk), and fructose, all of which are found in fruits and honey. The disaccharides are sucrose (a combination of glucose and fructose found in table sugar, bananas, green peas, and sweet potatoes), lactose (a combination of glucose and galactose found in milk), and maltose (a combination of two glucoses used in candy flavor and brewing beer). Many adults, especially Asian Americans and African Americans, suffer from lactose intolerance. In other words, undigested lactose is not absorbed and remains in the gastrointestinal tract, resulting in bloating, a large amount of gas, and abdominal cramping. This malady can be treated through a diet that is high in protein, high in carbohydrates, low to moderate in fat, and high in calories. The polysaccharides are composed of many monosaccharide molecules and are categorized as: (1) glycogen (which is synthesized in the liver and muscles and serves as a reserve source of blood glucose), (2) cellulose (found in many vegetables but indigestible by humans), and (3) starch (found in plant seeds, cereal grains, and some vegetables).

Carbohydrates are broken down into their components, and the metabolism of glucose is the most significant source of energy. (Glucose is the *only* energy source used by brain cells and acts as the most common energy "currency.") Four calories are produced per gram of carbohydrates. If carbohydrates are not abundant in the diet, protein and fat have to be metabolized to produce needed energy. Carbohydrates must be constantly replenished in the blood, either by eating or by breaking down glycogen that is stored in the liver and muscles.

Carbohydrates are important in a child's diet and should comprise approximately 60 percent of total caloric intake. Foods rich in carbohydrates include rice, pasta, noodles, bread, breakfast cereals, and potatoes. Many vegetables, fruits, and fruit juices are primarily carbohydrates. Although candy and cookies are sources of carbohydrates, the refined sugar they contain contributes to tooth decay and gum disease and does not provide additional nutrients; they also contain a high proportion of fat. Fruits, vegetables, juices, and milk make healthier snacks, but even these foods contain sugar. Thus, the individual should brush and floss immediately after the meal or at least rinse out the mouth with water. Brushing and flossing before bedtime are especially important in reducing tooth decay.

Dietary Fiber. Dietary fiber is a generic term for nondigestible carbohydrates (including cellulose, lignin, and pectin) found in plants; it has important health benefits in childhood, especially in promoting normal laxation (bowel movements). In addition, consuming fiber as part of the diet may help reduce the risk of heart disease, some cancers (such as colon cancer), obesity, hemorrhoids, and diverticular disease. The National Cancer Institute recommends a daily intake of 20 to 30 grams (g) with an upper limit of 35 g per day. A new recommendation from the American Health Foundation proposes that a reasonable goal for dietary fiber intake during childhood and adolescence may be the child's age plus 5 g per day, or the "age plus 5" rule (FDA 2002).

Despite intensive efforts by nutritionists, manufacturers, and others in the health care industry to promote the virtues of fiber, intakes remain below the recommended level. From 1989 to 1991, children consumed 11.8 g of fiber per day, or 88 percent of the "age plus 5" recommendation. Research has established that diets low in fat and high in fiber-containing grain products, fruits, and vegetables can reduce some types of cancer. Unfortunately, U.S. diets tend to be high in fat and low in grain products, fruits, and vegetables. The dietary goals promoted by the U.S. Food and Drug Administation (FDA) and other federal government agencies and health professional organizations recommend decreased consumption of fats; maintenance of desirable body weight; and an increased consumption of fruits, vegetables, and grain products (FDA 2002).

PROTEINS

Protein means primary, which suggests that **proteins** are essential nutrients. No organism can live, and almost no biological process can take place, without protein. A protein molecule is composed of smaller structures called *amino acids.* Eight amino acids (nine in infants) are termed *essential,* which means they must be provided by the diet; the remainder are termed *nonessential,* which means they are synthesized by the body. (All twenty amino acids are required by the body for proper nutrition.) These amino acids are building blocks necessary for performing many body functions. Proteins are present in every cell, in enzymes, and in body secretions. Proteins provide calories but also serve other important and complex functions. They help build new cells and tissues in growing children; repair damaged tissues; maintain tissues that are already built; and play a role in the manufacture of blood, enzymes, hormones, and human milk. Even antibodies, which combat infection, are synthesized from proteins in response to infectious agents.

Proteins provide four calories per gram. Proteins should comprise about 10 to 12 percent of a child's total caloric intake. Most children require approximately 60 g of protein daily. Milk and meat products (including poultry) are excellent sources of protein.

If a person eats a vegetarian diet, enough protein must be ingested to support normal growth and development. This requires **complementary protein ingestion,** a dietary strategy that ensures that each food supplies some amino acids that the others lack. For example, corn is deficient in the amino acids isoleucine and lysine, so it is often eaten with beans (which lack the tryptophan and methionine found in corn); similarly, wheat is deficient in lysine, so it may be combined with beans for nutritional completeness. Cereal grains, vegetables, and fruits contain vegetable protein, which must be augmented by other protein sources, as in tortillas and beans combined. Peanut protein is combined with wheat, oats, corn, rice, or coconut, and soy protein is combined with corn, wheat, rye, or sesame. Nonmeat sources of protein include soybeans, dried beans, nuts, and dairy products. In order for the appropriate nutrition to be achieved, however, the complementary foods must be eaten at the *same* meal.

LIPIDS

Lipids are an important part of our diet and are required for good health. **Lipids** are organic compounds that do not readily dissolve in water; based on their solubility, they are classified into triglycerides (neutral fats), phospholipids, steroids, and other lipoids. The energy of *triglycerides* provides much of the stored energy of the body, and the fat deposits insulate body organs against changes in environmental temperature and protect the organs and underlying tissues by acting as a shock absorber. Fats serve as carriers for absorption of the fat-soluble vitamins (A, D, E, and K), all of which are lipids. As food, they provide flavor and even contribute to satiety because the rate at which a meal is emptied from the stomach is related to the fat content, and the higher the fat content of a meal, the slower the food empties from the stomach.

Phospholipids are an essential component of all cell membranes and thus are ubiquitous throughout the human body. *Steroids* include cholesterol and its derivatives, such as vitamin D, the sex hormones (estrogen, progesterone, and testosterone), and hormones that regulate various body functions. *Other lipoid substances* include the prostaglandins, which are derived from fatty acids and have roles in such key functions as regulating blood pressure and gastrointestinal motility, and the lipoproteins, which transport cholesterol and fatty acids in the blood. Two major lipoproteins are high-density lipoprotein (HDL) and low-density lipoprotein (LDL), both of which carry cholesterol (discussed in further detail on page 491). A third type is very-low-density lipoprotein (VLDL), which transports triglycerides.

Triglycerides (Neutral Fats). The triglycerides, or neutral fats, are commonly called **fats** (which are solid at room temperature) and **oils** (which are liquid at room temperature). They are a group of chemical compounds that contain fatty acids, often in very long strands, and are the most concentrated source of usable energy in the body. Some fat is needed in the diet to supply essential fatty acids to build new fat molecules, and these fat molecules are stored in deposits throughout the body, including a layer just below the skin, where they can be accessed when energy is needed for growth or body maintenance.

There are two main types of fatty acids: saturated and unsaturated (the latter is further broken down into monounsaturated and polyunsaturated fatty acids). All fatty acids are molecules composed mostly of carbon and hydrogen atoms. A **saturated fatty acid** has the maximum possible number of hydrogen atoms attached to every carbon atom, so it is said to be saturated with hydrogen atoms; there are only single bonds between the carbon atoms. Some fatty acids have a double bond between two of the carbons and thus lack a pair of the hydrogen atoms found in saturated fatty acids; these double-bonded carbons are called units of unsaturation (since some hydrogen atoms are missing). If only one pair of hydrogen atoms is missing, the molecule is a **monounsaturated fatty acid;** if more than one pair of hydrogen atoms is missing, the molecule is a **polyunsaturated fatty acid.** Two types of polyunsaturated fatty acid, omega-3 and omega-6, are identified on the basis of where these double bonds and missing hydrogen atoms occur. The more saturated a fat is (i.e., the more hydrogen atoms and the fewer the double bonds between carbon atoms that it has), the more solid it is at room temperature.

Recently a new term has been added to the fat lexicon: **trans fatty acids.** These are byproducts of partial hydrogenation, a process by which some of the missing hydrogen atoms are put back into polyunsaturated fats during food processing. Some of the hydrogenated fatty acids take on a straighter structure as hydrogen atoms are added on diagonally opposite ends of the double carbon bond: these are the trans fatty acids. The straightened fatty acids pack more tightly together, so the resulting hydrogenated vegetable oils (such as vegetable shortening and margarine) are solid at room temperature.

Saturated fatty acids are mostly found in foods of animal origin such as animal fat, beef, butter, chicken eggs, and whole milk. Unsaturated fatty acids are mostly found in foods of plant origin, including vegetable oils (corn, olive, soybean, peanut, and safflower oils) and some seafoods. Olive and canola oils are particularly high in monounsaturated fats; most other vegetable oils, nuts, and high-fat fish are sources of polyunsaturated fats.

Cholesterol. All the cholesterol the body needs is made by the liver. It is used to build cell membranes and brain and other nervous tissue. Among other functions, cholesterol helps the body produce steroid hormones needed for the regulation of blood sugar, salt and water balance, production of bile acids needed for digestion, and reproduction.

A person's cholesterol number refers to the total amount of cholesterol in the blood. Cholesterol is measured in milligrams per deciliter (mg/dl) of blood. (A deciliter is a tenth of a liter.) Doctors recommend that total blood cholesterol be kept below 200 mg/dl; the average level in adults in this country is 205 to 215 mg/dl. Studies in the United States and other countries have consistently shown that total cholesterol levels above 200 to 220 mg/dl are linked with an increased risk of coronary heart disease.

Cholesterol is transported in the bloodstream in large molecules of fat and protein called **lipoproteins.** Cholesterol carried in low-density lipoproteins is called **LDL-cholesterol;** most cholesterol in the blood is of this type. Cholesterol carried in high-density lipoproteins is called **HDL-cholesterol.** LDL-cholesterol and HDL-cholesterol act differently in the body. A high level of LDL-cholesterol in the blood increases the risk of fatty deposits forming in the arteries, which in turn increases the risk of a heart attack; thus, LDL-cholesterol has been dubbed the bad cholesterol. Some very recent though not universally accepted studies have suggested this risk of LDL-cholesterol causing fatty acid deposits in the arteries increases if the LDL-cholesterol has undergone a chemical change known as oxidation. On the other hand, an elevated level of HDL-cholesterol seems to have a protective effect against heart disease, so HDL-cholesterol is often called good cholesterol. A common misconception is that people can improve their cholesterol numbers by eating good cholesterol; however, in food, all cholesterol is the same. In blood, whether cholesterol is good or bad depends only on the type of lipoprotein (HDL or LDL) that is carrying it.

Recommended Blood Levels of Lipoproteins and Triglycerides. In 1992, a panel of medical experts convened by the National Institutes of Health (NIH) recommended that individuals should have their HDL levels checked along with their total cholesterol. According to the National Heart, Lung, and Blood Institute (NHLBI), part of NIH, a healthy person who is not at high risk for heart disease and whose total cholesterol level is in the normal range (around 200 mg/dl) should have an HDL level of more than 35 mg/dl and an LDL level of less than 130 mg/dl in order to minimize the risk of heart disease.

The NIH panel also advised that individuals with high total cholesterol or other risk factors for coronary heart disease should have their triglyceride levels checked along with their HDL levels. NHLBI considers a triglyceride level below 200 mg/dl to be normal. It is not clear whether high levels of triglycerides alone increase an individual's risk of heart disease. However, they may be an important clue that someone is at risk of heart disease for other reasons. Many people who have elevated triglycerides also have high LDL or low HDL levels. People with diabetes or kidney disease—two conditions that increase the risk of heart disease—are also prone to having high triglycerides.

Health Implications and Diet. The vital roles of lipids are sometimes overlooked because of the association of fats with cardiovascular problems. Most people are aware that high levels of saturated fat and cholesterol in the diet are linked to increased blood cholesterol levels and a greater risk for heart disease and certain cancers. In countries where the average person's blood cholesterol level is less than 180 mg/dl, very few people develop atherosclerosis or have heart attacks. In many industrialized countries where diets are heavy with meat and dairy products (and thus contain a lot of saturated fats) and a lot of people have blood cholesterol levels above 220 mg/dl, coronary heart disease is the leading cause of illness and death and there is a high rate of certain cancers that have been linked to high fat intake. Blood lipids are major risk factors for heart disease, and their concentrations are modulated by both genetic and environmental factors. Among the latter, dietary habits (most specifically the consumption of large quantities of dietary fat and cholesterol) play an important role.

However, high-fat diets and high rates of heart disease don't inevitably go hand-in-hand. More Americans are now eating less fat, less saturated fat, and fewer cholesterol-rich foods than in the recent past, and fewer people are dying from the most common form of heart disease. Still, many people continue to eat high-fat diets, the number of overweight people has increased, and the risk of heart disease and fat-related cancers remains high.

Fat, whether from plant or animal sources, contains twice the number of calories of an equal amount of carbohydrate or protein (9 calories per g of fat as compared with 4 calories per g of protein or carbohydrate). By the time a person reaches the age of two, fat should comprise only 30 percent of the total calories consumed. (Infants and young children should not restrict dietary fat intake.) The upper limit on the grams of fat in a diet will depend on the actual amount of calories needed, and cutting back on fat can help reduce the number of calories consumed. For example, at 2,000 calories per day, the suggested upper limit of calories from fat is about 600. Sixty-five g of fat contribute about 600 calories (65 g of fat $\times$ 9 calories per g = 585 calories). On the Nutrition Facts label (see Figure 17.1), 65 g of fat is the Daily Value for a 2,000 calorie intake.

Fats contain both saturated and unsaturated (monounsaturated and polyunsaturated) fatty acids. Saturated fat raises blood cholesterol more than other forms of fat do. Reducing saturated fat to less than 10 percent of the total calories will help lower blood cholesterol level; on the Nutrition Facts label, 20 g of saturated fat (9 percent of caloric intake) is the recommended Daily Value for a 2,000 calorie diet. The fats from meat, milk, and milk products are the main sources of saturated fats in most diets. Many bakery products are also sources of saturated

Calories

Total calories are listed, as well as calories from fat. So in a serving of this product, 120 of the 260 calories are from fat. To calculate percent calories from fat, divide the calories from fat (120) by the total calories (260) per serving and multiply by 100.
120 ÷ 260 = .46
.46 x 100 = 46% of the calories are from fat.

Nutrition Facts

Serving Size: 1 cup (228g)
Servings Per Container: 2

Amount Per Serving

Calories 260 Calories from Fat 120

% Daily Value*

Total Fat 12g	20%
Saturated Fat 5g	25%
Cholesterol 30mg	10%
Sodium 660mg	28%
Total Carbohydrate 31g	10%
Dietary Fiber 0g	0%
Sugars 5g	
Protein 5g	

Vitamin A 4%	•	Vitamin C	2%
Calcium 15%	•	Iron	4%

* Percent Daily Values are based on a 2,000 calorie diet. Your daily values may be higher or lower depending on your calorie needs:

		Calories:	2,000	2,500
Total Fat	Less than		65g	80g
Sat Fat	Less than		20g	25g
Cholesterol	Less than		300mg	300mg
Sodium	Less than		2,400mg	2,400mg
Total Carbohydrate			300g	375g
Dietary Fiber			25g	30g

Calories per gram:
Fat 9 • Carbohydrate 4 • Protein 4

Serving Size

Similar food products now list similar portion sizes, which makes nutritional comparisons between products easier. Serving sizes are listed in common household (i.e., cups) and metric (i.e., grams) measures. The serving size listed now reflects amounts of food people typically eat.

% Daily Value

% Daily Value shows how a food fits into the overall daily diet based on a daily intake of 2,000 calories. Use these values as a guide to see if a food is high or low in a nutrient and to compare similar food products.

Daily Value Footnote

Some labels provide Daily Values, the recommended intakes of the nutrients listed for both a 2,000 and 2,500 calorie intake. Your daily values may be higher or lower depending on your calorie intake.

Calorie Conversion Information

Some labels provide the number of calories in one gram of fat, carbohydrate, and protein.

Figure 17.1
Interpreting Nutrition Labels

fats, and vegetable oils supply smaller amounts as well. Polyunsaturated and monounsaturated fats do not promote the formation of artery-clogging fatty deposits the way saturated fats do. Both kinds of unsaturated fats reduce the levels of LDL-cholesterol when they replace saturated fats in the diet; however, today many researchers believe that polyunsaturated fats may simultaneously decrease the beneficial HDL-cholesterol levels. For example, omega-6 polyunsaturated fatty acids have been found in some studies to reduce both LDL and HDL levels in the blood. Linoleic acid, an essential nutrient (one that the body cannot make for itself) and a component of corn, soybean, and safflower oil, is an omega-6 fatty acid. Partially hydrogenated vegetable oils containing polyunsaturated trans fatty acids may raise blood cholesterol levels, though not as much as saturated fat.

Edible oils rich in monounsaturated fats, such as olive and canola oil, tend to lower LDL-cholesterol without affecting HDL-cholesterol levels. The fats in most fish are low in saturated fatty acids, and fish such as mackerel and salmon (as well as soybean and canola oil) contain omega-3, a polyunsaturated fatty acid that lowers LDL and triglyceride levels and is under investigation for its possible potential to decrease the risk of heart disease in certain people. Some nutrition experts recommend eating fish once or twice a week to reduce heart disease risk. Dietary supplements containing concentrated fish oil are not recommended, however, because there is insufficient evidence that they are beneficial and little is known about their long-term effects (Mayfield 1999).

The body makes the cholesterol it requires and supplements this supply with cholesterol from food sources. Many people are confused about the effect of dietary cholesterol on blood cholesterol levels because, at first glance, it seems reasonable to think that eating less cholesterol would reduce a person's cholesterol level. In fact, eating less cholesterol has less effect on blood cholesterol levels than eating less saturated fat. However, some studies have found that eating cholesterol increases the risk of heart disease even if it doesn't increase blood cholesterol levels (Mayfield 1999).

The Nutrition Facts label lists the Daily Value for dietary cholesterol at 300 mg. Because dietary cholesterol comes largely from animal sources, many of which are also high in saturated fats, an individual generally can keep cholesterol intake at or below this level by eating more grain products (the less processing, the better), vegetables, and fruits, and by limiting intake of animal-based products.

Research focusing on the effects of different combinations of dietary fats and cholesterol on plasma lipid levels and removal of cholesterol from cells indicates that, when consuming diets low in cholesterol, the lipid levels in blood are better in subjects consuming high levels of oleic acid (a monounsaturated fatty acid found in almost all natural fats and promoted in the Mediterranean diet) than in those consuming low-fat diets. (The Mediterranean diet promotes the use of monounsaturated fatty acids, olive oil, and seafoods.) However, when people consume high cholesterol diets, the difference between diets containing high or low fat disappears. This suggests that reducing the intake of dietary cholesterol is an adequate initial recommendation to lower blood lipids, and, once this goal has been achieved, a diet rich in oleic acid may offer more cardiovascular protection than one low in total fat (Blanco-Molina et al. 1999).

What, then, *is* a healthy diet? Several medical societies have recommended reducing dietary intake of total and saturated fats and cholesterol; however, there is no total agreement, and some investigators suggest that emphasis should be placed on reducing the intake of saturated fat rather than total fat. Now, however, the advice is simply to reduce dietary intake of all types of fat (Mayfield 1999). Select foods that are lower in total fat, saturated fat, and cholesterol, which means eating fewer foods of animal origin (such as meat and whole-milk dairy products) and replacing those dietary calories by eating more grain products, fruits, vegetables, low-fat milk products or other calcium-rich foods, and more beans, lean meat, poultry, fish, and other protein-rich foods.

WATER

In considering nutrition, water is often overlooked, but it is second only to oxygen in importance to body functioning. A person can survive longer without food than water; there can be no life without water.

Water is an essential component of body structure. It also acts as a solvent for minerals and other physiologically important compounds. In the body, it transports nutrients to and waste products from the cells and water helps regulate body temperature. Water comes from fluids and solids in the diet and also is produced by the metabolic processing of energy nutrients within the tissues. Foods high in water content include fruits and vegetables; foods with low water content include meat. The amount of activity and the climate are important factors influencing the amount of water a person needs. Because children usually participate in more physical activities, they perspire more and therefore need more water than do many adults. Water is also lost through exhaled air. The recommended daily intake is the equivalent of six to eight glasses of water. Much of this is gained from solid foods.

MINERALS

The body needs organic compounds, such as carbohydrates, fats, and proteins, for proper nutrition, but it also needs inorganic materials such as minerals. These inorganic elements are present in the body in small amounts, but they play a vital role in nutrition. The major minerals needed by the body are calcium, phosphorus, potassium, sulfur, sodium, chloride, and magnesium. Food sources for these major minerals are:

> **calcium**—milk, cheese, sardines, salmon, green vegetables
>
> **phosphorus**—milk, cheese, lean meat
>
> **potassium**—oranges, bananas, dried fruits
>
> **sulfur**—eggs, poultry, fish
>
> **sodium**—table salt, beef, eggs, cheese
>
> **chloride**—table salt, meat
>
> **magnesium**—green vegetables, whole grains

Health Highlight
WATER CONTENT OF VARIOUS FOODS

Below are some interesting facts about the water content of foods we eat.

Breads: Most breads contain about 38 percent water.

Dairy Products: Soft cheeses contain around 58 percent water, hard cheeses contain approximately 38 percent, butter and margarines contain around 16 percent, and low-fat spreads are around 50 percent water. Milk contains 90 percent water, cream contains between 48 to 79 percent.

Fish and Shellfish: The water contents of various fish are similar, with cod, haddock, lemon sole, and trout consisting of 75 percent water and shellfish consisting of up to about 85 percent.

Fruit: Most fruits are 75–80 percent water, melons contain a higher percentage of water (90 percent) than other fruits.

Jams: Honey contains 23 percent water, while fruit jams contain 30 percent. Reduced-sugar jam has greater water content; marmalade contains 28 percent water.

Poultry and Meats: Most meats contain 50 percent water, while poultry generally contains around 60–65 percent.

SOURCE: React 1999

Water Content of Various Vegetables, Fruits, Nuts, and Seeds

Food Type	Percent of Water Content	Food Type	Percent of Water Content
Vegetables		Cherries	82
Asparagus	93	Cucumbers	93
Bok choy	87	Dates (fresh)	55
Celery	93	Figs	79
Endive	94	Grapes	79
Garlic root	64	Grapefruits	91
Green cabbage	90	Honeydew melon	94
Kale	65	Huckleberries	78
Lettuce	94	Lemons	85
Onion root	64	Lychees	82
Parsley	79	Mangoes	83
Watercress	91	Mulberries	85
Nuts and Seeds		Nectarines	80
Almonds	26	Okra	90
Brazil nuts	15	Olives (sun ripened)	70
Coconuts	35	Oranges	84
Coconut water	92	Pears	83
Macadamias	18	Persimmons	80
Pine nuts	15	Plums	84
Sunflower seeds	15	Prickly pears	79
Walnuts	25	Prunes (dried)	35
Fruits		Raspberries	83
Apple	84	Strawberries	89
Apricots	87	Tangerines	87
Avocados	75	Tomatoes	94
Bell peppers	93	Watermelons	94
Blackberries	82		
Cantaloupe	93		

SOURCE: Irishwizards Council 2003

Other mineral elements, known as **trace elements** and required in lesser amounts, are iron, zinc, selenium, magnesium, copper, iodine, fluorine, chromium, molybdenum, and cobalt.

Minerals function in the body in several ways. After the organic compounds have been oxidized, minerals remain to form actual body parts. For example, calcium, magnesium, and phosphorus are components of the bones and teeth. Minerals also act as regulators by contributing to the water and electrolyte balance of the body and are necessary to certain body functions, such as the transmission of nerve impulses. Minerals contribute to the osmotic pressure of body fluids and to the maintenance of neutrality—the acid–base balance of the blood and body tissues. Finally, they make possible the normal rhythm in the heartbeat.

Elevated amounts of some minerals may cause health problems. For example, elevated levels of sodium are associated with high blood pressure and cardiovascular disease.

Sodium. Salt and other sodium compounds are used to preserve, flavor, and stabilize other ingredients when food is being processed; they also occur in smaller amounts in unprocessed food. As a result, most processed food already contains the amount of sodium the Nutrition Facts label recommends for daily intake. It lists a Daily Value of 2,400 milligrams (mg) per day for sodium—the amount is contained in 6 g of salt; in household measures, one level teaspoon of salt provides about 2,300 mg of sodium.

In the body, sodium plays an essential role in the regulation of fluids and blood pressure. Studies of diverse populations have shown that a high sodium intake is associated with higher blood pressure. Although there is no way at present to tell who might develop high blood pressure from eating too much sodium, individuals can reduce their risk of high blood pressure by reducing their consumption of sodium. Typically, sodium-restricted diets can range from below 1,000 mg to 3,000 mg a day (FDA 1995). Fresh fruits and vegetables have very little sodium. Use herbs and spices to flavor food, and read the Nutrition Facts label to compare and help identify foods lower in sodium (Table 17.1 on page 498 provides some low sodium alternatives).

Other factors may interact with sodium to affect blood pressure, so reducing sodium intake alone may not be sufficient to control high blood pressure. Consuming less salt or sodium is not harmful and therefore can be recommended for the healthy normal adult.

Iron. A lack of essential minerals can cause malnutrition. For example, iron deficiency anemia is a major health problem in the United States and Canada and even more so in the rest of the world. Health care experts have identified iron as a priority category for nutrition monitoring. Individuals whose diets are deficient in iron will experience chronic fatigue, sensitivity to cold, edginess, depression, sleeplessness, susceptibility to colds and infections, and functional impairments in work performance, behavior, and intellectual development. This deficiency occurs most frequently in infants, adolescent males, and females during childbearing years (Hales 1999, 167).

Data show that less than half of preschoolers met their iron recommendations. The majority of primary school children (64 percent) and male adoles-

Table 17.1   *Low Sodium Alternatives*

If you find yourself continually eating more than 100 percent of the Daily Value for sodium each day, consider these low sodium alternatives. For labeled items, check the % Daily Value for sodium; try to select foods that provide 5 percent or less per serving.

Instead of:	Eat:
smoked, cured, salted, and canned meat, fish, and poultry	unsalted fresh or frozen beef, lamb, pork, fish, and poultry
regular hard and processed cheese	low-sodium cheese
regular peanut butter	low-sodium peanut butter
salted crackers	unsalted crackers
regular canned and dehydrated soups, broths, and bouillons	low-sodium canned soups, broths, and bouillons
regular canned vegetables	fresh and frozen vegetables and low-sodium canned vegetables
salted snack foods	unsalted tortilla chips, pretzels, potato chips, and popcorn

SOURCE: FDA 1995

cents (71 percent) met their iron recommendations, and their average intakes exceeded their respective recommendations. Only 21 percent of female adolescents met their recommended iron intake, and their average intake fell below the recommended intake by 16 percent (USDA 1999).

VITAMINS

No group of nutrients has captured the imagination of the public more than vitamins. Vitamins were discovered fairly recently, when physicians sought the cause of certain diseases, such as scurvy. They concluded that the chemical compounds called *vitamins* can make a great deal of difference to health. These vitamin-related discoveries led people to equate good nutrition with vitamins, and some even thought vitamins contained the essential element for life.

Vitamins are organic compounds required by every part of the body to maintain health and prevent disease. They are classified as either fat-soluble or water-soluble vitamins. Unlike minerals (such as calcium, which is integrated into bones), vitamins do not become part of the body. Only small amounts of vitamins are needed, but these must be provided by the diet because the body is not able to synthesize them in the required quantities for proper nourishment and body function. Vitamins foster growth, promote the ability to produce healthy offspring, maintain health, aid in the normal function of the digestive tract and appetite, and help maintain immune system functions.

Even though there is little proof that taking more vitamins than are recommended can help, many people look to vitamin supplements as a safety net in case they are not getting sufficient vitamins through their diets. This practice of taking megadoses of vitamins, especially in supplement form, may actually harm rather than help (Hales 1999, 167–168). Overdosing on vitamins can cause serious side effects: loss of coordination, nausea, rashes, diarrhea, and fatigue. Excess amounts of fat-soluble vitamins, stored in the body, can reach toxic levels. Even water-soluble vitamins, taken to extreme, can be dangerous. The key is moderation and a well-balanced diet featuring a range of healthful, vitamin-rich foods.

Food sources for some of the vitamins are:

A—liver; whole milk; butter; dark green, leafy vegetables

C—citrus fruits, broccoli, tomatoes, potatoes

D—eggs, liver, fortified milk

E—margarine, salad dressing

K—egg yolk, liver, milk, cabbage

thiamin (B_1)—pork, beef, liver, eggs, fish, whole grains, legumes

riboflavin (B_2)—milk, green vegetables, cereals

pyridoxine (B_6)—pork, milk, eggs, legumes

B_{12}—seafood, meats, eggs, milk

niacin—milk, eggs, fish, poultry

folic acid—spinach, asparagus, broccoli, kidney beans

biotin—milk, liver, mushrooms, legumes

Fat-Soluble Vitamins. Fat-soluble vitamins dissolve in fat and are found in the fatty parts of food and body tissues. They are stored in the body until needed, so it is not necessary to consume them every day. The fat-soluble vitamins transported by lipids through the body are A, D, E, and K. Vitamin A is important in promoting growth and health of body tissues as well as enhancing the function of the immune system. This vitamin also enhances vision by helping the retina function properly, permitting us to distinguish between light and shade and to see various colors distinctly. A form of vitamin A is used by dermatologists to treat acne and other skin disorders. Overdoses of vitamin A may result in yellowish, dry, scaly skin and dry, irritated eyes.

Vitamin D is essential for calcium absorption and thus is needed to prevent and cure rickets, a deficiency disease in which bones fail to harden. Vitamin E is an activator in certain enzyme reactions, and it protects vitamins A and C from being used up too quickly. Vitamin K is essential for the synthesis of prothrombin, a substance needed for normal blood coagulation.

Water-Soluble Vitamins. Water-soluble vitamins dissolve in water and are associated with the watery parts of food and body tissues. These vitamins are not stored by the body. Excess amounts are usually excreted in the urine and, therefore, should be provided in the diet on a regular basis. The water-soluble vitamins include the B vitamins and vitamin C (ascorbic acid). The B vitamins are essential to daily human nutrition. Known as the B-complex group, they help body systems combat stress and maintain energy reserves. The B-complex group consists of vitamin B_1 (thiamin), vitamin B_2 (riboflavin), vitamin B_3 (niacin), vitamin B_5 (pantothenic acid), vitamin B_6 (pyridoxine), vitamin B_{12} (cobalamin), folic acid, and biotin.

Thiamin is necessary for carbohydrate metabolism. It aids in the release of energy from food. Riboflavin helps body cells use oxygen, promotes tissue repair, and helps the nervous system function properly. Niacin is essential to growth; without niacin, thiamin and riboflavin could not function properly in the body. Pantothenic acid helps increase vitality and influences glandular functions. Pyridoxine is necessary for healthy teeth and gums and helps maintain normal body cholesterol. Further, it aids in the production of antibodies. Cobalamin works in conjunction with folic acid and iron to build normal blood cells and prevent pernicious anemia. Folic acid aids in the proper growth and reproduction of blood cells and contributes to healthy skin. Biotin is necessary for the proper use of fats, carbohydrates, and protein and helps produce antibodies. Vitamin C is vital in preventing scurvy, in the formation and maintenance of collagen (the cementing material that holds cells together), in the normal metabolism of some amino acids, and in the function of the adrenal glands.

Antioxidants

Chemical reactions occur continuously in the world around us and in our bodies. One of the most common types of reaction is oxidation. Some more familiar and visible examples of the damage caused by oxidation include rust, brittle rubber, and food spoilage. In our bodies, the energy-yielding reactions within cells are also **oxidation reactions,** that is, they are reactions in which either an oxygen atom adds an electron to or a hydrogen atom removes an electron from a substrate (a group of atoms or molecule)—the net result is a substrate that has had a partial or complete loss of a negatively charge particle, an electron. Two partially charged atoms or groups of atoms, one positively charged and the other negatively charged, now exist. Any atom or group of atoms that has an unpaired electron is called a **free radical,** or oxidant. Because electrons typically function in pairs, the free radicals are very prone to binding to other substrates in an effort to regain this paired status. When this happens in the human body, there is potential for a great deal of damage.

In the human body, this problem is mostly avoided because oxidation reactions are paired with reduction reactions so that the reduction reactions pick up the electrons that are lost during the oxidation reactions. Our bodies actually rely on these reactions occurring properly all the time. Whenever our bodies use glucose (recall this is the most common energy-containing molecule in the body), it is oxidation that releases the energy for our bodies to use. When more energy is needed than can be supplied by glucose in the blood, then our bodies start to tap into the stored energy supplies—especially those stored as fat. Oxidation of triglycerides, notably the fatty acid components, provides this energy. (Our bodies also oxidize glycogen, a different form of glucose storage found in muscle.)

When the free radicals are not incorporated immediately into other reactions, they may bind to inappropriate molecules or atoms and disrupt their normal function. For example, partially charged atoms or molecules often exist temporarily as intermediate steps in chemical reactions, so chemical reactions that are essential for normal body function may be interrupted if a free radical binds to one of the charged intermediates.

Oxidation and the resulting free radicals accelerate the aging process and contribute to organ and tissue damage. LDL oxidation has been linked to atherosclerosis (and thus contributes to heart disease). Oxidation processes contribute to the development of cancer. As research continues, free radical damage from oxidation appears more likely to be associated with chronic conditions; and, based on these findings, scientists are realizing that antioxidant supplementation (with vitamins C, E, and A) is essential (Saari 2002). **Antioxidants** act as scavengers by binding to free radicals, thus preventing them from causing damage.

The body uses many protective mechanisms against the damage caused by oxidation in the aging process. This protection includes a variety of enzymes that destroy free radicals, as well as food components, such as the antioxidant vitamins C and E and beta-carotene (a precursor of vitamin A). These defenses, in particular the antioxidant enzymes, weaken with time, and research indicates that good nutritional practices may help to defend against this decline (Saari 2002). Diets particularly rich in the antioxidant vitamins and bioflavonoids (the colored compounds in fruits and vegetables) may have cooperative effects to alter, reverse, or forestall the negative effects of aging. Therefore, it is important to examine the impact of the antioxidants contained in different foods on various neuronal and behavioral parameters known to change with age and determine whether their course can be altered. Several studies document the influence of dietary and synthetic antioxidants on normal, pathological age-related, and oxidative stress-induced behavioral changes in human and animal subjects (Cantuti-Castelvet, Shukitt, and Joseph 2000).

Another possible way to minimize free radical damage is by eating foods that boost antioxidant defenses. Vitamin C is found in fruits and vegetables. Beta-carotene is found in carrots, cantaloupe, dark green leafy vegetables, and vegetable-based soups. Vitamin E is found in vegetable oils, wheat germ, nuts, and green leafy vegetables, natural foods likely do not provide too much of these vitamins, but large doses of vitamin C or vitamin E used as a dietary supplement may actually promote free radical damage.

Trace minerals—copper, zinc, and selenium—act as antioxidants because they are necessary components of specific antioxidant enzymes and thus are essential to life. Organ meats such as liver, seafoods, nuts, and seeds are good dietary sources of copper and selenium. Zinc is found in meat, liver, eggs, and seafood. Trace minerals, like vitamins, should be consumed in proper amounts. Large amounts not associated with enzymes may promote free radical formation.

Follow these guidelines to potentially slow the aging process by preventing free radical damage. The recommended intake for vitamin C is 75 mg per day for women and 90 mg for men. Smokers need an additional 35 mg per day. For vitamin E, 15 mg per day (as alpha-tocopherol) is recommended. No specific amount is recommended for beta-carotene other than eating fruits and vegetables; beta-carotene supplements are not advised. For copper, 1.5 to 3 mg per day is recommended. For zinc, the recommended amount is 15 mg per day for men and 12 mg per day for women. The suggested amount of selenium is 55 micrograms (μg) per day (Saari 2002).

Nutritional Needs

About fifty different nutrients are needed to maintain health. No food contains all the nutrients needed, not even milk, which is highly regarded in our society. Therefore, a variety of foods are required to satisfy nutritional needs. One way to assure this variety and to establish a balanced diet is to select foods each day from the types identified in the Food Guide Pyramid (see Figure 17.2) by the USDA. The Food Guide Pyramid emphasizes foods from five food groups shown in the three lower sections of the pyramid. It includes nutritional goals for a diet that is adequate in protein, vitamins, minerals, and dietary fiber (without excessive amounts of calories, fat, saturated fat, cholesterol, sodium, added sugars, and alcohol) and usability goals for a guide that is practical and useful to consumers.

Unlike earlier guides such as the Basic Four, which recommended a foundation diet designed to prevent nutrient deficiencies, the Food Guide Pyramid specifies food choices for the total diet because both nutrient adequacy and excesses are of concern. The specific nutrient levels targeted are the Recommended Dietary Intakes (RDIs) for protein, vitamins and minerals, and levels of food components such as fat, saturated fat, cholesterol, sodium, and fiber recommended by the USDA's Dietary Guidelines for Americans and by consensus reports of authoritative health organizations. Consistent with the RDI, these goals apply to diets consumed over a reasonable period of time—a week, for example.

The Food Guide Pyramid builds on previous food guides, using familiar food groups as an organizing framework. Foods are grouped not only by their nutrient content, but also by the way they are used in meals. Serving sizes are expressed in household measures and in amounts commonly eaten. Recognizing that nutrient and energy needs vary considerably by age, sex, and activity level, the Food Guide suggests ranges in the numbers of servings from each food group, so that everyone in a household can meet their needs from one basic menu. Expected nutrient levels attained in food choice patterns suggested by the Guide are realistic because they are based on selection of commonly used foods, rather than depending on foods that are unusually rich in certain nutrients but are infrequently used (oysters as a source of zinc, for example). Finally, the Guide allows flexibility for consumers to eat in a way that suits their taste and lifestyle, while meeting nutritional criteria. Both RDI and Food Guide Pyramid serving recommendations are by convention expressed on a daily basis; daily menus vary around these standards to allow flexibility in food choices. Rather than prescribe specific low-fat foods (such as nonfat milk), the Guide permits consumers to

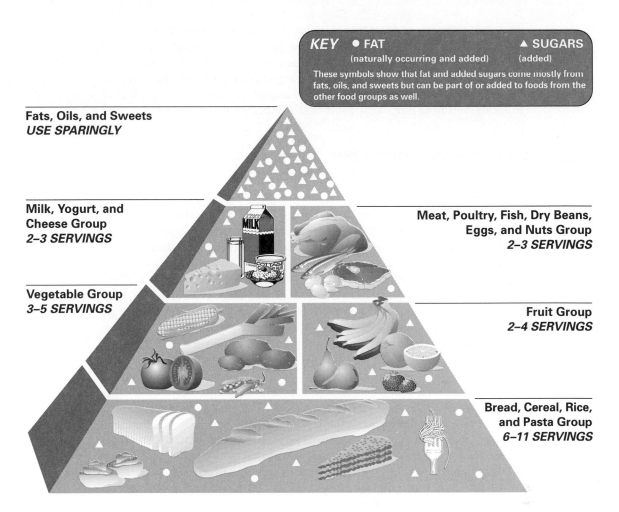

Fats, Oils, and Sweets
USE SPARINGLY

Milk, Yogurt, and Cheese Group
2–3 SERVINGS

Vegetable Group
3–5 SERVINGS

KEY ● FAT ▲ SUGARS
(naturally occurring and added) (added)
These symbols show that fat and added sugars come mostly from fats, oils, and sweets but can be part of or added to foods from the other food groups as well.

Meat, Poultry, Fish, Dry Beans, Eggs, and Nuts Group
2–3 SERVINGS

Fruit Group
2–4 SERVINGS

Bread, Cereal, Rice, and Pasta Group
6–11 SERVINGS

Figure 17.2
The USDA Food Guide Pyramid

decide which foods they prefer as sources of fat and added sugars, while keeping their total fat intake to no more than 30 percent of calories.

Nutritional Needs for School-Age Children

Caloric needs vary widely for elementary school children. They should eat at least the lower number of servings from each of the five major food groups daily. Most children will need more calories for growth and activity; they should eat larger portions of foods from the major food groups and some nutritious snacks while following the percentages of each nutrient as recommended by the FDA. Go easy on fatty and sugary foods from the Food Guide Pyramid's tip, such as butter, margarine, salad dressings, candies, and soft drinks, but don't forbid them. Have these as occasional treats, not everyday fare. Many children gain unwanted weight due to a sedentary lifestyle. Encourage physical activity, including outdoor play, to promote strength and fitness.

Characteristics of the Types of Food

Fruits are usually good sources of vitamins A and C, carbohydrates, and fiber. Citrus fruits are especially good sources of vitamin C. Two to four servings daily (at least one of which provides vitamin C), each about equal in size to an orange, are recommended.

Vegetables are usually good sources of vitamins A and C, carbohydrates, and fiber. Vegetables are low in calories if served without added fat. Dark green, leafy vegetables such as spinach, kale, collard greens, mustard greens, and broccoli are high in calcium and vitamins A and C. Orange vegetables such as carrots, sweet potatoes, and squash are also high in vitamin A. Three to five servings of vegetables daily (at least one of which provides vitamin A), each about equal in size to a small potato, are recommended.

Dried beans and peas are high in protein and iron. This food type also includes nuts, lentils, peanut butter, and tofu. They are usually low in cost and can be prepared a variety of ways. Nuts and peanut butter are high in fat and therefore high in calories. A combined total of two to three servings per day from this group and/or the meat, poultry, fish, and eggs group is recommended.

Meat, poultry, fish, and eggs are high in protein and iron. Lean meats, poultry without skin, and most fish are lower-calorie choices. A serving of this group is 3 ounces. A combined total of two to three servings per day from this group and/or the dried beans and peas group is recommended.

Bread, cereal, and pasta are high in iron, carbohydrates, and some B vitamins. Although the actual amount of protein is small in each serving, if many grain foods are eaten each day, part of the daily need for protein can be met. However, if these are the only sources of protein, they need to be combined with nuts and legumes to fulfill the needs for the required essential amino acids. Whole-grain products contain more fiber, vitamins, and minerals than refined products. Six to eleven servings daily, each about equal to the size of a slice of bread, are recommended.

Milk and cheese are good sources of calcium and protein. Low-fat milk and cheese made from low-fat milk are lower-calorie choices. These low-fat products have the same amount of vitamins and minerals but a lower percentage of fat. Two to three servings are recommended daily for this food group.

Sweets and fats are added to other foods, thus increasing the number of calories. These other foods supply few nutrients for the calories they contain. Beverages such as alcohol and soft drinks are included in this group. There is no recommendation for foods in this group; they should be used sparingly.

Daily Values

Another guide to proper nutrition are the Daily Values (DVs), formerly known as the Recommended Dietary Allowances (RDAs). These are basic dietary guides for the population as a whole and are designed to maintain good health. These recommendations have been set specifically as determined by the climate and general energy needs of the U.S. population. Statistics were obtained from large groups of people living in the United States to establish the criteria for the recommended allowances. The Daily Values are only estimates of nutritional needs, but they are useful for dietary planning to ensure proper amounts of various nutrients.

Food Problems

Problems concerning food have been a part of human life from the earliest times. In past ages, crop failures have led to famine and war. Even today, starvation kills hundreds of thousands of children and adults in very poor nations each year. Although there is also poverty in the United States, few children actually face the threat of starvation. Unfortunately, this does not mean that our nation does not have food problems. Many Americans are undernourished or malnourished. Overweight and obese individuals are also common.

UNDERNUTRITION

Typically, an undernourished person is also underweight, but this is by no means always the case. **Undernutrition** implies that the individual is not getting enough nutrients. This can occur even if the person is consuming more than enough calories. Thus, personal weight is not necessarily an indication of nutritional status. In the United States, malnutrition (an imbalance of proper nutrients) due to undernutrition is most likely to occur in infants, children, and adolescents, when nutritional requirements for tissue growth and development are high. When one is undernourished, the available proteins and carbohydrates are depleted, and the body begins to burn fat reserves. This process is known as *ketosis*. Undernutrition may cause blood sugar imbalances, lower basal metabolic rate, produce dehydration, provoke heart irregularity, inhibit growth, delay maturation, limit physical activity, and interfere with learning (Donatelle and Davis 1998, 274–275). The causes of undernutrition are many; poverty and lack of nutrition education are two major factors. Many Americans are undernourished because they resist changing nutritionally deficient eating habits and patterns. Other practices dictated by cultural taboos, religious beliefs, and cultural patterns also sometimes lead to nutritional health problems. Occasionally the cause is physiological. A poorly functioning body might fail to use nutrients supplied to it. For example, a disease such as hyperthyroidism can affect growth regardless of the quality of diet.

Psychological factors can also lead to undernutrition. Hurried meals in haphazard settings may be harmful because of the type and amount of food as well as how the food is eaten. The noise and confusion that often accompany rushed meals can affect proper digestion.

Anorexia Nervosa. An inaccurate perception of one's own nutritional state can bring on health problems such as anorexia nervosa. Anorexia nervosa literally means loss of appetite, but this is a misnomer: A person with anorexia nervosa is hungry, but he or she denies the hunger because of an irrational fear of becoming fat. Self-starvation, food preoccupation and rituals, compulsive exercising, and often an absence of menstrual cycles in women typically characterize anorexia nervosa. She may occasionally binge on large quantities of a particular food then make herself vomit and may regularly use large quantities of laxatives. (If these bingeing and purging behaviors are dominant, then she is diagnosed with bulimia.) This condition is more than a simple eating disorder: It refers to a distinct psychological disorder in which a drive for thinness and a fear of fatness result in life-threatening emaciation and a host of other problems. Untreated, anorexia can be fatal. It is not a fad that the victim will outgrow if left alone. The most common cause of death in a long-time anorexic is a low level of potassium in the blood, which can cause an irregular heartbeat; other causes of death are starvation, infections due to poor nutrition, dehydration from overuse of laxatives, and suicide due to depression. It occurs primarily in adolescents and may affect both sexes, but most often it is girls who become anorexic.

The central features of anorexia nervosa are difficult to specify because the disorder emerges over time as a complex mixture of the relentless drive for thinness, the effects of starvation, and commonly associated psychological disturbances (such as low self-worth and mistrust of others). A significant weight loss is one of the cardinal features of anorexia. The anorexic individual approaches weight loss with a fervor, convinced that her body is too large. Lost weight is viewed as an accomplishment. The fact that slenderness is highly valued in our culture contributes to these attitudes held by anorexics. This drive for thinness is coupled with an extreme fear of becoming fat. This phobic fear of weight gain may express itself as excessive anxiety over any weight increase. An anorexic individual also has a distorted body image—unable to recognize her appearance as abnormal. She will insist that her emaciated figure is just right or even too fat (USDA 1998).

Anorexics are typically compulsive, perfectionistic, and very competitive. The anorexic sometimes suffers from a low self-image due to a feeling of incompetence, so she becomes consumed with losing weight to demonstrate to herself and others that she is in total control. Therefore, if a friend, parent, or teacher admonishes the anorexic for looking too thin, the anorexic may take this as a compliment, for it means others are aware of his or her disciplined approach to weight loss. Therapy consists of psychological counseling and family therapy, as well as steps to improve nutrition.

The long-term effects of anorexia include psychological problems such as obsessions, compulsions, paranoia, social withdrawal, and depression. They may become irritable, hostile, indecisive, depressed, defiant, and resistant to change. The arguments with parents and other authorities over eating habits become power struggles for control. Starvation can interrupt normal brain–body functions such as sleep, maintenance of proper blood pressure, muscle weakness, immunity to disease, and sexual drive. Vomiting disrupts the potassium–sodium balance necessary for proper functioning of nerves and muscles (including the heart) and produces enamel erosion, tooth degeneration, and lesions in the esophagus. Table 17.2 on page 508 shows the warning signs and problems associated with anorexia nervosa.

Bulimia. Bulimia, sometimes called bulimia nervosa, is characterized by recurring periods of binge eating, during which large amounts of food are consumed in a short period of time—sometimes as many as 20,000 calories during the course of a single binge. The bulimic is aware that his or her eating is out of control. He or she is fearful of not being able to stop eating and is afraid of being fat. The bulimic usually feels depressed and guilty after a binge. Frequently, purging (through self-induced vomiting, abuse of laxatives and/or diuretics, or periods of fasting) follows the binges. The bulimic's weight is usually in a normal or somewhat above normal range; it may fluctuate more than ten pounds due to alternating binges and fasts. Table 17.2 shows warning signs and problems associated with bulimia.

Treatment. Treatment can save the life of someone with an eating disorder. Friends, relatives, teachers, therapists, dietitians, peer support groups, and physicians all play an important role in helping the ill person start and stay with a treatment program. Encouragement, caring, and persistence, as well as information about eating disorders and their dangers, may be needed to convince the ill person to get help, stick with treatment, or try again.

HUNGER AND LEARNING

Hunger is a physiological and psychological state that occurs when food needs are not met satisfactorily. Research has shown that hunger definitely has an effect on learning behavior. Hunger increases nervousness, irritability, and disinterest in a learning situation. Students who are hungry will demonstrate a lack of interest in what is being taught and an inability to concentrate.

Hunger and malnutrition lead to weakness and illness. A variety of avitaminoses (vitamin deficiency disorders) can result from malnutrition. A person's development and brain function can be severely affected by hunger. Malnourished individuals are also more susceptible to infections, which can further lead to impaired growth.

LIFESTYLE HABITS AND OBESITY

Obesity is prevalent among children and adolescents in the United States. Evidence gathered over the past three decades indicates that it is increasing. Data show that 13 percent of children ages six to eleven years and 14 percent of adolescents ages twelve to ninteen years in the United States are overweight. This is nearly double for children and triple for adolescents from twenty years ago. Overweight children, especially adolescents, are likely to become overweight or obese adults at risk for serious health problems such as type II diabetes, hypertension, heart disease, stroke, and some types of cancer. Over the past

Table 17.2   *Characteristics of Eating Disorders*

Eating Disorder	Warning Signs	Physical Problems	Psychological Problems
Anorexia nervosa	■ deliberate self-starvation with weight loss ■ intense, persistent fear of gaining weight ■ refusal to eat, except tiny portions ■ continuous dieting ■ denial of hunger ■ periodic bingeing and vomiting ■ compulsive exercise and hyperactivity ■ abnormal weight loss ■ sensitivity to cold ■ absent or irregular menstruation ■ increased hairiness	■ malnutrition ■ serious heart, kidney, and liver damage ■ intestinal ulcers ■ ruptured stomach ■ tears of the esophagus ■ dehydration ■ tooth/gum corrosion ■ exhaustion ■ insufficient blood sugar inhibits learning ■ delayed physical maturation ■ cessation of menstruation	■ depression ■ shame and guilt ■ mood swings ■ low self-esteem ■ withdrawal ■ perfectionism ■ impaired family and social relationships ■ "all or nothing" thinking
Bulimia	■ preoccupation with food ■ frequent binge eating, usually in secret, followed by vomiting and fasting after bingeing ■ abuse of laxatives, diuretics, diet pills, or drugs to induce vomiting ■ compulsive exercising ■ swollen salivary glands and pancreas ■ broken blood vessels in the eyes	■ malnutrition ■ serious heart, kidney, and liver damage ■ intestinal ulcers ■ ruptured stomach ■ tears of the esophagus ■ dehydration ■ tooth/gum corrosion	■ depression ■ shame and guilt ■ mood swings ■ low self-esteem ■ withdrawal ■ perfectionism ■ impaired family and social relationships ■ "all or nothing" thinking

twenty years, hospital costs for childhood obesity-related diseases have soared from $35 million in 1979 to $127 million in 1999.

Poor eating habits and inactive lifestyles, rather than heredity, are contributing to the prevalence of obesity among children and adolescents, particularly African Americans and Hispanics. Poor dietary patterns include increased intake of sugars in sweetened soft drinks, foods, and meals of high energy, low nutrient density, and large portion sizes. Researchers suggest that intake of soft drinks may promote obesity because of their high glycemic index (ability to raise blood sugar). Milk, on the other hand, which was once commonly consumed, may protect against obesity because of its low glycemic index.

Only 2 percent of U.S. children ages two to nineteen years meet the Food Guide Pyramid serving recommendations for all five major food groups. When the diets of young children ages two to nine were compared to the Healthy Eating Index, which is a measure of overall diet quality, 81 percent had diets that needed improvement (National Dairy Council 2003a).

Many children are less physically active than recommended; physical activity tends to decline in adolescence. Children are spending more time on sedentary activities such as television viewing and video games and less time on physical activity at home and at school. From 1991 to 1999, the percentage of students attending daily physical education classes at school dropped from 42 to 29 percent. According to the School Health Policies and Programs Study 2000, only 8 percent of elementary schools, 6.4 percent of middle/junior high schools, and 5.8 percent of senior high schools provide daily physical education. Only 71 percent of elementary schools provide regularly scheduled recess for kindergarten through fifth grade.

The health risks of obesity, such as degenerative diseases and shorter life span, may not be of immediate concern to elementary school students, but there are many other reasons for maintaining a healthy weight. Obesity can be considered a physical handicap at any age because it affects physical activity. Also, overweight students face many emotional problems. In a society where thinness is emphasized, overweight students may be shunned, ridiculed, stared at, and rejected socially. As a result, overweight students may lose their sense of self-worth and withdraw from others. A complicating problem occurs when overweight students find satisfaction in nothing else except eating, which causes them to gain even more weight, further alienating them from peers.

Being overweight becomes a health problem when the person is 15 to 20 percent above normal weight. Of course, body build and an individual's lean-to-fat ratio also have to be taken into consideration. Different people gain weight in different places in the body. Those who typically gain weight in the lower portions of the body (hips and thighs, usually females) do not have as many health risks posed as those who gain weight in the upper body (abdomen, usually males). A person might have a stocky build and be over the desired weight for his height and age, but the percentage of body fat might be within the normal range. More often than not, however, obesity is self-evident.

WEIGHT CONTROL

Weight reduction demands self-discipline and commitment. An overweight individual must accept personal responsibility for the condition. If an emotional problem is the cause, that problem must be treated first to ensure long-lasting success at weight control because the overweight condition is only a symptom of a deeper problem. Before any weight loss plan is implemented, a physician should be consulted.

Obese persons must consume fewer calories than they expend daily, but this is easier said than done. Dieters should use a diet that is similar to the one to which they are accustomed so they do not feel as restricted and tempted to quit dieting. Other techniques that have helped people lose weight are to:

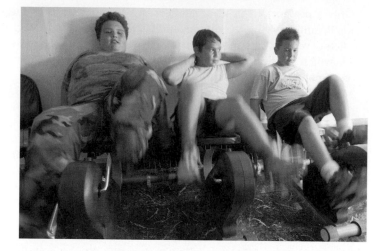

Obesity is a preventable condition among children and youth in the U.S.

- arrange to eat in one place only
- remove all unnecessary fat when cooking and eating meat
- avoid gravies, use herbs and spices for seasoning instead
- start meals with filling, low-calorie dishes such as soup or celery sticks
- eat fresh fruit instead of canned fruit
- eat regular meals—missed meals may make you even more hungry during the day
- eat raw vegetables for snacks
- eat baked, broiled, or boiled foods without adding fat
- use a salad-sized plate rather than a dinner plate so the portions look larger
- cut food into small bites and eat slowly
- brush the teeth after each meal; sometimes the aftertaste of food can stimulate the appetite
- exercise moderately and regularly
- develop hobbies; sometimes people substitute food for friends and outside activities

Care should be taken not to lose weight too rapidly. Rapid weight loss may result in exhaustion, kidney problems, dehydration, reduced cardiovascular output, decreased strength, decreased growth, and decreased endurance.

One point that should be kept in mind regarding an individual's weight is ideal weight versus average weight. Some weight tables will provide data on average weight; but, as noted earlier, trends for the average American child are moving toward overweight. Ideal weight tables should be used as the standard for evaluating weight.

Further, weight alone should not be the total issue. The child's body fat (or lean-to-fat ratio) is even more critical. If a child is "big boned," he or she may appear overweight, yet his or her body fat may be very acceptable. Conversely, a child with small bones may weigh within an acceptable range but actually have a body fat percentage that is unacceptable. Also, if a person couples a dieting program with an exercise program, that person may be losing fat and gaining muscle. Since muscles weigh more than fat, the result may not be lost pounds but rather lost fat—a healthy condition. However, since most dieters are concerned only with how much they weigh, they may be disappointed that they are not losing weight. Again, the focus for a dieter should be on the lean-to-fat ratio, not on weight alone.

THE ROLE OF THE TEACHER

Teachers should provide accurate information concerning nutrition and teach students how to make wise decisions in order to help prevent their undernourishment. They need to emphasize the importance of eating a good breakfast and lunch, as well as encourage sociability among students when they are eating. Teachers can help the students enjoy the taste, smell, color, and texture of food and thereby increase interest in it. In addition, teachers have an excellent chance to be exemplary role models by eating the right foods in the right way while at school.

THERAPY AND COUNSELING

Weight reduction is usually more successful when using a "buddy system" or peer support groups. Teachers can help by getting together several students who have a similar goal of weight reduction and having them eat together and share their concerns and problems. Teachers can also educate obese and overweight students about proper nutrition and encourage physical activity. To nurture the emotional health of the obese student, teachers need to offer security and acceptance without pitying or overprotecting the student. Being supportive will produce much better results than constant harassment or criticism. Trying to reduce the student's anxiety while helping build self-esteem and independence are also important.

Other Food-Related Issues

FOOD QUACKERY

Obese individuals may understand the need to diet but may want to do so as painlessly as possible. Such individuals are vulnerable to fad diets advertised to help a person lose weight quickly. Some of these fad diets are restricted in variety, expensive, useless, and sometimes even detrimental to health. Most fad diets are directed at adults, rather than children, of course, but children are impressionable. It is important to put these diets into proper perspective. The fact is that most people who are overweight do not need to read a book on what to eat to lose weight. Simply eating somewhat less of everything will usually produce results, if the diet is followed conscientiously.

Food quackery is by no means confined to diet books or diet clinics that employ dubious methods. The whole natural and health foods industry is considered quackery by many nutritional experts. Both of these areas prey on natural fears and uncertainties about foods and nutritional requirements. There is no accepted legal definition of what natural foods actually are and no way to keep entrepreneurs from selling granola, dried fruits, and so on at inflated prices, all the while hinting that these products are somewhat healthier for a person to eat. So-called health foods, such as bee pollen and algae extracts, fall into the same category. Such foods are not harmful to health, but they are no better than foods obtained from ordinary sources. Advocates of natural, organic, and health foods claim that additives or pesticide residues in regular foods can cause disease or even lower the nutritional value of the food, but these claims may be highly exaggerated. By and large, the FDA and other supervisory agencies do a good job in preventing possibly harmful or unsafe foods from reaching the market. Teachers can help students become informed consumers of food products and develop a good knowledge of nutritional principles. But nutrition should not become an obsession, as it is with many food faddists. Students should also be taught to recognize the difference between nutrition and food panacea.

FAD DIETS

Many overweight and obese individuals (an estimated 20 percent of men and 40 percent of women in the United States) are trying to lose weight. Although it took several months and years to put on the extra weight, many of them are looking for a quick way to lose that weight. This attitude results in choosing quick-weight-loss diets that are not effective and may be harmful.

Some choose metabolic products, such as herbs or caffeine, to lose weight. Herbs have not been shown to speed the loss of fat, and caffeine shows little promise as a weight-loss aid.

Others go on very-low-calorie diets, which severely restrict nutrients and can result in serious metabolic imbalances. Weight can be lost on this type of diet, but much of the weight lost will be lean protein tissue and/or water, not fat. This results in harm to the muscles (including the heart), loss of essential vitamins and minerals through the water loss, and dizziness and fatigue. Further, if one cuts calories, this slows the metabolism; and once this person goes off the diet, the metabolism remains slow and the body continues to use few calories—and the pounds come back.

Liquid protein diets (low-carbohydrate diets) operate on the theory that insulin is controlled and therefore more fat is burned. With this type of diet, ketosis (ketones formed and released into the bloodstream) will result. Ketosis will increase blood levels of uric acid, a risk factor for gout and kidney stones. There is no research evidence that carbohydrates lead to fat storage and weight; and further, the excessive protein in this diet can damage the kidneys and cause osteoporosis.

Over-the-counter diet aids act as mild stimulants and suppress the appetite, usually by providing fiber and thereby providing a feeling of fullness. The FDA has found no evidence to support fiber as an aid in weight control or as an appetite suppressant.

Prescription drugs, such as Redux and Pondimin (fen-phen), curb hunger by increasing the level of serotonin in the brain. These were intended for the obese, but were banned in 1997 after the FDA found strong evidence that they could seriously damage the heart.

Some people try crash diets to lose a moderate amount of weight in a very short period. These types of diets can damage several body systems, and have been proved not to work because most of these individuals regain their weight. This yo-yo dieting causes many health problems and shortens lifespan. The best way to lose weight is to lose weight slowly (no more than one-half to one pound a week), eat properly and in moderation, and exercise (Floyd, Mimms, and Yelding-Howard 1988, 307–309).

FOOD LABELING

A tremendous amount of nutritional information is available today, but many Americans are still misinformed and confused about the foods they buy and eat. Some FDA regulations have resulted in improved labeling designed to give a listing of nutrients in the product and to make the information on food labels more meaningful to consumers (see Figure 17.1 on page 493). For example, ingredients are listed on the label in order, beginning with the largest quantity. Typically, the label provides nutritional information based on one serving of the food product rather than on the entire can or package.

Manufacturers must use nutritional labeling when they add any nutrient to packaged food or when they make some nutritional claim for their products. Labeling is also meant to stop unsupported generalizations and fraudulent statements. Nutritional labeling of food products is being sought for nearly all foods. This would be difficult for some foods, such as fresh fruits, but labeling of all food products would be beneficial to the consumer.

In 1993 the FDA revised food labeling regulations and replaced the RDAs with DVs. These translated into the most significant change on the new food labels. The main difference between the RDAs and DVs is that DVs provide the percentage of recommended daily amounts of vitamins, minerals, total fat, saturated fat, cholesterol, sodium, carbohydrates, fiber, sugar, and protein. The DV label, which applies to healthy individuals, is a better guide toward planning a daily diet.

The new label reference value, DV, comprises two sets of dietary standards: Daily Reference Values (DRVs) and Reference Daily Intakes (RDIs). Only the DV term appears on a food label, though, to make label reading less confusing. DRVs have been established for macronutrients that are sources of energy (fat, saturated fat, total carbohydrate [including fiber], and protein) and for cholesterol, sodium, and potassium, which do not contribute calories but are known to influence health status.

DRVs for the energy-producing nutrients are based on the number of calories consumed per day. A daily intake of 2,000 calories has been established as the reference. This level was chosen, in part, because it approximates the caloric requirements for postmenopausal women. This group has the highest risk for excessive intake of calories and fat.

DRVs for the energy-producing nutrients are calculated as follows:

- fat based on 30 percent of calories
- saturated fat based on 10 percent of calories
- carbohydrate based on 60 percent of calories
- protein based on 10 percent of calories
- fiber based on 11.5 g of fiber per 1,000 calories

Because of current public health recommendations, DRVs for some nutrients represent the uppermost limit that is considered desirable. The DRVs for total fat, saturated fat, cholesterol, and sodium are:

- *total fat:* less than 65 g
- *saturated fat:* less than 20 g
- *cholesterol:* less than 300 mg
- *sodium:* less than 2,400 mg

Under regulations from the FDA of the U.S. Department of Health and Human Services and the Food Safety and Inspection Service of the USDA, food labels include:

- formats that enable consumers to quickly find the information they need to make healthful food choices
- information on the amount per serving of saturated fat, cholesterol, dietary fiber, and other nutrients of major health concern
- nutrient reference values, expressed as % Daily Values, that help consumers see how a food fits into an overall daily diet
- uniform definitions for terms that describe a food's nutrient content—such as "light," "low-fat," and "high-fiber"—to ensure that such terms mean the same for any product on which they appear
- claims about the relationship between a nutrient or food and a disease or health-related condition, such as calcium with osteoporosis and fat with cancer (helpful for people who are concerned about eating foods that may help keep them healthier longer)
- standardized serving sizes to make nutritional comparisons of similar products easier
- declaration of total percentage of juice in juice drinks

Nutrition Education

In emphasizing sound nutrition to students, teachers need to make sure that the learning opportunities provided are interesting and personalized. Students should be taught to make responsible food choices. The home and school have to work together to make the nutrition education of the student a success.

THE SCHOOL LUNCH PROGRAM

School lunch programs began with the enactment of the National School Lunch Act in 1946. This federal legislation provided surplus agricultural commodities and federal funds to local school districts for the purpose of providing nutritious meals to children through a school lunch program. Federal government management of this program is the responsibility of the USDA.

The National School Lunch Program (NSLP) provides nutritionally balanced, low-cost or free lunch to more than twenty-seven million children each school day and also provide snacks to children who are in afterschool programs. NSLP mandates that the meals provided must meet federal nutrition requirements. Through this program, children receive information on making healthy food choices and the cafeteria staff receives training and technical support (USDA Food and Nutrition Service Public Information 2002a).

Though the school lunches provided through federal programs may be nutritious, several factors prevent children from eating wisely at school. Many schools offer foods that are not as nutritious but are sold in competition to the regular school lunch. Also, many schools sell soft drinks and snacks through vending machines, and some children consume these instead of the regular cafeteria meal. Many of the foods sold in competition with school meals are low in nutrient density and high in fat, added sugars, and calories. These competitive, less nutritious foods can contribute to diet-related health risks, as well as send messages that contradict what is taught in the health education classroom (National Dairy Council 2003b).

The educational impact of a lunch program can be important if it is used correctly. For students who bring their lunches from home, teachers need to provide several examples of nutritious sack lunches (for example, a sandwich including some type of lean meat and lettuce on whole-wheat bread, banana, raisins, and milk).

The cafeteria can be used as a place in which to help students learn table manners, sitting posture, and appropriate social behavior. The planning, preparation, and serving of meals by the cafeteria staff can also provide excellent learning opportunities for students.

Summary

- Although food is basic to human existence, food choices often have little to do with good nutrition.
- Socioeconomic factors, personal preferences and habits, cultural customs, and religious beliefs are all determining factors in the food we select.
- The eating habits of American students are often poor. This is due primarily to the habits of their parents, hurried lifestyles, and lack of nutrition education.
- Snacking can be improved to help supplement an otherwise poor diet.
- The development of positive lifetime eating habits in students is a critical issue.
- Food's basic function is to provide nutrients to the body.

- All foods have specific caloric values.
- The USDA's Food Guide Pyramid and the Daily Values can be used to plan a healthy diet.
- Food problems abound among students.
- Hunger and malnutrition affect a student's growth and learning.
- The number of overweight students is increasing.
- Pressure from peers to be thin or to look good in order to be accepted encourages anorexia and bulimia. These conditions are physical and emotional disorders. Sometimes therapy and counseling are needed to correct these problems.
- Food quackery preys on the fears and uncertainties people have regarding foods.
- Students should be taught to distinguish between truth and misleading statements.
- Food labels are provided on most foods to help determine the nutritional value of a food.
- Students should be taught to make responsible choices about food.
- Teachers and parents have to work together for nutrition education to be successful.

DISCUSSION QUESTIONS

1. Describe why U.S. diets are often insufficient even though we live in an affluent country.
2. What factors determine one's selection of foods?
3. Discuss the importance of complex carbohydrates in the diet.
4. Discuss some healthy ways to snack to enhance your diet.
5. List the food sources for proteins.
6. Differentiate between saturated and unsaturated fats.
7. Describe the importance of water to the body structure.
8. What beneficial roles do minerals play in body function?
9. Discuss the role of antioxidants in enhancing health.
10. Describe the use of the USDA's Food Guide Pyramid in selecting proper foods.
11. Discuss the typical characteristics of a person with anorexia.
12. Describe obesity as an emotional and physical disorder.
13. How can food labels be helpful to consumers?
14. Discuss the importance of the school lunch program.

CRITICAL THINKING QUESTIONS

1. What strategies should school administrators use to encourage children to eat more nutritious and balanced meals and snacks while at school?
2. Devise a strategy that will help young children interpret food labels properly.

3. Compare the relative benefits and disadvantages of selling nonnutritious foods from vending machines in schools.

4. Consider the typical diet of Americans as described in the text. What economic factors contribute to this type of diet?

5. What would you consider the ideal diet plan?

WEB SITE ACTIVITY

Go to *www.nationaldairycouncil.org/lv104/nutrilib/digest/dairydigest_736b.html*, the Web site of the National Dairy Council. Find out more information about U.S. school children's eating habits and physical activity patterns and their influences upon children's health and obesity patterns.

WEB SITES OF INTEREST

The Centers for Disease Control and Prevention (CDC): *www.cdc.gov*
The CDC is an agency of the U.S. Department of Health and Human Services. It is one of eight federal public health agencies within the Department of Health and Human Services. Its mission is to promote health and quality of life by preventing and controlling disease, injury, and disability.

United States Department of Agriculture (USDA): *www.usda.gov*
This is the home page for the USDA, the organization that gives us the Dietary Guidelines for Americans, among other nutrition-related information.

Food and Drug Administration: *www.fda.gov*
It is the FDA's job to see that the food we eat is safe and wholesome, the cosmetics we use won't hurt us, the medicines and medical devices we use are safe and effective, and that radiation-emitting products such as microwave ovens won't do us harm.

The National Heart, Lung, and Blood Institute's Obesity Education Initiative, "Achieve Your Healthy Weight!": *www.nhlbi.nih.gov/health/public/heart/ obesity/lose_wt/ wtl_prog.htm*
This Web site provides information on how to lose and control weight, guidelines on treating overweight and obesity, assessment of overweight and obesity, and principles of safe and effective weight loss.

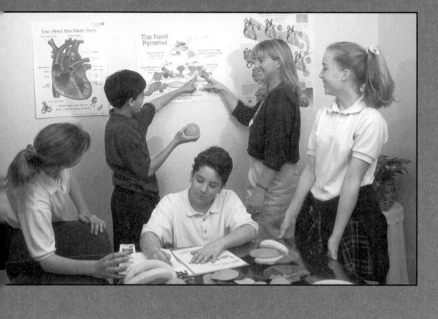

CHAPTER EIGHTEEN

Strategies for Teaching Nutrition

Students need to internalize nutrition information and recognize its relevance to their health. To help the students do this, teachers should present learning opportunities that relate nutritional information to the students' daily lives.

VALUED OUTCOMES

After doing the activities in this chapter, the student should be able to express and illustrate the following guidelines:

- Nutrition plays a vital role in human development.
- There is a close relationship between dietary practices and overall health.
- The taste, sight, and smell of foods sometimes dictate food behavior.
- Nutritional status may affect self-image.
- Food serves several functions in meeting body needs.
- Food fads and fallacies can affect an individual's food behavior.
- Caloric intake should be balanced with energy needs.

- There are many individual and ethnic variations in food behavior.
- Physical, psychological, and social factors affect personal food behavior.
- There are healthy and unhealthy ways of losing weight.
- A good breakfast is important for growing and learning.
- Food is an important part of our lives.
- Food nutrients can be classified as carbohydrates, lipids, proteins, water, minerals, and vitamins.
- Eating a variety of carefully selected foods is the best way to ensure that the body receives the proper amounts of the nutrients it needs.
- The Food Guide Pyramid can serve as an aid in planning balanced, nutritious meals.
- The lack of certain nutrients can lead to certain diseases.

- Being underweight or overweight can lead to physical and emotional problems.
- Maintaining a proper weight is an individual responsibility, but others can help if there is a weight problem.
- Even a person who does not have a weight problem can be malnourished.
- Simple foods can be nutritious and provide a well-balanced diet, if properly selected.
- Trying new and different foods can be fun.
- Junk foods, such as candy and soft drinks, can cause health problems if consumed regularly.
- Many people in the world do not have enough to eat.
- Food labels can provide useful nutritional information.
- Money spent for food should be spent wisely.

REFLECTION

The Surgeon General of the United States has called our attention to the problem of childhood obesity in our country. As you read through this chapter, and as you select strategies for your classroom, reflect on how you can help students reduce their risk of obesity.

A Flexible Approach to Nutrition

Teachers have the responsibility of helping students learn the basic principles of nutrition so that they will understand the important relationship between nutrition and health and increase their skills in solving food- and nutrition-related problems. The concept of nutrition is quite abstract to younger elementary school children and is often seen as connected with, yet divorced from, eating. Your job in teaching nutrition is to make that concept more concrete to your students by presenting learning opportunities that relate nutritional information to daily life. In other words, you must personalize the information so that students will internalize it and recognize its relevance to their health.

Avoid a rigid, by-the-rules approach, and do not reduce nutrition education to a set of rules. Not only will a rule-based approach make nutrition seem grim, but it will also cause students to reject sound principles as unrealistic. Help students to understand the motivations for choosing and eating certain foods and that some of these motivations have little to do with the amount of nutrients to be attained from that food. For example, a person might be choosing a certain midafternoon snack because it was the one always offered by his or her parents. But that snack might not be as nutritious as another readily available snack.

Children and adults will change their habits only when they personally recognize the importance of doing so. Do not expect changes overnight. Encourage introspection, and foster positive decision-making skills. Act as a role model for changes you wish to bring about. Respect differences in tastes, likes, and dislikes.

Shown to the right of each activity title in this chapter is the suggested grade level(s) for which the activity might be appropriate. However, many of the suggested activities could be modified for use at various grade levels. Many of the strategies in this chapter reference the Food Guide Pyramid; it can be found on page 503. When doing activities in which students are asked to taste or consume foods (milk, cheese, peanut butter, etc.), be sure to confirm that students are not allergic to those foods.

Value-Based Activities

WHAT'S HEALTHY?
Grades (4–5)

Valued Outcome: The students will be able to decide which breakfast foods are healthful and which are not.

Description of Strategy: Divide the class into groups of four to six students. Have the students get out two sheets of paper for the group. On one sheet of paper, write Nutritious; on the other sheet of paper, write Not Nutritious. Have the group decide what a nutritious breakfast is and write it down. Label the foods by their food groups as given on the Food Guide Pyramid. Then have them make up a breakfast that is not nutritious and label the foods by their food groups. Have a group discussion about their answers. After the discussion, do the same concept for lunch and dinner.

Materials Needed: paper and pencils for each student

Processing Question: Why is it important to eat a nutritious breakfast?

HEALTHY FOOD VOTING
Grades (K–5)

Valued Outcome: The students will be able to determine if their favorite foods are healthy or unhealthy.

Description of Strategy: Start by asking the students what their favorite foods are. List them on the board. After making these lists, make two separate columns and label one Healthy and the other Unhealthy. Then call out the list of favorite foods, and have the students vote whether each of the foods should go in the Healthy or the Unhealthy column.

Materials Needed: board and markers

Processing Question: How can I change my diet if most of my favorite foods are unhealthy?

NUTRITION SENTENCE COMPLETION   Grades (4–5)

Valued Outcome: The students will be able to complete nutrition-related statements with their own feelings and beliefs.

Description of Strategy: Create a handout of the following statements. Have the students complete the handout with phrases that come to mind immediately on hearing the key phrase beginning the statement:

- The most important meal of the day for me is . . .
- Eating a good breakfast is . . .
- My favorite foods are . . .
- Eating right means . . .
- I think that my present diet is . . .
- Between-meal snacks should be . . .
- One problem about nutrition for me is . . .

Materials Needed: handouts and pencils for each student

Processing Question: Who can help you determine what is included in a good breakfast and/or snack?

RANK-ORDERING FAVORITE FOODS   Grades (3–5)

Valued Outcome: The students will be able to clarify their values regarding their favorite foods.

Description of Strategy: Have each student prepare a list of three or four favorite foods or dishes from each section of the Food Guide Pyramid. Then tell the students to rank-order each food or dish, with the most favorite being labeled "1." Now have the students compare their lists. What class preferences seem to emerge? What are some individual preferences? Follow with a discussion of personal likes and dislikes.

Materials Needed: paper and pencils for each student

Processing Question: Do several of the students have the same favorite foods as you do? If they do not, why do you think that is true?

VALUES CONTINUUM   Grades (4–5)

Valued Outcome: The students will be able to explain how different eating lifestyles can affect one's nutrition.

Description of Strategy: Pass out continuum sheets (see the example below). One end of the continuum represents a lifestyle in which every meal is eaten at home under relaxed conditions. The other end of the continuum represents a lifestyle in which every meal is eaten outside the home under hurried or hectic conditions. Have each student place an X on the continuum that represents his or her assessment of eating lifestyle. Follow with a general discussion of how eating lifestyle may affect growth and development as well as emotional state.

All meals eaten at home
(relaxed conditions)

All meals eaten outside
the home (hectic conditions)

Materials Needed: continuum sheets and pencils for each student

Processing Question: How does a hurried or relaxed eating lifestyle affect the digestion of the food we eat?

WHAT'S FOR LUNCH?   Grades (3–5)

Valued Outcome: The students will be able to analyze the nutritional quality of their school lunches.

Description of Strategy: Have the students write down and analyze their school lunches for three days. After three days, have the students share what they thought about the school lunches. Discuss which food groups were poorly represented and which food groups were well represented. Have the students give their own opinions about the school lunches. As an instructor, make sure good things are said as well as bad.

Materials Needed: none

Processing Questions:

1. Did you enjoy these lunches?
2. Were you able to eat the types of foods you enjoy?
3. Did your analysis determine that your lunches were healthy? Unhealthy?

FOOD POLL   Grades (3–5)

Valued Outcome: The students will be able to choose a response to several opinion questions related to food.

Description of Strategy: Discuss the typical secret voting procedures for political elections in the United States. Determine a food-related issue involving your school—for example, should breakfast be served in your cafeteria every school day? Choose representatives to discuss different sides of the issue. Prepare ballots with the candidates' names. Allow the candidates to debate. Allow the students to register to vote, enter a voting booth, and vote according to the procedures in your state.

Materials Needed: voting ballots, ballot boxes, registration table, pens, voting booth

Processing Question: Why did you vote the way you did?

NUTRITION SELF-PORTRAITS   Grades (K–2)

Valued Outcome: The students will be able to draw a picture that describes how the foods they eat help them become healthy.

Description of Strategy: Have each student draw a picture of himself or herself in the center of a piece of paper. Then have the students draw around their pictures all kinds of nutritious foods that they like to eat. Display the self-portraits around the room.

Materials Needed: paper and crayons or markers for each student

Processing Questions:

1. Why is it important to eat nutritious foods?
2. How do nutritious foods enhance our health?
3. What activities could we do besides eating nutritious food to keep us healthy?

Decision Stories

Follow the procedures outlined in Chapter 4, pages 80–83, for presenting decision stories.

WHAT TO DRINK?   Grades (K–2)

Al has just come inside from playing a game of football with his friends and is very thirsty. He opens the refrigerator and finds water, soda pop, and fruit juice.

Focus Question: Which would be best for Al to drink? Why?

JOHN AND BRAD'S SACK LUNCH   Grades (K–2)

John and Brad are best friends and have been friends since kindergarten. They are both in the second grade and always sit together at lunch. They both bring their lunch to school with them every day. Brad is always jealous of John because John always has a better-looking lunch. John's typical lunch consists of a bologna sandwich with lots of mayonnaise, chips, a candy bar, a soda, and sometimes hard candy. Brad's lunch usually consists of a turkey sandwich with mustard, baby carrots, fruit, milk, and sometimes a granola bar. Brad doesn't understand why his lunch never looks as good as John's.

Focus Questions:

1. Whose diet is healthier? Why?
2. Which person do you think has more energy? Why?

SOURCE: Dietz and Stern 1999

SNACK TIME   Grades (K–5)

John came home from school hungry. His mother told him that dinner would be late, so he could have a snack. She told him to go to the kitchen and get a piece of fruit to eat. But John remembered a candy bar that he had in his lunch box and thought of having that instead, even though he knew that the fruit would be better for him.

Focus Question: What should John do?

FAST FOOD   Grades (K–5)

Tim doesn't like the food they serve in the school cafeteria. Some of his friends go to a fast-food restaurant near the school instead. He would like to go with them, but he knows that his parents want him to eat in the cafeteria.

Focus Question: What should Tim do?

Dramatizations

EATING FOR SPECIAL NEEDS   Grades (4–5)

Valued Outcome: The students will be able to plan meals for people with special needs.

Description of Strategy: Have a couple of students in the class role-play patients in the hospital. Example: The first patient is a sixty-seven-year-old man who has no teeth and an ulcer. The second patient is a seven-year-old girl who has had her tonsils removed and has a sore throat. The third patient is a forty-five-year-old man who is overweight and has a serious heart ailment. Make or plan a breakfast, lunch, and dinner for all the patients and then discuss the results.

Materials Needed: none

Processing Questions:

1. Why do some people need to avoid or include certain foods in their diets?
2. What would happen to these patients if they ate or avoided certain foods such as foods that were hard to chew?

STAR SEARCH   Grades (K–5)

Valued Outcome: Students will be able to describe various nutrition problems.

Description of Strategy: Divide the students into groups of four to six. Have them make up a song, poem, dance, or skit about a nutritional problem, such as eating too much junk food or not eating foods from the Food Guide Pyramid. The students then present their work to the class, and the audience should try to guess what the problem is and then discuss it. At the end of the class, reward everyone with stickers or a snack.

Materials Needed: pencils and paper for each student, rewards

Processing Question: Why do so many people in our country have nutritional problems when we have such a plentiful supply of food? How can such nutritional problems affect our overall health?

GOOD AND HEALTHY SNACKS   Grades (K–5)

Valued Outcome: The students will be able to identify nutritious snacks.

Description of Strategy: Ask the students what snacks they like to eat that are good for them (most will respond with apple, orange, or banana). Ask a similar question about vegetables. Then teach students the following Snack Rap:

1. Apples, oranges, lettuce, cheese

   All good snacks, if you please

   Refrain: Five a day are what you need

   To grow up BIG and STRONG you see!

2. Apples, oranges, celery, cheese

   All good snacks, if you please

   (Refrain)

3. Apples, oranges, broccoli, cheese

   All good snacks, if you please

   (Refrain)

Options: The song may be done as a round, or movements may be added. For example, students jump on "BIG" and flex muscles on "STRONG." Additional movement can be added by preceding the song with:

   Come gather round, we will talk

   about good nutrition as we walk.

Materials Needed: none

Processing Question: How many servings of fruits and vegetables should we have every day?

SOURCE: Timpanelli 1999

SELLING A PRODUCT
Grades (4–5)

Valued Outcome: The students will create nutritional advertisements.

Description of Strategy: Divide the students into groups of three to five. Give each group a product (some products should be nutritious and others nonnutritious). Have each group work together to think of a way to sell the product, and then come up in front of the class and try to sell their products. Discuss the product and the food group to which it belongs.

Materials Needed: different food products for each group of students

Processing Questions:

1. Why do companies use advertisements to sell their products?
2. How should we evaluate such advertisements to make sure we make wise nutritional decisions?

FOODS THAT KEEP THE BODY HEALTHY
Grades (K–3)

Valued Outcome: The students will be able to identify certain foods that help keep the body healthy.

Description of Strategy: On butcher paper, draw an outline of three types of bodies: heavy, average, and thin. Have the students attach pictures to each body type that might result from a diet of these foods. Discuss with the students why an excess of certain foods can have a negative effect on the body. (It is important to point out that some diseases may also affect body shape, so diet *is not* the only factor that may be involved.)

To show the positive effect foods have on the body, have students role-play a race. Let two students who are going to run in a race role-play different ways of eating in preparation for the event. For example, one eats very nutritious light meals, whereas the other eats high-calorie junk food. Let the two students enact what they would feel like while running in the race.

Materials Needed: drawing of the three body types on butcher paper, pictures of body types from magazines

Processing Questions:

1. What effect does food have on our body build?
2. What effect does food have on our energy level?
3. What foods should you eat to prepare for a race or other endurance activity?
4. What effect would poor food choices have on one's endurance?

ROLE-PLAYING NUTRIENTS
Grades (K–3)

Valued Outcomes: The students will be able to describe the significance of nutrients, vitamins, and minerals through role-playing.

Description of Strategy: Assemble the students in cooperative groups. Assign each group a category—either nutrient, vitamin, or mineral. Then have each group research their category and dramatize characteristics of their category. The nutrient-category students may use food representations to dramatize characteristics of different nutrients; for example, for the carbohydrates in a fruit, the student could simulate planting, growing, harvesting, shipping, buying, eating, and digesting the food. Each group will present its dramatization to the class and explain why they chose to dramatize the way they did. They will explain the significance of their nutrient, vitamin, or mineral and its relationship to a healthy diet.

Materials Needed: none

Processing Questions:

1. What are the important characteristics of each category of nutrients, vitamins, and minerals?
2. Why is it important to know these characteristics?
3. What foods should you eat to prepare for a race or other endurance activity?
4. What effect would poor food choices have on one's endurnace?

CAFFEINE AND SLEEPING   Grades (K–5)

Valued Outcome: The students will identify one of the effects that caffeine has on the body.

Description of Strategy: Ask the students what they know about sleep. Introduce caffeine by showing the students pictures of chocolate, cola, tea, and coffee. Ask them if they know what the objects in the pictures have in common. Explain that each of the objects contains caffeine. Ask the students if they know what caffeine is. Explain that caffeine is a drug called a stimulant, so it speeds up the nervous system and makes a person jittery or hyperactive. Let the students know that when they eat or drink something that contains caffeine and it makes them hyperactive, it is hard to sleep.

Tell the students that they will play a role-playing game. Divide the class in half: one half will be the actors, the other half will be the guessers. Tell the actors the situation: they are at a friend's birthday party, and they will be spending the night. The friend's mom said that the students could eat as much chocolate and drink as much cola as they like, as a special treat. Give each actor a card that says one of the following: "You said 'No, thank you,' and only ate milk and cookies"; "You ate one piece of chocolate and drank half of a cola"; and "You ate as much chocolate and cola as you could." The actors will demonstrate trying to go to sleep, without saying what they did or didn't eat. After the actors have finished, it is the job of the guessers to decide how much caffeine each actor consumed.

Materials Needed: pictures of chocolate, cola, tea, and coffee; note cards of responses for the game

Processing Questions:

1. How does caffeine make people jittery and hyperactive?
2. What happens when you try to go to sleep after you've had too much caffeine?

CHOOSING FROM A MENU   Grades (K–5)

Valued Outcome: The students will be able to select foods from a restaurant menu.

Description of Strategy: Bring several menus from area restaurants or let students make menus. Have several students enact a situation in which they are seated in a restaurant and must make choices from the menu. Have others play the role of waiter or waitress to help guide the diner's choices.

Materials Needed: menus from restaurants, paper and pencils for each student

Processing Question: Why is it important to know how to order from a menu in a restaurant?

GARDEN PUPPET SHOW   Grades (K–3)

Valued Outcome: The students will be able to demonstrate different foods that are grown in the garden and be able to tell the benefit of each food to the body.

Description of Strategy: Let the students make puppets of different fruits and vegetables. Let them enact a scene in a garden in which the various foods tell what they will do for the body when they are eaten.

Materials Needed: paper lunch bag or cloth; craft items (construction paper, glue, wire, etc.) for each student

Processing Question: How do various garden-grown foods help our bodies function better?

DIETING PUPPETS   Grades (K–3)
AND EATING DISORDERS

Valued Outcome: The students will be able to demonstrate the problems some individuals have in gaining weight and losing weight.

Description of Strategy: Prepare several puppets, some to represent thin people trying to gain weight, others to represent overweight persons trying to lose weight, and some to represent persons with an eating disorder (anorexia nervosa or bulimia). Have the puppets sitting at a table during a meal and discussing why they are eating (or not eating) various foods.

Materials Needed: paper lunch bags or cloth and markers or crayons for each student

Processing Question: Why do some thin people try to lose more weight? How can such behavior affect that person's health?

NUTRIENTS ON TRIAL   Grades (4–5)

Valued Outcome: The students will be able to determine essential functions of the nutrients of the body.

Description of Strategy: Have the students conduct a mock court having nutrients on trial. Give the students situations in which the nutrients on trial are accused of not being useful to the body. The nutrients' defendants must defend their essential function in the body.

Materials Needed: judge's gavel and robe (optional)

Processing Question: What are the useful functions provided by each nutrient?

CAFETERIA SELECTION   Grades (K–5)

Valued Outcome: The students will be able to select a meal by choosing foods from each level of the Food Guide Pyramid.

Description of Strategy: Using food pictures, set up a "cafeteria line" from which students will choose a meal to place on a tray. Have students take turns being the cashiers—checking to see that choices include food from each level of the Food Guide Pyramid.

Materials Needed: food pictures from magazines, scissors, glue, paper

Processing Question: Why do we need foods from each level of the pyramid?

FOOD PUPPETS   Grades (4–5)

Valued Outcome: The students will be able to select foods that provide a balanced diet.

Description of Strategy: After discussing the foods from Food Guide Pyramid and the nutrients they provide, have the class make puppets representing various foods from the pyramid. Prepare a skit that explains how the foods work together to provide a balanced diet containing all essential nutrients, including water.

Materials Needed: paper lunch bag or cloth, markers or crayons, construction paper, and glue for each student

Processing Question: How can combinations of foods enhance our health?

STRANGER IN A STRANGE LAND   Grades (4–5)

Valued Outcome: The students will be able to discuss typical foods eaten in different countries.

Description of Strategy: Divide the class into small groups. Have each research the foods and dishes eaten in a different nation, such as Mexico, India, Malaysia, Germany, Japan, and Greece. Then have the students in each group prepare models or drawings of different typical dishes served in their assigned nation. You act the part of a traveler who has just arrived in the country and is very hungry. Ask about each dish the students have to offer. What is it made of? How is it prepared? How does it taste? How does one eat it? Follow with a general discussion of different ethnic foods.

Materials Needed: paper, markers, modeling clay, and paint for each student

Processing Questions:

1. How do other countries' eating habits differ from ours?
2. Why should we know about other cultures' dietary habits?

Discussion and Report Techniques

FOOD LABELS IN THE CLASSROOM   Grades (3–5)

Valued Outcome: The students will be able to identify the nutritional content of various foods.

Description of Strategy: Give each student several food labels. Then have each student read thoroughly all information given on the packaging and write down all nutritional information such as grams of protein, carbohydrates, and fat per serving. Use current health references (nutrition textbooks and brochures) to go over the six basic dietary requirements for maintaining a healthy body, which are carbohydrates, protein, lipids, vitamins, minerals, and water, and look for these dietary requirements on food labels. Make a classroom list of packaging and labeling techniques meant to attract the consumer; classify these appeals into categories such as good taste, low cost, convenience, and health. Under the health category determine which health factors are being considered (low in calories, no cholesterol, fiber, and no additives). Answer any questions that the students have regarding the food labels.

Materials Needed: Food labels brought in by students, brochures and textbooks on nutrition, overhead projector and pens or board and markers

Processing Questions:

1. How can attractive packaging often mislead or confuse the consumer regarding the nutritional value of the contents found within?
2. How important is it to read food labels carefully before consuming a product?

SOURCE: Teacher Store 1999; Roger 1994

THE INFLUENCE OF ADVERTISING ON FOOD CHOICES

Grades (3–5)

Valued Outcome: The students will be able to identify advertising techniques that influence consumers to buy food products.

Description of Strategy: Have the students cut out food advertisements from magazines and newspapers. Show the class a short tape that you have prepared of recorded food commercials. Then divide the students into groups of three to five. In the groups, have the students discuss the techniques used in the commercials and printed advertisements to try to sell the various food products. Have each group make a list of these techniques and share them in a class discussion. Record the students' answers on the board. After all responses have been recorded, discuss the following advertisement approaches: bandwagon, brand loyalty, testimonial (celebrity appeal), feel good appeal, overgeneralization, and reward appeal. Categorize the list on the board into these six approaches. Then give each group two products to advertise—one that is nutritious and another that is nonnutritious (such as a food with very high fat content). Direct the groups to create a magazine or newspaper advertisement or a thirty-second commercial to advertise both products and present the advertisements to the class. Conclude the lesson with a discussion of the advertising techniques used to advertise the various products.

Materials Needed: magazines, newspapers, paper, pencils, art supplies, and products (pictures or actual products) for each group; taped food commercials; television; VCR; and overhead projector and pens or board and markers

Processing Questions:

1. When creating your advertisements, did you use a different strategy to promote the different types of foods (nutritious versus nonnutritious)? What did or did not influence this difference?

2. Name three types of advertising techniques and give an example of each.

3. How are food advertisements produced to make you want to buy and eat that particular type of food?

4. Do you think food advertisements have enticed you to buy a food that you did not actually need?

SOURCE: Health Strategies, Inc. 2002

FUN WITH FOOD: THE FOOD GUIDE PYRAMID

Grades (3–5)

Valued Outcome: The students will be able to keep a food log and match the foods they have eaten to the correct categories in the Food Guide Pyramid.

Description of Strategy: Have the students talk about their favorite foods and the foods they commonly eat at home. Write some of them on the board. Then draw a food pyramid on the board. Have the students draw their own food pyramid and write the various foods listed on the board in the proper place on their pyramids. Instruct the students to use their pyramid to help make food choices.

Next, give each student a handout of the Food Guide Pyramid labeled with the proper group names and examples of what goes in each category. Include on the handout the number of servings of each food they should eat. Review the handout with the students and help them name the foods on the pyramid. Ask questions such as: What are the foods we need to eat the most of (cereal, bread, rice, pasta)? What are the foods we need to eat the least of (butter, margarine, oils, sweets)? Have students look at the pictures on the handout and read the names of the foods as they point to them. Refer back to the list of foods that the students ate at home and have the class try to figure out the foods that go into each category.

Divide the students into small groups (no more than three students in a group) and ask them to determine what foods make up a balanced meal for breakfast, lunch, and dinner. Have the students draw and label the foods that they choose. Encourage the students to consider food they eat at home or food they would like to eat at home. Prompt the students with questions to get them to evaluate the decisions they made on their menus. Ask these questions: Is your own diet out of balance? What would you do to change your diet to come up with a better balance? When the students are done completing their food pyramids, have them share the meals they created with the class. Display the meals around the room or on the bulletin board.

Materials Needed: board and markers or overhead projector and pens; paper, pencils, handouts of Food Guide Pyramid for each student; construction paper, scissors, glue, markers, and crayons for each group.

Processing Question: What is the Food Guide Pyramid? What types of foods go in each category?

SOURCE: Teacher Store 1999; Gassiott 1999

WOULD YOU LIKE A SNACK? Grades (3–5)

Valued Outcome: The students will be able to decide what are nutritious and nonnutritious snacks.

Description of Strategy: Have the students work in pairs or groups of three. Supply each group with one poster board and one marker. Have them label the first side of the poster Nutritious Snacks and the other side Nonnutritious Snacks. Have the partners decide on three nutritious snacks and determine to which food group each snack belongs. Then have them do the same for three nonnutritious snacks. Have a class discussion about the answers on their posters. After discussing the snacks, have all of the students write down on a sheet of paper a menu for a nutritious breakfast, lunch, and dinner. Then have them write down one breakfast, lunch, and dinner that is not nutritious. Once again, discuss these with the class.

Materials Needed: poster board, markers, and paper for each group; pencils for each student

Processing Questions:

1. Why should we eat nutritious snacks?
2. Why is it important not to eat nonnutritional snacks?

SOURCE: Emazing, Inc. 1999

NUTRITION   Grades (K–5)

Valued Outcome: The students will identify the six basic dietary requirements needed for maintaining a healthy body and how the body benefits from each of the nutrients.

Description of Strategy: Explain to the class that today's lesson is about being able to identify the six basic dietary nutrients needed for maintaining a healthy body and the benefits from each nutrient. Introduce the six basic dietary required nutrients (carbohydrates, proteins, lipids, water, vitamins, and minerals) and list them on the board. Tell the students some of the foods that contain many of the six basic nutrients; for example, pasta contains carbohydrates, peanut butter contains protein, ice cream contains fat (lipids), and so on. Pick students to go to the board three at a time and write a food under each category for the six nutrients. Each student will have an opportunity to write a food on the board. Explain the importance of each of the dietary nutrients in relation to its function in the body. Explain that they are the substances in food needed to support life functions. For example, fats are an important part of all cells, membrane structures in the body, and tissues; and proteins provide calories, build and repair body tissues, and function as enzymes, antibodies, and so on. (See Chapter 17.)

Materials Needed: overhead projector and pens or board and markers

Processing Question: Why is it important to consume each of the nutrients daily?

FOOD GUIDE COLLAGE   Grades (3–5)

Valued Outcome: The students will explain why the Food Guide Pyramid is a valid source of information about nutrition.

Description of Strategy: Have the students collect food pictures from magazines, newspapers, or grocery store advertisements. Ask students to find ten to fifteen pictures each. Collect all the pictures, place them in a pile, and mix them up. Organize students into groups of four or five. Give each group a poster board and an equal portion of the magazine pictures. Tell students to cut the poster board into the shape of a pyramid and paste the magazine pictures of food to make a collage, showing foods in each food group. (Have a large copy of the Food Group Pyramid displayed in class for use as a reference.) Each group will present their collage to the class and explain the different food groups.

You can extend this activity and create an assessment of the program by asking students to use the posters as a reference and draw a healthy meal on a paper plate.

Materials Needed: large copy of the Food Guide Pyramid for display; magazine, newspaper, and grocery store advertisements; poster board, glue or tape, crayons, and scissors for each group

Processing Questions:

1. Why is it important to eat a variety of foods?

2. In which category of the Food Guide Pyramid do you have difficulty meeting the recommended servings each day?

SOURCE: Health Strategies, Inc. 2002

NUTRITION   Grades (3–4)

Valued Outcome: The students will be able to explain the difference between their own eating habits and the eating habits of others.

Description of Strategy: Have the students write down their favorite ethnic food (Italian, American, Mexican, etc.), their overall favorite food, their favorite fruit, their favorite vegetable, and their favorite dessert. Explain why some of the foods are more nutritious than others, the different foods that each ethnic group cooks, and the nutritional value of those foods. Announce a category (e.g., favorite ethnic group), and have all the students with the same answer stand together. Do this until all the categories are completed. Then as a class, talk about everyone's favorite foods.

Materials Needed: paper and pencils for each student

Processing Question: Does everyone have the same tastes and favorite foods? Why or why not?

FOOD BASKET TURNOVER   Grades (4–5)

Valued Outcome: The students will be able to demonstrate knowledge of the essential groups of the Food Guide Pyramid.

Description of Strategy: Using masking tape, create the outline of a food pyramid on the classroom floor. Designate each area by a sheet of paper affixed alongside each section (the label should contain the name of the food group and the amount of servings suggested daily). Instruct students to brainstorm different foods that fit into each category of the Food Guide Pyramid and write them on a piece of paper. Have them include at least one food that they have never tried and one food that they dislike in each food group and place NT beside the food he or she has never tried and DL beside the food he or she dislikes. Compile a written list of foods (grouped by category) on the overhead, while the students name the food group in which it belongs.

Explain that the class will play a game called "Food Basket Turnover" to help them learn how many servings of each food group are necessary for a healthy diet. Have each student draw one food task card from a group of prepared task cards (each containing a picture of a different type of food), take the card, and move to the appropriate location on the classroom floor. After all task cards have been chosen, visually check for accuracy and declare, "Food Basket Turnover!" On this signal, the students return to their desks. Repeat the pyramid activity two additional times. Have students share orally with classmates one fact learned from their experience and participation in the Food Guide Pyramid activity.

Materials Needed: masking tape, paper and pencils, overhead projector and pens, large Food Guide Pyramid chart, food task cards (one per student, each with a picture of a specific food)

Processing Question: How is the Food Guide Pyramid helpful in planning our daily diets?

DIET AND ATHLETIC PERFORMANCE   Grades (5–6)

Valued Outcome: The students will be able to research and report on the relationship between proper diet and improved athletic performance.

Description of Strategy: Have the students research the relationship between proper diet and improved athletic performance. One suggestion is to have them interview a local high school athlete or coach for his or her own eating behaviors. Report the results to the class.

Materials Needed: references on diet and athletic performance

Processing Questions:

1. What effect does a nutritious diet have on athletic performance?
2. What effect does a poor diet have on athletic performance?
3. What types of foods should be eaten to enhance athletic performance?

FOOD JOURNAL   Grades (4–5)

Valued Outcome: The students will be able to describe their eating habits.

Description of Strategy: Have the students keep a journal of what they eat for one week, starting on a Sunday and ending on the following Saturday. (Provide them with charts such as the sample chart below.)

Date and Time	Foods	Servings	Place	With Whom

Have them bring this to class on the Monday after it is completed. In pairs, have students use the Food Guide Pyramid to decide the number of servings from each section that were eaten each day. The students should record this information on a separate sheet of paper. After the number of servings for each section for each day has been tallied, make a class graph showing the food groups and the number of servings eaten for any one day. (Decide which day you want to use. You may want to use one weekday and one weekend day to compare.) Use the graph to talk about how many students are eating the correct number of servings. Lead a discussion on what foods they need to eat more or less of to be healthier.

Materials Needed: pencil or pen and journals for each student, chart, a copy of the Food Guide Pyramid, materials to compile a class graph

Processing Questions:

1. In which areas of the pyramid did you eat enough, and in which did you not eat enough?

2. Why do we eat sometimes even when we are not hungry?

BREAKFAST BOOK   Grades (K–5)

Valued Outcome: The students will be able to explain how a healthy diet can increase the likelihood of physical and mental wellness.

Description of Strategy: If your school has a breakfast program, explain to the students that these meals are nutritionally balanced to provide the fuel needed to help their bodies work. Ask the students for suggestions, and make a "Healthy Breakfast List" on large chart paper. In order to have a nutritious breakfast, include food from at least three of the food groups. Some ideas are peanut butter on toast, yogurt, cereal with fruit, cold pizza, fresh or dried fruit, a glass of juice, a sandwich, and a glass of milk. Have the students write a Big Breakfast Book about the foods they like to eat for breakfast; include things such as what they like to eat, whom they eat with, how they feel when they do not eat breakfast, and so on. Have each student write or dictate his or her own words and illustrate them. Then bind all pages together into a book; let the students choose the title for their book. When the book is complete, read it to the class, let each student author read his or her own page to the class, or let the principal come in for an authors' reading. Display the book for the students to see.

Materials Needed: chart paper, pencils, markers or crayons, and paper for each student

Processing Question: Why is breakfast the most important meal?

SOURCE: Utah Education Network 1996, 1997b

FAVORITE FOOD CHART   Grades (K–1)

Valued Outcome: The students will be able to name their favorite foods.

Description of Strategy: Have a large piece of chart paper up on the board. Ask the students to think of all their favorite foods: foods their parents make, foods they eat at their grandparents' house, foods they order when they eat out, or foods they eat at their friends' homes. As the students name each food, write it down on the chart paper. Let them illustrate their words. They could look at all the words that begin with a particular letter. They could also look for letters in their names that appear on the chart. Ask the students which foods they think will be the best for their bodies.

Materials Needed: chart paper; pencils, markers, or crayons

Processing Question: What qualities of these foods make them your favorites? Is a food with these qualities necessarily good for you?

SOURCE: Utah Education Network 1996

FOODS FROM AROUND THE WORLD   Grades (4–5)

Valued Outcome: The students will be able to report on foods grown in different countries and regions.

Description of Strategy: Locate countries or regions on a world map. Have the students choose a particular country or region and research the history of a food or type of food from that country. Students will then present in oral, written, or pictorial form their information about the foods from a specific country.

Materials Needed: maps and geographical information about different countries, chart paper, and markers for students who choose the written or pictorial form

Processing Question: How does the preparation and type of food that you researched differ from American food?

DO YOU WANT TO EAT THIS FOOD?   Grades (5–6)

Valued Outcome: The students will be able to read and interpret food labels for various products.

Description of Strategy: Have the students compare the nutrition labels from various foods, such as waffles, potato chips, soup, yogurt, and ice cream. Have the students determine which they would rather eat according to the nutrition labels.

Materials Needed: food labels from various products

Processing Question: Why is it important to be able to understand food labels?

NUTRITION IQ   Grades (4–5)

Valued Outcome: The students will be able to test their nutrition knowledge by completing the worksheet.

Description of Strategy: Have each student complete a worksheet containing questions such as those in the following list. Have the students turn in their work or discuss the questions as a class.

True or False

T/F 1. You'll get proper nourishment if you just eat a variety of foods.

T/F 2. People who don't eat meat, poultry, or fish can still stay healthy.

T/F 3. Food eaten between meals can be just as good for your health as food eaten at regular meals.

T/F 4. Fresh vegetables cooked at home are always more nutritious than canned or frozen vegetables.

T/F 5. A high-protein, low-carbohydrate diet is ideal for losing weight.

T/F 6. When dieting, avoid starchy foods, such as bread and potatoes.

T/F 7. If you weigh what you should (according to accepted weight standards), you're getting proper nourishment.

T/F 8. Milk contains all the essential elements of a good diet.

T/F 9. Give a child all the foods he or she wants, and the child will never suffer from malnutrition.

T/F 10. Dark bread has the same caloric value as white bread.

T/F 11. Once a person stops exercising, muscle fibers change to fat.

T/F 12. Women in their childbearing years need more iron than men do.

Materials Needed: worksheets and pencils for each student

Processing Question: Why is it important to our health to have a good "nutrition IQ"?

BEING HEALTHY!   Grades (4–5)

Valued Outcome: The students will be able to explain the effects of a proper diet on their physical and mental health.

Description of Strategy: Have the students write down four to six sentences about how they feel mentally, physically, and emotionally when they eat nutritious foods. Then, have them do the same thing about how they feel when they eat nonnutritious foods. Write the three aspects of health on the board, and discuss the answers.

Materials Needed: pencil and paper for each student, board or overhead projector and markers

Processing Question: How can food affect your ability to learn?

GROCERY SHOPPING   Grades (K–3)

Valued Outcome: The students will be able to purchase foods efficiently from a "grocery store."

Description of Strategy: Tell the students that they are each to pretend they have $20. Have a variety of food labels set up on a table with their prices. Make note cards for fruits and other products for which you don't have labels. Tell the students that they need to purchase food for two people for three days. Have them shop for the food they'll eat by writing down the food item and its cost. Discuss the results by asking a variety of questions, such as: Who here has bought enough food for three meals a day? Who has bought something from each category of the Food Guide Pyramid?

Materials Needed: food labels, note cards representing fruit and other products without labels

Processing Questions:

1. Why is it important to plan a budget for buying food?
2. What can you learn about a food from reading the label?

HEALTHY BREAKFASTS   Grades (K–3)

Valued Outcome: The students will be able to explain why we need a good breakfast and will be able to choose healthy breakfast foods.

Description of Strategy: Give each student a magazine containing food pictures that he or she can cut out. The students will cut out enough pictures to create a balanced breakfast. They will glue these pictures onto a sheet of construction paper labeled "A Healthful Breakfast."

Materials Needed: magazines, glue, scissors, construction paper, and markers or crayons for each student

Processing Questions:

1. Why is breakfast called the most important meal of the day?
2. What types of foods are good to eat at breakfast?

EATING FOR HEALTHY TEETH   Grades (K–5)

Valued Outcome: The students will be able to identify foods that are good for the teeth.

Description of Strategy: Share the following information with the students. Unhealthy foods are foods that stick to your teeth and/or contain a lot of sugar. Healthy foods can include those foods, like apples, that can help clean your teeth as you eat them. Other healthy foods for teeth include foods high in calcium and phosphorus. Remind students that even healthy foods can promote tooth decay if trapped food is not removed from teeth by flossing and brushing, since bacteria can grow in food left on and around teeth.

Have students bring in at least ten pictures—drawn or cut out of magazines and glued or taped onto paper—of healthy and unhealthy foods for our teeth. Have them label each picture healthy or unhealthy.

Write Healthy and Unhealthy on the board and provide examples for both categories. Then divide the class into groups of three or four. Say, "Please work as a group. Copy the chart and words off the board. As a group, complete the chart by listing healthy foods for teeth under the Healthy side and the unhealthy foods under the Unhealthy side." Walk around the room to monitor for understanding. Allow time for them to complete the assignment. When all groups

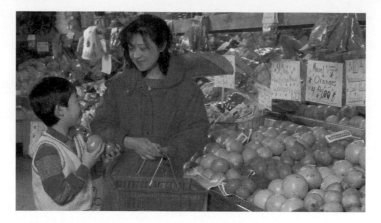

A field trip to the grocery store is an excellent strategy for teaching nutrition.

have finished, have the class help you complete the chart on the board. Have them explain why they put certain foods under certain categories. Have students review the labels they put on their magazine pictures. Should any of these labels be changed?

Materials Needed: board and markers or overhead projector and pen; magazines, glue or tape, paper, and pencils for each student

Processing Questions:

1. What are the healthiest foods to eat for our teeth?
2. What foods will hurt our teeth?

HEALTHY WEIGHT

Grades (4–5)

Valued Outcome: The students will be able to explain the benefits of being at a healthful weight.

Description of Strategy: Write the following menus on the board and ask the students which lunch is more nutritious.

Menu 1: skim milk, bran muffin, fruit salad, broiled chicken, whole-grain rice, beans

Menu 2: chocolate milkshake, cheeseburger, french fries, chocolate chip cookies

Then list the seven diet goals on the board:

1. Eat a variety of foods.
2. Be at a healthful weight.
3. Eat few fatty foods.
4. Eat more fiber.
5. Eat less sugar.
6. Use less salt.
7. Do not drink alcohol.

Have the students write the diet goals on a 3×5 index card. They should keep the index card with them and refer to it at mealtimes until they have memorized the goals. This will help them become accustomed to considering the diet goals when selecting foods. Discuss each diet goal. For example:

- *Eat a variety of foods.* Ask students to identify the food groups and give the number of servings from each group that should be eaten daily.

- *Be at a healthful weight.* Explain that your body works best when you are at the weight that is right for you. Let the students know that the doctor can tell them if they are at a healthful weight. Explain to the students that they can make wise choices to help them be at a healthful weight and how important it is to exercise and eat properly balanced meals.

Materials Needed: board and markers or overhead projector and pen, 3×5 index cards

Processing Questions:

1. Why should you follow the seven diet goals?
2. What are some ways nutrients help your body?
3. Why is it important to be at a healthful weight?

CLASSIFYING NUTRITIOUS AND NONNUTRITIOUS SNACKS

Grades (K–2)

Valued Outcome: After completing the week's activity centers, the students will be able to categorize healthy and unhealthy snacks.

Description of Strategy: Introduce each center as follows:

"Today, class, we are starting a new week, and the topic is nutrition. All our centers will be related to nutrition.

"First we have the Book Center. There are many books to read and look at. There will also be a couple of books you can listen to.

"Next we have the Block Center. Here I encourage you to use your imagination and relate something you build to healthy and unhealthy snacks.

"Next we have the Writing Center. Here you can make your own nutrition journal by tying some decorative paper together. Today's topic is to draw or tell about the snacks that you like to eat.

"Next we have the Cooking Center, where you can mix your own healthy snack. After you mix together the appropriate ingredients, you can take your mix to the eating area and enjoy it. You will be mixing things like Chex cereal, pretzels, peanuts, raisins, and popcorn in a little bag and shake it all together. Then it is ready to eat.

"Next we have the Art Center. In art today we are going to make a collage of nutritious (good for you) and nonnutritious (not so good for you) snacks. Look through the magazines and find pictures of either nutritious snacks or nonnutritious snacks. Then glue them on your piece of paper. Try choosing only pictures of nutritious and nonnutritious snacks for your collage.

"In the Math Center, you will sort the pictures of snacks into two piles of nutritious and nonnutritious snacks.

"In the Language Arts Center, there is a worksheet, and on the worksheet there are both nutritious and nonnutritious snacks. Color the nutritious snacks.

"In the Science Center, you will taste nutritious and nonnutritious snacks and chart how well you liked each snack. Then as a class we will look at the results to see who liked what the best.

"In the Game Center there will be several games to play, such as Xs and Os, Hangman using the Alphabits cereal, and the usual games that are there.

Materials Needed: nutrition books, building blocks, decorative paper, crayons or markers, nutritious and nonnutritious snacks; sandwich bags, magazines, construction paper, glue, title cards, worksheet for Language Center that has pictures of both nutritious and nonnutritious foods; Alphabits cereal

Processing Question: What types of food provide the healthiest snacks?

SCHOOL CAFETERIA MENUS   Grades (4–5)

Valued Outcome: The students will be able to write sample menus incorporating a variety of foods from the school lunch program.

Description of Strategy: Have the school dietitian bring various cafeteria menus to class and show how a variety of foods is incorporated into them. Have the students write sample menus incorporating a variety of food characteristics for the school lunch program.

Materials Needed: pen and paper, copies of the Food Guide Pyramid (optional for each student)

Processing Question: Does your school lunch menu have foods from each category of the Food Guide Pyramid?

WEIGHT MANAGEMENT PROGRAMS   Grades (6–8)

Valued Outcome: The students will be able to learn healthy weight reduction methods.

Description of Strategy: Invite a leader of a weight reduction group that stresses balanced nutrition in its program to discuss the effect and health implications of prolonged overeating and crash diets. Have students submit questions on index cards in advance to be answered by the resource person.

Materials Needed: index cards for each student

Processing Questions:

1. What are the dangers of dieting improperly?
2. Why are fad diets so popular?

CANDY MACHINES IN THE SCHOOLS DEBATE

Grades (3–5)

Valued Outcome: The students will be able to debate whether candy machines should or should not be installed in the school cafeteria.

Description of Strategy: Should candy machines be placed in the school cafeteria? Have two debate teams argue the issue. Act as moderator and keep the debate on track. Then follow with a general class discussion.

Materials Needed: none

Processing Questions:

1. Why are candy machines present in some schools?
2. Does the presence of such machines encourage poor eating habits on the part of some students?

FOOD LABEL ACTIVITY

Grades (5–6)

Valued Outcome: The students will be able to identify and report on regulations concerning labeling food.

Description of Strategy: Have the students research the regulations concerning labeling of packaged foods and present their reports either orally or in writing. Individualize the activity by having each student prepare a report on a specific food product. Then have the student discuss his or her findings in class, explaining what information is contained on the label of the package for his or her product. Later, put all the packages on display so that students may examine them.

Materials Needed: various packaged foods

Processing Questions:

1. Why do packaged foods have labels?
2. How can such labels help us eat healthier?

DIET MODIFICATION

Grades (4–5)

Valued Outcome: The students will be able to compare diet modifications.

Description of Strategy: Give the students a problem such as modifying diets for athletes or planning inexpensive party menus. Have them consult at least three different sources of information. Compare the conclusions that might be reached from the information derived from the three sources.

Materials Needed: references on diets

Processing Questions:

1. How do professional nutritionists help us eat more healthily?

2. Why is it important to plan the meals for events such as those listed in the Description of Strategy?

BRAINSTORMING ABOUT NUTRITION   Grades (K–5)

Valued Outcome: The students will be able to brainstorm concerns about the school food service program.

Description of Strategy: Organize students into several groups. Have them identify students' concerns about the school food service program and brainstorm potential solutions to the problems they have identified. Have them summarize their ideas and present them to the school dietitian.

Materials Needed: paper and pencils for each student

Processing Questions:

1. How would you rate your school food service program?

2. What barriers to effectiveness do most school food service programs face?

PYRAMID ESSAY   Grades (4–5)

Valued Outcome: The students will be able to identify foods from the Food Guide Pyramid that they like the least and the best.

Description of Strategy: After a discussion of the Food Guide Pyramid, have the students write a short essay about the food group they like the best and the least, along with their favorite and least favorite foods in the groups.

Materials Needed: a poster of the Food Guide Pyramid, paper and pencils for each student

Processing Questions:

1. What is the purpose of the Food Guide Pyramid?

2. Which levels do you like the most? The least?

Experiments and Demonstrations

SAY CHEESE   Grades (K–5)

Valued Outcome: The students will be able to compare and contrast the taste and texture of various cheeses. The students will be able to determine that cheeses are part of the dairy section of the Food Guide Pyramid.

Description of Strategy: Display a variety of cheeses such as cheddar, colby, blue, Swiss, mozzarella, Monterey Jack, etc. Have students compare and contrast the cheeses regarding the texture, taste, and smell. Give each student a handout

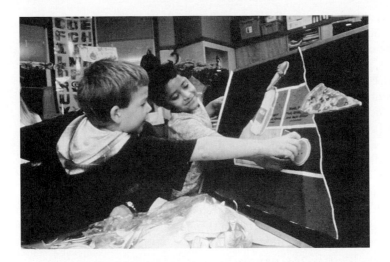

Hands-on activities enhance the learning of health concepts.

that lists the different cheeses. Have the students fill in the three columns (texture, smell, and taste). Have students write down if the cheese is soft, hard, crumbly, or smooth to touch. Next, have the students describe the way the cheese smells. Last, have the students write down if the cheese is peppery, sharp, tangy, or buttery when they tasted it. After the students have tasted, felt, and smelled the cheeses, have them compare the results to see which cheeses are similar and which ones are different. Graph the students' results on the board. Follow the activity with a discussion about why cheese belongs in the dairy section of the Food Guide Pyramid.

Materials Needed: a variety of cheeses, handout for each student listing types of cheeses

Processing Questions:

1. Which type of cheese did you like the best?
2. Did you find any cheeses that tasted the same?
3. What food category of the Food Guide Pyramid does cheese belong to?

SOURCES: American Dairy Association 2002; National Dairy Council 2003

FATTY FOODS   Grades (4–5)

Valued Outcome: Students will be able to list benefits and drawbacks of eating fatty foods and will identify foods that are high in fat through experimentation.

Description of Strategy: Divide students into groups. Have each group make a chart about the benefits and drawbacks of including fatty foods in their diets. Discuss the answers that the groups listed. Be sure to talk about fat as a necessary nutrient for the body. Point out that fat helps us by giving us energy and by keeping our skin and hair healthy, insulating our body to protect us from heat and cold, and cushioning parts of the body such as our bottoms and the soles of our feet. Also mention that excess fat can lead to heart, lung, and joint problems, so we do not need very much fat. The top of the Food Guide Pyramid includes fats, oils, and sweets. This means that very little of this group should be part of our diets.

Have the students test various foods (for example, corn or potato chips, sunflower seeds, pecans, peanut butter, mayonnaise, cheese, butter, margarine, lettuce, celery, cooked pasta, potatoes, tomatoes, oranges, apples, bananas, carrots, chocolate chips, coconut, and cooked rice) to find out their fat and oil content. Have the students cut brown paper sacks into squares and draw circles on the paper. Label each circle with a specific food. Then have them break off a piece of that food and rub it on the paper within the circle. Allow the paper to dry completely. Foods that are high in fat/oil will leave translucent spots where they were rubbed on the paper. Have the students make a chart with two columns. Label one column Foods Containing Fat/Oil, and the other column Foods with Little or No Fat/Oil and list the foods they tested under the appropriate column. Have the class discuss the results of the experiment and any foods that surprised them with their fat and oil content.

Materials Needed: notebook paper, pencils, brown paper sacks cut into square pieces, foods to test

Processing Questions:

1. What are two benefits and two drawbacks of including fat in your diet?

2. Were you surprised by the amount of fat/oil in any of the foods? Which ones and why?

SOURCE: Health Strategies, Inc. 2002

LET'S BE HEALTHY! Grades (K–4)

Valued Outcome: The students will be able to explain how to use good habits and make wise choices for good health. They will see how exercise, regular bathing, and good personal hygiene pay off in the future. They will also describe how they can have strong bones, a nice complexion, and healthy teeth.

Description of Strategy: Post the Food Guide Pyramid in front of the classroom. Tell the students how important it is to eat right. Tell them about each of the food groups.

- *Fats, Oils, and Sweets*—includes fried foods, sugary foods
- *Dairy Group*—includes cheese, butter, ice cream, yogurt
- *Vegetable Group*—includes broccoli, lettuce, spinach, carrots
- *Meat Group*—includes pork, steak, beef, beans
- *Fruit Group*—includes apples, oranges, tangerines, cantaloupes
- *Bread Group*—includes rolls, cereal, crackers, pasta

Have the students work in groups of three. Tell them that they need to measure one cup of Kix, one cup of Cheerios, and one cup of Chex and pour them into a large bowl. Tell the students to now add two cups of pretzels and two cups of raisins. Let the students know this is healthy for an in-between meal snack. Have each student choose a magazine and cut out pictures of a toothbrush, cup, a soft drink, comb, hairbrush, and spoon or fork. Paste the pictures on a piece of construction paper and have the students draw an X through each picture. Title the poster "Things I do not share." Now cut out pictures of things the students can share; paste them on another piece of construction paper and label it "Things I can share." Teach the students the following song for when they brush their teeth so they will be more excited about brushing.

> This is the way we brush our teeth,
> Brush our teeth,
> Brush our teeth.
> This is the way we brush our teeth,
> So early in the morning!

Materials Needed: Food Guide Pyramid for display; boxes of Kix, Cheerios, and Chex; raisins; pretzels; magazines; scissors; glue; markers for each student

Processing Question: How can we learn to make the right food choices?

SOURCE: U.S. Department of Education 2002, 2003

OUR BODIES NEED WATER   Grades (4–5)

Valued Outcome: The students will measure and physically see how much water is recommended each day. Through tracking and recording their water intake, the students will see if their intake meets the daily requirements (eight fluid ounces per day).

Description of Strategy: Make the following statements about water and the ways it helps your body: Water in blood lets it flow through the body, carrying nutrients and oxygen. Water helps cool our bodies when we sweat. Water helps our bodies remove wastes. The body needs at least a quart of water each day to replace water that it uses.

Group the students in pairs. Each pair needs either a four-ounce glass, an eight-ounce bottle of water, a sixteen-ounce thermos, or a thirty-two-ounce pitcher of water. Each group also needs a quart container filled with water. Have the groups measure out how many of their containers equals one quart of water. Record their answers on the board. Display a picture of bottled water, watermelon, fruit juice, celery, lettuce, and tomato. Ask students which foods are sources of water (all of them). Have students cut out pictures of foods that are sources of water. Have each student make a collage. Show them how much a quart of water is in a clear container. Ask them if they drink that much every day.

Materials Needed: one container for each pair of students (available container sizes should be four, eight, sixteen, and thirty-two ounces), one quart of water for every two students; board and markers or overhead projector and pen; pictures of various drinks and foods for display; magazines, scissors, construction paper, glue for each student

Processing Questions:
1. Why is water important to us?
2. Do you drink enough water?

SOURCE: Health Strategies, Inc. 2002

IS IT HEALTHY OR NOT?   Grades (K–5)

Valued Outcome: The students will be able to determine if a group of foods comprises a healthy meal.

Description of Strategy: Set up several meals on a table. Have a highly nutritious meal, a nonnutritious meal, a somewhat nutritious meal, etc. Divide the class into groups of four. Have the groups go to each meal and look at them, but tell students they must work individually. Give them five to seven minutes at each station and have them guess whether the meal is nutritious. Tell them that they are not allowed to talk to anyone. Have them write whatever comments they want about the meal. Then have the groups get together and discuss what they wrote. Have a group discussion about every meal. Let the groups explain what they wrote and why.

Materials Needed: food (or pictures of food set on plates), plates, glasses, utensils

Processing Question: What criteria do you use to decide whether or not a meal is nutritious?

FATS AND THE HEART   Grades (3–5)

Valued Outcome: The students will be able to describe the effects of a poor diet on the heart.

Description of Strategy: Have a picture of the heart on the wall. Point out the different valves. Explain how the blood enters and leaves the heart. Ask a variety of questions about the heart. Show the fact that eating too much junk food that contains fat can block one of the valves. When a valve is blocked it can cause the heart to beat abnormally. If the heart doesn't beat normally, it can stop and this can cause a heart attack. Show students a section of hose or pipe that has been cut open lengthwise (to simulate a blood vessel) and has a piece of chewed gum or some putty stuck to an inside wall (to simulate a fatty deposit, or plaque). Point out that blocked blood vessels can also trigger a heart attack. Bring in pieces of fat. Try to get a pound of fat (or suet) so students can see what it looks like when you gain a pound of fat.

Materials Needed: picture of the heart (must show interior structures), hose or pipe cut lengthwise, piece of chewed gum or putty, a pound of fat (suet)

Processing Questions:

1. How do nutritious foods help the heart function better?
2. How do nonnutritious foods harm the functioning of the heart?

COMPLETE PROTEINS   Grades (4–5)

Valued Outcome: The students will be able to describe complete proteins.

Description of Strategy: Explain how complete proteins contain just the right amounts of all nine essential amino acids. Animal sources of protein (meat, fish, eggs, milk, and milk products) contain complete proteins. Plant sources of protein (dried beans, peas, nuts, breads, and cereals) contain incomplete proteins. These are low in one or more essential amino acids. Have index cards made that have the names of foods that provide incomplete proteins written on them ("Beans," "Rice," "Grains"). Take two blank cards and put them together. Label this "Complete protein." Then take one incomplete protein card and add another incomplete protein card to show how to make a complete protein, such as "Beans and Rice." Explain the fact that this method of combining foods to make a complete protein is what most vegetarians do because they don't eat meat.

Materials Needed: index cards with labels as described in Description of Strategy

Processing Questions:

1. What role does protein play in our diet?
2. What would happen to the body if we did not eat enough of the right kind of proteins?

EATING FEWER FATTY FOODS   Grades (K–5)

Valued Outcome: The students will be able to identify fatty foods, different kinds of sugars, and salt content of various foods and follow a plan to eat fewer of all three food types. They will be able to identify sources of fiber by reading cereal box labels and follow a plan to eat more fiber.

Description of Strategy: Place a piece of bacon and a slice of an apple on a brown paper grocery bag to demonstrate how the bacon leaves a grease spot but the apple does not. Explain to the students that fats such as that which left the grease spot can collect on arterial walls. Then, using empty cereal boxes, have the students read the cereal labels to determine which cereals contain sources of fiber. Instruct the students to create a name for a cereal that tells the consumer that the cereal contains fiber.

Write the following words on the board: *glucose, sucrose, maltose, fructose, lactose,* and *corn syrup.* Explain that these are words for different kinds of sugar. Add the word *sodium* and explain that this word is used for salt. Have the students pretend they are sugar and salt detectives. They are to read labels at home to find what kinds of foods contain sugars and salt and should make a list of five foods that contain sugars and five foods that contain salt.

Materials Needed: slices of bacon, an apple, empty cereal boxes, chalkboard and chalk or overhead projector and pen

Processing Questions:

1. Why should we eat more fiber? How does that make us healthier?
2. Why should you keep your arteries clear of fat? What else could you do to keep them clear of fat? (exercise)
3. Why should you eat less sugar?
4. Why should you use less salt?
5. Why is it important to read food labels?

DIFFERENCES IN MILK   Grades (K–5)

Valued Outcome: The students will be able to compare the taste of various milk products.

Description of Strategy: Display a collection of milk products: whole, skim, evaporated, condensed, powdered, chocolate, buttermilk, etc. Compare the various milk products regarding taste, smell, feel, consistency, and appearance. Discuss what the different types of milk are used for and ask why consuming dairy products is so important.

Materials Needed: variety of milk products

Processing Questions:

1. What purposes does milk serve in our diet?
2. Which type of milk is most nutritious for children under age two? Which is most nutritious for people over age two? Why is there a difference?
3. Which type of milk do you prefer?

GROCERY STORE   Grades (K–5)

Valued Outcome: The students will be able to select foods from a group that will fit in the various categories of the Food Guide Pyramid.

Description of Strategy: Tell the students you are going to build a grocery store in your classroom. In order to do this activity, have them bring clean empty food containers from home. Provide a table where the containers may be displayed. This will promote a desire to be aware of the foods we eat and to see the large variety of foods available to us. After the containers are collected, divide them into the food groups found on the pyramid. Divide the class into small groups, and let them go shopping in the grocery store. When they return to their desks, have them sort the food according to the Food Guide Pyramid groups.

Materials Needed: empty food containers, Food Guide Pyramid for display

Processing Question: Were you able to select foods from all the Food Guide Pyramid categories?

SOURCE: Utah Education Network 1997b

FOODS EATEN IN THE CAFETERIA   Grades (3–5)

Valued Outcome: The students will observe various foods eaten by students in the school cafeteria.

Description of Strategy: Have the students observe the kinds and amounts of foods eaten by students in the school cafeteria. Record the information by grade level, if possible, on an observation form (see the following example). This activity can be followed with the next activity, "Food Waste".

Sample Observation Form	
Servings of Meats	
Servings of Vegetables	
Servings of Fruits	
Servings of Grains	
Servings of Dairy	

Materials Needed: observation form and pencils or pens for each student

Processing Questions:

1. Do most students in your school eat healthy lunches in the cafeteria?

2. Does your school lunch program offer various alternatives for eating?

FOOD WASTE   Grades (3–5)

Valued Outcome: The students will identify foods that are wasted by the students in the school cafeteria.

Description of Strategy: The previous activity "Foods Eaten in the Cafeteria" could be followed up with a food waste survey to determine which foods are not eaten from each food group. Have the students observe what types of food and how much are discarded into the trash cans by students. Then, using a chart like the one shown below, make a graph of the information and present arguments to increase selection of the food groups that are not chosen or eaten often.

Food Waste Observation Survey	
Meats Disgarded	
Vegetables Disgarded	
Fruits Disgarded	
Grains Disgarded	
Dairy Disgarded	

Materials Needed: food waste survey, graph paper and pencils or pens for each student

Processing Questions:

1. Do you think a lot of foods are wasted in your cafeteria?

2. What types of food are wasted the most?

3. What environmentally healthy act can be done with the wasted food?

FOOD PREPARATION

Grades (4–5)

Valued Outcome: The students will be able to prepare a food in a variety of ways to illustrate ways to vary their diet.

Description of Strategy: Have students conduct a hand-on activity in which they prepare one specific food in several different ways. (Students may need to decide on different ways to prepare the food on one day, then make the food on another day to allow ingredients to be gathered.) Have them evaluate their perceptions of the food prepared in each way.

Materials Needed: a quantity of a specific type of food (for example, different types of pasta or tuna fish), additional ingredients for different recipes

Processing Question: Why is it important to know different ways to prepare the same type of food?

FOOD AND THE FIVE SENSES

Grades (3–5)

Valued Outcome: The students will be able describe how the five senses affect food selection.

Description of Strategy: Use a food, such as an apple, to teach about the senses. Cut the apple, and ask the students how the apple looks different on the outside and inside (using sight). Give everyone a chance to smell an apple that has been cut and one that is whole. Which has more of an odor (smell)? Have the students determine if the apple is warm or cool, soft or firm, light or heavy (touch). Have students bite into an apple and describe the sound (hearing). Have the students describe whether the taste was sweet, bitter, or salty (taste). (This activity may be done with a variety of foods.)

Materials Needed: apples

Processing Question: How do the various senses work together to enhance our enjoyment of foods?

Puzzles and Games

FOOD GUIDE PYRAMID RELAY

Grades (K–5)

Valued Outcome: Students will be able to place foods into the correct groups on the Food Guide Pyramid.

Description of Strategy: Place an oversize version of the Food Guide Pyramid, labeled with the six food groups, at the front of the room. Tape an envelope below each of the food groups. Have the class discuss each food group and name foods that would be in each group. Write each food mentioned on two index cards (one on each of the two colors). Place the two index cards in two separate paper bags (one color always in one bag and the other color always in the other bag). Now divide the class into two teams. Have the teams line up single file. When you say "Go," the first person of each team goes to the front, takes out one of the index cards from the team bag, and then puts the food in the proper food group envelope on the Food Guide Pyramid (no help is allowed or the card will not count). The next person goes when the person in front of him or her passes the front start line (defined on the floor by a piece of tape). When all of the index cards have been placed in the envelopes and the final person passes the start line, the team is done. The team that finishes first earns five points. Now open the Food Guide Pyramid envelopes. Each team gets two points for each correct answer (the difference between teams can be seen by the color of the index cards). The team with the most points wins!

Materials Needed: oversized version of the Food Guide Pyramid, labeled with food groups; envelopes; tape; two sets of index cards (different colors); markers; two paper bags

Processing Questions:

1. What are two foods from each of the food groups on the Food Guide Pyramid?
2. In what food group do each of these foods belong: apples, peanut butter, carrots, Snickers candy bar, butter, rice, fish, potatoes, lettuce, cereal? (*Hint:* a food may belong in more than one food group.)

SOURCE: Sanden 1997

FOOD GUIDE PYRAMID BINGO   Grades (K–5)

Valued Outcome: The students will be able to place foods in the proper group by using the Food Guide Pyramid.

Description of Strategy: Hand out the bingo cards to the students. Each card will have six columns across it, labeled to represent the six categories of the Food Guide Pyramid. The spaces below the columns will have the name of a food that is in that food category. Draw index cards with the names of various foods on them, and read them aloud to the students. The students will then place a button, bean, or token over the names of the foods on their cards. The student who reaches six categories across wins since he or she now has the number of food categories represented to have a reasonably balance meal. Let the person who wins lead the next game.

Materials Needed: bingo cards (as described above); tokens, beans, or other counters for each student; index cards with various names on them

Processing Questions:

1. Which food group should you have the most of in a day?
2. Why is it important to have more of this category than any other?

NUTRIENT GAME

Grades (K–5)

Valued Outcome: The students will be able to display knowledge of the nutrients by grouping them properly.

Description of Strategy: Make up six big poster-board cards, each with one of the six nutrients (carbohydrates, lipids, proteins, water, vitamins, and minerals) on it. Then write names of different foods onto index cards, allowing one card for each student. Give the nutrient cards to six students and the food cards to the remaining students. Have the students with the food cards walk around and try to group themselves to the appropriate nutrient group. No one is allowed to speak in this game, and students should try to work as fast as they can. The group that gathers first wins. Everyone in their group must belong to that nutrient, or they are disqualified.

Materials Needed: six poster-board cards, one for each of the six nutrient groups; index cards with names of different foods (one per student)

Processing Question: Why is it important to include a variety of nutrients in our diet?

ALPHABET GAME

Grades (3–5)

Valued Outcome: The students will be able to spell the names of foods and nutrients correctly.

Description of Strategy: Divide the students into three groups. Write the letters of the alphabet onto index cards (some letters may be repeated) and give a set to each group. Ask the students a question such as "This nutrient is responsible for building new cells and tissues in growing children." The group must work together to think of an answer and then spell the word correctly (protein). Each student should have only one letter in his or her hand. The group should be standing in a straight line with the word spelled correctly. The group who can do this first wins.

Materials Needed: three identical sets of index cards with letters of the alphabet written on each card, a list of questions

Processing Question: What is the function of each nutrient?

LEARNING THE FOOD GUIDE PYRAMID

Grades (3–5)

Valued Outcome: Students will be able to describe the Food Guide Pyramid.

Description of Strategy: Divide the class into groups of four to five students. On each table have some magazines, paper bags, six poster boards or pieces of construction paper, scissors, and glue. Each student should have his or her own paper bag. Have each group label one poster board for each category of the Food Guide Pyramid. Then have them cut out pictures of different foods from the magazines and place them in their bags. Have the students exchange bags with each other. Tell them to remove the different foods from the bag and paste each on the correct poster board according to the category in the Food Guide Pyramid in which it belongs. Once the students finish, have each group show their poster boards. At the end of class, hang the posters around the classroom.

Materials Needed: magazines or grocery store advertisements, scissors, glue, poster boards or construction paper for each group; paper bags for each student

Processing Questions:

1. What are the categories in the Food Guide Pyramid?
2. Why is it important to know the various categories in the Food Guide Pyramid?
3. Which foods did you have trouble placing in the proper category? Why?

WHAT KIND OF FOOD AM I? Grades (3–5)

Valued Outcome: The students will be able to guess types of food from clues.

Description of Strategy: Say "Now we are going to play the 'What kind of food am I?' game." Tape the name of a food on each student's back. "No one is allowed to tell you what your food is, and you are not to tell anyone the name of his or her food." Once everyone has become a food, start the game. Call the students up to the board one at a time. Have them turn around so their classmates can see the food. One at a time, the classmates will start describing the food—which food group the student belongs to, the shape, color, or size, or even other foods it might taste good with or be found in. After each hint, the student may guess which food she or he is. After the student guesses his or her food, write it on the board under the correct category. Allow students to keep their food tags.

Materials Needed: tape, paper for food tags for each student

Processing Question: What types of clues (characteristics) about foods will help identify those foods?

LABEL SCAVENGER HUNT Grades (3–5)

Valued Outcome: The students will be able to identify certain foods just by reading the food labels.

Description of Strategy: Give several food labels (that have been removed from the products) to groups of students. Have them try to determine what food each of the ingredient labels is describing. Points can be awarded to the groups on the basis of guessing the correct food from the labels.

Materials Needed: food labels

Processing Question: How can the information from food labels help us to identify foods?

FOOD ALPHABET

Grades (K–3)

Valued Outcome: The students will be able to list the names of foods for each letter of the alphabet.

Description of Strategy: Divide the students into teams, and assign each team a number of letters of the alphabet. For example, one team can be assigned letters *A* through *E,* the next team letters *F* through *J,* and so on. Challenge each team to write down at least one food for each letter assigned to the team.

Materials Needed: pen and paper for each team

Processing Question: What are the names of foods that start with each letter of the alphabet?

CULTURAL FOODS GAME

Grades (3–5)

Valued Outcome: The students will be able to recognize food cards representing foods from different cultures and identify the country of origin.

Description of Strategy: Paste or draw pictures of different ethnic foods in the center of an index card. Write the name of the food at the top of the card. The player must recognize the country when he or she sees the name of food. Suggested number of cards is thirty for two to four players, more for larger groups.

How to Play:

1. Shuffle the deck of index cards well.

2. Deal five cards to each player face down.

3. The player on the dealer's left draws one card from the deck. He or she may either keep the card or discard it right side up next to the deck. If the card is kept, the player must discard another (the player must have five cards in his or her hand at all times).

4. The opponent(s) may either take the card that is right side up or draw from the deck and then discard a card.

5. The game continues until a player has five different cultures of food represented by his or her cards.

6. The player lays down his or her hand for the opponent(s) to see and check. If correct, he or she is then declared the winner.

   Variation: Players can decide to play for one culture of food, in which case six cards should be made for each of five cultures. When a player sees the first five cards he or she is dealt, he or she can decide which country is best represented (by the most cards) in his or her hand. This will determine which country he or she plays for, and he or she will try to get a "set" of five cards for that country. The first player to get a set is the winner.

Materials Needed: one package of 3×5 index cards, pictures of at least six different foods from countries studied (Foods from Mexico, France, China, Germany, Italy, and Hawaii are especially interesting.)

Processing Questions:

1. What are some foods from other countries that are different from ours?
2. Why is it important to know about other cultures' foods?

WHEEL OF FOOD   Grades (K–5)

Valued Outcome: The students will be able to participate in a game identifying certain foods from the Food Guide Pyramid.

Description of Strategy: This game is set up like "Wheel of Fortune." The spinner spins the wheel indicating from which food category the secret word will be chosen. One student will act as the host; the remainder of the class will take turns being the player(s) and serving as card holders. Students serving as card holders will be given the correct cards to spell out a food name. The blank sides of these cards will be held toward the class until the card holder is instructed by the host to turn the card. Remind the students that the food they will be trying to spell out will come from the food category chosen. This first team, or student, chooses a letter; if the letter is in the word, they continue. If the first team/student is incorrect, the second team/student gets a turn and so on. The team to turn or guess all letters and spell the name of the food is the winner.

Materials Needed: wheel with the six categories from the Food Guide Pyramid; cards arranged in sets that spell out names of different foods; Food Guide Pyramid for display

Processing Questions:

1. What are the different categories of foods within the Food Guide Pyramid?
2. Why is it important to know the foods within each category?

BALANCED MEALS   Grades (4–5)

Valued Outcome: The students will be able to name at least two reasons why eating vegetables is important, name the six food groups, and select and construct a balanced meal.

Description of Strategy: This game has two parts. In the first part—"The Balance Game"—students identify whether a meal is balanced or not. Then in the second part—"Meals on Wheels"—the students identify whether the balanced meal provides the daily amounts needed in a healthy diet.

Show the students six plates, each containing a different meal (construct the food from paper or cut out pictures from magazines). Have students decide if each meal is balanced. Instruct them to clap if it is or to rub their head if it is not. The game is played with a makeshift balance. If the meal is balanced, do not move the balance, but if the meal is not balanced, adjust the balance so that it is uneven. This is designed to visually show the students what a *balanced* meal is.

After completing "The Balance Game," use an interactive bulletin board titled "Meals on Wheels" to decide if each meal contains the proper daily amounts of nutrients. Write the names of the food groups in a different color on a wheel (refer to the Food Guide Pyramid). Give the students colored stickers that correspond to the colors of the food groups. Have them break down each meal into individual food groups. For every item in the meal, place a colored sticker on the wheel in the appropriate food group. Then have the students add up the number of stickers in each category to see if they had the daily amounts that they needed in order to have healthy meals that day.

Materials Needed: paper food to represent six meals, poster-board balance scale that can be tipped, wheel with names of the six Food Guide Pyramid categories written in different colors and stickers in corresponding colors

Processing Question: What does it mean for a meal to be balanced?

FOOD MEMORY   Grades (3–5)

Valued Outcome: The students will be able to explain how a healthy diet can increase the likelihood of physical and mental wellness.

Description of Strategy: Play a memory game with the class. Display four pictures of foods from one of the five major Food Guide Pyramid groups and a food choice from the fats and sugar group. Ask the students to name the foods. Choose one student and have him or her stand up and turn around so that he or she does not see the pictures. Then have the student name at least two pictures of the nutritious foods from memory. Repeat this activity using foods from different groups and different students. If this is too easy, use five or six pictures to play the game. Explain that these foods are nutritious, and our bodies need them to be healthy.

Materials Needed: pictures of foods from the Food Guide Pyramid

Processing Question: Why is it important to eat a variety of foods from the Food Guide Pyramid?

SOURCE: Utah Education Network 1997a

MYSTERY BAG   Grades (K–5)

Valued Outcome: The students will be able to identify foods using the sense of touch.

Description of Strategy: Make a mystery bag (for example, a simple drawstring bag). Fill the bag with different foods. Have one student at a time come to the bag, reach in, and try to identify one of the foods without breaking any. The student may pull the food out of the bag and show the class then will decide into which section of the Food Guide Pyramid the food belongs.

Materials Needed: drawstring bag, different foods, Food Guide Pyramid for display

Processing Question: Were you able to identify foods by touch instead of smell and taste?

SOURCE: Utah Education Network 1997b

EGG HUNT

Valued Outcome: The students will be able to determine which snacks are healthy and comply with the Food Guide Pyramid.

Description of Strategy: Review with the students the Dietary Guidelines for Americans discussed in Chapter 17. Insert one printed guideline each into colored plastic egg like fortunes hidden inside fortune cookies. Hide the filled eggs around the classroom or outside in the school yard. Provide students with paper lunch bags, crayons, markers, glue or tape, and illustrations of nutritious foods. Include a variety of foods that are familiar to most students, representing each of the categories in the Food Guide Pyramid. Omit foods with high sugar and fat content. Invite students to decorate their paper bags using handmade drawings and illustrations of the nutritious foods from the pyramid that they would like to eat. Direct students to return to an assigned starting point when time is called. Students will open their eggs and remove the nutrition message. Read aloud messages while serving nutritious snacks to reinforce the Food Guide Pyramid concepts covered in this lesson.

Materials Needed: Guidelines for Healthy Eating, Food Guide Pyramid for display, colored plastic eggs (enough to put one guideline in each egg), small slips of paper (each with one guideline written on it), paper lunch bags for each student, crayons, markers, glue or tape, pictures of nutritious food, nutritious snack foods

Processing Question: How can you tell if a food is nutritious?

SOURCE: Geiger and Wills 1998

Other Ideas

FIELD TRIPS

Valued Outcome: The students will be able to participate in a field trip relating to food or dairy products.

Description of Strategy: Arrange to take the class on a field trip to a dairy, bakery, food processing plant, or other nutrition-related operation. Be sure to prepare your class thoroughly for the trip before they go. Discuss the nature of the operation that they will see. Explain the processes they will observe, and have the students prepare a list of questions they will want to ask.

Materials Needed: none

Processing Question: How do the processes of food preparation vary in the different nutrition-related operations?

POSTER CONTEST

Grades (3–5)

Valued Outcome: The students will be able to construct a poster using topics concerning all aspects of food.

Description of Strategy: Each week assign a theme for individual posters, using such topics as the Food Guide Pyramid, table manners, essential nutrients, and so on. Post the completed art in the classroom or in the school cafeteria.

Materials Needed: poster board, art supplies to construct posters

Processing Questions:

1. How do such signs serve as reminders for good food-related behavior?

2. What are some essential messages that should be related through such signs?

Resources

WEB SITES

Abramson Cancer Center of the University of Pennsylvania
www.oncolink.upenn.edu

Administration on Aging
www.aoa.dhhs.gov

Agency for Healthcare Research and Quality
www.ahcpr.gov

American Academy of Family Physicians
www.aafp.org

American Cancer Society
www.cancer.org/docroot/home/index.asp

American Dietetic Association:
Your Link to Nutrition and Health
www.eatright.org

American Medical Association
www.ama-assn.org/ama/pub/category/1947.html

American Social Health Association
www.ashastd.org

Centers for Disease Control and Prevention:
Data and Statistics
www.cdc.gov/scientific.htm

Centers for Disease Control and Prevention:
National Center for Chronic Disease Prevention
and Health Promotion
www.cdc.gov/nccdphp/sgr/sgr.htm

Centers for Disease Control and Prevention:
The CDC prevention guidelines database
http://wonder.cdc.gov/wonder/prevguid/prevguid.shtml

Department of Applied Health Science,
Indiana University
www.drugs.indiana.edu/health/k-12.html

Family Health Productions
www.abouthealth.com

Food and Drug Administration
www.fda.gov

MedicineNet, Inc.
www.medicinenet.com/script/main/hp.asp

National Institute on Aging
www.nia.nih.gov

Office of Disease Prevention and Health Promotion
www.odphp.osophs.dhhs.gov

ParentsPlace.com
www.parentsplace.com

Psychiatric Times. Eating disorders in males
www.psychiatrictimes.com/p950942.html

U.S. Department of Agriculture, Food Safety and
Inspection Services
www.fsis.usda.gov

VIDEOS

Nutrition and exercise (Grades K–5)
Presents details about food groups, fiber, vitamins, cholesterol, weight control, disease prevention, exercise, and energy metabolism. Helps students understand the Food Guide Pyramid. Available from Sunburst Communications, 101 Castleton Street, P.O. Box 40, Pleasantville, NY 10570. (25 minutes, Item 2439)

Real people:
Coping with eating disorders (Grades 5–12)
Gives viewers revealing insights into eating disorders by documenting the stories of three young people—an anorexic, a bulimic, and a compulsive overeater. Interweaving their stories, a specialist discusses the pattern, symptoms, and treatment of eating disorders. Available from Sunburst Communications, 101 Castleton Street, P.O. Box 40, Pleasantville, NY 10570. (27 minutes, Item 2299)

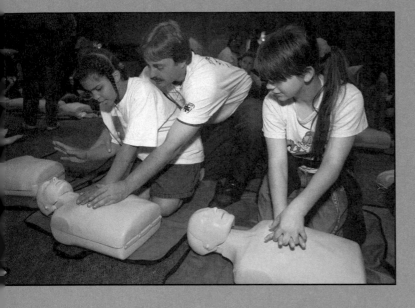

CHAPTER NINETEEN

Injuries:
Accident and
Violence
Prevention

As a teacher, your involvement in safety education is imperative because of the number of accidents that occur while the child is at school.

VALUED OUTCOMES

After reading this chapter, you should be able to:

- discuss the difference between intentional and unintentional injuries
- discuss the major human and environmental causes of accidents
- describe the characteristics of an accident-prone person
- discuss young people's attitudes toward violence
- list the ways for a child to protect him- or herself against violence

- list the ways for a child to protect him- or herself against adult and stranger abuse
- describe why risk-taking is a necessary evil
- discuss the major parts of a school safety program
- contrast a positive approach to safety education with a negative approach
- discuss the growing violence problem in U.S. society

REFLECTIONS

As you read through this chapter, reflect upon the dangers to personal safety found in your environment—including the possibilities of both intentionally and unintentionally inflicted injuries. As you reflect upon these dangers, you will become more aware of strategies that can be employed to protect your personal safety and that of the people around you.

Children, Accidents, and Violence

Children are especially susceptible to *unintentional injuries,* mainly because they are unaware of dangers. According to the National Center for Injury Prevention and Control (NCIPC) injuries and death caused by injuries continue to present a major challenge. Unintentional injuries are the leading cause of death in children, and almost one-fourth of all school-aged children experience an injury that is severe enough to require medical attention or to cause them to miss school (NCIPC 1999).

THE VIOLENCE EPIDEMIC

The epidemic of youth violence that initially came to public attention in the 1980s is far from over. The problem is pervasive and ongoing. As arrest rates for young people committing homicide and other violent crimes skyrocketed from 1983 to 1993, Congress and many state legislatures attempted to quell the dramatic rise in the number of murders committed by young people by passing tougher gun-control laws and trying juveniles in adult courts. Although overall arrest rates began to decline by the mid-1990s, by 1999 violent crime rates once again increased and, in fact, rivaled those of 1983.

In 1998, youths accounted for one out of six arrests for all violent crimes. (This share has decreased about 16 percent in recent years.) By 1999, arrests of young people for all crimes totaled 2.4 million; 104,000 of these were arrests for such violent crimes as aggravated assault (69,600), robbery (28,000), forcible rape (5,000), and murder (1,400). Even though the 1999 arrest rate for violent youth crimes was the lowest in the 1990s, it was still 15 percent higher than it was in 1983.

It is not surprising that the violence during this era was accompanied by an increase in youth carrying and using weapons. Instant access to weapons (especially firearms) often resulted in violent or deadly acts that resulted in arrests. As weapons carrying declined, so did arrest rates (although the decline in arrest rates was not uniform for all types of violent crimes).

Despite the decline in arrest rates, the amount of underlying violent behavior in youth appears to have increased in recent years. This could reignite a resurgence in the incidence of weapons carrying that poses a grave threat for another epidemic of youth violence (Satcher 2001).

The Need for Safety Education

Fortunately, most accidents that happen to children are not serious or fatal. Unfortunately, accidents occur often enough to make safety an extremely important part of elementary health instruction. As a teacher, your involvement in safety education is imperative because of the number of accidents that occur while the child is at school. Your efforts, combined with those of the school administration, can make a difference. It is very important for teachers to comply with and periodically review school district policies concerning safety and first-aid procedures.

The number of accidents among children is unnecessarily high. Although accidents will always occur, given the nature of children, accidents don't just happen. In most instances, they are caused by human error or carelessness, and these factors can be positively influenced by safety education. Children do not have to learn safe behavior through trial and error; they do not have to continue having accidents in order to recognize the importance of safety. They can be taught the elements of safety in a positive way that will result in fewer accidents of all types, both at school and away from school. As a teacher of health education, this should be one of your major goals.

This chapter presents an overview of the elements of safety education and violence prevention. Topics include risk taking and safety procedures, positive characteristics of safety, accident prevention, violence and violence prevention, types of accidents, violence in schools, and the school safety program.

Safety and Risk Taking

We take risks in almost any of our activities, from going to school or work in the morning, to cooking or eating a meal, to engaging in daily tasks and recreational activities. If safety were our only concern, logically many of these efforts would have to be curtailed: One could be hit by a truck while crossing the street, choke on a piece of food, or suffer a fatal injury while at work or at play. What is an acceptable degree of risk depends on the needs and desires of the individual and the activity. Some adults, for instance, make their living by engaging in highly risky activities—race drivers, deep sea divers, law enforcement officers, and so forth. Such individuals are often held in high esteem and even glamorized by the rest of the population, demonstrating that risk taking is viewed positively in our society.

Fostering Safety Behavior

Children develop an unrealistic view of risk taking from viewing the glamorous aspects, and this attitude may tempt them to enter into situations that are potentially very hazardous. This, combined with natural curiosity and energy, can greatly increase the chance of serious accidents. Part of your job in teaching safety education is to make children aware that unnecessary risk taking is not socially endorsed behavior, and that it is important to safely prepare for necessary activities in which there are some risks involved. This cannot be accomplished, however, by simply providing your students with a list of safety don'ts. Children, especially younger children, should be emphatically warned of dangers in the environment. However, the "don't" approach to safety education, when used exclusively, is negative, and not likely to influence behavior permanently.

A POSITIVE APPROACH TO SAFETY

You are more likely to influence children's behavior toward safer personal practices when you take a positive approach. Emphasize that safety is largely a matter of individual choice and responsibility. Although an acceptance of risk is a part of living, embracing risk without recognizing and accepting the possible consequences is not wise. In considering role models, point out that even adults who make their living in the most hazardous of ways do all they can to minimize the risk involved.

As in all areas of health education, stress the importance of personal decision-making skills. Accidents happen not because of chance or fate, but because of the inherent risk involved in the activity combined with the possibility of human error. When children understand and internalize this concept, they will be in a better position to enhance their own personal safety. By recognizing their own choices and responsibility, they will begin to be better able to assess the risk involved in a given activity and to take steps to minimize the possibility of making errors when engaged in that activity.

To become mindful of safety, a person must become analytical. What are the risks involved in the activity contemplated? What can be done to lessen those risks? After determining the probable answers to these questions, the individual can then act accordingly. The process of becoming analytical about decision making begins in childhood. You can do much to help children develop analytical decision-making skills by providing a variety of learning opportunities that require them to think before they act.

Of course, you cannot expect a child to have the analytical skills of a competent adult, and therefore you must also supervise children's activities to prevent needless accidents. This supervision should take place in the classroom, gymnasium, cafeteria, hallways, and playground. As much as possible, however, relate your supervision to individual decision-making skills. Always keep a positive approach to safety.

Accident Proneness

Certain people are more prone to accidents than others. Statistics indicate that people who have had one accident are more likely to have another one than those who have not had any previous accidents. The accident-prone person may be impulsive, drawn to adventure and excitement, or always in search of immediate pleasures. This type of individual does not like to plan ahead and may harbor resentment against authority figures. The rebellion may be a response to a strict upbringing in childhood. He or she usually cannot tolerate discipline, including the self-discipline caution requires.

Characteristics of an accident-prone person may include aggression and overactivity. Although statistically boys are three times more likely than girls to have an injury-prone personality, studies show that other possible factors include:

- **Economic status**—Over a three-year period, a group of economically deprived children at a summer camp had a disproportionately high number of accidents.
- **Personal characteristics**—Cognitive abilities and personality traits may play a role; extroverts, for example, have more accidents than introverts.
- **Transient states**—These have to do with illness or mood. Illness is likely to make people more accident prone, either because they are not physically capable of performing the tasks they are trying to do, or because their illness makes them lose concentration. Similarly, mood can have an effect on concentration and a person's ability to think clearly (Sturt 2003).

Accidents

TYPES OF ACCIDENTS

Accidents involving schoolchildren can be classified into six categories: school, traffic, recreational, home, personal, or disaster. Disaster situations include floods, hurricanes, tornadoes, and earthquakes. Because these are general emergencies involving a large segment of the population, they will not be detailed here.

Health Highlight

HEALTHY PEOPLE 2000

UNINTENTIONAL INJURIES REVIEW

BY U.S. SURGEON GENERAL

- Seven of the 26 separate objectives have met the year 2000 targets, and 11 more have made substantial progress. But almost a third of the objectives have shown little or no progress.

- Injuries are still the leading cause of death for everyone under age 44.

- The death rate due to injuries for men is more than twice that for women.

- Almost half of the deaths are motor vehicle related, but motor vehicle crash death rates are down—almost 20 percent—due in part to the increased use of seat belts and child restraint seats.

- The rate of alcohol-related motor vehicle deaths has been cut by almost 40 percent.

- The death rate from drowning has declined, and the fire-related death rate has met its Healthy People 2000 target.

- There has been more success in preventing fire-related deaths: The death rate for young children has been cut in half.

- The overall rate of drowning deaths declined by about 30 percent over the past decade.

- Substantially fewer children were seen in emergency rooms for nonfatal poisonings—this statistic is well below the year 2000 target.

SOURCE: Sondik 1999

School Accidents. Most school accidents occur in physical education classes, during playground activities, and in sports contests. These activities expose the students to greater levels of risk, and many of these injuries can be attributed to lack of proper equipment (NCIPC 1999). Plan carefully to ensure maximum safety. First of all, the teacher in charge should make sure that sports and playground equipment are in good condition and suitable for the activity. Work closely with school administrators, other faculty members, and the school custodians. Equipment that is not in use should be stored so that it does not interfere with the ongoing activity. Swings and other play equipment should be inspected regularly. The playground should also be routinely inspected for hazards, such as broken glass and damaged fencing, before children are allowed to play. Metal playground equipment that is standing in the sun should be checked before children use it in order to avoid potential burns.

Next, be sure that all physical activities are properly supervised by an adequate number of faculty members. Some schools now require teachers supervising playground activities during school to stand and watch children carefully rather than completing paperwork or other distracting activities. Teachers should confine all activities to designated areas and make sure that the activity of one group of children does not interfere with that of another group. Keep any activity you are supervising well ordered, and watch for signs of fatigue. When a child becomes tired, the chances for an accident increase. Finally, when your students have finished the activity, make sure that equipment is properly stored. Lock all equipment cabinets to prevent unauthorized, unsupervised use.

Safety in the hallways, stairways, cafeteria, and other parts of the school outside the actual classroom should be maximized by teacher supervision. Stress the importance of polite, considerate behavior rather than simply demanding that students follow rules. Hall monitors should not function as prison guards. Work with school administrators and custodians to keep the school environment free of potential hazards. Stairways should have banisters and adequate lighting. Water fountains should have the appropriate amount of water pressure—not too low to cause children to bump their teeth and not too much to cause water to spill on the floor. Spills of any sort should be wiped up promptly, and litter should be removed. Doors to maintenance areas should be locked.

In the classroom itself, make sure that you also maintain a safe environment. Keep equipment and supplies stored until they are needed. Supervise all activities closely. If you prepare any experiment or classroom demonstration that could be hazardous, do not take unnecessary risks. For example, if a demonstration involves the use of a sharp object or a chemical, do not have students help you. Also, be especially careful with any electrical apparatus.

A safety concern that has received considerable attention in the schools is the danger of asbestos. Asbestos was widely used as an insulating material in schools for many years and in other commonly occurring items, such as brake linings in cars. Asbestos is considered a danger to health only if the insulation is disturbed regularly through contact. If this happens, fibers that can block breathing passages will be released into the air.

The asbestos minerals have a tendency to separate into microscopic particles that can remain in the air and be easily inhaled; persons occupationally exposed to asbestos have developed several types of life-threatening diseases, including lung cancer. Although the use of asbestos and asbestos products has dramatically decreased, they are still found in many residential and commercial settings and continue to pose a health risk to workers and others (National Institute for Occupational Safety and Health 2002). Many school systems are replacing asbestos with safer types of insulation.

Carrying of weapons is a major contributor to accidents at school (NCIPC 1999). This topic will be addressed in further detail on pages 574–575.

Traffic Accidents. Going to and from school accounts for few school accidents. This is surprising when one considers the potential dangers that children face as pedestrians, bicyclists, and bus and auto passengers. The low accident rate speaks well for school safety patrols and pedestrian and bicycle safety programs. Nonetheless, traffic accidents do occur, and they are often serious. Help your students recognize the importance of following established safety procedures when they are pedestrians, bicyclists, and vehicle passengers.

As pedestrians, children should understand how to interact with motor vehicles. Traffic laws are designed not only for operators of motor vehicles, but also for pedestrians. Each has an obligation to the other, a point you should stress. Help younger children learn the meaning of traffic signs and signals, and explain the reasons behind traffic regulations. Youngsters usually do not appreciate the physical principles involved in the operation of a motor vehicle and

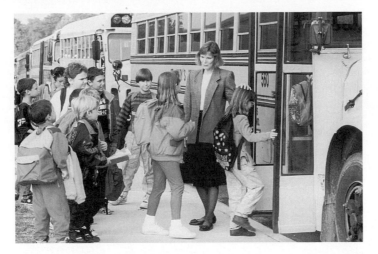

Being safe in and around the school bus is an important part of a student's life.

do not understand that a car cannot stop immediately or that the child can see the car much better than the driver can see him or her. Further, children often become so engrossed in their own activities that they simply do not consider the vehicular traffic around them. They may dart into the street after a ball without thinking.

Bicycle safety should also be emphasized. Children often assume that traffic laws and regulations apply only to motorized vehicles. They see themselves not as operators of vehicles—which they are—but rather as mounted pedestrians. To some degree, this is a values-related issue and must be approached as such because children do not see themselves as being irresponsible when they fail to heed traffic regulations.

Most children are regular passengers on school buses and in family vehicles. Because of the large numbers of children being transported to and from schools in buses and cars, children need to become aware of proper safety practices in buses and cars. Drivers of school buses are responsible for supervising students during their ride. Cooperate with drivers in establishing firm guidelines for safe student behavior while loading, riding, and unloading the buses. Unruly students can easily distract a driver so that an accident results. Make clear the possible consequences of unruly behavior, and point out that the well-being of many people can be affected by poor behavior. Also provide instructions for safe behavior. Children should enter the bus in an orderly manner and move to their seats quickly and carefully. They should remain seated during the ride. Books, lunch boxes, and other objects should be kept out of the aisles. Windows should remain closed unless the driver opens them. If windows are opened, children should not stick their arms or heads out or throw objects out the windows. Finally, students should remain well clear of the bus when it is approaching the bus stop and after they have been dropped off.

As automobile passengers, children should also be aided in developing safety practices. Emphasize that even though it may look easy, driving a car requires the full attention of the driver. Children should not distract the driver and should not lean out of windows. Stress the importance of wearing safety belts

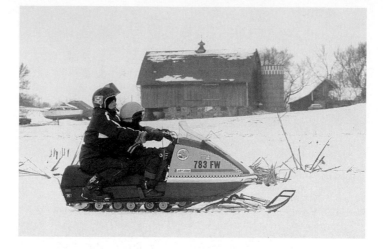

Teach about forms of recreation popular in your area, such as snowmobiling, skiing, hunting, and fishing.

and using child safety or booster seats, even if the parents of some children do not regularly use them.

In the United States, many states in now require the use of safety belts by passengers. Many other states are considering such legislation. Not wearing a safety belt is essentially irrational behavior. Excuses given for not using safety belts are varied. Some drivers find them constricting or uncomfortable. Others say that they are not needed for short trips. A few claim to fear being trapped inside the vehicle in case of an accident. None of these reasons hold up. The truth is that people refuse to wear safety belts either because of laziness or because of a belief that somehow preparing for an accident by wearing a belt will actually allow an accident to take place. This type of reasoning for not wearing a belt is a psychological device called *denial*.

Recreational Accidents. A large portion of recreational accidents happen to children in and around water. Thus, water safety should be an important component of the instruction that you provide. All children should be taught to swim at an early age. This is something that you can encourage by getting parents and students involved in organized recreational programs.

Even if children know how to swim, however, the danger of accidental drowning always exists. Most drownings happen to people who are not dressed for swimming, which implies that they were not planning to be in the water. Victims usually fall into the water, whether in a home pool, from a boat, or by a river or lake. Emphasize to your students that any body of water should be treated with respect and caution, including a flooded drainage ditch. In your discussion of water safety, include the rules for boating safety, such as always wearing a life vest.

Camping and hiking activities contribute to many recreational accidents. Falls from cliffs and other high places result in hundreds of fatalities and injuries each year. Stress the importance of being cautious in unfamiliar terrain.

Skateboards also cause many recreational accidents among children. The popularity of skateboards is high, as is the number of resulting accidents.

Health Highlight
WINTER SPORTS SAFETY

Make sure children are safe when they toboggan, skate, or ski by keeping these factors in mind:

- Children can strangle on a cord or scarf, so use a neck warmer instead of a scarf, and take the cords and drawstrings off their clothes.
- Keep children warm. Dress children in layers, and make sure their heads and necks are covered by hats and neck warmers. Watch for frostbite!
- To avoid sunburn on sunny days, be sure they are wearing sunscreen on their face and ears.
- Check your children's equipment to make sure that it fits properly and is in good condition.

When tobogganing or sledding:

- Make sure children wear a helmet.
- Choose a hill that is away from roads and parking lots.
- Choose an area where there are no rocks, trees, fences, or other dangers in the path.

- Teach children to slide down the middle of the hill, climb up the side, and watch for other sledders coming down the hill.
- Teach them to move out of the way quickly when they get to the bottom.

When skating:

Children should wear a helmet. If skating on lakes or rivers, make sure the ice is smooth and at least 10 centimeters or 4 inches thick. Never skate near open water.

- Children should skate in the same direction and at the same speed as the crowd.
- Skaters who cannot keep up with the crowd should move to the side.
- When playing hockey, only wear an approved helmet. Replace hockey helmets at least every 5 years.

SOURCE: Product Safety, Health Canada 1999

Emphasize the need to wear proper protective equipment. Also note that skateboards should not be used on streets. A collision between a car and a child on a skateboard can be fatal for the child.

Your treatment of recreational safety should also include any forms of recreation popular in your area. See the Health Highlight box above for examples of precautions to take during various outdoor recreation activities.

Home Accidents. "There's no place like home" implies that home is a pleasant place to be. Unfortunately, there's also no place like home for accidents. More accidents happen in the home than in any other place, partly because most people spend a great deal of time at home.

The leading cause of death in the home is fire. Most home fires occur in the kitchen and bedroom. For the latter, smoking in bed is often the cause. Home safety, including fire safety, is primarily a parental responsibility, but you can help by making your students aware of possible hazards. Work with parents and children to ensure that every family has a fire safety and fire evacuation plan.

For younger children, emphasize the danger of playing with matches or with the kitchen stove. Encourage parents to install smoke detectors and to keep cookware handles turned toward the back of the stove. Teach children what to do if a fire breaks out in the home, especially at night. Too often, frightened children seek shelter in a closet or other enclosed area rather than fleeing, and some will be frightened by the sight of a firefighter dressed in turnout gear. Follow

Health Highlight

HOME ALONE!

An increasing number of children spend time at home alone while their parents are working. For this reason, certain rules should be followed to ensure the personal safety of these children:

1. Always keep the doors locked, and never permit a stranger to enter the house.
2. Become familiar with appropriate ways to respond on the telephone (for example, never say that you are home alone).

3. Know how to use the telephone to summon help (for example, parent's work numbers) in an emergency (for example, fire or a stranger at the door).
4. Know the emergency telephone numbers in the community (for example, police and fire department).
5. Have a trusted neighbor you can call or go to if you become scared or upset.

SOURCE: Miller, Telljohann, and Symons 1996, 202

each fire drill in school with a discussion of home fire drills. Every member of the family should know the evacuation route and an alternative route if the primary one is blocked by smoke or flames.

Poisoning is another common home accident, especially among younger children. Explain the dangers of ingesting any substance, such as medicines, food that may have gone bad, and household chemicals. Make sure that parents understand the dangers of accidental poisoning from such substances as aspirin, and encourage them to keep a list of emergency procedures on hand and the telephone number of the local poison control center.

Electrical appliances are a common source of home accidents. Make sure that children understand the danger of playing with any electrical device. Also discuss how electrical overloads can lead to home fires and how electrical appliances can electrocute someone if they are knocked into water.

Your instruction in home safety techniques should include specific recommendations, such as not leaving toys or other objects on stairs or sidewalks, and wearing protective eye equipment when using power tools or lawn equipment. Encourage parents to do all they can to keep the home a safe environment for themselves and their children. For example, you may wish to prepare a checklist for students to take home to their parents. Discussion of items on the checklist can provide a valuable learning experience for all involved.

Just as a family should have a home evacuation plan in case of fire, it should also have a general disaster plan. Encourage students and their parents to work out a plan for any disaster that might hit their community. Depending on the locale, disasters might include earthquakes, floods, tornadoes, or blizzards. Each family member should know what to do in case a disaster strikes, including knowing the name and phone number of someone who does not live in the immediate vicinity and who may act as a contact person in the event of a major disaster.

School Violence: An Overview

Schools should be safe and secure for all students, faculty, and staff so teaching and learning can occur. Contrary to the image of pervasive violence in schools that is projected by the popular media, more violence occurs against children and youth away from rather than at school. According to the National Center for Educational Statistics (NCES), in 1999, students were more than two times more likely to be victims of serious violent crime and seventy times more likely to be murdered away from school (NCES 2001, 2002a). The NCIPC finds that less than 1 percent of all homicides to children five to nineteen years of age occur in or around school grounds (NCIPC 2002).

The total nonfatal victimization rate and the percentage of students being victimized at school generally declined between 1992 and 1999. However, the prevalence of some types of crimes at school has not changed. For example, between 1993 and 1999, the percentage of students in grades 9 through 12 who were threatened or injured with a weapon on school property within the prior twelve months remained at about 7 to 8 percent (NCES 2001). Nevertheless, students seem to feel more secure at school now than they did just a few years ago. There has been a decline in the percentage of students who reported avoiding school for their own safety and who reported the street gangs at their schools (NCES 2001). Unfortunately, however, violence, gangs, and drugs are still present in schools today.

CHILDREN'S EXPOSURE TO VIOLENCE

The debate about the connection between children's exposure to violence and the number of violent crimes committed by children is heated, ongoing, and currently inconclusive. It is undeniable, however, that many of America's children consume a steady diet of verbal and physical violence that begins early in life with cartoons and video games, and continues throughout life with movies, other popular media, and even the evening news. (Numerous reports state that children in the United States spend more time watching television than attending school.)

While the evidence for a correlation between exposure to media violence and committing violent acts may be inconclusive, it has been posited that children who are abused often become abusive and violent themselves. An increasing number of children who are not victims of abuse or violence often commit violent acts due to boredom or a need for control.

Sometimes, simply engaging parents to take an interest in their child's behavior and welfare is more than half the battle in stopping school violence. But more and more parents work outside the home, which makes them less accessible to school officials. Some parents are tired of dealing with their child's problems and simply give up trying. Unfortunately, these attitudes cross all socioeconomic strata. But parents who abuse their children or who fail to provide guidance and discipline can be assured that they are likely contributing to the spread of school violence.

In generating statistics on school violence, researchers generally survey students and teachers regarding several key areas, including:

- violence at school as opposed to away from school
- prevalence of threats or intentional injury
- physical fighting
- bullying
- violent acts involving teachers

The NCES provides an extensive breakdown of such statistics by student characteristics (gender, age, race/ethnicity, and so on) and by type of crime. Below are some statistical highlights from students and teachers surveyed in recent years. You may find it interesting to compare the national NCES statistics to those in your local area.

VIOLENCE AGAINST STUDENTS AT SCHOOL AND AWAY FROM SCHOOL

Violence at school and while going to and from school can lead to stress, injury, and impeded student achievement overall. Fortunately, as these statistics for the year 2000 show, the victimization rate for serious violent crime at school and away from school generally declined from 1992 to 2000.

- Students ages twelve through eighteen were victims of about 128,000 violent crimes at school (rape, assault, and robbery, for example) and about 373,000 violent crimes away from school.
- Students were victims of about 700,000 nonfatal violent crimes (that is, serious violent crime plus simple assault) at school, and about 921,000 away from school.
- The rate of serious violent crime at school and away from school was higher for males than for females. No difference was found in the rates of serious violent crime at school among students living in urban, suburban, and rural areas.
- Whether at school or away from school, younger students (ages twelve through fourteen) were victimized by serious violent crime at a rate no different from older students (ages fifteen through eighteen).

THREATS OR INTENTIONAL INJURY ON SCHOOL PROPERTY

The percentage of students threatened or intentionally injured on school property is a critical measure of school safety. The percentage of students in grades 9 through 12 who were threatened or injured with a weapon on school property in the twelve months prior to the survey has fluctuated in recent years and thus provides no clear upward or downward trend.

- From 1993 to 2001, between 7 and 9 percent of students in grades 9 through 12 reported being threatened or injured with a weapon on

Health Highlight
YOUTH RISK BEHAVIOR SURVEY

Developed in 1990, the Youth Risk Behavior Surveillance System (YRBSS) monitors health risk behaviors that contribute to the leading causes of death, disability, and social problems among youth and adults in the United States, including behaviors that contribute to unintentional injuries and violence. The YRBSS includes the Youth Risk Behavior Survey (YRBS) of representative samplings of 9th through 12th graders at the national, state, and local level. The YRBS is conducted every 2 years by the Centers for Disease Control and Prevention to determine, among other things, whether health risk behaviors increase, decrease, or stay the same over time. The YRBS provides data on high school students in public and private schools in the United States.

■ 35.7% of high school students reported being in a physical fight in the past 12 months and 4% of students were injured in a physical fight seriously enough to require treatment by a doctor or nurse.

■ 17.3% of high school students carried a weapon (e.g., gun, knife, or club) during the 30 days

preceding the survey.

■ 4.9% of high school students carried a gun during the 30 days preceding the survey.

Regarding school-related violence, the 1999 YRBS found that:

■ 14.2% of high school students had been in a physical fight on school property one or more times in the past 12 months.

■ 7.7% of high school students were threatened or injured with a weapon on school property during the 12 months preceding the survey.

■ 6.9% of high school students carried a weapon on school property during the 30 days preceding the survey.

■ 5.2% of students had missed 1 or more days of school during the 30 days preceding the survey because they had felt too unsafe to go to school.

SOURCE: NCIPC 2002

school property. In 2001, males were more likely than females to report being threatened. Students in lower grades were more likely to be threatened or intentionally injured than were students in higher grades.

■ In 1999 and 2001, no difference was detected in the race/ethnicity of students being threatened or injured with a weapon on school property.

PHYSICAL FIGHTING

While the percentage of students who reported fighting on or off school property has declined from 1993 to 2001, this form of violence is still a health risk for students on and off campus. The following statistics are for 2001.

■ Thirty-three percent of students in grades 9 through 12 reported that they had been in a physical fight anywhere in the last twelve months. About 13 percent of all students said that they had been in a physical fight on school property.

■ Forty-three percent of males and 24 percent of females said they had been in a fight anywhere; 18 percent of males and 7 percent of females said they had been in a fight on school property. Of ninth- through twelfth-grade students, those in lower grades reported being in more fights than students in higher grades anywhere and on school property.

- No difference was detected by race/ethnicity in the percentage of students who reported being in fights on school property.

BULLYING

Although we don't typically think of bullying as an act of violence, it can contribute as much as does violent crime to a climate of fear and intimidation. Students ages twelve though eighteen were asked if they had been bullied at school. Here are the results for 2001.

- Eight percent of students reported that they had been bullied at school in the last six months, compared to 5 percent in 1999.

- Both males and females were likely to be victims of bullying.

- The percentage of students who reported that they had been bullied increased between 1999 and 2001 for each racial/ethnic group (Caucasian, Hispanic, and non-Hispanic) except for African Americans, which held at about 6 percent in 1999 and 2001, repectively.

- There were few differences among racial/ethnic groups in the percentage of students who reported being bullied, except for Caucasian students who were more likely than African-American students to report being bullied.

- Students in lower grades were more likely to be bullied than were students in higher grades.

VIOLENCE AGAINST TEACHERS

Most teachers feel safe in their schools during the day, but after school hours they may not (especially in urban areas). Strict teachers who insist students adhere to rigorous standards are most at risk of being victimized. Data collected in the 1993/1994 and 1999/2000 school years on threats and physical attacks against elementary and secondary teachers by students clarifies this problem (NCES 2002b).

- The percentage of elementary and secondary teachers threatened by a student with injury declined (9 percent versus 12 percent, respectively).

- Teachers in central city schools were more likely to be threatened with injury or physically attacked than were teachers in urban fringe or rural schools. No differences were detected in the percentage of teachers being threatened or attacked when urban fringe and rural schools were compared.

- African-American teachers were more likely to be threatened than were Caucasian teachers in 1999/2000, but the prevalence of teachers attacked by students did not vary according to the teachers' racial/ethnic backgrounds.

- In 1999 to 2000, secondary school teachers were more likely than elementary school teachers to have been threatened with injury by a student from their school, but were less likely than elementary school teachers to have been physically attacked by a student.

- Public school teachers were twice as likely as private school teachers to be threatened with injury and attacked by students in school in 1999 to 2000.

- Teachers in public central city schools were four times more likely to be targets of threats of injury and about three times more likely to be targets of attacks than teachers in private central city schools in 1999 to 2000.

THE GOOD NEWS!

Now for the good news: Most children have never committed violent acts. In fact, the 80–15–5 rule generally applies:

- Eighty percent rarely break the rules or violate principles.

- Fifteen percent break the rules somewhat regularly by refusing to accept classroom principles/restrictions.

- Five percent are chronic rule breakers who are out of control most of the time and may commit acts of violence in school and in the community.

STRATEGIES TO PREVENT SCHOOL VIOLENCE

The most common school security measure used requires school staff, in particular teachers and security staff, to monitor students' movements in and around the school. Equally effective, and less costly than guards, is the use of students' parents as monitors and teachers' aides. Youth are less likely to misbehave or engage in violent acts if parents from their neighborhood are highly visible.

Institutionalization of discipline and dress codes is another strategy used to curb violence. These codes should be developed collaboratively by administrators, teachers, parents, and students. Schools must be sure that the rules created have a purpose and that they explicitly tell students what kinds of behavior are acceptable and how the school will deal with students who break the rules.

Some school communities seek to counter lack of effective parenting by establishing tutoring programs and providing mentors for students. The mentors are community volunteers from business, service organizations, colleges and universities, churches, and retiree organizations. Some schools have established counseling programs for students; however, most elementary schools do not have them, and most high school counselors have 350 to 400 students each.

Another form of counseling is the widespread use of conflict resolution strategies to defuse potentially violent situations by persuading those involved to use nonviolent means to resolve their differences. Schools that have adopted conflict resolution strategies are trying to teach young people new ways of channeling their anger into constructive, nonviolent responses to conflict. Some schools use students as a conflict resolution team to help maintain order in the school by counseling their peers and intervening in disputes among students. Conflict resolution teams also help by encouraging peers to talk through their problems and by training other students to use conflict resolution strategies.

Schools should strongly consider the establishment of crisis centers for students who commit violent acts or threaten violence. Crisis centers should not be used for long-term interventions, but rather as in-school areas where students can be sent to "cool off" and to receive on-the-spot counseling.

Some schools and communities have made efforts to reduce the number of property crimes by providing part-time employment for students during the school year and full-time employment during the summer months. The goals of these work programs include building self-esteem and a sense of responsibility, learning the value of money and the importance of getting a good education, and staying in school until graduation.

Another strategy being used by an increasing number of schools is extending the number of hours that the school is open; students can participate in organized activities such as sports, gymnastics, crafts, art, music, and tutorial programs.

Several urban school districts have organized youth collaboratives. These collaboratives focus on school dropout prevention and the preparation of youth for the work force. These groups promote the need to provide coordinated services for youth and families. With the business community, school districts seek to address the needs of students at risk of educational failure through the combined efforts of the city government, health, law enforcement, education, social service agencies, and the religious community.

Efforts to prevent violence in schools must involve teachers at every step of the process. Whether or not through formal communications channels, all teachers should be aware of the discipline problems that occur in their school. Strategies designed to eliminate or reduce such problems will not work unless teachers are involved in the design and implementation of programs to establish a safe, orderly environment in the school. Faculty members who are aware of what is going on in the school and of strategies to address problems are apt to become actively involved in supporting schoolwide efforts to correct the problem. It is also important for teachers to be able to discuss any major discipline problems they are having with students in their classrooms. These discussions can be part of regular monthly faculty meetings or special sessions.

Critical to the elimination of violent acts in schools is support for teachers' efforts to address discipline problems. Since teachers are the front line, it is paramount that they receive support from their administration. Administrators must provide teachers and other school staff with the assurance that violent students will be dealt with swiftly and firmly, and that teachers will receive support in their efforts to maintain an orderly classroom.

To maintain a safe and orderly classroom conducive to teaching and learning, a teacher must set forth both academic and behavioral expectations for the classroom. It is very important for them to establish control on the first day of school and maintain it steadily thereafter. Students are perceptive: They quickly become aware of teachers who are not in control of their classrooms. Being in control does not mean being rigid or being a tyrant; it means asserting authority and demanding and getting respect. Teachers also must ensure that the behavior standards are followed—and they must do so in a manner that is fair but firm and consistent. Students who fail to comply with the discipline standards must be dealt with quickly and firmly.

Equally important, and often a factor ignored in discussions about discipline and violence in schools, is the academic side of the issue. Classrooms where the academic objectives are unclear are fertile for disruptive student behavior and perhaps violence. This does not mean that every student should be seated quietly at a desk with a book open or busy filling in the blanks on a form. It does mean that the lessons have been carefully planned to elicit maximum teaching and learning. It means students are actively engaged in learning activities—sometimes in groups. It means using strategies to ensure that students comprehend what is being taught and are able to demonstrate their learning. It means insisting that all students strive to meet the academic as well as behavioral standards for the class and assisting those who have difficulty doing so.

Disruptive or violent behavior in the classroom is a way for some students to mask their frustration and anger over their academic deficiencies. The fact that all students do not acquire knowledge the same way must be reflected in the teacher's instruction. Applied strategies of effective teaching, along with lesson plans that respond to students' cultural diversity and learning styles, can significantly reduce instances of potentially disruptive or violent behavior in our nation's schools.

PERSONAL SAFETY

Becoming a victim of violent behavior or sustaining an unintentional injury can harm your health as much as any of your own unhealthy behavior. Intentional injuries reflect violence committed by one person acting against another person. According to the National Center for Health Statistics (2001), the categories of intentional injuries include homicides, physical assault, sexual assault, rape or attempted rape, physical fighting, weapon carrying, and suicide.

Unfortunately, many children suffer from injuries inflicted on them by adults, sometimes parents or relatives of the children and sometimes by strangers. Children need to be taught to trust their feelings when they do not feel right about a person or a situation. For example, being touched by an adult, and the touch feels uncomfortable, the child needs to know to inform another adult. Emphasize to children that they have a right and a responsibility to determine when and how they wish to be touched. Teach them to assert their own personal space, or privacy. They need to be taught to keep their distance from people who make them feel most uncomfortable.

Each child should be taught to be more aware of his or her surroundings—that is, be aware if someone is following him or her. Walk in the middle of the sidewalk, and try to walk with someone else. Stay away from dark places when alone. Tell them it is all right to scream if they are approached by someone intending to do them harm.

Health Highlight

ABOUT SCHOOL HEALTH POLICIES AND PROGRAMS STUDY

School Health Policies and Programs Study (SHPPS) is a national survey periodically conducted to assess school health policies and programs at the state, district, school, and classroom levels.

School Policy and Environment

- 60.4% of states and 50.6% of districts provided model policies on accident or unintentional injury prevention to districts or schools during the 2 years preceding the study

- 58.3% of states and 77.1% of districts have policies on the inspection or maintenance of playground facilities and equipment; during the 12 months preceding the study, 94.8% of elementary schools performed inspection and maintenance on their playground facilities and equipment

- 90.0% of states and 89.9% of districts have policies on the protection of students and staff from environmental hazards such as asbestos, pesticides, or chemicals in labs and workshops; during the 12 months preceding the study, 94.4% of schools performed inspection and maintenance for these hazards

- 82.0% of states and 80.0% of districts have policies on the inspection or maintenance of special classroom areas, such as chemistry labs, workshops, and art rooms; during the 12 months preceding the study, 80.8% of schools performed inspection and maintenance of these areas

- 46.9% of states, 97.1% of districts, and 97.8% of schools have a policy prohibiting physical fighting by students

- 98.0% of states, 99.1% of districts, and 96.1% of schools have a policy prohibiting weapon possession or use by students

- 28.6% of states, 62.5% of districts, and 64.9% of schools have a policy prohibiting gang activities

- 83.7% of states and 68.7% of districts provided model policies to schools on violence prevention during the 2 years preceding the study

SOURCE: National Center for Chronic Disease Prevention and Health Promotion 2002

The School Safety Program

Instruction in safety education should be only one part of your school safety program. The total program should consist of these components:

- providing instruction by and for faculty, staff, and students
- planning and implementing safety procedures
- providing safe transportation, including bus travel, walking, and bicycle safety
- establishing accident reporting and record-keeping procedures
- making sure there is liability insurance protection for staff
- providing emergency health care for all people attending or employed by the school
- creating a safe environment

The responsibilities of each person involved in the safety program should be defined by the school. Additionally, the school should instruct each person

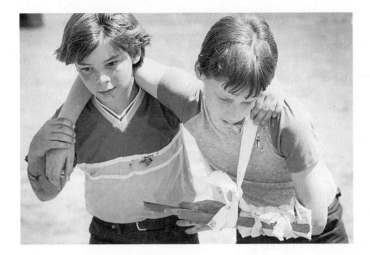

Children should have some knowledge of first aid procedures to be of help in emergency situations.

regarding specific duties or responsibilities. Supervision should be provided for all school activities, including travel to and from school, physical education, playground time, and after-school gatherings.

Some schools have established school safety councils to develop rules, policies, and procedures for safe living within the school and for school activities. Safety councils provide excellent learning opportunities and allow for student involvement. For example, a school safety council could do a needs assessment or accident survey for the school. This procedure makes the students and others involved aware of the accident situations in their school environment, thus helping to prevent future accidents.

Generally, any accident that causes a student to miss school, go home from school, or that involves property damage should be reported. Some schools have specific forms for reporting any type of accident in or around the school. Accident reports can provide data for studying accident trends in the school environment. They are also valuable in the event of lawsuits filed against the school.

First-Aid Skills

First aid means just that: providing aid before more qualified medical help can be obtained. Adults and children alike should have some knowledge of first-aid procedures so they can help an accident victim in an emergency. Often such knowledge can make the difference between life and death in extreme cases. However, first aid should never be dispensed casually—and not at all if more qualified help can be obtained quickly. As a classroom teacher, you should learn basic first-aid procedures and instruct your students in them. Most often, first-aid procedures are used in common incidents involving cuts, nosebleeds, sprains, and so on.

Begin your own preparation by checking with the school administration and medical personnel to determine established procedures for handling medical problems and emergencies. This is extremely important as far as liability is concerned and cannot be stressed too strongly. In most instances, you will probably be told not to offer any medical assistance except under clearly life-threatening circumstances or when there is no possibility of obtaining more qualified assistance. In some instances, however, administering first aid may be acceptable and provided for in the school safety program.

Keep in mind that first aid is not treatment; instead, it is protection of the victim until treatment can be given. The purpose of first aid is to offer emergency care, prevent further injury, lessen the victim's pain, and ward off unnecessary complications, such as shock. While this is being done, help should also be sought. (More information about first aid can be found in Appendix A.)

EMERGENCY SITUATIONS

The best way to prepare yourself to handle an emergency medical or accident situation is to become qualified to handle emergencies. If you are not qualified, you should become qualified by taking a first-aid and CPR (cardiopulmonary resuscitation) class through the American Red Cross, National Safety Council, and/or American Heart Association. You will gain hands-on experience in dealing with a variety of situations and will have a chance to practice basic first-aid skills before you actually have to use them.

Summary

- Elementary school children are subject to many injuries, some intentional and some unintentional.
- Accidental deaths are the leading cause of death for this age group, but deaths and injuries from violence are on the rise.
- Children are becoming involved in violent behavior in increasing numbers, both as perpetrators and victims.
- Safety education that covers both safety and violence prevention should be a vital part of health instruction.
- Safety education will help students to increase their awareness of the potential for and cause of accidents; provide them with factual knowledge about safety; help them adjust to new, unfamiliar environments; and heighten their potential for living full, productive lives.
- Positive, safe behavior should be seen by the students as an important part of living.
- The emphasis in safety education should be on positive attitudes and values.
- Learning opportunities in safety should be designed to help students recognize potentially hazardous situations, develop a sense of responsibility for their own safety and others', and make wise decisions regarding their behavior.

- Do not provide safety instruction that is limited to accident statistics, safety rules, or scare tactics. Instead, stress that living is much more enjoyable when a person is safe.
- Teach the students how to prevent violence in their own lives and how to respond if they are faced with violence.
- As the teacher, you should set a good safety model for your students.
- The classroom and other parts of the school environment should be examples of safe, efficient places to work and live.
- Be aware of your responsibility as a teacher regarding liability in various school situations.
- Because so many accidents happen to children while they are attending school, you should learn basic first-aid skills and CPR to treat injuries resulting from accidents.
- Students should learn how they can be of help in emergency situations.

DISCUSSION QUESTIONS

1. Describe the factors that lead to a disproportionate number of accidental deaths among children.
2. Discuss the reasons for some people taking risks in our society.
3. How can we teach children to assume a positive approach to safety?
4. Describe the emotional makeup of an accident-prone individual.
5. Discuss the ways to make a playground safer for children.
6. Describe the proper behavior for a child while riding on a school bus.
7. Discuss the steps to take when confronted by someone who is threatening to attack you.
8. Enumerate the rules for children to follow to ensure their personal safety from strangers.
9. Discuss the first-aid procedures to follow in a breathing emergency.
10. Discuss the types of educational programs designed to prevent violent behavior.

CRITICAL THINKING QUESTIONS

1. Consider the case of an automobile accident in which a driver runs into the back of another automobile when the roads are wet and visibility is low. How much of this type of unintentional accident would you attribute to human factors and how much to environmental factors?
2. Explain your willingness to take the risk to perform daily tasks, such as driving or riding to work and school, crossing a busy street, and walking through a parking lot.
3. Compare the response of students who are taught safe behavior from a positive point of view versus a negative point of view.

4. Do you think that some individuals have more accidents than others because of coincidence? Or, do you think that each of those individuals' inordinate amount of accidents can be explained by emotional factors (for example, accident proneness)?

5. Considering your own personal beliefs, character, and past experience, what do you think would be the best approach for you to take if someone is threatening to attack you? What preventive steps would you be willing to take to prepare yourself for such an event?

6. Despite having training in first aid and crisis procedures (such as hurricanes, etc.), some people are concerned that they would panic in such a situation. Detail some steps to take to prevent such a panic reaction.

7. Design what you would consider a feasible school safety plan to prevent intentional and unintentional injuries.

WEB SITE ACTIVITY

Visit the SafeUSA Web site (*www.cdc.gov/safeusa/mission.htm*) and click on "Safety at School." What are the safety procedures for Playground Safety?

WEB SITES OF INTEREST

The National Safety Council: *www.nsc.org/gen/informa.htm*
The mission of the National Safety Council is "to educate and influence society to adopt safety, health and environmental policies, practices, and procedures that prevent and mitigate human suffering and economic losses arising from preventable causes."

esafety.com: A Parenthood Safety Web Site: *www.esafety.com/esafety_cfmfiles/ index.cfm*
Provides resources for parents regarding safety procedures for young children.

Education World: *www.education-world.com/help/about.shtml*
Makes the Internet easier for educators to use. Includes a search engine for educational Web sites only. Creates a home for educators on the Internet where they can gather and share ideas and easily find lesson plans and research materials.

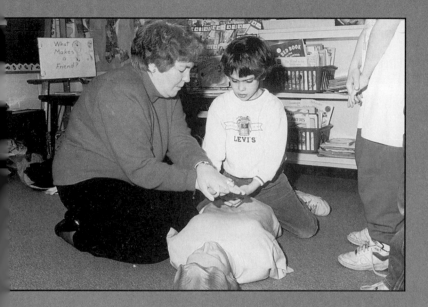

CHAPTER TWENTY

Strategies for Teaching about Injuries: Accident and Violence Prevention

If there is one area of health education that has lagged behind, it is safety and accident prevention.

VALUED OUTCOMES

After doing the activities in this chapter, the student should be able to express and illustrate the following guidelines:

- Each person is to a large degree responsible for his or her own personal safety.

- Peers exert a tremendous influence over safety practices.

- Obedience to safety rules enhances the quality of life.

- Risk taking is a part of living, but unnecessary risk taking greatly increases the risk of harm to oneself and to others.

- The degree of risk in any particular activity can often be determined by analytical thinking.

- Rules and procedures for safe behavior help prevent accidents in the home, school, and community.
- Hazardous conditions should be corrected whenever possible.
- There are many people and community agencies who can help when accidents occur.
- Elementary school children have more fatal accidents than any other age group.
- More than half of all accidents involving children happen at school.
- Playground rules are important for safe activities.

- Elementary students need to practice safe behavior in traffic.
- Home and school fire escape routes should be practiced frequently.
- Acting without thinking often results in an accident.
- Basic first-aid skills are important for everyone.
- Improper first aid can do more harm than good.
- Safety is not just a matter of luck.
- Safe behavior must be learned.

REFLECTIONS

As you utilize the strategies in this chapter, reflect on how you can emphasize assuming personal responsibility in one's safety and risk-taking behavior. Also, consider how each of these strategies can emphasize taking a positive approach to safety behavior as opposed to using scare tactics.

Fostering Safety Behavior

Progress has been made in virtually every area of health education in the previous century, including disease prevention, environmental sanitation, and nutritional habits. If there is one area of health education that has lagged behind, however, it is safety and accident prevention. Safety education has lagged behind partially because many teachers and organizations tend to teach safety education in a negative way, emphasizing rules and a list of "don'ts" for the students to follow. Also, some educators and organizations utilize scare tactics in safety, but these tactics have very little long-term value in changing behavior.

Many laws have been passed, especially in the area of traffic safety. Some states are passing mandatory safety belt and stiffer drunk driving laws. These laws should help save more lives on the road; however, despite these and other legislative safety efforts, thousands of Americans die or are injured each year because of needless accidents. The situation will not change significantly until Americans reject an attitude of apathy toward safety and adopt a lifestyle of safe behavior.

Shown to the right of each activity title in this chapter is the suggested grade level(s) for which the activity might be appropriate. However, many of the suggested activities could be modified for use at various grade levels.

Value-Based Activities

SAFETY HABITS BELIEFS   Grades (K–5)

Valued Outcome: The students will define their knowledge of safety habits.

Description of Strategy: Before spending time discussing safety rules and habits, have the students complete a series of statements that show how they feel when it comes to safety. Prepare a handout using the list below for suggested statements to include. On a volunteer basis, discuss the values implicit in the statements on the handout.

1. I wear a helmet when I ride a bicycle because _____.
2. I can avoid falling by _____.
3. I think the most dangerous type of safety violation is _____.
4. The safest place to walk is _____.
5. I always swim with an adult present because _____.
6. The most important thing I can do when mowing the lawn is _____ _____.
7. The best thing I can know when there is a fire is _____.
8. The best place for poisons to be kept is _____.
9. In case of an emergency, I need to know how to call the local emergency numbers because _____.
10. I always fasten my safety belt in the car because _____.
11. I think the most important thing that I can do to try to remain safe is _____.
12. All students should be required to participate in disaster drills (for fire, tornado, hurricane, etc.) because _____.
13. To me, safety education means _____.
14. Accidents are the result of _____.
15. As a pedestrian, I should know _____.

Materials Needed: handouts and pencils for each student

Processing Questions:

1. Why do we need safety rules and regulations?
2. If we don't follow rules, what might happen?
3. Why did you select what you did for the most important thing you can do to try to remain safe?
4. How can your attitude toward safety improve your safety?

SAFETY VOTING   Grades (K–5)

Valued Outcome: The students will be able to respond to safety-related statements based on their values.

Description of Strategy: Have your students raise their hands to agree or disagree with the following statements:

- Some accidents are caused by people showing off.
- All the medicines in my house are stored in a safe place.
- Some medicines can be taken without parents' permission.
- I know the number of the local poison control center.
- I read labels on all medications before I take them.
- It is important to wear a safety belt even on short trips.

Materials Needed: none

Processing Question: What variables help you determine your values about safety practices?

STRANGER SAFETY   Grades (K–3)

Valued Outcome: The students will be able to make safe decisions about interaction with strangers.

Description of Strategy: Pose a series of statements to the students and have them respond by giving thumbs up for "OK to do" and thumbs down for "not OK to do." Show a picture card of each situation as you make each statement. Some example statements you might use are:

- I would accept candy or gifts from someone I did not know.
- I would accept a ride from someone I did not know.
- I would talk to my mother's friend.
- I would let someone I did not know into my house.
- I would help someone find his or her puppy, even if I did not know that person.
- I would talk to my school counselor.
- I would tell someone I have met on the Internet where I go to school.

Materials Needed: large cards of people involved in activities correlated with the statements

Processing Questions:

1. Why are some of these behaviors dangerous and other behaviors safe?
2. What should you do if a stranger approaches you?

Valued Outcome: After a class discussion about water safety, the students will be able to categorize the listed behaviors as safe or unsafe and write two of their own water safety rules.

Description of Strategy: Lead the class in a discussion about water safety. To begin, ask the students "How many of you like to swim?" Then, "Do any of you swim at a pool or a lake where there are lifeguards? Who can tell me one thing a lifeguard does?" Answers will vary.

Next, lead a class discussion using prompts: "Why does a lifeguard sit on such a high chair/stand?" (so he or she can see the whole pool area) "Why would a lifeguard need to be able to see everyone?" (to keep everyone safe and make sure everyone is following the rules) "What should you do if you hear the lifeguard blow his or her whistle?" (stop what you are doing and give the lifeguard full attention) "What are some of the pool rules?" (do not run on deck, no pushing each other in or under water, no diving in the shallow end of the pool, get out of the pool when the lifeguard tells you to) "Why do they have these rules?" Go through each one: No running because someone could fall and get hurt on the deck or fall into the water; it is dangerous to horseplay in water because someone could drown; no diving in shallow water because the diver could hit his or her head on the bottom of a pool and be injured or drown; and get out as soon as the lifeguard gives the instruction because there is most likely a danger such as lightning, or the pool water has been contaminated (with vomit, feces, etc.)

Explain to the students that following pool rules keeps them, others, and the lifeguards safe. Wrap up this part of the discussion by having the student recall some fun things they can do at a pool (swim, float, talk to their friends, play a water sport, go down a water slide, etc).

After the discussion, do the following activity. Give each student the following items: two paper plates, one with a sad face and one with a happy face, two blank slips of paper, and slips of paper with the following statements written on them (each slip should contain one statement):

- Play tag on the pool deck. (unsafe)
- Play with a beach ball in shallow water. (safe)
- Take turns with a friend holding each other under the water. (unsafe)
- Ignore the lifeguard's whistle if I am sure it is not directed at me. (unsafe)
- Cannonball into the deep end if the area is clear. (safe)
- Dive off a diving board after checking that the area is clear. (safe)

At the front of the room, place an additional set of plates and a master set of statements to sort later. At their desks, have the students sort the slips of paper into safe (happy) and unsafe (sad) piles. Then have the class sort the master slips together by reading each statement aloud and asking the students which plate it should go on. Then, have the students write their own safe or unsafe behaviors on the blank slips of paper. Have each student read his or her statement aloud before placing it on the appropriate plate. Be sure to have them write their names on the back so you will be able to evaluate what they have learned.

Materials Needed: two paper plates per student and one teacher set (one with a happy face and one with a sad face), pencils and slips of paper with statements for each student

Processing Questions:

1. What are two safe and two unsafe behaviors?

2. What is the most important rule to remember when at the pool?

Decision Stories

The teacher and students will follow the procedures outlined in Chapter 4, pages 80–83, for decision stories.

FIRE! Grades (K–5)

Marilyn is alone in her house. She goes into the hallway on the second floor and sees flames coming from the room down the hall. The flames are between Marilyn and the only staircase to the downstairs part of the house.

Focus Question: What should Marilyn do?

THE HILL Grades (K–5)

George and Mario like to ride their bikes to school. There is a hill on the way to school. Near the top of the hill, there is a stop sign, but if they stop, getting over the hill is difficult. George usually stops, but Mario never does. George has to get off his bike and start again. Mario kids him about this and calls him a chicken. George does not want to seem a coward to his friend, but he knows that he should stop for traffic signs.

Focus Question: What should George do?

SHOW AND TELL Grades (K–2)

Valerie and Davina are in the same second grade class. One day during lunch, Davina tells Valerie she has something to show her when they are back in the classroom. After lunch, while the teacher is busy talking to another student and they are putting away their lunch boxes, Davina pulls out a gun from her backpack to show Valerie and says, "I found this in my dad's room. Isn't it cool?" Valerie knows guns are dangerous because their teacher had a police officer talk to the class about gun safety. Valerie knows that she should not touch guns and that guns are not allowed at school.

Focus Questions:

1. What should Valerie do?

2. Why are guns dangerous?

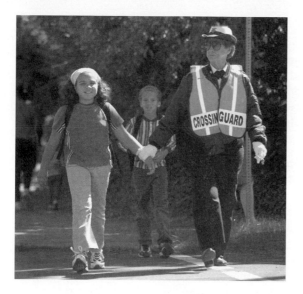

Students need to be safe pedestrians.

AROUND THE NEIGHBORHOOD   Grades (K–3)

Joseph and Eli are best friends in the same third grade class. Sometimes Eli plays at Joseph's house, and Joseph often plays at Eli's house after school. Many times they like to ride their bikes around Eli's neighborhood. There is a lot of traffic on Eli's street, and Joseph and Eli know they should always wear their helmets. In class, they have learned about bike safety and what they should do to be safe. Joseph always wears his helmet, but Eli does not. Eli says, "Helmets are for babies, and I don't play with babies." Joseph doesn't want to argue with Eli or lose his friendship.

Focus Questions:

1. What should Joseph do?
2. What could Joseph say to Eli to convince him to wear his helmet?

SAFETY BELTS   Grades (K–5)

Jaime's friend, Warren, and Warren's parents came to Jaime's house to take Jaime and Warren to a party. When Jaime got into their car, he noticed Warren and his parents were not wearing their safety belts, and the one at his seat was hard to find. Jaime had been taught always to wear his safety belt, but he was afraid he would embarrass Warren and his parents if he were the only one in the car to wear his safety belt.

Focus Question: What should Jaime do?

THE RAFT

Jason and his friends are playing by a river near their home. Some of the boys decide to build a raft. They are going to use it to cross the river. They find some wood on the river bank and start making the raft. But it doesn't look too sturdy to Jason. When the time comes to put the raft in the water, Jason has his doubts. What if the raft falls apart while the boys are on it? Jason knows how to swim, but swimming might be difficult with his clothes on—and he is not sure the others can swim.

Focus Question: What should Jason do?

THE STRANGER

Beth and her sister Harriet are walking home from school. Just then a car pulls up by the curb. The driver is a man Beth and her sister have never seen. He asks them their names, and they tell him. Then the man says that he is a good friend of their father. He says that their father has asked him to pick them up and take them for a ride. The stranger offers to buy the girls some ice cream, too.

Focus Question: What should Beth and her sister do?

THE FIRST REAL PARTY

Maria is a shy girl and is rarely invited to parties. Sam, a friend at school, asked Maria if she would like to come with him to a party this Friday night. Maria accepted, thinking this would be her chance to get to know some more people. At the party, some of the kids were smoking and drinking. Sam wanted Maria to smoke and drink, too. He said this would help her come out of her shell.

Focus Question: Should Maria smoke and drink at the party?

MEDICINE

Cristina is getting over a cold. It is nothing serious, but she stayed home from school for two days. Now she is back. Her cold is almost gone, but she is still coughing. At lunch, Cristina sits with her friend Pam. Pam has been taking medicine for an infection. "It's really good stuff," Pam says to Cristina. "I'll bet it would make your cough go away just like that. Why don't you try some?"

Focus Question: What should Cristina do?

EMERGENCY CARE

Mary came home from school and found her grandmother lying at the foot of the stairway unconscious. She could not wake her.

Focus Questions:

1. Who should Mary call?
2. What else should she do for her grandmother?

Dramatizations

DISASTER DRAMA   Grades (3–5)

Valued Outcome: The students will be able to learn first-aid procedures to use during a disaster.

Description of Strategy: Have the students enact a mock disaster. Set up the classroom as if a tornado or hurricane had hit the area, and the students are the only trained first aiders who can help. Assign some students to be victims with a variety of injuries (provide descriptions of injuries and symptoms on index cards), and the other students will play the parts of emergency care personnel who will perform first aid for the victims.

Materials Needed: first-aid kits, bandages, cards with descriptions of injuries and symptoms

Processing Questions:

1. How can you help during a disaster?
2. What first-aid skills would you need to know?

SCHOOL BUS BEHAVIOR   Grades (K–5)

Valued Outcome: The students will be able to identify proper conduct on a bus.

Description of Strategy: Divide students into groups. Give each group a situation that has happened on the bus. Have students decide what should be done.

> **Case 1:** Two students are fighting.
>
> **Case 2:** Two students are sitting on the same seat; one student wants the window up, the other student wants the window down.
>
> **Case 3:** A student is holding his arms and head out of the window.

Materials Needed: none

Processing Question: Why is it important to behave well on the school bus?

LOOKING FOR HAZARDS   Grades (K–5)

Valued Outcome: The students will be able to identify hazardous areas in the school setting.

Description of Strategy: Assign students to visit various classrooms, such as gym, looking for hazards. Have them report the findings to the class then return to the same classroom in one week to see if the hazard still exists.

Materials Needed: form for each student that lists rooms in the school

Processing Questions:

1. What safety hazards are typically found in schools?
2. What can students do to help eliminate these hazards?

PHONING FOR HELP Grades (K–5)

Valued Outcome: The students will be able to learn the proper technique for using the phone during an emergency situation.

Description of Strategy: In many emergency situations, assistance can be obtained by telephoning the proper authority or agency. Stress the importance of knowing who to call and what to say on the telephone. Have the students prepare a list of emergency telephone numbers for their area, including those of the fire department, the poison control center, and so on. Then have them role-play emergency situations. One student plays the part of the telephone operator or official. Another student then phones for help. Point out that information given over the telephone should be stated clearly and accurately. Let each student role-play the part of an emergency caller at least once. Follow the activity with general discussion of proper use of the telephone.

Materials Needed: telephone book, pencils and paper for each student

Processing Questions:

1. Do you know the phone numbers of your local fire department, etc.?
2. What information should you give over the phone in case of an emergency?

SAFETY PUPPET SHOW Grades (K–2)

Valued Outcome: The students will be able to demonstrate their ability to react in emergency situations.

Description of Strategy: Have students make or use puppets (such as "Safe Susan" and "Hazardous Harry") to perform safety-related skits. Topics could include disaster situations, handling medical emergencies, fire safety, recreational safety, and safety in the home.

Materials Needed: paper bag or cloth for making puppets and markers for each student

Processing Questions:

1. Why is it important to plan ahead for disaster situations?
2. How can you help your family during a disaster?

COMMERCIALS FOR SAFETY Grades (3–5)

Valued Outcome: The students will be able to prepare a script on different safety hazards.

Description of Strategy: Discuss public service safety messages that students may have seen on television. Then have students prepare individual thirty-second or one-minute scripts that offer safety advice on specific safety hazards. Some students may want to work in small groups to dramatize the situation under discussion. Others may want to use props, such as an electrical appliance, to demonstrate a safety concept. Encourage imagination.

Materials Needed: props as per the individual student or group

Processing Questions:

1. What safety messages have you seen on television?
2. How do they help prevent accidents?

SAFETY ATTITUDES   Grades (3–5)

Valued Outcome: The students will be able to role-play positive and negative attitudes concerning safety.

Description of Strategy: Attitudes play a large part in safety behavior. Have students role-play people with positive and negative attitudes while participating in several activities (such as bicycling or playing ball). *Positive* attitudes include consideration, maturity, courtesy, and honesty; *negative* attitudes include selfishness, impatience, childishness, competitiveness, showing off, daydreaming, and unnecessary risk taking.

Materials Needed: none

Processing Questions:

1. How can one's attitude about safety cause or prevent an accident?
2. What are examples of positive safety attitudes? of negative safety attitudes?

Discussion and Report Techniques

MEDIA CRIME QUIZ   Grades (7–8)

Valued Outcome: The students will be able to explain the media's portrayal of youth violence and its effect on society's perceptions toward young people.

Description of Strategy: Give the students the following quiz (answers are provided in parentheses):

1. In terms of crime, how old is a "youth"? (between twelve and seventeen years of age)
2. When you see stories about youth in the news—or read stories about them in the newspapers—what types of stories come to mind? (Crime-related stories or ones connected to violence will likely dominate student responses.)
3. When you hear stories about teens and violence in the news, how does it make you feel? (Answers will vary; many students may feel offended that youth are often portrayed in a negative light; some may feel that these stories reflect reality.)
4. Do you ever see youth like yourselves and your friends in the media?
5. Why is there so little emphasis on stories about regular kids, and so much emphasis on negative stories about kids?

6. How do media stories about youth and crime affect your perceptions and attitudes on this issue?

7. How do media stories affect your parents' perceptions and attitudes?

8. The term *media myth* is used to describe the media's continued portrayals of images and information that are not based on fact. A media myth is created when whole groups of people are misrepresented because the extreme actions of a few of them dominate the media. Can you think of any examples of groups of people who have been affected by media myths?

9. What media myths have been created regarding youth?

10. Do you think media myths about youth have ever affected how you have been treated?

Materials Needed: quiz for each student

Processing Question: Did your perceptions of youth crime change after taking the quiz?

SOURCE: Media Awareness Network 2003

DRUG SAFETY   Grades (3–5)

Valued Outcome: The students will be able to determine healthful and harmful things that people put in their bodies.

Description of Strategy: Have students make a list of things that are harmful to their bodies. After students have made their lists, have them look through magazines and cut out pictures of things that will keep their bodies healthy and things that will harm their bodies. Have students compare the pictures with their lists. On the same sheet of paper, have students answer the following questions:

- What might happen if you took medicine that was not for you?
- What might happen if you took too much medicine?

Tell students they should only take medicine prescribed by a doctor or medicine given by their mom or dad. Tell them that medicine can be very harmful and even deadly if taken incorrectly. Talk to students about peer pressure. Tell them that sometimes their friends may try and talk them into doing something they know is wrong or something they don't feel comfortable about. Tell students that it is okay to say "No." Ask the students to write their responses to the following questions on the same sheet of paper they have been using.

- What would you do if your friend offered you a cigarette?
- What if your friend told you that his or her mom and dad were at work and your friend wanted you to come over after school and drink one beer just to try it. What would you do?

Materials Needed: notebook paper, pencils, and magazines for each student

Processing Question: How do you feel when you see other people abusing a drug?

WHAT IF?   **Grades (3–5)**

Valued Outcome: The students will be confronted with a variety of threats and develop safety tips on how to be prepared for dangerous situations.

Description of Strategy: Begin with a large pad of paper with one safety tip written on the top of each page. Divide the class into groups. Have the groups write when the tip would be useful and list everything the group knows about the subject within a given time limit. Then bring the class together to discuss the subjects and the tips. Several pre-selected students will then act out the scenarios listed below.

1. What if you are walking home and believe someone is following you? What can you do?

2. What if an older kid on an elevator threatens you? How can you keep a safe distance from this person?

3. What if your sister pinches you every time you make her mad? How can you set boundaries and get her to respect them?

4. What if you are home alone and someone comes to the door? What safety measures does a child home alone need to know?

5. What if your ride is late picking you up after sports practice, and everyone else has left? How can you stay alert and safe?

Materials Needed: large pad of paper, markers, tape to hang the paper, and prepared questions for follow-up

Processing Questions:

1. What are four rules to follow when you are home alone?

2. What are some ways to protect your safety at school?

SOURCE: Chaiet and Russell 1998

CHEMICAL SAFETY IN THE HOME   **Grades (3–5)**

Valued Outcome: The students will have a more detailed knowledge about the dangers of home chemicals, and they will have helpful advice on what to do in case of an emergency.

Description of Strategy: Divide the students into groups. Provide each group with a top view of a home with each room labeled (kitchen, bathroom, etc.), and ask them to write in each box what hazardous chemicals they think might be found in that room. Use this activity to assess the students' depth of knowledge.

Have the students use the Internet to research useful information on household chemicals, which can be found at *www.epa.gov.* Point out the dangers of exposure to certain chemicals, such as antibacterial cleaners (*www.epa.gov/pesticides/kids/hometour/products/disinf.htm*), biological chemicals found in household plants (*www.epa.gov/pesticides/kids/decoys/plants.htm*), insect sprays (*www.epa.gov/pesticides/kids/hometour/products/ispray.htm*), oven cleaners (*www.epa.gov/pesticides/kids/hometour/products/oclean.htm*), and other products, which can be accessed via *www.epa.gov/pesticides/kids/hometour.htm.* Have the students come up with their own ideas on a sheet of paper about what to do in case of an emergency involving chemicals. Have them look up useful information on what to do if an accident happens at their home in the case of exposure through their skin, eyes, mouth (swallowing), or breathing the hazardous chemicals. Have them look up this information at *www.epa.gov/pesticides/kids/hometour/ accident.htm*. Show the students the listing of emergency phone numbers in their local phone book.

Materials Needed: top view of room layout of a house (one for each group), pencils for each student, computer with Internet access, and a local telephone book

Processing Questions:

1. How, when, where, and why are there accidents at home?

2. Why do people underestimate the dangers of exposure to household chemicals?

3. How can you prevent an accident from occurring, and if one does occur, what should you do?

SOURCE: U.S. Environmental Protection Agency 2002

ALLERGIES   Grades (3–5)

Valued Outcome: The students will identify what causes allergies, the most common allergic reactions, what triggers allergic reactions, and what to do if you experience an allergic reaction.

Description of Strategy: Allergies are common, so have the students write down if they have any allergies, what allergens cause them, and what their reaction is to them. Give the class a homework assignment that requires them to use the Internet to look up as much information as they can on allergies and how to handle an emergency allergenic episode (first-aid procedures). Assign each student a specific part of the topic, so no two students' information is the same. Suggest these three Web sites for their use.

> *www.the allergyreport.org/reportindex.html* (current articles about allergies or information on management of allergic diseases)
>
> *www.foodallergy.org/questions.html* (food allergies and the body's reaction to allergies)
>
> *www.ivillagehealth.com/conditions/respiratory/articles/0,11299, 165874_174569,00.html* (asthma, triggers, etc.)

Have the students bring their information to class, then divide them into groups according to relative topic (e.g., all the students who researched allergic reactions in one group, those who researched first-aid procedures in another group), and have the groups present their information in a format using a heading and bullets on one piece of paper. Have every student take notes, then, if time permits, have them all practice the proper first-aid procedures.

Materials Needed: paper and pencils for each student, computer with Internet access

Processing Questions:

1. If you are allergic to spinach and you ate some spinach, what possible reactions could you have?

2. What should you do if a classmate has an allergic reaction? What are the proper first-aid procedures?

SOURCES: iVillage 2000

HOME-ALONE SAFETY   Grades (K–5)

Valued Outcome: The students will be able to write from memory two safe or unsafe behaviors associated with home-alone safety.

Description of Strategy: As an introduction to this lesson, have students indicate orally whether the following statements are true or false. After each statement, give the correct answer and ask a student who answered correctly to explain why his or her answer is correct. (This will give you an idea of focus areas for subsequent lessons and expose the class to home-alone safety awareness.)

True or False

T/F   1. If the door is open or unlocked when I arrive home alone, I should go in and check things out.

T/F   2. It is okay to give out information to adults on the phone.

T/F   3. I can watch television or talk on the phone with my friends.

T/F   4. If someone knocks on my door, I should open it.

T/F   5. I should shut and lock the doors to my house.

T/F   6. I can play outside as long as I stay near the house or in my yard.

After the class discussion, have each student write about two safe or unsafe home-alone safety behaviors.

Materials Needed: paper and pencils for each student, master list of quiz questions

Processing Questions:

1. Why would you not answer the door when you are home alone?

2. What if the person knows your name and your parents' names or says your mom or dad asked him or her to come?

3. What should you do if your door is already open and unlocked when you arrive home?

SCHOOL SAFETY

Grades (3–5)

Valued Outcome: The students will be able to list school safety rules.

Description of Strategy: Have students work in groups of three. Have students list safety rules they should follow at school. Examples include no running in the halls, put supplies away when finished, share, wait your turn in lines and on playground equipment, follow all school bus safety rules, and follow the teacher's instructions. Have the groups share their answers with the rest of the class, and write the responses on the board or on an overhead transparency.

Have each student write and illustrate a short book on school safety. Have them go through the writing process of prewriting, drafting, editing, revising, rewriting, and publishing. After their story has been through the writing process, have them write their story on the pages in a booklet or type them into the computer and then illustrate it. Display the books in the classroom or, if possible, the library. (Since the students will take their stories through the writing process, this activity will take several days to complete.)

Materials Needed: computer or sheets of white paper folded into a booklet for each student; crayons, pencils, notebook pages, colored pencils or markers for each student; overhead projector and pen

Processing Question: How do school safety rules benefit you as an individual?

FIRST-AID KITS

Grades (3–5)

Valued Outcome: The students will be able to describe what goes into a first-aid kit.

Description of Strategy: Explain to the students that there have been many scrapes and cuts in the classroom and that you think they need to make a classroom first-aid kit. Ask the students what they think a first-aid kit can be used for and why it is important for people to have one. Discuss why first-aid kits are important and the situations in which they can be used.

Divide the class into groups of three or four. Have each group suggest what should go in the class first-aid kit and why. After each group has a list of items, have one person from each group tell what items are on their list. (Write items on the board or overhead as they are read.) Once each group has finished, discuss each item and any other item that was missed.

Show the students a variety of first-aid supplies, and discuss whether each one should go in the kit. Demonstrate how each item is used, and then place the first-aid items in the kit. At the end of the discussion, the class first-aid kit will be complete.

Materials Needed: paper and pencils for each student, board and markers or overhead projector and pen, first-aid supplies in box

Processing Question: Why is it important to have a first-aid kit in each classroom?

SOURCE: P. E. Central 2000a

DON'T TOUCH THAT!   Grades (3–5)

Valued Outcome: The students will be able to determine the difference between safe and unsafe items and situations found at home.

Description of Strategy: Discuss the safety hazards that are found in and around a house. Explain that many accidents occur at home. Have each student make a page with newspaper and magazine clippings of accidents that have occurred in people's homes. Then have students write a sentence explaining how the accident happened and how it could have been avoided. Put all the papers together to construct a class scrapbook.

Materials Needed: scrapbook; newspapers, magazines, pictures, glue or tape, pencils or pens for each student

Processing Question: What steps can you take to prevent home accidents?

PREVENTING SCHOOL VIOLENCE   Grades (6–8)

Valued Outcome: The students will be able to recognize and explain that violence is learned and that we often learn it through what the media show us. Students will also be able to identify nonviolent scenarios and be able to reconstruct a violent situation into a nonviolent situation.

Description of Strategy: Before beginning this activity, you may want to send a letter to parents explaining the assignment. Assign students to watch television shows one evening (perhaps allow a week for students to complete this assignment), looking specifically for violence that is depicted in the shows that they typically watch. Ask each student to choose the situation that was the most severe in the show he or she watched and answer the following questions:

- What is the name of the television show you watched?
- How many violent situations did you see?
- What was the violent situation?
- What kind of person performed the crime and why?

After the students have answered these questions, have them use their answers to rewrite the violent situation or situations in a nonviolent way and share their revised scenarios with the class. There must be no violence in the dialogue at all.

Materials Needed: television at home, pens or pencils and paper for each student

Processing Question: What effect does the violence on television shows have on youth in our society?

SOURCE: P. E. Central 2000b

Valued Outcome: The students will be able to identify the correct action to take in emergency situations.

Description of Strategy: Each of the following items describes an emergency that was handled incorrectly. Read each item. Identify the incorrect action, and tell why it was incorrect. Explain what you would do in the situation.

- Leroy was hit in the head by a moving swing and was knocked unconscious. Since it was a very hot day, his friend Eddie moved him into the shade before going for help.

- While Liz was babysitting for the Jacksons, two-year-old Timmy drank some liquid from an unlabeled bottle. When Liz found him, Timmy was pale and sweaty, with stains from whatever he drank around his mouth. Liz immediately gave him some syrup of ipecac to make him vomit. Then she called the poison control center.

- While José and Ben were sledding, José was thrown from his sled, hitting his head on a rock. Although conscious, he felt nauseated and too dizzy to walk. Before going for help, Ben covered José with his coat and gave him some hot chocolate from their thermos to keep him warm.

- Nancy and Kayla were in the park, eating hamburgers and talking. Kayla, who had been lying on her back while she ate, suddenly jumped up and made strange wheezing sounds as if she couldn't breathe or speak. Nancy saw that Kayla was probably choking and ran to get some water for her.

Materials Needed: none

Processing Question: Why is it important to know the correct action to take in emergency situations?

DISASTER DEMONSTRATION　　　　　　　　　　　**Grades (K–5)**

Valued Outcome: The students will be able to demonstrate proper behaviors during various disasters.

Description of Strategy: Assign groups of students to demonstrate the proper behaviors during various emergency situations, such as a tornado, hurricane, earthquake, and an armed intruder. (Be sure to include whatever types of disasters are more likely to occur in your geographic area.) Have them give instructions to the other students, and actually carry out the drill.

Materials Needed: none

Processing Questions:

1. What types of disasters could occur in your area?

2. Does your family have a plan to follow if such a disaster occurs?

DRINKING AND DRIVING   Grades (3–5)

Valued Outcome: The students will be able to describe activities of various organizations that deal with drinking and driving.

Description of Strategy: Have students work in groups of three to four. Assign each group to report on the activities of a group that is involved with promoting alcohol awareness (such as Students Against Drunk Drivers [SADD], Mothers Against Drunk Drivers [MADD], and local law enforcement agencies) or report on your state's drunk driving laws. A related activity could be to have the class establish a SADD chapter in the school.

Materials Needed: resources for students to research their topic

Processing Questions:

1. Is there a SADD or MADD chapter in your town?
2. How have these groups tried to reduce drunk driving in your state?

SAFETY BELT DEBATE   Grades (4–5)

Valued Outcome: The students will be able to debate the topic of whether or not safety belts should be worn.

Description of Strategy: Choose two teams of students to research the use of safety belts in automobiles. One team should argue that wearing safety belts, even for short trips, can save lives and prevent needless injuries in case of an automobile accident. The other team should present reasons why many people don't bother or refuse to wear safety belts. Have the class decide which argument is more based on fact.

Materials Needed: resources for students to research their topic

Processing Question: Why is it important to wear a safety belt every time you ride in a car?

HOLIDAY SAFETY DIARY   Grades (K–5)

Valued Outcome: The students will be able to list hazards that occur during holidays.

Description of Strategy: As a class, identify major holidays, and list them on the board or on an overhead transparency. Have students make a list of accidents or safety hazards that occur more often during each holiday and ways in which those accidents could be reduced or prevented.

Materials Needed: overhead projector and pen or board and markers, pencils and paper for each student

Processing Questions:

1. How can holiday disasters be prevented?
2. If such a disaster cannot be prevented, how can we plan in order to reduce the number and severity of accidents?

NUCLEAR DISASTER EVACUATION   Grades (3–5)

Valued Outcome: The students will learn the specifics of a nuclear disaster evacuation.

Description of Strategy: Have a local safety official discuss the various reasons for an evacuation during a nuclear disaster. Also, have them detail exactly how evacuation routes were planned for their specific town.

Materials Needed: none

Processing Questions:

1. Do you have any nuclear power sources near your home?

2. Are you familiar with the evacuation routes in the event of a nuclear disaster?

Experiments and Demonstrations

CUTS, SCRATCHES, AND ABRASIONS   Grades (3–5)

Valued Outcome: The students will demonstrate a basic knowledge of cuts, scratches, and abrasions and what to do if they get one.

Description of Strategy: Begin the class by walking into the room with a bandage on your arm. Ask the students what they think is wrong with your arm. Explain to the students that you cut your arm, and you had to try to make it better.

Explain to the students what a cut, scratch, and abrasion are and how they might happen. Cuts are deeper and caused by sharp objects like knives, scratches are shallow and caused by sharp objects like a fingernail or thorn, and abrasions are caused when large areas of skin are rubbed away. Tell the students the steps to follow to help your cut heal: apply pressure to stop the bleeding, clean the cut with water, apply antibacterial cream (if approved by school and if needed), and put a bandage on the cut. Show the students a picture of someone with stitches and explain that stitches may be needed if a cut is very deep. Review these steps with the students a few times, and make sure they all understand what they are doing.

Tell students to find a partner and practice cleaning and putting an adhesive bandage on the cut. Have plenty of bandages available for the students to practice with. While the students are practicing, walk around the room and make sure students are doing it properly. Have the students come up one at a time and perform the techniques for you while all the other students continue to practice.

Materials Needed: soft cloths, antibacterial cream, different types of bandages, picture of a cut with stitches

Processing Questions:

1. What is the difference between a cut, a scratch, and an abrasion?

2. What is the proper technique for cleaning and bandaging a cut?

3. What materials are needed to treat a cut?

STRAINS AND SPRAINS

Valued Outcome: The students will demonstrate the basic knowledge of sprains and strains and what to do if they have one.

Description of Strategy: Begin the class by walking into the room with a splint or air cast on your ankle. Ask the students what they think is wrong with your ankle. Tell them that it is sprained (but not really). Explain to the students how you get a sprain or strain. Sprains are caused when the ligaments that reinforce a joint are stretched or torn. Strains, also called "pulled muscles," occur when a muscle is overstretched or torn by overuse or abuse; the injured muscle may become inflamed, and adjacent joints are usually immobilized. Tell the students what to do if they think they have hurt their ankle: They should not move it and should tell an adult what has happened. They may have to go to the doctor. If you have a sprain or strain, you may have to wear a splint or temporary cast.

Explain to the students that RICE is a mnemonic that stands for Rest, Ice, Compression, and Elevation. Explain to the students why each of these steps is important. Have the students draw and color a picture of them following the RICE method. While they are doing that, call them up individually and have them tell you what RICE stands for.

Materials Needed: a splint or temporary cast, paper and crayons for each student

Processing Questions:

1. What is the difference between a sprain and a strain?
2. What is the proper technique for taking care of the sprain or strain?

BACKPACK SAFETY

Valued Outcome: The students will demonstrate basic knowledge of backpacks and how to use them safely.

Description of Strategy: Begin the class by having the students pack their backpacks as if they would be going home for the day. Walk around to make sure that the students pack everything that they normally take home in their backpack. Ask them if they think that their backpacks are too heavy. Tell the class that a backpack should weigh only 10 percent of their own body weight. Let the class take turns measuring how much they weigh and how much their backpack weighs, and then tell them if their backpack is too heavy. Explain to the students that a heavy backpack can cause your back, shoulders, and neck to ache. The weight can cause damage to the disks that are between the vertebrae in your back and can also do damage to your nervous and circulatory systems. You may have problems for the rest of your life if you do not follow the safety tips for using a backpack.

Tell the students that there are many ways to make sure that their backpacks are safe. They can make sure they get a backpack with two shoulder straps and a waist strap, put the heaviest things closer to their back, and do not carry anything that is not necessary. Backpacks should not be carried over just one shoulder; use both shoulder straps. They could also get a backpack that has wheels or one with a lot of pockets that can spread out the weight. Have the students draw a picture of themselves with their backpack using one of the safety tips. Call the students up while they are working on their picture and have them explain why the improper use of backpacks can be bad for your health.

Materials Needed: a scale, paper and markers for each student

Processing Questions:

1. How can backpacks cause back pain?
2. What are some ways to prevent backaches from backpacks?

SIDEWALK SAFETY   Grades (K–5)

Valued Outcome: The students will be able to identify and choose safe traffic behavior.

Description of Strategy: Set up streets and crosswalks in your classroom using masking tape on the floor. Let the students play the roles of crossing guard, stop sign, and traffic light. You play the roles of car, motorcycle, bicycle, and pedestrian. Use props and costumes to demonstrate safe traffic scenes: the light is turning red, the crossing guard stops traffic, proper direction of traffic movement, approaching a stop sign etc.

Teach students to stop, look, and listen when they are going to cross a road. They should look left, right, and then left again for oncoming vehicles. If the roadway is clear, then they should walk quickly (not run) straight across the road, using crosswalks if they are available. Remind them to cross streets with an older sibling or adult if possible, since younger children do not have the necessary experience or sufficiently developed nervous systems to correctly estimate vehicle distance and speed.

Materials Needed: masking tape, crossing-guard sash, hand-held stop sign, traffic light prop (a box with two sides showing a green light and two sides showing a red light)

Processing Questions:

1. Where should you walk if you are a pedestrian in this situation?
2. What would be the safe thing to do if you were driving a car in this situation?
3. Why is it safer to walk in the direction that is opposite to that of the traffic on your side of the road?

SOURCE: WGBH Play and Learn with Arthur 2003

PERSONAL SAFETY IN THE COMMUNITY—
ROLE-PLAY   Grades (K–3)

Valued Outcome: The students will be able to demonstrate ways they can protect their personal safety at home, at school, and in recreational areas such as the park or play area.

Description of Strategy: Set up the classroom to represent a community with the school, a home, a park, and a sidewalk/road area. Use two to four chairs as a car and one chair as a bicycle. Have students find a seat in the section designated as the school, while you discuss the importance of personal safety. Pick students out of the class, and have them help you illustrate certain points such as walking with a partner rather than alone to the park or from home. Ask students to volunteer telling why a situation would or would not be risky.

After you have covered the main points of personal safety, have each class member draw a card out of a box. Each card contains the student's location in the community and a role to play, such as teacher located in the classroom at the school. Each geographic area of the community works together to present a skit to the class of one safe behavior and one unsafe behavior in their assigned area. After each skit is complete, ask the students to volunteer ideas for other things they could have done as a skit. If time allows, the students can draw a new card and act out some of the skits suggested during discussion.

Materials Needed: cards listing various role-play situations, a box, chairs, barriers to section off classroom, signs identifying the sections of the "community," sheets of paper taped to the floor to identify sidewalk, masking tape

Processing Questions:

1. What are some ways you can protect yourself while at school?

2. What are some ways you can protect yourself while playing outside?

3. Why is it better to walk with a partner rather than alone outside of school?

SOURCE: yoursafety.ca 2003; University of Northern Iowa 2003

BIKE SAFETY   Grades (K–5)

Valued Outcome: The students will practice correct bicycle safety, identify correct and incorrect bicycle safety, and identify road signs/signals.

Description of Strategy: As a class, discuss the different road signs (such as stop and yield signs). Demonstrate safety signals while riding a bicycle, and have students imitate them. Have students divide into groups and give them a skit cue card that will instruct them on which safety signal they should give, which response they should make to a road sign, and whether it should be performed correctly or incorrectly, (e.g., incorrect left turn). Ask the group to demonstrate putting on helmets, getting on their "bikes," and demonstrate what the cue card says. Have each group honk a bicycle horn to get a turn to guess what the group's role-play was. The group that wins goes next. This continues until everyone has gone or all the cue cards are demonstrated.

Materials Needed: examples of road signs, five bicycle horns (as buzzers), helmets (optional), skit cue cards, chairs to represent bicycles

Processing Questions:

1. What do the different road signs mean?

2. What are some correct and some incorrect bicycle techniques?

3. Why is it important to wear bicycle helmets?

SOURCES: Tennessee Department of Safety 2003; University of Oklahoma Police Department 2003

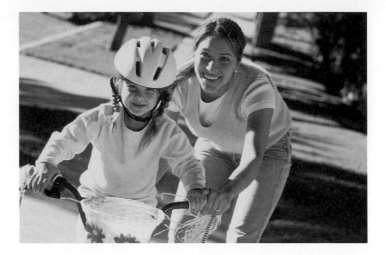

Learning to be safe while riding a bicycle can prevent many accidents.

FIRE SAFETY AT HOME   Grades (K–5)

Valued Outcome: The students will be able to evaluate a situation involving fire and smoke and decide the best way to exit a building.

Description of Strategy: Have the students discuss what they already know to do when a fire happens in school and at home. Most students only practice the school drill twice a year and never at home, so it will be important to go through the school procedure before the actual drill occurs so that they know what to do. Have the students help you make a fire plan using a school map and procedures just for your classroom. After the discussion and plans are made, have students quietly practice entering and exiting the building. When outside, find your special spot to meet and tell the students as they walk outside to make a chain and do not let go until all are in the meeting spot and class roll has been taken. Practice this several times until the students feel comfortable.

After the students have practiced entering and exiting the building, have them help you set up two houses (a one story and a two story) in the classroom. Assign some students to the houses and others to the audience. The students will describe their plan for escape from their home and then demonstrate it for the audience. If the students want, they can set up special situations such as fire in the hallway on the first floor or other obstacles. Once each group has practiced escaping out of the homes, ask the students to practice stop, drop, and rolling in the event their hair or clothing catches on fire.

Some points to keep in mind include:

- Using the back of your hand, feel the surface of any closed door you must open during your escape. If the door is hot, find a different way out.

- Toxic gases may be low across the room, and smoke may be up higher. Crouch down or crawl on hands and knees in smoke-filled rooms.

- *Do not hide* inside the building.
- Take the easiest and fastest exit out of a building if it is not blocked. Try the door first (instead of the windows).

Materials Needed: blankets, mats/small pieces of carpet, chairs or sturdy tables to make the homes

Processing Questions:

1. What is the best measure of protection when there is a lot of smoke in the house or classroom?
2. Why is it important to have a special meeting place?
3. Why is it important to have plans at home and at school?

SCHOOL BUS SAFETY   Grades (K–3)

Valued Outcome: The students will be able to identify the danger zones around the school bus and how to safely board and unboard the school bus.

Description of Strategy: As a demonstration, you will get off the bus and look both ways, and then walk three steps or more away from the bus, safely out of the road. Have each student get off the bus following your demonstration; then practice picking them up, making sure they are watching the danger zones. After all the students are on your bus, explain to them what the emergency exit in the back is for and that the bus driver will give them instructions to go out that door; they should not go out without the driver instructing them to do so. Have the students walk with you out to a school bus provided by a local school bus driver. Show the students the danger zones (such as the front of the bus and the back of the bus).

At the end ask for students to partner and show the class at least one element of bus safety (for instance, walking to the bus, walking three steps away from the bus, sitting straight up with feet facing the front of the bus, not leaning out the window or across the aisle to the people across from you, etc).

Materials Needed: school bus

Processing Questions:

1. What are the danger zones around the school bus?
2. Why is it important to look both ways before getting off the school bus and then to walk at least three steps away from the bus?
3. When should you use the emergency exit?
4. What are some examples of proper school bus behavior when the bus is in motion?

SOURCES: National Highway Traffic Safety Administration 2003

BASIC WATER SAFETY/REACHING ASSISTS   Grades (4–5)

Valued Outcome: The students will discuss basic safety rules for swimming pools or lakes and perform various reaching assists to help a distressed swimmer.

Description of Strategy: In preparation, consult your local American Red Cross or swimming pool for additional safety rules and to borrow equipment that may not be available from your school. Have the students tell the safety rules that they already know. Write them on the board or an overhead transparency and explain why each is important and why it should be followed. Go over any safety rules that the students did not mention and why each is important.

Explain what a distressed swimmer is and again emphasize safety rules. Ask the students what they would do if they encountered a distressed swimmer, and emphasize getting help in that situation. Explain reaching assists, and give a demonstration using a shepherd's crook or reaching pole. Ask the students what else could be used for a reaching assist, and then demonstrate the use of arms and legs and any other equipment for reaching assists.

Have the students practice reaching assists in pairs, starting with arms and legs and then using various pieces of equipment. Review reaching assists and safety rules and how they are related. Finish with a summary of the safety rules.

Materials Needed: chalkboard and chalk or overhead projector and pen, masking tape to outline a swimming pool on the floor, shepherd's crook or reaching pole, any other rescue equipment

Processing Questions:

1. Why is it necessary to demonstrate reaching assists?
2. What are some basic water safety rules?
3. How are these two components related?

TOOL SAFETY   Grades (3–5)

Valued Outcome: The students will become familiar with proper tool safety.

Description of Strategy: Bring a variety of tools, appliances, and common implements to class, and discuss the safe use of each. Demonstrate items that are appropriate to your age group. These might include scissors, knives, hand tools, small electrical appliances, gardening equipment, and kitchen equipment.

Materials Needed: hand tools, small kitchen tools, electrical appliances, scissors, knives, gardening tools

Processing Questions:

1. What tools, appliances, and implements do your parents or guardians use around the house and/or yard?
2. What are the possible safety problems that might accompany the use or misuse of these tools?

THE HUG OF LIFE

Valued Outcome: The students will be able to demonstrate the Heimlich maneuver.

Description of Strategy: Have a trained representative from the American Heart Association or American Red Cross demonstrate the proper use of the Heimlich maneuver. Emphasize that this is only a mock demonstration, and be careful not to apply too much pressure.

Materials Needed: none

Processing Questions:

1. How does the Heimlich maneuver work to help a person who is choking?
2. How is this procedure conducted differently for children and adults?

RESUSCITATION ANNIE

Grades (3–5)

Valued Outcome: The students will learn mouth-to-mouth resuscitation.

Description of Strategy: If you have a CPR (cardiopulmonary resuscitation) mannequin available, demonstrate the proper technique for mouth-to-mouth resuscitation. Contact your local chapter of the American Heart Association or American Red Cross for assistance in presenting this demonstration. The students must be heavy enough to do proper chest compressions.

Materials Needed: CPR mannequin

Processing Questions:

1. How does resuscitation help a victim of a breathing problem?
2. Can you perform these procedures?

FIRE EXTINGUISHERS

Grades (3–5)

Valued Outcome: The students will be able to learn the proper techniques of using a fire extinguisher and be able to identify the classes of extinguishers.

Description of Strategy: Show the students how to operate the extinguisher. Identify the different classes of extinguishers. (You may wish to contact your local fire department on current maintenance procedures required for fire extinguishers.)

> **Class A:** used for wood, paper, or textile fires
>
> **Class B:** used for oil, grease, or paint fires
>
> **Class C:** used on electrical equipment

Materials Needed: fire extinguishers from each class

Processing Questions:

1. Does your family have a working fire extinguisher in your home?
2. Do you know how to use the extinguisher?

Puzzles and Games

FIRE SAFETY BINGO   Grades (K–2)

Valued Outcome: The students will be able to identify several fire safety rules.

Description of Strategy: Review fire safety rules. Pass out bingo cards and M&Ms. Explain the rules of the game:

- Questions will be read aloud to students.
- Students must raise their hand in order to answer a question.
- If a student answers a question correctly, he or she will place an M&M on one of the squares on his or her bingo card.
- The game ends when a student has completely filled his or her card and yelled "fire safety"!
- The game can be repeated as many times as time permits.
- Students may eat their M&Ms when the game has ended.
- Added incentives, such as additional computer time, could be added for the winners.

Materials Needed: list of questions and answers dealing with fire safety, bingo cards with nine blank squares and M&Ms for each student

Processing Question: What fire safety rules can you practice in your home?

SOURCE: Governale 2000

RESCUE 911   Grades (K–5)

Valued Outcome: The student will be able to explain how to handle emergency procedures.

Description of Strategy: Begin by asking the students if they know the number to call in an emergency. (Note: dialing 911 will connect the caller with an emergency dispatcher, but the 911 center that takes the call may not be a local center. It is critical for the caller to be prepared to give the full address, including city *and* state, to which the emergency personnel should go. Check what is available in your area.) Discuss when the number should be called (for example, fire, stranger in the home, unconscious person) and why it is important to call 911 in an emergency. Explain that the 911 center will contact the emergency personnel who can assist in the problem (for example, police, firefighters, ambulance). Demonstrate the information that should be given to the 911 dispatcher (name, street address, city, state, type of emergency), then have students practice dialing the telephones (make sure they are not plugged in) and giving their own home information to the "dispatcher."

Tell the students they are going to play a rescue game. They are going to pretend there is a fire, and everyone in the building needs to be rescued. Form two equal teams, and have them sit behind a restraining line. Have them imagine they are in a burning house. Each team has two or three rescuers who each have a carpet square. The rescuers are standing on the fire safe spot—an area marked off by you. On command—Rescue 911—the rescuers run to the burning house and rescue each person one by one. Rescuers may need to work in teams to remove larger students. The rescuer must pull the victim to safety, but do not allow students to recklessly pull too hard on the limbs of other students. *Make sure you review proper ways to move individuals and emphasize that a safe rescue is what is important.* "Victims" must remain sitting or kneeling on the carpet square through the entire rescue. This continues until everyone on the team is rescued. Tell students not to worry about which team wins. The true fun is getting your turn to rescue.

Materials Needed: push-button and/or rotary style telephones (optional)

Processing Questions:

1. What is an appropriate situation in which to call 911? What are some inappropriate situations?

2. Why is it helpful to post the full address in a visible location near each telephone in the building?

SOURCE: P. E. Central 2000c

SAFE ROUTE HOME   Grades (K–5)

Valued Outcome: The students will be able to determine the safest route home from school.

Description of Strategy: Have students map out a safe route to their home from their school. The students should have their parents or guardians provide input to help chart the safest route. Ask them to identify an alternative route to use in the event of a problem with the safest route.

Materials Needed: pencils and paper for each student

Processing Questions:

1. How do you travel from school to home?

2. If you walk or ride your bicycle, do you have a safe route planned?

3. If you walk from the school bus stop to your home, do you have a safe route planned?

Other Ideas

TRAFFIC SAFETY OBSTACLE COURSE   Grades (K–5)

Valued Outcome: The students will learn the importance of traffic signs.

Description of Strategy: Set up a simulated obstacle course on the playground (or in a parking area that has been blocked off to traffic) illustrating such traffic hazards as busy intersections, unmarked intersections, and so on. Mark each potentially hazardous part of the course with traffic safety signs, including speed limit signs, yield signs, and pedestrian signals. Have some students wear appropriate bicycle safety gear and go through the course on bicycles, while others play the part of pedestrians. (You may wish to review bicycle safety rules at this time. If bicycle helmets are to be shared, provide plastic liners for the helmets.) Discuss the importance of following traffic safety signs, signals, and regulations.

Materials Needed: poster board, markers, scissors, construction paper, bicycles and bicycle safety gear, plastic sheets or bags to line bicycle helmets that will be shared

Processing Questions:

1. Why is it important to practice negotiating traffic obstacles?
2. What dangerous activities by students cause accidents in traffic situations?
3. How can you help eliminate some of these dangerous activities?
4. How do traffic signs prevent accidents?

FIELD TRIPS   Grades (K–5)

Valued Outcome: The students will be able to inspect a fire station or other safety-related agency or equipment and learn how it operates.

Description of Strategy: If feasible, take the class on a field trip to the local fire station or other safety agency outlet (ambulance or police car might visit the school, etc.). Prepare the class thoroughly for what they will see, and have them write down a list of questions they wish to ask those in charge.

Materials Needed: pencils and paper for each student

Processing Questions:

1. What items are available to help deal with specific emergencies?
2. How does each safety agency help the public prevent accidents?

Resources

BOOKS

Bourgeois, P., and B. Clark. 2000. *Franklin's bicycle helmet.* Scholastic: Canada.

Chaiet, D., and F. Russell. 1998. *The safe zone: A kid's guide to personal safety.* New York: Morrow Junior Books.

WEB SITES

General Health

American Cancer Society: *www.cancer.org*

American Medical Association:
Adolescent Health Links
www.ama-assn.org/ama/pub.category/1979.html

Bike police: *www.ou.edu/oupd/bikesafe.htm*

CDC Prevention Guidelines Database
http://wonder.cdc.gov/wonder/prevguid/prevguid.htm

ERIC Clearinghouse on Information & Technology, Syracuse University
http://askeric.org/cgi-bin/printlesson.cgi/Virtual/Lessons/Health/Safety/SFY0016.html

The Life Education Network: *www.lec.org*

National Program for Playground Safety
www.uni.edu/playground/home.html

Tennessee Department of Safety: Bus Safety
www.nhtsa.dot.gov/kids/bussafety/index.htm

Tennessee Department of Safety: Tennessee Driver License Handbook and Study Guide
www.state.tn.us/safety/cntents/html

Educational and Community-Based Programs

Washington State Department of Health, Office of Minority Health Resource Center: *www.doh.wa.gov*

Occupational Safety and Health

American Industrial Hygiene Association
www.aiha.org

CDC National Institute for Occupational Safety and Health: *www.cdc.gov/niosh/homepage.html*

CDC Scientific, Surveillance, and Health Statistics, and Laboratory Information
www.cdc.gov/scientific.htm

CDC WONDER: *wonder.cdc.gov*

DOL Mine Safety and Health Administration
www.msha.gov

Occupational Safety and Health Administration
www.osha.gov

U.S. Department of Labor: *www.dol.gov*

Safety and Accident Prevention

American Academy of Orthopaedic Surgeons, Prevention of Injuries
www.aaos.org/wordhtml/press/prevent.htm

Consumer Product Safety Commission
www.cpsc.gov

Driver's Support: *www.veta.se*

National Highway Transportation Safety Administration: *www.nhtsa.dot.gov*

National Program for Playground Safety:
www.uni.edi/playground/home.html

National Safety Council: *www.nsc.org*

Travelers' Safety
werple.mira.net.au/%7Ewreid/bali_p2h.html

U.S. Fire Administration: *www.usfa.fema.gov*

Safety and Violence Prevention

Public Broadcasting Station
http://pbskids.org/arthur/grownups/activities/play_learn/sidewalk_safety.html

ChildFun, Inc.: Child Fun Family Web Site
http://childfun.com/themes/safety.shtml

Violent and Abusive Behavior

CDC National Center for the Injury Prevention and Control: *www.cdc.gov/ncipc/ncipchm.htm*

Hawaii: *www.hawaii.gov/health/index.html*

Massachusetts
www.magnet.state.ma.us/dph/dphhome.htm

Pavnet Online: *www.pavnet.org*

General Sites

American Medical Association: *www.ama-assn.org*

MedicineNet: *www.medicinenet.com*

Medscape: *www.medscape.com*

Oncolink: *www.oncolink.upenn.edu*

ParentsPlace.com: *www.parentsplace.com*

Links Only

Hardin Meta Directory of Internet Health Sources
www.arcade.uiowa.edu/hardinwww/md.html

VIDEOS

Real people: Violence in the family
Designed to offer understanding and real help to teens who live in the estimated one out of four families in which violence occurs. Interweaving

continued

first-person accounts by teens who grew up in violent homes, dramatic stories, and interviews with experts, program helps viewers learn coping skills and distinguish between what is normal family life and what is not. Available from Sunburst Communications, 101 Castleton Street, P.O. Box 40, Pleasantville, NY 10570. (33 minutes, Item 2642)

Resolving conflicts

Provides an introduction to conflict resolution by demonstrating essential techniques. Shows students that when they express themselves clearly and listen carefully, they improve their ability to solve problems, are able to take greater responsibility for themselves, and get better at getting along in and out of school. Available from Sunburst Communications, 101 Castleton Street, P.O. Box 40, Pleasantville, NY 10570. (24 minutes, Item 2488)

Student workshop: Solving conflicts

Designed as a hands-on workshop in conflict resolution skills. Minidramas raise problems students will recognize from their own lives, giving them practical help with their school, peer, and home relationships. Available from Sunburst Communications, 101 Castleton Street, P.O. Box 40, Pleasantville, NY 10570. (26 minutes, Item 2448)

Student workshop: What to do about anger

Designed as a hands-on workshop in anger management skills to help children get along better with friends, family, and authority figures. Program teaches students the difference between angry feelings and angry behavior; how to handle anger by controlling how they act; and how to deal with angry energy in safe, positive ways. Available from Sunburst Communications, 101 Castleton Street, P.O. Box 40, Pleasantville, NY 10570. (34 minutes, Item 2628)

Threat of a gang fight

Introduces three eighth-grade girls who were in the middle of peer mediation when one started calling the other names and threatening a fight. The argument escalated but was short-lived. Each side of the story was told and evaluated, and the girls settled their disputes. The mediators, however, felt that a follow-up will be necessary in the future. Available from Aquarius Productions, Inc., 5 Powderhouse Lane, P.O. Box 1159, Sherborn, MA 01770.

Understanding Violence

Describes violence in children and the atmosphere in which they grow up. Clearly points out that exposure to violence is detrimental to a child's mental health and explores the role of media in children's perception of violence. Explains the importance of teaching children social skills, conflict resolution through peer mediation, and the use of energy in a constructive way. Available from Films for the Humanities & Sciences: P.O. Box 2053, Princeton, NJ 08543-2053. (27 minutes, Item BVL5996)

What can we do about violence:
Part 1: Juveniles locked up

Features Bill Moyers and emphasizes the importance of early intervention. Based on a California juvenile system, the video examines and interviews several men and women ages thirteen to twenty-four who describe their disturbing life experiences (including abuse as children and lack of family support) and how they turned to gangs and violence. Available from Films for the Humanities & Sciences: P.O. Box 2053, Princeton, NJ 08543-2053. (56 minutes, Item BVL5483)

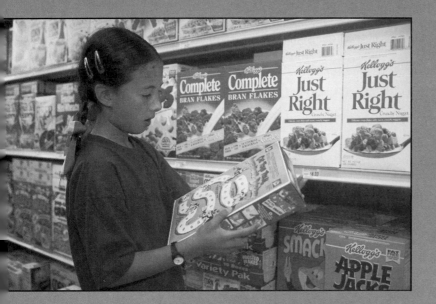

CHAPTER TWENTY-ONE

Consumer Health

The most violent element in
society is ignorance.

—Emma Goldman

VALUED OUTCOMES

After reading this chapter, you should be able to:

- analyze the role of advertising in consumer purchases
- list various advertising approaches
- discuss how quackery affects health care
- state criteria for selecting a health care professional
- state criteria for selecting a health care facility
- list the rights of the consumer
- discuss private and governmental agencies that help protect the consumer

Over the past decade people have become increasingly concerned about their quality of health care. Health consumers are asking questions of their health care providers, seeking second opinions, and sometimes choosing to forgo treatments. As you reflect upon this chapter, see if you can identify several guidelines or principles that health care consumers might keep in mind when selecting products or services.

A Nation of Consumers

We are all consumers. A consumer is anyone who selects and uses products to fulfill personal needs and desires. Consumer products range from the clothes we wear, to the foods we eat, to the over-the-counter (OTC) drugs we buy for self-medication. Consumer services include those provided by physicians, dentists, and other medical professionals. In this chapter, we examine the area of **consumer health,** which is defined as the intelligent purchase and use of products and services that will directly affect one's health. At first, this may seem only a small percentage of consumer goods and services, but in fact many more are health related than may be supposed. For example, buying a car may not seem to be a health-related matter, but it is, at least in part. One car might be safer than another vehicle because it is equipped with dual airbags, antilock brakes, and side-impact protection that are not in the other model.

This chapter cannot discuss all aspects of consumer health, only the more directly health-related issues. We also look at consumer psychology and how various forces attempt to manipulate consumer attitudes and behavior. In addition, we discuss consumer rights, consumer-oriented legislation and government agencies, and the role of the teacher in consumer health education. Some of the information may seem to be very adult oriented, but if children are going to be wise consumers as adults, the process must begin in the elementary school years.

Advertising and Consumer Behavior

Everyone has consumer needs and desires. From childhood, we are barraged with advertising that attempts to foster these needs and desires so that one blurs into the other. A need becomes a desire, and a desire is perceived as a need. Our economic system is built on supply and demand, and producers do all that they can to nurture a growing demand.

This manipulation of consumer psychology and behavior begins in early childhood, often by means of Saturday morning television commercials aimed specifically at young children. Typical products promoted are toys, candy, and breakfast cereals. As children grow older, the products change, but the message is still one of persuasion. In fact, the methods used to advertise the products are quite sophisticated. By law, advertising of any kind may not be false or misleading. The advertising agencies do an excellent job of stimulating desire and creating a belief about need.

Businesses spend billions of dollars each year on advertising; more money is spent on advertising health products than on any other category of items. Prescription drug manufacturers now spend more than $1 billion per year to advertise in magazines, newspapers, and on television. This is in addition to the several billion dollars spent each year promoting prescription drugs to physicians (Barrett, Jarvis, Kroger, and London 2002). A great deal of psychological research goes into advertising so that the target group—whether children, teenagers, homemakers, young adults, or older adults—can be effectively reached. The entire point of this endeavor is to get consumers to buy a particular product or engage in a specific activity. Advertising seeks not to inform, but to persuade.

There are dozens of different brands of products from which to choose. In many ways, the U.S. consumer is fortunate to have so many choices. Competition for the consumer dollar also stimulates the development of better and more efficient products and services. Consider the level of quality that would be available if only one brand of each type of product or service were offered. By providing us with so much choice, however, our economic system also makes it more difficult to make informed decisions about purchases. Many of the products on the market are virtually indistinguishable from one another as far as quality and effectiveness are concerned. Price may be the only difference, and even that may not be much of a factor. For example, all brands of aspirin are basically the same in quality and effectiveness, regardless of advertising claims to the contrary (Cornacchia and Barrett 1993).

Because the purpose of advertising is to persuade, most advertising contains little informational content. Even that which appears to be informational is carefully selected so that the product being advertised will appear to be uniquely better in some way. Certainly, no manufacturer could be expected to state, "Our product is no different from our competitors' products, but please buy ours anyway."

Advertising Approaches

Advertising is a sophisticated kind of manipulation. Advertising experts understand that, despite the lack of information conveyed about the actual merits of a product, consumers can be convinced that one particular brand should be sought out from among the dozens of very similar products on the market. The reason for this is that advertising seeks to appeal to the irrational, not the rational, aspects of human psychology. By making a particular product sound more appealing, *for any reason,* an advertiser can increase the market share of the

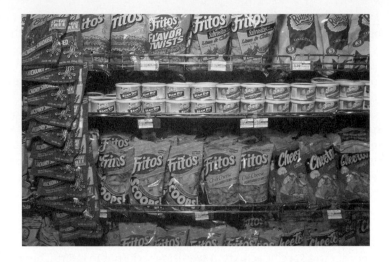

Packages and advertisements can be powerful stimuli. Students should be made aware of this.

product. This can be done in a variety of ways, almost all of them noninformational in nature. It is important to remember that the same appeals are used on children as on adults. Table 21.1 contains some of the most common advertising techniques.

Many advertisers combine the approaches mentioned in Table 21.1 with visual and/or emotional imagery. Whether in a magazine advertisement or television commercial, the visual aspects of the advertisement are just as important as the written or spoken message. If the visual message of the commercial is pleasant, the reader or viewer will more likely associate positive thoughts with the product. Students should be made aware of the powerful stimuli provided by advertisements. Consumers must learn to recognize that there is a great deal of puffery in almost any commercial or advertisement, regardless of the approach used to convey the message. Often there is little difference in effectiveness between one health product and another, and price is not a big factor either. We are all manipulated by advertising, and even if a person actually feels better about using one product over another, usually there is no difference in health consequences whether Brand X or Brand Y is selected. For children and adults, what is important to their consumer health is to develop an understanding of how advertising seeks to manipulate them so that when more serious health problems arise, they will not be deceived by advertising claims. Perhaps most important, the limited effectiveness of all OTC drugs and self-medication must be recognized.

Table 21.1   Common Advertising Techniques

Techniques	Appeals	Questions to Ask
bandwagon	Typical phrases: *everyone uses, nation's leading, used by millions, preferred by most, used for more than twenty years*	Is it really true? Who says?
costs	cost-effective, costs less than competition	Is the cost really less? What is the quality?
effectiveness	Typical phrases: *most effective, relieves pain, relieves itch, protects, easy to use*	What is the evidence? How long is it effective? Does it really work?
endorsements/testimonials	use of actors, athletes, dentists, physicians to promote	What are their qualifications to endorse the product?
scientific appeal	use of phrases such as *many doctors recommend* or *hospital tested*	Is the information accurate? What evidence? Where did the information come from?
slogans/humor	humorous lyrics, cartoon characters, phrases such as *Morning Mouth*	Does the product really work?
snob appeal/superiority	famous person or use of phrases such as *people who know*. Use of words *long-lasting, natural, extra strength*. Contains some ingredient from Europe, etc.	Does the person really know? What is the real implication of the words used? Does it work as claimed?
social	makes you more attractive, smell better, more socially acceptable	Does the product really work?

Other Influences on Product and Service Choices

Consumer decisions are influenced not only by advertising, but also by an individual's level of education, family beliefs, religion, socioeconomic status, community, and personal goals. A host of other factors may be involved, including one's physical and emotional needs, motives, and personality (Corry 1983). People may model their buying patterns and selections after those of family members, friends, or peers. The more status or importance that the person being modeled has, the greater his or her influence.

With all these influences, it might seem that a person can hardly be blamed for sometimes making poor choices about consumer health products and services. But this denies personal responsibility. Not everything can be blamed on advertising or outside influences—people often make harmful health decisions quite independently of either. They may use advertising claims to shore up these decisions, for example, by relying on OTC products in an attempt to cure ill health when they actually know that they should be seeking more effective medical treatment. Such individuals are only too willing to create a false sense of security or relief by accepting advertising claims uncritically or by enlarging on such claims themselves in order to find easy answers where no such answers exist. In the final analysis, consumers can make informed choices if they want to do so. As with other aspects of wellness, each individual must accept self-responsibility. Consumers can then seek out information on products and services, analyze each on its own merits, and make better decisions accordingly.

Consumer Myths and Misconceptions

Some consumer health myths might be classified as folk beliefs. Although not based on any scientific facts, many of these myths are widely believed. In some instances, belief in certain of these myths can lead to unwise consumer health decisions. For example, a belief that so-called organic or natural foods are somehow better than regular produce available in stores can lead to wasteful spending on overpriced specialty products. Some consumer health myths are believed because the person is desperate for relief. Sufferers of arthritis, which is an incurable condition at present, may wear a copper bracelet in the hope that perhaps the myth about the curative properties of copper really has some truth to it. They may also spend money on mud baths or other worthless forms of supposed therapy. Since some of these treatments do provide relaxation, leading to a feeling of temporary relief, they are not entirely without value. But consumers who place their faith in them are deluding themselves as to long-term benefits.

Consumer misconceptions also lead to wasteful spending and, occasionally, to actual harm to health status. Perhaps the most common misconception is that producers manufacture only products that are needed; therefore, if a product is on the market, it must be fulfilling a need. In fact, many products are marketed to create a need that does not actually exist. For example, many mouthwashes, tonics, and other nostrums provide few health benefits. However, most consumers believe that any product that continues to be sold must be meeting a real need. Constant advertising reinforces this misconception through sheer repetition. Even the better educated are often ignorant about consumer health information and hold many misconceptions. For example, when college students were surveyed concerning their knowledge of health care, only 49 percent responded correctly to a series of questions on the subject. Of this same group, 42 percent believed that health articles printed in popular magazines were always checked for scientific accuracy before publication.

Clearly, consumers must become better informed if they are to make wise consumer health decisions. They must recognize the negative impact that myths and misconceptions can have on personal health. They must also become more aware of how advertising seeks to manipulate consumer behavior and learn to reject appeals to emotion in favor of facts and accurate information. Obtaining factual information about health products and services is not always easy. By law, advertisers must tell the truth about their products, prove the claims they make, be specific about any guarantee or warranty, and avoid making misleading statements. In addition, the advertising code subscribed to by most business advertisers puts forth similar guidelines. However, most products are still made to sound more effective than they really are. It is ultimately the consumer's responsibility to see through this misleading advertising and make wise decisions accordingly. To accomplish this, children and adults must strive to become intelligent health consumers. Cornacchia and Barrett (1993, 10–11) offer six guidelines for intelligent consumers:

1. The intelligent consumer is well informed and knows how to make sound decisions.

2. The intelligent consumer seeks reliable sources of information.

3. The intelligent consumer is appropriately skeptical about health information and does not accept statements appearing in the news media or advertising at face value.

4. The intelligent consumer is wary of inept practitioners, pseudopractitioners, and pitchmen in the business and medical worlds and can identify quacks and quackery.

5. The intelligent consumer selects practitioners with great care and questions fees, diagnoses, treatments, and alternative treatments.

6. The intelligent consumer willingly speaks out by reporting frauds, quackery, and wrongdoing to appropriate agencies and law enforcement officials.

Quackery

There are many models of medical treatment. Some of them are valid and time tested; some are new and their advocates are working to gain acceptance. Others, however, do not seek scientific validation and, in fact, avoid scientific inquiry. The first category of medical models includes conventional medicine practiced by physicians who are licensed and certified in their fields. The second category includes such approaches to health care as biofeedback and holistic health, which may be of value in treating certain health conditions. The third category is quackery, the use of worthless approaches that often promise miraculous results.

Quacks usually try very hard to appear scientific. Their offices may closely resemble conventional physicians' offices, even to the framed degrees (but often from diploma mills) on the walls. They may dress as physicians, in a white laboratory coat or with a stethoscope around their neck, employ scientific-looking gadgets, and use scientific-sounding language to explain their supposed treatments. But it is all a sham, and a quack will always find an excuse for not permitting the form of quackery to be subject to independent scientific scrutiny.

Although some quacks may sincerely believe in the efficacy of their treatments, most are simply out to victimize the consumer to make money.

Quackery flourishes in the United States for a variety of reasons. The primary reason is ignorance. Many Americans do not know the difference between legitimate and illegitimate medical practitioners. Anyone who claims to be a doctor or a healer is taken at face value. Another reason quackery exists is that quacks often promise cures or relief that legitimate medical practitioners cannot offer. For those suffering from incurable diseases, the false hope that quacks hold out may seem irresistible. Since nothing else can help them, they turn to quacks in desperation. People also sometimes consult quacks because they hope to get around the high cost of legitimate medical attention; the quack promises a quick and inexpensive cure. In other instances, people turn to quacks because they wish to avoid surgery or other involved legitimate medical treatment. Some individuals may not realize the difference between scientifically proven methodologies and legitimately trained professionals versus those who are trained in treatments that are outside this body of knowledge. Still, of course, many people actually believe the deceptive claims made by quacks (Payne and Hahn 2002).

If quacks cannot effect cures, why do so many people continue to have faith in them? In some instances, quacks do seem to provide relief or cures. In such cases, the patient may be a hypochondriac with no actual physical problem. If the person believes that help is being provided, the problem disappears. In cases where an actual problem does exist, the natural healing powers of the body may be responsible for a cure attributed to a quack. Finally, temporary relief or remission may be mistaken for a cure.

Not only is the consumer's pocketbook shortchanged in quackery treatments, medications, and devices, but people's health can be undermined. Quackery delays proper treatment and increases the possibility of a more serious outcome. Using good sense and seeking information from physicians or some reputable agency is a good start to finding proper information (Greenberg and Dintiman 1992, 491). Some nonprofit agencies that may be able to help provide reliable information and referrals include the Consumer's Union, American Cancer Society, Arthritis Foundation, American Heart Association, American Lung Association, American Medical Association, American Dental Association, and the Better Business Bureau.

Health Care

The U.S. health care delivery system continues to evolve. Rising medical care costs, as well as the ever-increasing number of uninsured or underinsured individuals, are significant factors contributing to many of the proposed changes. The reasons for increasing health care costs include current reimbursement practices, increasing technology, and rising physicians' fees and other health care salaries (which are in part due to increasing litigation and litigation insurance costs). Another factor in high health care costs, particularly in hospitals, is the cost of care for the poor, uninsured, and underinsured. The poor and the elderly are the ones who suffer most from the current health care delivery system. Government programs such as Medicare and Medicaid help, but for many individuals the portion of the bills not paid by these programs is still financially overwhelming.

The vast majority of Americans cannot afford the costs of medical care without some form of health insurance. Health insurance is a contract between an insurance company and either an individual or a group for the payment of medical costs. Health insurance usually requires the individual or group to pay a premium to the insurance company each month. The insurance company then pays for all or part of the health care costs, depending on the type of coverage provided.

MEDICAL INSURANCE

As fees for medical and health care services continue to climb, it is more important than ever to have adequate medical insurance. A typical plan may pay 80 percent of medical costs, with the individual responsible for the remaining 20 percent. Premiums for this coverage are paid by employer contributions and employee pay deductions. Group insurance plans typically have a deductible that the insured is responsible for paying before costs are covered by the insurance company.

Basic health insurance includes benefits for hospital, surgical, and medical expenses. Some plans will include provisions for dental and vision coverage. The extent of benefits differs from contract to contract. Individual employees (self-employed) may purchase insurance that covers these areas, but today most workers are covered by a group plan at their place of employment.

In addition, most insurance plans will offer what is called comprehensive coverage that is designed to offset large medical expenses resulting from serious illness or injury. These programs are designed to take over where basic insurance plans stop coverage. Comprehensive insurance coverage usually covers every type of medical situation prescribed by a physician for both in and out of the hospital. Examples of potential services covered include office visits, nursing care, physical therapy, emergency ambulance service, prescription drugs, prosthetic appliances, and psychiatric care.

GOVERNMENT HEALTH INSURANCE

Two examples of government insurance plans are **Medicare** and **Medicaid**. Medicare is financed by Social Security taxes and is designed to provide health insurance for people sixty-five years and older, the blind, severely disabled, and those requiring specialized treatments such as kidney dialysis. Medicaid is underwritten by federal and state taxes. It provides limited health benefits for people who are eligible for assistance from two programs: Aid to Families with Dependent Children and Supplementary Security Income.

Health Maintenance Organization. A health maintenance organization (HMO) is a health plan that contracts with providers for prepaid, comprehensive care for its members. Members are required to obtain care from providers within the HMO. Different models for HMOs include the group model, the individual practice association (IPA) model, the network, and the staff model.

- *Group model*—an HMO in which the organization contracts with provider group practices
- *IPA model*—a type of HMO in which the organization contracts for services with a variety of providers from both individual (solo) and group practices
- *Network model*—an HMO in which the organization contracts with a provider network providing multispeciality care at varied locations
- *Staff model*—an HMO that directly hires its own providers and pays them on salary, rather than on a dynamic scale influenced by the number of patients they see or procedures they perform

Preferred Provider Organization. Preferred provider organizations (PPOs) are fee-for-service plans. The PPOs contract with a group of providers who agree to negotiated fees for services. These fees are usually 15 to 29 percent lower than standard fees. Clients/patients can use services from any provider they wish but will pay a higher percentage of the cost if they use a non-PPO provider. The plan usually includes a deductible paid by consumers before they are eligible for benefits. The main advantages of this model are that a referral is not required and there are more physicians from which to choose.

Point of Service. A point of service (POS) plan is an insurance plan in which subscribers use approved providers who have agreed to accept fixed copayments. The primary care physician is the coordinator of the system by referring patients to a specialist if deemed necessary. This form of health insurance option provides comprehensive care coverage and permits smaller deductibles in cases of accident or unexpected illnesses.

WHEN TO SEEK HEALTH CARE

Sometimes it is difficult to determine when to seek health care attention. Some people tend to wait too long before seeking health care, while others may seek help unnecessarily. For many, the ability to tolerate discomfort determines whether or not they seek help. Health care decisions are largely personal and based on the perceived severity of the symptoms. Being in tune with one's body and having knowledge of the signs and symptoms of illness can help someone make the decision to seek or wait to get medical attention.

Several symptoms indicate the need for medical attention. Blood present in urine, feces, vomit, sputum, or other body fluids indicates the need for medical advice. Pain in the abdomen, especially when accompanied by nausea, may indicate a wide range of conditions, ranging from appendicitis to pelvic inflammatory disease—all of which need a physician's attention. A stiff neck

Health Highlight

RESPONSIBILITIES OF THE HEALTH CARE CONSUMER

- To identify the qualities one wants in a health care provider and one's individual philosophy and goals regarding health; then to choose a provider based on these factors.
- To utilize health care resources appropriately and in a responsible manner. This includes becoming familiar with one's own insurance coverage, including the benefits and limitations of coverage.
- To schedule appointments in advance, informing the receptionist if the provider needs to address more than one health care problem. Acute problems are often accommodated with an appointment either the same day the client calls or the following day. One should even call before going to the provider's office when emergencies arise, because the provider may prefer to have the client seen in the emergency room at a hospital.
- To check into the health care setting on time or before the appointment time. If unable to keep an appointment, call to cancel or reschedule.

- To utilize time with the provider efficiently by being an accurate historian regarding the concern being addressed, past medical and family medical information, and any medications taken currently or in the past.
- To participate in decisions regarding care, openly expressing any concerns or questions.
- To comply with care agreed upon with the provider, including instructions for medications or other treatment prescribed for home, and follow-up appointments/phone calls.
- To address continued concerns (those not resolved in discussions with the provider) formally with the medical director or administrative manager of the facility.
- To choose and maintain a primary care provider with whom one is willing to openly address personal health care issues.
- To ultimately accept responsibility for lifestyle choices and habits that may impact one's health status.

SOURCE: Health with WebMD 2000

accompanied by fever may indicate meningitis, which may be lethal if left unattended. And obviously, any disabling injury requires prompt medical assistance (Anspaugh, Hamrick, and Rosato 2002).

Presence of fever is another area of concern when someone is deciding to seek medical care. A fever is an indication that the immune system is working to fight an infection. If left untreated, a fever may damage various body organs and structures. Self-treatment in the form of aspirin, acetaminophen, or ibuprofen usually lowers temperature. However, if there is no improvement in twenty-four to thirty-six hours, or if a low-grade temperature continues over an extended period, a physician should be consulted. Fever in children should always be discussed with a physician.

SELECTING A HEALTH CARE PROFESSIONAL

Nearly everyone should have a primary-care physician. If a medical emergency arises, a person can seek help immediately from a trusted health care professional who knows the patient's history. Just as important, by having a personal physician or other health care professional, a person can better maintain good health by means of regular checkups or consultations with the provider about

Health Highlight

HEALTH CARE SPECIALISTS

Name of Specialist	Field of Specialty
Medical Specialists	
Allergist	Allergic conditions
Anesthesiologist	Administration of anesthesia (for example, in surgery)
Cardiologist	Coronary artery disease; heart disease
Dermatologist	Skin conditions
Endocrinologist	Diseases of the endocrine system
Epidemiologist	Investigates the cause and source of disease outbreaks
Family practice physician	General care physician
Gastroenterologist	Stomach, intestines, digestive system
Geriatrician	Diseases and conditions of the aged
Gynecologist	Female reproductive system
Hematologist	Study of blood
Immunologist	Diseases of the immune system
Internist	Treatment of diseases in adults
Neonatologist	Newborn infants
Nephrologist	Kidney disease
Neurologist	Nervous system
Neurosurgeon	Surgery of the brain and nervous system
Obstetrician	Pregnancy, labor, childbirth
Oncologist	Cancer, tumors
Ophthalmologist	Eye disease and treatment
Orthopedist	Skeletal system
Otolaryngologist	Head, neck, ears, nose, throat
Otologist	Ears

health concerns. A health care professional should be selected carefully. Some suggestions for doing so are listed here.

1. Choose your physician while you are in good health. If you wait until a medical crisis arises, you will have to rely on whomever you can find. Having a physician you trust and feel comfortable with *before* a crisis will lessen anxiety in a crisis.

2. To locate physicians who are accepting new patients, telephone the local county medical society. (You can find the number in the telephone book yellow pages.) If you are not sure what kind of physician you need, such as a specialist or a general practitioner, the medical society can also offer some initial advice. Generally you will be given the

Name of Specialist	Field of Specialty
Pathologist	Study of tissues and the essential nature of disease
Pediatrician	Childhood diseases and conditions
Plastic surgeon	Use of material to rebuild tissues
Primary-care physician	General health and medical care
Proctologist	Disorders of the rectum and anus
Psychiatrist	Mental illnesses
Radiologist	Use of X rays
Rheumatologist	Diseases of connective tissues, joints, muscles, tendons, and so on
Rhinologist	Nose
Surgeon	Treats diseases by surgery
Urologist	Urinary tract of males and females and reproductive organs of males

Dental Specialists

Dentist	General care of teeth and oral cavity
Endodontist	Diseases of tooth below gum line (performs root canal therapy)
Orthodontist	Teeth alignment, malocclusion
Pedodontist	Dental care of children
Periodontist	Diseases of supporting structures
Prosthodontist	Construction of artificial appliances for the mouth

Other Specialists

Chiropractor	Emphasizes the use of manipulation and adjustment of body structures to treat disease
Naturopathic physician	Emphasizes lifestyle and dietary therapies in the prevention and treatment of disease
Optometrist	Examines and tests eyes for visual defects and prescribes vision correction lenses
Osteopath	Emphasizes structural integrity of the body; uses manipulation along with medical therapies
Podiatrist	Care and treatment of the foot
Psychologist	Study of human behavior

names of two or three physicians you can call. A local hospital can also be a good source of information about physicians who are accepting new patients.

3. Select a board-certified family practitioner for a family physician, a pediatrician for children, and a gynecologist for females (see the Health Highlight box above for other types of specialists).

4. Check the credentials of physicians you are considering. Don't be afraid to ask questions about how the person is keeping current in the field.

5. Get details about office hours, emergency care, whether house calls will be made, and so forth. Also try to determine how long a patient usually has to wait before seeing the doctor.

6. Determine the fee schedule for checkups and different types of treat-ment. Doctors often base their fees on recommended prices recorded in a fee schedule book produced by the American Medical Association. The fees are recommended ranges, not fixed prices, and a physician may charge on the high or low end. Keep in mind that the most expensive physician is not necessarily the best.

7. Choose a physician who is able to communicate with you in terms you can understand. You have a right to know what is going on during any treatment, and the doctor has an obligation to keep you informed. Re-gardless of their medical skills, however, some physicians are better communicators than others.

8. Choose a physician with whom you feel comfortable. The doctor's age, sex, and personal manner may all be factors that make you more com-fortable or less comfortable. Set up an appointment to talk with the pro-fessional to see whether he or she is willing to communicate openly and honestly.

9. Choose a physician in whom you can have confidence. Even if the per-son is highly qualified and well thought of in the profession, you may be put off by some personal quality.

10. Change physicians if you are not satisfied with the way you are being treated. Find a doctor with whom you feel comfortable.

Ask questions! The more questions you ask, fewer mistakes occur, and the more power patients have in the doctor–patient relationship (Devita 1995).

CHOOSING A HEALTH CARE FACILITY

If given a choice, few people would select the use of an emergency room (ER) or hospital. Unfortunately, most people will need the services of these facilities at some time. Consequently, knowing what to consider when choosing a health care facility should be weighed long before it is needed.

ERs should be used only in an absolute emergency; most ERs are under-staffed, overcrowded, and harried. If the ER personnel view a particular situation as less serious, the patient will probably have a longer wait than someone in an acute state. Tests that may be needed are more difficult to arrange, and the cost for an ER visit is higher than the cost of a visit to a physician's office.

When there is time to select a hospital, it is wise to discuss with your physi-cian the options that are available. Many times, physicians hold admitting priv-ileges at more than one hospital. Every attempt should be made to find out as much as possible about the hospital. Some possible questions to consider in-clude the following.

Why does your physician use this hospital?

What is the patient-to-nurse ratio?

What are the room rates?

What are the costs of laboratory services, X rays, and so on?

How frequently does the hospital perform the procedure you require?

What is the history of malpractice charges against the hospital?

Can you tour the hospital?

What are your rights as a patient?

Choosing a hospital is serious business. Don't be afraid to ask questions.

Health-Related Products

Americans spend billions of dollars each year on health care products ranging from OTC drugs to cosmetics. Many of these products are used to help relieve symptoms, aid in curing illnesses, and provide cosmetic effects. Unfortunately many products are not needed, don't provide the advertised effect, and may have the potential to harm health.

OVER-THE-COUNTER DRUGS

There are more than one-half million OTC health care products. These vary widely from mouth washes to pain relievers. In fact, some of the most beneficial OTC drugs can also create problems. For example, pain relievers such as aspirin and ibuprofen (a nonsteroid anti-inflammatory drug) can damage the lining of the stomach, which can lead to ulcers and other problems. Large doses have been associated with kidney damage. Another pain reliever, acetaminophen, also relieves pain and reduces fever and is the drug of choice for relieving pain in children. However, with heavy doses, the drug can cause bleeding and liver damage. Both of the above-mentioned pain relievers should be taken with food and a full glass of water to reduce irritation to the lining of the stomach.

Two other frequently used OTC products also provide good examples of potentially hazardous use. Nasal sprays relieve congestion by shrinking the blood vessels in the nose. If used for too long, more and more spray is required to maintain effectiveness and the vessels begin to swell, which worsens the congestion. This is called the rebound effect. Prolonged use can result in bleeding and partial or complete loss of the sense of smell. Another product that holds potential misuse problems is laxatives. Many people, especially the elderly, consider a daily bowel movement necessary. Chronic use of laxatives destroys much of the flora in the intestinal tract, making constipation even worse. Bulk laxatives are better than regular laxatives, but exercise and a high-fiber diet are much safer alternatives for promoting normal defecation.

COSMETIC PRODUCTS

Many health care products are intended to be used externally. Some of these have little effect but, due to massive advertising campaigns and misconceptions about their effectiveness, are extensively used.

Skin Products. Some products are designed to prevent or cure acne, rejuvenate skin, prevent body odor, or protect against excessive sun exposure. Acne

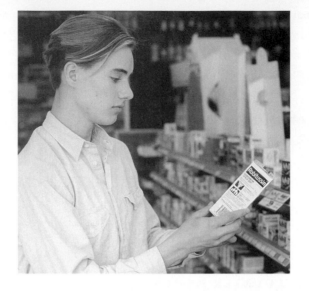

All OTC products must be checked carefully for possibly harmful ingredients.

products, in conjunction with washing the face with a mild soap, may help control the condition. OTC skin rejuvenators have never been shown to be effective at actually changing skin properties, regardless of the claims that are made. A moisturizer can help with the dry skin associated with aging, although it does not actually change the skin. Retin A, a prescription drug, does seem to help delay skin deterioration and restore a more youthful appearance for those individuals who can use it, but it irritates the skin and may result in peeling, blotching, or other undesirable side effects. Deodorants and antiperspirants can help control body odor, but no product can prevent sweating in extremely hot weather or during exercise (nor is this desirable because sweating is the body's primary means of cooling itself). Regular washing is essential if the bacteria and other odor-causing substances are to be removed.

Hair Products. Hair products run the gamut from removing hair to restoring, cleaning, and coloring the hair. There are several products designed to remove hair. Shaving can be used in almost all circumstances and is a safe method of hair removal except for the risk of cutting oneself. Tweezers can be used to pluck unwanted hair but present some danger of infection because the adjacent skin may not be clean. Chemicals can be used to soften and remove hair at the root; wax can be warmed and used to tear hair from the roots as it hardens on the skin; and a fine pumice stone can be used to prevent hair from growing above the skin. Although these products are usually safe, if sometimes painful, there is always the possibility of skin reactions, irritations, and infections. A dermatologist should be consulted if any symptoms appear.

Most hair-restoring products do not work—many products advertised in the media have not been proven to be effective. A drug invented by the Upjohn Company called Minoxidil (Rogaine) does seem to grow limited amounts of hair in some people. Rogaine can now be purchased over-the-counter; however, it has never been shown to totally restore hair (Propecia 1998, 26). Surgery can replace lost hair, but it is extremely expensive, painful, and may take a year or two to complete. Certainly, before considering surgery, the person should consider multiple medical opinions.

Hair-cleaning products are generally safe. There are a wide variety available, and personal preference is usually the primary criterion for selecting a particular product. Some people may have allergic reactions to hair products, but this tends to be atypical. Most people consider dandruff a hair problem, but it is actually a scalp problem in which the scalp sloughs off dead skin cells. If hair is washed daily, dandruff is not usually a problem, so it is unnecessary to purchase a special hair product to help fight dandruff—any hair-cleaning product will serve to remove the flakes. People with a severe problem may wish to use an antidandruff shampoo, however. The Food and Drug Administration (FDA) considers antidandruff shampoos to be a drug. These products can help control dandruff but cannot cure it. Dandruff may be the result of a social or psychological problem but usually poses no medical or health threat unless it is a symptom of psoriasis, seborrhea, or dermatitis, which require a physician's attention.

Hair-coloring products should be used with caution since many of these products can cause skin irritation or harm the eyes upon direct contact. These products are used for cosmetic reasons only. Consequently, care should be used by testing the product on a small area of the hair prior to covering all the hair with the product.

Oral Products. Oral products include toothpaste, mouth washes, and gargles. There are many toothpaste products that, when used with dental flossing, serve to protect against tooth decay. Living in an area where the water supply contains fluoride also helps prevent dental cavities. A toothpaste with fluoride should be used. It is unwise to purchase toothpastes with whiteners since they contain abrasives that damage the teeth.

Mouth washes and gargles do little to eliminate unpleasant odors or treat a sore throat. Since unpleasant odors do not develop in the mouth but are carried from the intestines to the lungs and exhaled, these products can only mask smells. Bad breath also may be a symptom of other conditions such as infections, tumors, or diabetes (Cornacchia and Barrett 1993). In fact, excessive use of mouth wash can actually dry the mucous membranes, making a sore throat even more irritated.

Consumer Rights and Protection

One of the basic premises of wellness or high-level health is that individuals should be responsible for their own health behavior. This is certainly true for consumer health. With so much competition for every dollar spent, and with so much available to buy, consumers need to guard against wasteful spending on products and services of dubious value. For the most part, consumers do not protect themselves properly through informed consumer health behavior. Fortunately, government agencies and private organizations have stepped in to establish consumer rights and offer some protection. On 15 March 1962, President

The following is a brief list of some of your rights as a consumer in the health care system. It is the responsibility of each of us to make sure we are not denied these rights.

■ We have the right as a parent to stay with our children during tests and treatments, provided there is no interference with the medical treatment or child abuse is not suspected.

■ We have the right to request that a relative or friend accompany us during a test, treatment, or hospitalization.

■ We have the right to see our medical records if the state in which we live so allows. State laws vary on this issue.

■ We have the right to emergency care whether or not we have insurance.

■ We have the right to refuse to sign any form. The provider can also refuse to provide treatment in the absence of your signed authorization.

■ We have the right to a second opinion, but our doctor can also stop treating us for challenging him or her.

■ We have the right to leave the hospital at any time, even against medical advice or without paying the bill.

■ We have the right to refuse or stop any treatment.

■ We have the right to an itemized, detailed bill for all medical services.

■ We have the right to know the results of all tests unless the doctor has reason to believe that the information will be harmful.

John Kennedy sent to Congress his "Special Message on Protecting the Consumer Interest" (Cornacchia and Barrett 1993). The message stated that additional legislative and administrative actions were required to assist consumers in the exercise of their rights. Kennedy outlined these rights:

■ *Right to safety*—to be protected against the marketing of goods that are hazardous to health or life

■ *Right to be informed*—to be protected against fraudulent, deceitful, or misleading information or advertising

■ *Right to choose*—to be assured that consumer interests will receive full and sympathetic consideration in the formulation of government policy on consumer matters

In 1970 and 1971, Mary Gardiner Jones of the Federal Trade Commission and consumer activist Ralph Nader further extended the definitions of consumer rights to include these rights:

■ the right to expect quality of design, workmanship, and ingredients in products and services

■ the right to be charged fair prices

■ the right to receive courteous and respectful treatment from firms

■ the right to expect consumer products and services whose use by the consuming public is consistent with the values of a humane society

■ the right to redress of legitimate grievances related to purchased products and services

These consumer rights, of course, are meaningless unless they are backed up with the power of legislation. Over the years, hundreds of federal, state, and local laws have been passed to ensure the rights of consumers and to protect consumers from fraudulent or harmful products and services. An example of a federal agency that seeks to protect the rights of the consumer is the FDA. In 1998, the FDA sent 1,589 warning letters, 3,736 products recalls, 25 seizures, 8 injunctions, 41,575 import detentions, and 373 criminal prosecutions (Nordenberg 2000).

CONSUMER PROTECTION AGENCIES

Many federal agencies work to protect the consumer. One of the most active of these agencies is the FDA. Responsibilities of the FDA include periodic inspection of foods, drugs, devices, and cosmetics. The agency demands proof of the safety and effectiveness of any new drug before it is marketed and has the power to recall possibly unsafe drugs or other substances from the market. The FDA also enforces the law against illegal sales of prescription drugs; investigates therapeutic devices for safety and truthfulness of labeling claims; and checks importation of foods, drugs, devices, and cosmetics to ensure that they comply with U.S. laws.

Another government agency, the Federal Trade Commission (FTC), is responsible for eliminating unfair or deceptive practices in commerce that curtail competition. In other words, this agency prevents the free enterprise system from being suppressed by fraudulent trade techniques or by a company creating a monopoly on a product or service. The FTC has the authority to stop the dissemination of advertisements of foods, drugs, devices, or cosmetics when such action is in the best interest of the consumer. Also, if a label on a product is misleading, the FTC can order the withdrawal of that product from the shelves.

The Consumer Product Safety Commission, established by the federal government in 1973, protects the public against unreasonable risks of injury from products. This commission oversees the enforcement of the Flammable Fabrics Act, the Federal Hazardous Substances Act, and the Poison Prevention Packaging Act, among many others. Under these acts, the Consumer Product Safety Commission is responsible for regulating the manufacture for sale of all highly flammable wearing apparel and fabrics. This is especially helpful for the consumer, because the majority of fabrics used in today's clothing burn quite easily.

In January 1964, President Lyndon Johnson established the President's Committee on Consumer Interests. This committee was replaced by the Office of Consumer Affairs in 1971. The main purpose of this office is to act as a consumer voice in the presidential administration, but it also coordinates all governmental activities in the field of consumerism; conducts investigations on consumer problems; handles consumer complaints; facilitates communication on consumer affairs between the government, business, and the consumer; and helps disseminate helpful information to the consumer.

Various department-level organizations within the federal government also aid the consumer. The U.S. Department of Commerce encourages industry to avoid packaging proliferation that can lead to consumer confusion in shopping. This department can request mandatory packaging standards. The Department

Health Highlight
CAN A WEB SITE BE TRUSTED?

With the amount of information exploding onto the World Wide Web, the question arises whether the information found at a site can be trusted to be scientifically accurate and truthful. It is important to remember that the Internet is filled with good/bad, true/false, complete/incomplete, and even dangerous information. To help determine if the information can be trusted, ask the following questions:

- Where does the information come from? Reputation counts. Information from established medical institutions or government agencies can usually be trusted.

- Does the site reflect more than one opinion? Quality sites will often feature a variety of perspectives.
- How often is the information updated? Good Web sites update at least monthly, sometimes weekly.
- Does the site promote products or procedures? Do not trust sites that rely on anecdotal records and testimonials to promote their products. Be suspicious of sites that dwell on the shortcomings of mainstream medical practice.

of Labor provides the consumer price index, the measure of changes in the nation's economy and currency, and also surveys employment trends and studies prices of various commodities. The U.S. Department of Agriculture (USDA) inspects meat and food animals before slaughter to prevent any diseased meat from reaching the stores. The USDA establishes grades of meat to help the consumer in identifying the different levels of quality. The U.S. Postal Service investigates any incidence of mail fraud and regulates attempts to sell worthless or harmful merchandise or medicines through the mails. There are also many trustworthy Web sites that seek to protect the consumer (see Health Highlight box above).

PRIVATE AGENCIES

Many private agencies also assist the consumer by providing accurate, unbiased information about products or by attempting to eliminate fraud and deception by businesses. For example, Consumer's Union publishes *Consumer Reports,* a magazine that provides impartial information about products; it informs the consumer about the best buys and the most reliable products. *Consumer Reports* also helps the consumer by interpreting advertising on many products.

Better Business Bureaus are private, nonprofit, business-supported groups that help the consumer mediate misunderstandings between customers and businesses. These groups provide information about a company, help resolve complaints against companies, foster ethical advertising and selling practices, alert consumers to bad business practices, and provide the media with informational materials on consumer subjects. Better Business Bureaus have no legal powers, but they can arbitrate between consumer and business. When illegal practices are discovered and a business refuses to cooperate, the matter is turned over to the appropriate law enforcement agency. These bureaus are one of the more important sources of help to which consumers may turn when they need assistance, especially with regard to health products and devices (Cornacchia and Barrett 1993).

Many cities have chambers of commerce that are supported by businesses in that community. These organizations publish a business consumer relations code of ethics. Their work is quite similar to a Better Business Bureau in that they act as liaisons between the consumer and business. They also protect the consumer by attempting to eliminate fraudulent business practices.

Even with all these government and private agencies working to protect the consumer, however, it remains the individual's responsibility to be informed about products and services in order to increase the probability of satisfaction when purchasing a product.

Teaching Consumer Health Education

Consumer health education teaches students to learn to make wise decisions about buying and using products and services, especially in health-related areas (Corry and Galli 1985). Children need to become knowledgeable about consumer rights and consumer responsibilities. They (like their adult counterparts) have rights as outlined earlier in the chapter, but rights are balanced with responsibilities. These responsibilities include seeking out accurate information about products and services, being skeptical of advertising claims, recognizing the differences between needs and desires, and making wise consumer choices. This process must begin early in life and be fostered throughout the elementary school years. Even though the information presented in this chapter may seem more appropriate for adults, the concepts that lead to becoming an effective consumer as an adult are instilled in each child early in life.

The most effective way that all consumers, regardless of age, can protect themselves in the area of consumer health is through preventive health care. By learning about proper nutrition, exercise, and health care, students can avoid the need for many consumer health products such as tonics, diet products, or some other worthless health product or service.

When it comes to teaching consumer health education, the importance of critical thinking cannot be overemphasized. Children must recognize that, just because a product is advertised on television or in a newspaper, it is not necessarily worthwhile or useful. They should learn to see how wants can be fostered artificially. In addition, they should learn not to accept advertising claims or promises without thinking about them critically. Children need to understand that much of what is said in a commercial or print advertisement is meaningless. For example, a product may be touted as new or improved. Is new necessarily better? Improved in what way? If a product is advertised as being "25 percent more effective," students should ask, "More effective than what?" Generally, no answer to these questions can be found.

The intent of consumer education is not to teach students *what* to buy, but rather *how* to buy. Students should be encouraged to get the facts, comparison-shop, consider the consequences of all purchases, and budget their money the same as any wise adult would do. By learning the importance of wise consumer behavior, students can incorporate the concepts taught into their own value system. Finally, students should be informed of their rights as consumers and what recourse they have if they are victimized in the marketplace. All consumers have legal rights. Exercising these rights can help put an end to deceitful health care practices and services as well as worthless health care products.

Summary

- A consumer is anyone who selects and uses goods and services.
- Consumer health education is concerned with those products that directly or indirectly affect personal health.
- Consumers become aware of available products primarily through advertising.
- Advertising seeks to influence consumer psychology and behavior by confusing wants with needs and by fostering desires.
- Many advertisements for health products seek to give the impression that the products are more effective than they actually are.
- Consumers are persuaded to buy a product because of a variety of appeals.
- Quackery is widespread in the United States despite legal measures designed to prevent it.
- Resorting to a quack can prevent a person from getting proper or even life-saving treatment.
- Many people today either are not insured or are underinsured.
- Private insurance companies, HMOs, and government plans help meet needs and reduce costs but do not fill the needs of all citizens.
- A physician and health care facility must be selected with care.
- Private and government agencies help protect consumer rights, evaluate the quality and effectiveness of health-related products, and police business practices.
- The primary responsibility of each consumer is to become knowledgeable when making health-related consumer decisions.
- Helping students learn to become informed, wise consumers is a vital part of teaching consumer education.

DISCUSSION QUESTIONS

1. How does advertising manipulate consumer psychology and behavior?
2. Discuss the most typical advertising approaches.
3. Describe the influences, other than advertising, that affect consumer behavior.

4. List and discuss some common health-related consumer myths.

5. Discuss the teacher's role in combatting consumer misconceptions.

6. Discuss the role of Better Business Bureaus in protecting consumers' rights.

7. What are some considerations that should be made when selecting a physician?

8. What are some of the agencies that help protect the health consumer?

CRITICAL THINKING QUESTIONS

1. What types of myths and misinformation develop concerning consumer health issues? Why?

2. Discuss the preparations you would make before a doctor's appointment.

3. How much help do you think you get from government consumer protection agencies? What responsibilities do you have in protecting yourself against quackery or fraud?

4. What guidelines would you develop for acceptable advertisement of health-related OTC products?

WEB SITE ACTIVITY

After reading this chapter, reflect on the many types of consumer health issues that might concern an individual. Select one of the suggested Web sites, and explore it to determine if you were correct in seeking the type of information you desired from that particular site.

WEB SITES OF INTEREST

American Board of Medical Specialists: *www.ama.assn.org*
Publishes the Compendium of Certified Medical Specialties, *a list of physicians by name, specialty, and location.*

The American College of Surgeons: *www.facs.org*
Identifies doctors who have passed a peer-reviewed evaluation and are staying current with the latest developments in their field.

Consumer Reports: *www.consumer report.org*

U.S. Consumer Gateway: *www.consumer.gov/#spcc*
Source of consumer information.

Medicare: *www.Medicare.gov*
U.S. Government site for Medicare.

Citizens for Health: *www.citizens.org*

Mayo Clinic Health Oasis: *www.mayohealth.org*
Useful, understandable health information.

Health with WebM.D.: *www.adam.excite.com*
Provides information on a variety of health consumer issues.

Quackwatch: *www.quackwatch.com*
Provides source for ongoing investigations in the areas of quackery and reliable publications and reports on illegal marketing.

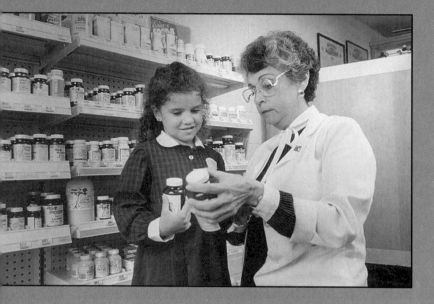

CHAPTER TWENTY-TWO

Strategies for Teaching Consumer Health

One human frailty is to
believe what we are told by
others.

—Warren E. Schaller and
Charles R. Carroll

VALUED OUTCOMES

*After having done the following activities, the
student should be able to explain and illustrate the
following statements:*

- Health care products and services should be used
  only when needed.

- It is important to obtain accurate information
  concerning health care products and services.

- Not all products and services are worthwhile or
  necessary.

- Advertising seeks to persuade rather than to inform.

- Many advertising claims are inflated or misleading.

- Family, friends, and peers influence one's choice of
  products and services.

- Labels on all health care products should be read carefully, and the directions should be followed closely.
- The existence of widespread quackery in health care products and services must be recognized.
- There are many ways to spot quack products and services.
- Quack products and services are useless and/or dangerous.
- Medical attention should be obtained only from qualified and recognized professionals.
- Many government and private agencies work to protect the consumer.
- Federal, state, and local laws enforce the rights of the consumer.
- The best way to make wise consumer decisions is to become informed about the facts concerning products and services. Making wise consumer decisions is ultimately a personal responsibility.

REFLECTIONS

As you read through the activities found in this chapter, reflect on the many choices students must make as consumers. What concepts should be emphasized in helping students become aware of their options and how to make informed decisions? Select one concept and describe the types of activities at each grade level that would best illustrate the concept.

Establishing Consumer Behavior Patterns

The patterns established in childhood of appraising, selecting, and using consumer products and services can influence a person's physical, psychological, and social well-being for a lifetime. To choose wisely requires accumulating knowledge and formulating attitudes about different kinds of products and services. Students must learn that products and services differ in quality, cost, and intrinsic value. They must also recognize how advertising and social forces influence ideas about needs and desires. Above all, they must understand that the responsibility for making wise consumer decisions ultimately is a personal one.

Consumer health pertains to products and services that either directly or indirectly relate to personal health. Most directly health-related products and services include over-the-counter (OTC) medications, cosmetics, and medical and dental treatment. Broadly speaking, however, almost any product or service purchased can in some way be health related. For example, choice of foods has a bearing on nutrition. Choice of clothing relates not only to physical needs, but also to psychological expression of personality. Choice of discretionary purchases, ranging from toys to jewelry to stereo equipment, affects income available for necessities.

In this chapter, both the rights and the responsibilities of the consumer are emphasized. A variety of suggestions for learning activities will assist you in helping students establish responsible consumer behavior patterns.

Health Highlight

A THOUGHT ON GENERIC DRUGS

Substantial savings to consumers can be obtained through the use of generic drugs. Generic drug sales have increased dramatically since 1984 when the U.S. Congress passed the Drug Price Competition and Patent Term Restoration Act. The Food and Drug Administration (FDA) issues guidelines to ensure that generic drugs retain the same quality and potency as brand-name drugs. Almost 80 percent of generic drugs are produced by brand-name firms in their manufacturing plants. The FDA's Office of Generic Drugs conducts reviews and approves generic drugs for marketing. What does this suggest to you concerning generic drug use?

Shown at the right of each activity title in this chapter is the suggested grade level(s) for which the activity might be appropriate. However, many of the suggested activities could be modified for use at various grade levels.

Value-Based Activities

Valued-based activities are designed to help students develop their critical thinking skills, personalize information, and establish those concepts that are conducive to high-quality wellness. You can design a variety of activities that are value based, depending on the content being discussed. Some suggestions follow.

WHY DO I BUY?   Grades (4–6)

Valued Outcome: The students will be able to identify the reasons they purchase various products.

Description of Strategy: Each student should think of a product that he or she buys from time to time. It can be any sort of product, not necessarily a health-related one. Ask the students the questions below. Have them explain and discuss the answers they give. How do they relate their decisions to their values?

- How does advertising convince consumers to buy a product?
- If your friends use a certain product, would you use it also?
- Does cost affect what you buy?
- If you didn't like a product, but it was the only kind available, would you buy it?
- If you had your choice of two products, one in a bright, colorful box and one in a plain box, which would you buy?
- Would you buy a product because your family likes it?

- Does the quality of a product matter?
- Would you try several brands to find one you like?
- Do you tell other people about products you like/buy?
- What kind of products would you buy because of an associated name; in other words, because of who wears them or whom they represent?

Materials Needed: none

Processing Questions: none

ASSESSING ATTITUDES   Grades (4–6)

Valued Outcome: The students will be able to analyze why they purchase products.

Description of Strategy: Create a handout from the following list of statements, and pass it out to the students. Have students assess their own attitudes about each one. By doing so, the students will become more aware of why they make choices.

		Agree	Disagree	Not Sure
1.	Most television commercials give accurate information about the product advertised.	____	____	____
2.	If my friends have a certain product, I usually want to buy that product, too.	____	____	____
3.	I only buy products that I need.	____	____	____
4.	Advertisers must tell the truth.	____	____	____
5.	Only products and services that are useful are sold.	____	____	____
6.	I sometimes buy things that I don't need.	____	____	____
7.	There is not much point to saving money.	____	____	____
8.	Sometimes I buy things without knowing very much about how good they are.	____	____	____
9.	Health care products are always safe to use.	____	____	____
10.	The products I buy for myself can affect my health.	____	____	____

Materials Needed: handout for each student

Processing Questions:

1. What seems to be most important in determining why you buy a product?
2. Are there products you buy that perhaps you could do without?
3. Are any of the products you buy potentially harmful to you?
4. Do all the products you buy seem to be as good as you thought they would be?

BUDGET DIARY

Valued Outcome: The students will develop insight into the reasons they purchase products.

Description of Strategy: Have each student keep a notebook diary of all purchases made for a week or longer. Every purchase made should be recorded in the diary, along with the reasons for that purchase. Money spent on food, snacks, toys, video games, school supplies, transportation, books and magazines, pet supplies, hobbies, and health care products should all be recorded. Explain to the class that the amount of money each student spends is not as relevant as how the money is spent. After the diaries have been completed for the assigned time period, have each student analyze his or her purchases and answer the processing questions below. Answers to these questions should be written out so that students can clarify their thoughts better and come to personal conclusions about their patterns of consumer behavior. On a volunteer basis, have students explain to the class what they learned from this activity. Follow this with a general discussion.

Materials Needed: notebook diary for each student

Processing Questions:

1. What items did you buy that brought you a great amount of pleasure?
2. What items did you buy that disappointed you?
3. Do you think that you spent any money unwisely? Why?
4. Does this diary suggest ways that you could budget your spending money better? How?
5. What does this diary tell you about your consumer habits? Are there patterns in the way you spend your money?

I'M A WISE CONSUMER BECAUSE. . .

Valued Outcome: The students will be able to identify their positive purchasing habits.

Description of Strategy: Ask each student to complete the following statement in a written paragraph of twenty-five words or less: "I'm a wise consumer because. . . ." Each answer should be based on actual behavior or attitudes. Discuss each student's response in a general class discussion. Ask students to explain on what values their statements are based.

Materials Needed: none

Processing Questions:

1. What makes you a wise consumer?
2. What do you consider before buying a product?
3. What consumer tips did you learn from others in your class?
4. How can these tips help you in the future?

Valued Outcome: The students will be able to identify factual health-related information.

Description of Strategy: Create a handout from the following questions and give a copy to each student. Ask him or her to place a checkmark in the blank under the appropriate answer.

	Agree	Disagree	Not Sure
1. Raw eggs are more nutritious than cooked eggs.	_____	_____	_____
2. Eating an egg a day is harmful.	_____	_____	_____
3. Fish and celery are brain foods.	_____	_____	_____
4. Frozen orange juice is less nutritious than fresh.	_____	_____	_____
5. All fruits and vegetables should be eaten raw.	_____	_____	_____
6. It is dangerous to leave food in a can that has been opened.	_____	_____	_____
7. Drinking too much water will make you retain fluid.	_____	_____	_____
8. Drinking ice water causes heart trouble.	_____	_____	_____
9. If one vitamin pill a day is good, two are better.	_____	_____	_____
10. Meat is fattening.	_____	_____	_____
11. Toast has fewer calories than bread.	_____	_____	_____
12. Special diets help people with arthritis.	_____	_____	_____
13. Acupuncture is a reliable method of treating illness.	_____	_____	_____
14. Cooking with an iron skillet increases the amount of iron in the food cooked.	_____	_____	_____
15. Cooking with aluminum pots and pans may increase the likelihood of getting Alzheimer's disease.	_____	_____	_____

Materials Needed: handout for each student

Processing Questions:

1. What are some additional statements you have heard concerning health fact or fiction?
2. Why does misinformation begin concerning health?
3. Why is misinformation about health issues a problem?
4. How does misinformation concerning health issues begin?
5. How is misinformation concerning health issues disseminated?

WHAT IS REALLY HAPPENING?   Grades (6–8)

Valued Outcome: The students will be able to identify the amount of time companies spend in attempting to influence consumer spending and habits.

Description of Strategy: Assign the students to watch television for one hour. Ask them to keep track of the amount of time spent in advertisements during the hour. Provide a chart such as the one shown below for their record keeping.

Television Viewing Form

Name of Program	Number of Minutes of Program	Type of Commercial	Number of Seconds/Minutes
1.			
2.			
3.			
4.			

Total Minutes of Programs _____   Total Seconds/Minutes for Commercials _____

Materials Needed: stopwatch, calculator, viewing form for each student

Processing Questions:

1. How much time was devoted to advertising?
2. To whom did the advertising appeal: children, young adults, and/or grown-ups?
3. What type of product was on most of the commercials you saw?
4. What message was each commercial trying to get across?
5. Did you think all the commercials were truthful?

TECHNIQUES THAT SELL   Grades (6–8)

Valued Outcome: The students will identify the strategy utilized in attempting to sell a particular product.

Description of Strategy: After reviewing the various strategies used to sell products, divide the class into groups of three to five students. Assign each group a different selling strategy. Have them review media such as magazines, newspapers, radio, and television to find examples of their strategy. If possible, have them record or provide examples of their technique.

Materials Needed: magazines, newspapers, radio, television, and tape recorder or video cassette recorder for each group

Processing Questions:

1. Were you able to find all the techniques discussed?
2. Why are there so many different techniques?

3. What technique(s) were used most often?

4. What type of technique appeals to you?

5. Why does that particular technique appeal to you?

WHAT IS IN THERE? Grades (6–8)

Valued Outcome: The students will realize the many drugs that they have in their household.

Description of Strategy: Ask the students to request a parent to review the different drugs found in their household. With adult supervision, each student should list the drug and the main ingredient of each drug and its intended purpose. Students can then research any ingredient they don't understand or research that drug on the Internet. Provide a chart such as the one shown below to list the different drugs.

Drug Chart

Name of Product	Main Ingredient	Purpose of Drug

Materials Needed: copy of drug chart for each student, computer(s) with Internet access

Processing Questions:

1. What type of drug(s) were most often found in your house?

2. Do some of the drugs serve the same purpose?

3. How many of the ingredients did you not know the effect of?

4. Did any of the ingredients of the various products have the potential to interact with one another?

WHERE IS THE HELP? Grades (5–8)

Valued Outcome: The students will be able to discuss agencies that can help protect consumers.

Description of Strategy: Ask the students to investigate the following agencies to determine the types of services/protection they can offer the consumer:

> Better Business Bureau (BBB)
> Small Claims Court
> Consumer Product Safety Commission (CPSC)
> Food and Drug Administration (FDA)
> Federal Trade Commission (FTC)

Have them list the types of services offered by each. Prepare a handout from the following information and have each student complete the form.

Where Is the Help?

Directions: Indicate which agency(ies) could provide help with the problems listed below:

a. BBB
b. Small Claims Court
c. CPSC
d. FDA
e. FTC

Agency

_____	1. Your new toy truck has small pieces that your younger sister might swallow.
_____	2. Food purchased at your local store was found to have worms and was spoiled.
_____	3. You are looking for information on a new drug.
_____	4. Your mom has purchased a product that is labeled as hamburger, but it does not look or smell like hamburger—your mom suspects it was mislabeled.
_____	5. Your new CD player gives you a slight shock every time you turn it on.
_____	6. Your dad takes his car to the serviceman for repair. But the car still does not work, and the serviceman says it is not his fault.
_____	7. Your deodorant has caused you to break out.
_____	8. Your family wants to check out a local company before doing business with it.
_____	9. You see an advertisement that is false or misleading.

Materials Needed: copy of worksheet for each student

Processing Questions:

1. Do some of the agencies cover a variety of complaints and issues?
2. Which agencies can respond most quickly to a consumer complaint?
3. What are the responsibilities of the consumer before purchasing a product or service?

WHAT IS BEST? Grades (5–8)

Valued Outcome: The students will be able to identify the major OTC pain relievers and discuss differences between them.

Description of Strategy: Introduce the concept that there are several types of OTC pain relievers. Ask the students to identify by brand name products that they know help to relieve pain, fever, and headaches. Write their responses on the board or on an overhead. Introduce the notion that each of these products has an active ingredient (drugs such as acetaminophen, acetylsalicylic acid, ibuprofen, naproxen). Have the students research which of the products they identified are in each of the four categories of active ingredients. Ask them to identify similarities, differences, and potential dangers associated with each type of product and record them on a chart similar to the one below.

Drug Chart

Name of Product	Main Ingredient	Purpose of Drug

Materials Needed:
chart listing the various pain relievers, drug books or computer access to Internet, overhead projector and pen or board and markers

Processing Questions:

1. Are any of the medications potentially harmful?

2. Do some of the drugs require a higher dose than others? Did all the drugs provide pain relief for the same amount of time?

3. Were all the medications safe for children to take?

4. Did any of the products offer different benefits or advantages?

Decision Stories

Follow the procedures outlined in Chapter 4, pages 80–83, for presenting decision stories such as these.

BROKEN PROMISES   Grades (1–3)

Ricardo saw a model car advertised on television. It looked like a fun toy. He saved up his money and bought the model. But when he opened the package, the car didn't look as well made as it did on television. He started playing with it, and the car broke. He was angry and disappointed. He felt like throwing the car away, but it had cost a lot of money.

Focus Question: Was it Ricardo's fault that the car broke?

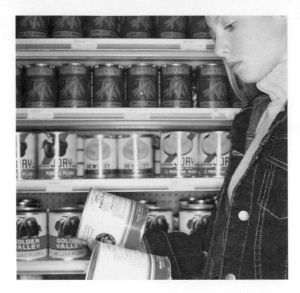

Wise consumers read labels carefully and compare brands before purchases.

VITAMINS FOR VERA?   Grades (2–4)

In her health class, Vera has been learning about the importance of vitamins for good health and growth. She wonders if she is getting enough vitamins because sometimes she feels tired and worn out. One day, Vera's mother asks her to go to the grocery store to buy some milk. While at the store, Vera sees a shelf with many different kinds of vitamin pills on it. She has some money of her own with her. Maybe she should buy some vitamins so she might feel healthier.

Focus Question: What should Vera do?

MUNCH OR LUNCH   Grades (4–6)

Miguel likes to play video games at the arcade. He spends a lot of his money playing Munchman, his favorite video game. He is getting better and better at it, but playing Munchman often leaves him without any money for other things. His parents give him lunch money every day. Up to now, he hasn't spent this money on anything except lunch. But maybe he could cut a few corners. Maybe he could buy less for lunch and use the rest of the money to play video games.

Focus Question: What should Miguel do?

MUSIC, MUSIC, MUSIC   Grades (5–8)

Marsha likes music. She spends a lot of her money buying tapes and CDs. One day, Marsha sees an advertisement for a CD club in a magazine. For only ten dollars she can buy any three of her favorite CDs through the mail. Marsha sends off a money order, and in a few weeks her three selections arrive. She is very pleased. The CDs are great, and for ten dollars they are a real bargain. However, the next month three more CDs arrive in the mail, but Marsha didn't order them. Still, there is a bill for twenty-five dollars along with the CDs.

1. Does Marsha have to pay for the new CDs?
2. How can she find out about her consumer rights in this matter?
3. What should she do differently in the future

SHAMPOO OF THE STARS   Grades (4–6)

Ling's friends have been telling her about a new shampoo called Hairdoyoudo. They say that it makes their hair feel soft and look pretty. Ling has also seen the product advertised on television. A famous young model with beautiful hair says that she uses it. Ling would like to use Hairdoyoudo, also, but her mother buys another brand of shampoo that is less expensive and seems to work fine. Ling asks her mother to buy Hairdoyoudo, but she refuses, saying it is overpriced. Ling is very upset since she wants her hair to look as nice as her friends' hair. But how can that be if she has to use another shampoo?

Focus Question: What should Ling do?

SPOTS AND SHAUN   Grades (6–8)

Shaun has acne. He is very embarrassed about his spots and blemishes. One day he sees an advertisement for a new acne medication in a magazine. The advertisement promises a miracle cure within thirty days. The product has a money-back guarantee, but it can only be purchased by mail. The advertisement also says that the product has a secret ingredient that no other product has. It sounds like just what Shaun has been looking for, even if the product costs $12.95 a tube.

Focus Question: Should Shaun order the product?

Discussion and Report Techniques

HOW ARE YOUR HEALTH HABITS?   Grades (6–8)

Valued Outcome: The students will be able to evaluate their health to determine what lifestyle changes they might make.

Description of Strategy: Have students develop and conduct a survey of health habits at their school. Answers should be either yes or no and should include questions dealing with superstitions and personal health habits. For example: Have you ever bought a product just because you saw it advertised on television or in a magazine? Have you ever ordered anything through the mail and been disappointed with the merchandise? Do you take vitamins? Tally the results and post them on a bulletin board. Also, post the medically correct answers so students can assess their own knowledge, or lack of knowledge, concerning health issues.

Materials Needed: a list of possible questions to be asked in the survey (enough questions should be provided to help students start the project)

Processing Questions:

1. What did you discover from the survey?
2. How should you change any negative lifestyle habits you identified?
3. What positive health habits did you identify?
4. What additional information would you like?

HEALTH AND BIG BUSINESS   Grades (6–8)

Valued Outcome: The students will work in groups to design a health-related business and present their plans to the class.

Description of Strategy: Invite guest speakers in the health field to describe their business operations and the service they provide to the community. Include local health officials, nurses and/or doctors, aerobics instructors, university health professors, fitness and wellness personnel, and health club personnel. Working in large groups, have the students study and design their own health-related businesses. Have each group present its program to the class via lecture, bulletin board, poster board, and so forth for class review and discussion.

Materials Needed: materials to be determined by students

Processing Questions:

1. What health areas do you think would be most profitable from a business perspective?
2. What kinds of problems did you find when trying to set up a business (expenses, finding qualified personnel, obtaining equipment, and so on)?
3. Why did you choose your specific area to set up a business?

DECIPHERING WHAT WE EAT   Grades (6–8)

Valued Outcome: The students will use nutrition labels to plan a healthy meal.

Description of Strategy: Have the students bring package labels to class that list the ingredients and the nutritional values of various food products. In groups, have the students decide which of the foods they eat are really good for them and explain why or why not. Have students make note of added ingredients, such as salts, sugars, and hidden fats they may not be aware of eating. Using the labels in each group, have students plan a meal that will provide 33 percent of their daily needs without acquiring too much fat, cholesterol, or simple sugars.

Materials Needed: labels for various food products

Processing Questions:

1. Were there any foods that surprised you regarding the amount of fat, sugar, or other added ingredients they contain?

2. Do you have any suggestions for getting the nutrients you need without adding ingredients that might not be as healthy?

3. Can you eat in a manner that is nutritious and still eat appetizing food?

HEALTH MYTHS   Grades (4–6)

Valued Outcome: The students will make a collection of health myths and state why they are accurate or inaccurate.

Description of Strategy: Students can research and collect health myths such as "Feed a cold and starve a fever," "Toads cause warts," and "An apple a day keeps the doctor away." Develop a bulletin board or scrapbook listing and illustrating the adages as well as whether they are true or false. Discuss the scientific accuracy for the sayings that may have relevance and why people continue to follow such beliefs today.

Materials Needed: list of myths, construction paper, markers, glue

Processing Questions:

1. Are all health myths completely false?

2. Why do you think people first developed these myths?

3. Why do people continue to believe these myths today?

HEALTH NEWS   Grades (5–8)

Valued Outcome: The students will gather current health information and present it in newspaper form.

Description of Strategy: Have students research, develop, and publish a copy of a newspaper dealing with health issues. Included in the paper should be articles, cartoons, editorials, advertisements, and human interest stories written by the students. If students are using the Internet to research medical information, remind them to be wary of the source of the information and to rely only on reputable sources such as the Centers for Disease Control and Prevention, the American Heart Association, etc.

Materials Needed: sources containing health information such as magazines and newspapers

Processing Question: What did you learn about health that you did not know before?

HEALTH PROMOTION AGENCIES

Grades (6–8)

Valued Outcome: The students will learn what health promotion agencies are responsible for specific activities.

Description of Strategy: Create a handout similar to the Teaching in Action box below. The handout should have a list of agencies involved in health promotion programs and the description of each agency's function.

Materials Needed: handout for each student

Processing Questions:

1. What other agencies can you name?

2. What agencies do you think are most important to our personal protection?

TEACHING IN ACTION *Health Promotion Agencies*

Directions: Write the letter of the health promotion agency next to the description of its functions. Not all items in the lettered list will be used.

_____ 1. enforces laws for labeling and safety of cosmetics, medicines, and food

_____ 2. responsible for inspecting and grading meat and poultry

_____ 3. prevents false advertising from being sent through the mail

_____ 4. has offices all over the country to handle consumer complaints and keep track of businesses engaged in fraudulent practices

_____ 5. involved in examining and testing electrical devices to ensure safety in operation

_____ 6. in charge of coordinating federal efforts in the field of health care

_____ 7. promotes cancer research and educational programs dealing with all aspects of cancer

_____ 8. under the guidance of the United Nations, oversees programs dealing with disease, nutrition, and sanitation in all member countries

_____ 9. establishes regulations on the manufacture and sale of biological products, researches health problems and provides information to the public, and assists local and state health departments

_____ 10. within a specific political division, maintains clinics, laboratories, and staffs of nurses and other personnel to aid in the prevention and control of disease

a. BBB

b. Department of Health, Education, and Welfare

c. U.S. Postal Service

d. National Association for the Prevention of Blindness

e. Underwriters Laboratory

f. American Heart Association

g. American Cancer Society

h. Public Health Service

i. FDA

j. World Health Organization

k. U.S. Department of Agriculture

l. state and local health departments

Answers: 1. i 2. k 3. c 4. a 5. e 6. h 7. g 8. j 9. h 10. l

ADVERTISING:
DON'T BUY IT HOOK, LINE, AND SINKER   Grades (4–8)

Valued Outcome: The students will be able to understand the role of advertising in product purchases.

Description of Strategy: Create a handout from the questionnaire below and distribute it to the students. Ask students to bring various advertisements to class. Help them determine the types of appeal used in each advertisement and list them on the board. Then have students circle the appropriate letter to best complete the statement or question.

1. When a product's package says, "Free coupon inside," the advertising appeal being used is
   a. cost and rewards
   b. scientific appeal
   c. snob appeal
   d. testimonial or authority figure

2. People who purchase and use goods and services are called
   a. advertisers
   b. consumers
   c. researchers
   d. shopkeepers

3. Advertising is designed to do all of the following except
   a. entertain
   b. dissuade
   c. persuade
   d. promote

4. The most serious health-related effect of not understanding advertising techniques is
   a. dependence on a stimulant drug
   b. failure to seek proper treatment
   c. feelings of total frustration
   d. loss of one's self-respect

5. In evaluating an advertisement that features an endorsement by a famous person, the most important question should be
   a. How is this person qualified to judge the product?
   b. How much money is this person being paid?
   c. Does this person really like the product?
   d. Does this person use the product regularly?

Answers: 1. a   2. b   3. b   4. b   5. a

Materials Needed: copy of questionnaire for each student, board and markers or overhead projector and pen

Processing Questions:

1. What is the most important role advertising serves?

2. Why do famous people serve as spokespersons for various products?

3. Do any health products have potentially dangerous consequences?

THE LAWS OF ADVERTISING   Grades (5–8)

Valued Outcome: The students will be able to list at least three laws that protect consumers.

Description of Strategy: The students can learn about the laws that protect consumers against fraud or useless products and services. They can begin to learn about advertising laws by looking under "consumer protection" on the Internet, in the catalog system, or in the *Reader's Guide to Periodical Literature* at the library. Write the laws on the poster board and discuss.

Materials Needed: poster board, computer with Internet access, access to *Reader's Guide to Periodical Literature*

Processing Questions:

1. Why was it necessary to pass laws to protect us against fraud?
2. Do you think most consumers know about these laws?
3. What is the key to consumers being protected against fraud?

DO ONLY DUCKS QUACK?   Grades (4–6)

Valued Outcomes: The students will be able to describe quacks and quackery.

Description of Strategy: Develop a class discussion around the topic of quacks and quackery. Questions that can be used include:

- What is quackery?
- Why does quackery continue to flourish?
- Who are the people most likely to believe what quacks say?
- How can consumers be protected from quackery?
- What can be done if you think a legitimate physician is in error?
- Why would people give testimonials about products that have no proven value?
- In what areas of health concern would it be easiest to get people to buy products?

After the discussion, divide students into groups. Each group is to develop and build a pretend fraudulent medical device and/or medicine to present to the class. Have the students formulate advertisements to stimulate interest in their phony product. After completion, projects can be displayed in the classroom. Presentations can be videotaped.

Materials Needed: materials to build devices or to present medicines, poster board and markers for each group, videotaping equipment (optional)

Processing Questions:

1. Do you think fraudulent medicines and cures are very prevalent?
2. Should there be strong laws against people advertising phony remedies? Why or why not?

HEALTH OPTIONS?   Grades (6–8)

Valued Outcome: The students will identify different forms of treatment other than traditional medicine.

Description of Strategy: After dividing the class into small groups, have the students investigate alternative health care choices. The following could be included: acupuncture, chiropractic, faith healing, holistic health, homeopathy, visualization, laughter therapy, or positive self-talk. Reports are then given to the class. Students should discuss the scientific basis of each, the feasibility of trying alternative kinds of medical care, under what circumstances they might try an alternative form, and the intrinsic value of each method. A master list of alternative treatments may be given to the class to help the students choose their topics. Presentations can be videotaped.

Materials Needed: list of alternative health care choices to hand out to students, videotaping equipment (optional)

Processing Questions:

1. Would you try any of these alternative forms of treatment?
2. Do you think some or all of these alternative forms of treatment are useful?
3. What are some guidelines we should keep in mind when deciding if we might try an alternative treatment?

LABELS ARE IMPORTANT   Grades (5–8)

Valued Outcome: The students will learn how to read and interpret health care product and OTC drug labels correctly.

Description of Strategy: With the cooperation of parents, have each student analyze the information given on the package of a health care product or OTC drug. Use the processing questions below for the analyses. Students should prepare individual reports about what they find.

Materials Needed: labels from OTC drugs and health care products

Processing Questions:

1. What did you learn from reading the label that you did not know before?
2. Are any drugs safe for everyone to take?
3. Why do you think the warnings were placed on the product package or label that you brought in?
4. The labels of health care products and OTC drugs caution against using the product if you have certain allergies or medical conditions. What do you think would happen if you had an allergy or condition that may cause a reaction, but you took the drug or used the product anyway?

CONSUMER REPORTS   Grades (4–6)

Valued Outcome: The students will learn about comparison shopping and where to obtain product information that is free from advertising.

Description of Strategy: Older elementary school children can learn about how products and services are evaluated objectively by reading copies of *Consumer Reports* magazine. Get some back issues from the public library, and discuss the products tested. Note that this magazine does not carry any advertising.

Materials Needed: copies of *Consumer Reports*

Processing Questions:

1. Why do you think this magazine has no advertising?

2. Pick a product that you find particularly attractive, such as a car. After reading the comparison of it with similar products, are you convinced you like the product as well as you did before you read the product comparison?

3. What is the advantage of reading a magazine such as *Consumer Reports*?

WHERE CAN I GO FOR HELP?   Grades (6–8)

Valued Outcome: The students will learn about health care services offered in their community.

Description of Strategy: Have students research legitimate health care services available in the community and write reports on their findings. Community health care resources include private physicians, dentists, therapists, hospitals, clinics, health maintenance organizations (HMOs), telephone referral services, and so on. Keep a list of the type of services each student chooses, so that not too many will have the same topic. Have students discuss their resource in class. Students should seek information concerning eligibility for services, types of services, where the facility is located, the types of staff (personnel) employed, and the duties of the staff.

Materials Needed: list of the health care services offered in the community with headings for categories of services, phone numbers, and descriptions of services to be filled in by the student

Processing Questions:

1. Are there many health organizations in your community?

2. What services does your organization provide?

3. How do the various health services differ?

Dramatizations

NOW FOR THIS COMMERCIAL MESSAGE   Grades (5–8)

Valued Outcome: The students will be able to analyze commercials to determine misleading or overstated claims concerning health care products.

Description of Strategy: Ask the students to work together in pairs or small groups to reenact commercials they have seen on television for health care products or services. Let each group decide on the commercial they wish to reenact. Draw up a master list to avoid duplication. Have the students closely study the commercial of their choice at home. Then let them work together, rehearsing their reenactment. Each student should play a different role. For example, one student can recommend the product, and another student can act out trying out the product, as in many aspirin commercials. When the students are ready, have each commercial reenacted in front of the class. After the reenactment, the students who played the roles should explain what might have been misleading or overpromising about what they said or did. Videotaping will allow reuse of some of the commercials at a later time.

Materials Needed: videotaping equipment (optional)

Processing Questions:

1. What types of commercials seem to be the most misleading?

2. How do these commercials seem to overstate the effectiveness of the product?

3. What is misleading about the commercials you have just seen?

DR. I. M. A. QUACK   Grades (5–8)

Valued Outcome: The students will learn to recognize phony health and medical treatment claims.

Description of Strategy: Let each student come up with a quack product or service and try to convince the class that this product or service is actually of value. Encourage imagination. For example, one student might try to convince the class that magnetic energy can cure arthritis. Another might claim to have invented a product that will cure the common cold. Have the class listen to each presentation without interruption but then point out any fallacies of each presentation.

Materials Needed: a box containing props for role-playing

Processing Questions:

1. What were some of the statements made that might make us want to buy the product or service?

2. What made some of the presentations believable?

3. Can you identify some points we should keep in mind when selecting health care products or services?

FINDING A DOCTOR   Grades (2–4)

Valued Outcome: The students will be able to identify criteria for selection of a physician or a dentist.

Description of Strategy: After discussing the procedures that can be used for locating a qualified physician, have students role-play the techniques. For example, one student plays the part of a representative from the county medical society who recommends physicians who are accepting new patients. Another student calls on the telephone and asks for the names of such physicians, or one student can play the part of a doctor while the other plays the part of a prospective client. The latter should ask questions about availability of services, fees, qualifications of the doctor, and so forth.

Materials Needed: two telephones (optional)

Processing Questions:

1. Where would you look to help identify the location of a physician or dentist?
2. How would you contact a physician or dentist?
3. What questions would you ask before using the services of a health care professional?

COMPLAINTS   Grades (6–8)

Valued Outcome: The students will practice appropriate ways to complain about defective or ineffective health care products.

Description of Strategy: Have small groups of students role-play how they would act when complaining about a defective or ineffective health care product or service. One student should act the part of the disgruntled consumer, another the part of the seller, and a third the part of a consumer advocate or representative of a local Better Business Bureau or other consumer-oriented group.

Materials Needed: none

Processing Questions:

1. What are some agencies where consumers can seek help?
2. Where do you begin when filing a consumer complaint?
3. Who is ultimately responsible for protecting us in consumer issues?

MEDICINE SAFETY RULES   Grades (2–4)

Valued Outcome: The students will be able to list the rules for safely taking medicine.

Description of Strategy: After discussing the medicine safety rules detailed in the following list, divide the class into seven groups, and let each group develop a brief skit—two to five minutes—dramatizing each rule. The rest of the class will try to determine which rule is being acted out by each group.

- Don't take any medicine without asking an adult about it first.
- Only take medicines that you really need.
- Take only the medicine prescribed by your doctor especially for you.
- Never take more than one medicine at a time, unless your doctor tells you to do so. Different medicines may interact in a way that can be dangerous or even fatal.
- Don't take any medicine unless you are sure you know what it is.
- Throw away medicine that doesn't have a label or that has passed the expiration date.
- Keep all medicines out of the reach of younger children.

Materials Needed: medicine safety rules listed on poster board

Processing Questions:

1. Why are medicine safety rules so important?
2. Are there other medicine safety rules you could think of to help protect us?

Experiments and Demonstrations

IS THERE ANY DIFFERENCE?   Grades (3–6)

Valued Outcome: The students will taste different unlabeled cola drinks and try to determine what each one is.

Description of Strategy: Many products are indistinguishable once removed from their packaging. To demonstrate this, bring in some different brands of cola drinks. Pour small amounts of three or four different brands into paper cups, and have the students do taste comparisons. Let them try to guess which cup contains a particular brand.

Materials Needed: liters of several different colas, small cups

Processing Questions:

1. Do you have a favorite cola drink? Could you tell which one it was?
2. How much do you think advertising affects what you buy?

WHICH IS BETTER?   Grades (5–8)

Valued Outcome: The students will exchange consumer products such as shampoo or soap to determine if there are actual differences between them.

Description of Strategy: Ask students to bring a particular brand of shampoo or soap to school, making sure that the brands are not all the same. Then have students trade the products they now use with someone using another brand of shampoo or soap. Let each volunteer use the alternate product for a week or two and then report on the results.

Materials Needed: index cards or paper for each student for recording comments

Processing Questions:

1. Did the alternate shampoo or soap do just as effective of a job, or were differences noted?

2. Were any differences a matter of individual preference?

3. Are different products perhaps more or less effective for different individuals?

COMPARISON SHOPPING   Grades (4–6)

Valued Outcome: The students will learn to compare similar products from a cost perspective.

Description of Strategy: Have the students develop a list of five or six health care products, such as toothpaste, deodorant, soap, eye drops, dental floss, and antiseptic cream. Let each student comparison-shop for these items and report on which stores in the community sell each brand of product for the best price. This can be done either by visiting stores or by checking prices in newspaper advertisements. You may wish to have the students comparison-shop for specific brands that they normally use, or you may suggest that the students look for the cheapest and most expensive brand of each type of product. Compare the results in a class discussion.

Materials Needed: sheet for each student for listing products, price, and comments

Processing Questions:

1. Do the same products cost the same at various stores?

2. What is the difference in cost between the most expensive and the least expensive version of a certain item?

3. Is the most expensive product always the best? Is the least expensive product always the worst?

4. On what criteria should you base your purchases?

FOOD LABELING   Grades (6–8)

Valued Outcome: The students will read and record data contained on a food label.

Description of Strategy: Labeling of foods transported interstate is controlled by the FDA. According to FDA guidelines, food labels must be accurate, in English, and include information for each of the areas listed in the Teaching in Action box "Food Label Information Form." Have students select a food product (or you can assign one) and then fill in information for each area on the form. Discuss the questions below.

Materials Needed: copies of the Teaching in Action box "Food Label Informational Form" for each student

Name of product _____

Nutrition facts

Serving size: _____

Servings per container: _____

Amount per serving

Calories: _____   Calories from fat: _____

Percent daily value*

Total fat: _____   _____ %

   Saturated fat: _____   _____

Cholesterol: _____   _____

Sodium: _____   _____

Total carbohydrates: _____   _____

   Dietary fiber: _____   _____

     Soluble fiber: _____   _____

     Unsoluable fiber: _____   _____

   Sugar: _____   _____

Protein: _____   _____

Vitamin A: _____   _____

Vitamin C: _____   _____

Calcium: _____   _____

Iron: _____   _____

*Percent daily values are based on a 2000-calorie diet. Your diet values may be higher or lower depending on your calorie needs.

	Calories	2000	2500
Total fat	Less than	65 g	80 g
Saturated fat	Less than	20 g	25 g
Cholesterol	Less than	300 g	300 g
Sodium	Less than	2400 g	2400 g
Total carbohydrates	300 g	275 g	
Dietary Fiber	25 g	30 g	

Calories per gram

Fat: _____   Carbohydrates: _____   Protein: _____

Processing Questions:

1. How many times did you find salt and sugar listed in the product that you chose? (Remember, salt and sugar may be listed under different names.)

2. How many servings were contained in the package you selected?

3. How many additives and artificial ingredients were contained in your food product?

4. How does the product compare with a 2,000- or 2,500-calorie diet?

LISTEN CAREFULLY   Grades (4–6)

Valued Outcome: The students will increase their awareness of meaningless phrases used in advertising.

Description of Strategy: Tape some radio or TV commercials using either audiotape or videotape, and play them back for the class. First, play the commercial in its entirety, asking students to listen or watch for any misleading statements. Play the commercial again, this time stopping the tape to discuss statements such as "Now more improved than ever" or "America's number one choice!" Explain that these types of statements are especially meaningless since the comparison is not specifically stated. List these statements so the students can review them.

Materials Needed: audiotape or videotape of commercials, tape player or videocassette recorder and television, poster board, board and markers or overhead projector and pens

Processing Questions:

1. What types of statements do you find used most often?

2. How are certain statements misleading?

3. What are examples of other commercials on television or radio that are also uninformative or misleading?

Puzzles and Games

SCRAMBLED-UP HEALTH   Grades (4–6)

Valued Outcome: The students will learn discretion when using health care products or services.

Description of Strategy: Through various media, people are constantly being bombarded with ads about goods and services that supposedly improve health or appearance. Create a handout with scrambled words that name some items that should be considered with caution and discretion (see the Teaching in Action box "Beware of . . . "). Have students unscramble the words and write them in the blanks.

Materials Needed: handout of scrambled words for each student

Processing Questions:

1. Have you heard or read health claims that might not be truthful?

2. How can you determine if a health claim is accurate and truthful?

CONSUMER RIDDLES   Grades (3–6)

Valued Outcome: The students will solve these riddles about consumerism.

Description of Strategy: Use the following riddles on consumerism to assess student knowledge of consumerism.

- I am a fraud, but I sound like a duck. What am I? (a quack)
- An inflated advertising claim is a huff and a _____. (puff)
- My initials are BBB. I can help you if you have a consumer problem. What am I? (Better Business Bureau)

Materials Needed: riddles

Processing Questions:

1. What other riddles can you identify that illustrate an aspect of consumerism?

2. Can you think of an example for each of the riddles?

TEACHING IN ACTION *Beware of . . .*

1. religious faith _____. (rsleahe)

2. advertisements where the only "evidence" is _____ of other people. (nistmstoeie)

3. so-called doctors whose only degrees are from unaccredited or nonexistent _____. (tnisotsituin)

4. products that miraculously cause weight _____ such as "body wrapping." (odcruetin)

5. high-potency _____ that make extravagant claims about their effect. (ansivitm)

6. very expensive cures or remedies that may not be harmful by themselves, but are totally _____. (viftecefine)

7. overuse of medicines that may be _____ forming. (bahti)

8. medicines that may alleviate symptoms temporarily, but prevent a possibly sick person from seeking the _____ help that is needed. (oinspfolresa)

9. using medicine that has been _____ for someone else whose symptoms are similar. This is especially dangerous because the problems causing the sickness and how two people react may be entirely different. (rsiepcbdre)

Answers: 1. healers 2. testimonies 3. institutions 4. reduction 5. vitamins
6. ineffective 7. habit 8. professional 9. prescribed

SCRAMBLED WORDS   Grades (4–6)

Valued Outcome: The students will unscramble words relating to consumerism.

Description of Strategy: Have students unscramble each of following words, or provide a list of your own.

1. mocmlaceri (commercial)
2. qyuracek (quackery)
3. singiadevrt (advertising)
4. elagl githrs (legal rights)
5. aeetngura (guarantee)

Materials Needed: copy of words to unscramble for each student

Processing Questions:

1. Can you define all the scrambled words?
2. How does each word relate to consumerism?

CONSUMER HEALTH TIC-TAC-TOE   Grades (3–5)

Valued Outcome: The students will develop health-related questions and use them to beat an opposing team at tic-tac-toe.

Description of Strategy: This game can be played either by two players or by the whole class divided into two teams. Have each team come up with a health-related question for one of the tic-tac-toe squares. The opposing side or player tries to answer and to mark a particular square. The correct answer must be given. If an incorrect answer is given, no mark on the tic-tac-toe board is to be made. Each side plays in turn until there is a winner.

Materials Needed: health-related questions, poster board with tic-tac-toe grid for each group, two different colors of counters for each group

Processing Questions:

1. Can you correct all the answers that were missed?
2. What are some additional questions?

SHOPPING GAME   Grades (4–8)

Valued Outcome: The students will participate in a game to increase their knowledge of consumer spending.

Description of Strategy: Prepare a shopping game board as shown in the Teaching in Action box "Shopping Game Board." The game can be played by two to six players. Each player is given $200 in play money at the start. A "central bank" is given $100 in play money; this is where students place or remove money for their purchases or refunds. Participants roll dice in turn to determine the number of moves. The winner is the player with the most money at the end of the game. Play can continue until only one player has any money left. Let each

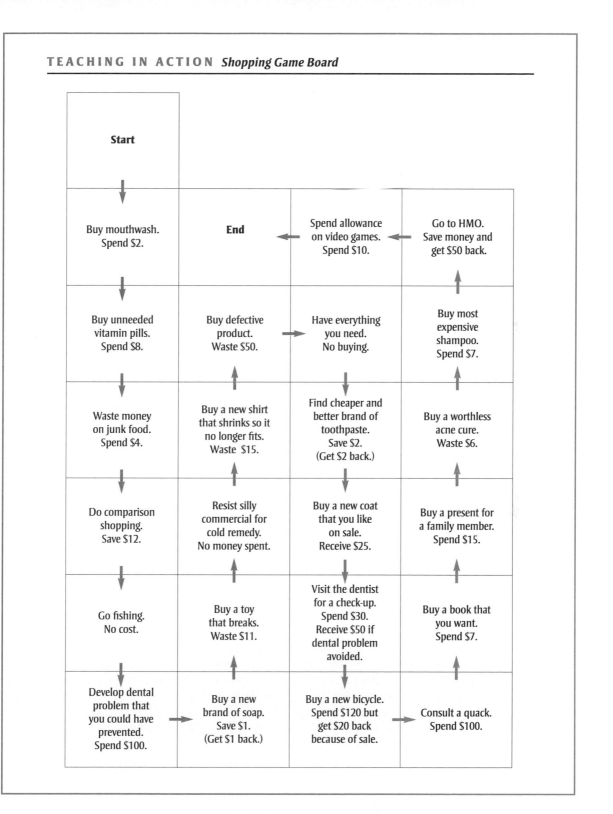

Start			
Buy mouthwash. Spend $2.	**End**	Spend allowance on video games. Spend $10.	Go to HMO. Save money and get $50 back.
Buy unneeded vitamin pills. Spend $8.	Buy defective product. Waste $50.	Have everything you need. No buying.	Buy most expensive shampoo. Spend $7.
Waste money on junk food. Spend $4.	Buy a new shirt that shrinks so it no longer fits. Waste $15.	Find cheaper and better brand of toothpaste. Save $2. (Get $2 back.)	Buy a worthless acne cure. Waste $6.
Do comparison shopping. Save $12.	Resist silly commercial for cold remedy. No money spent.	Buy a new coat that you like on sale. Receive $25.	Buy a present for a family member. Spend $15.
Go fishing. No cost.	Buy a toy that breaks. Waste $11.	Visit the dentist for a check-up. Spend $30. Receive $50 if dental problem avoided.	Buy a book that you want. Spend $7.
Develop dental problem that you could have prevented. Spend $100.	Buy a new brand of soap. Save $1. (Get $1 back.)	Buy a new bicycle. Spend $120 but get $20 back because of sale.	Consult a quack. Spend $100.

player decide to what extent he or she won or lost by the consumer decisions the game dictated. Follow with a discussion of options in buying products and services.

Materials Needed: copy of shopping game board (see Teaching in Action box) for each group of students, dice (one per group), play money ($200 per student and $100 in assorted denominations in the central store), game pieces such as buttons (one per student)

Processing Questions: none

Other Strategies for Learning

SLOGANS—DO THEY SELL?   Grades (5–8)

Valued Outcome: The students will discuss the impact of slogans on the health care products they purchase.

Description of Strategy: Create a handout similar to the Teaching in Action box "Slogans and Selling," and provide each student with a copy. You may wish to add or replace items with slogans that are popular in your area. Or, students can develop their own lists using magazines, videos, and television.

Materials Needed: handout for each student with slogans for various products

Processing Questions:

1. What other slogans you can think of?
2. Why do slogans influence what we buy?
3. Do any of the slogans provide you with actual information about the product?
4. Do you find that you purchase products more if you like and remember the slogan associated with it?

PACKAGING   Grades (4–6)

Valued Outcome: The students will recognize the importance of attractive packaging in influencing the purchase of a product and will design a package for a product of their own.

Description of Strategy: Some of the appeal of a product results from the way it is packaged. Have the students bring in empty packages from various health care products. Discuss the visual appeal of each one, then have the students design packages of their own for the products. First, they should try to design a package they think would be very appealing to consumers. Then they should design a package that would not appeal to consumers. These can be shown to other students for feedback.

Materials Needed: construction paper, glue, markers, empty health care product packages

Directions: Place the correct letter in the blank to the left.

_____ 1. We build excitement	a. Dairy Queen
_____ 2. The heartbeat of America	b. General Electric
_____ 3. You'll love this place	c. Campbell Soup
_____ 4. For the times of your life	d. Ford Motor Company
_____ 5. Taste it again for the first time	e. Pontiac
_____ 6. It pays to Discover	f. Burger King
_____ 7. We bring good things to life	g. Dr. Pepper
_____ 8. M'M! M'M! Good!	h. Mastercard
_____ 9. Hot Eats! Good Treats!	i. Chevrolet
_____ 10. The best things in life are free. For everything else there's _____	j. Kodak
_____ 11. Built _____ Tough	k. Kellogg's Corn Flakes
_____ 12. Just what the doctor ordered	l. Discover credit card

Answers: 1. e 2. i 3. f 4. j 5. k 6. l 7. b 8. c 9. a 10. h 11. d 12. g

Processing Questions:

1. Was it difficult to design a package that would help sell your product?

2. What did you find the most attractive—certain colors or designs or wording?

3. How much do you think packaging influences what you and your family buy?

THE PHARMACIST AND YOU   Grades (4–6)

Valued Outcome: The students will learn what a pharmacist does.

Description of Strategy: Have students visit a pharmacy, or invite a pharmacist to class to discuss his or her training and educational level and exactly what he or she does as a pharmacist. Students can work together to make a list of questions to ask the pharmacist about the job, how he or she likes it, his or her income level, the industry's view of the use of generic medications, and the decisions he or she makes in collaboration with both doctors and pharmaceutical salespeople. Questions can also be asked, or research done, into the history of pharmacy and how modern technology has enabled it to evolve into an exacting science today. Perhaps brainstorming with the students can help them generate questions of interest to the group.

Materials Needed: list of questions to be asked at interview

Processing Questions:

1. Would you be interested in a career in pharmacy?

2. What kinds of questions could a pharmacist help you answer about drugs and medications?

3. What is the most important thing a pharmacist does?

Resources

BOOKS

Being a wise health care consumer. 2000. Farmington Hills, MI: American Institute for Preventive Medicine.

Greenburg, S. 2002. *Physician's desk reference for nonprescription drugs.* 21st ed. Orodell, NJ: Medical Economics Data

PAMPHLETS

Consumer health. 2002. Santa Cruz, CA: ETR Associates.

Over-the-counter drugs: Harmless or hazardous? 1997. Broomall, PA: Chelsea House Publishers.

Your rights as a consumer. 1997. Broomall, PA: Chelsea House Publishers.

WEB SITES

American Cancer Society. *www.cancer.org*

Healthlinks. *www.hslib.washington.edu*

Health Resources. *www.1hr.com*

Mayo Clinic Health Oasis. *www.mayohealth.org*

National Center for Complementary and Alternative Medicines. *http://almed.od.nih.gov/nccam*

Prescription Drugs. *www.pharminfo.com*

U.S. Food and Drug Administration. *www.fda.gov*

VIDEOS

Supermarket persuasion:
What marketers know (Grades 6–8)
A video tour through the world of consumer manipulation at the grocery store. Available from The Learning Seed at *www.learningseed.com.* (24 minutes, Item 273)

Why ads work: The power of self-deception (Grades 6–8)
Describes how advertisements are carefully crafted. Available from The Learning Seed at *www.learningseed.com.* (21 minutes, Item 199)

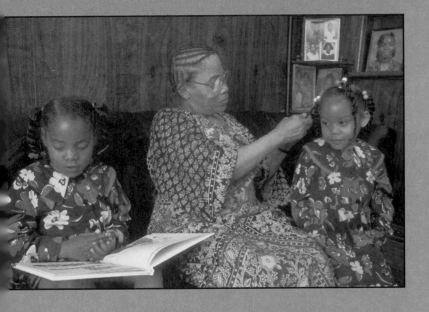

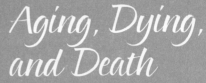

Aging, Dying, and Death

Aging is a normal developmental process . . . each of us is aging every day. Death should not be considered taboo . . . it should be seen as a natural part of our existence.

VALUED OUTCOMES

After reading this chapter, you should be able to:

- discuss aging as a normal part of the life cycle
- describe how ageism affects the elderly in our society
- describe the current demographic aspects of the elderly in the United States
- explain the factors that can help delay or retard the physiological changes that occur in aging
- list the reasons why elderly people have problems with nutrition
- describe Alzheimer's disease
- suggest intergenerational contact programs for school-age students and the elderly
- discuss the factors that will lead to better quality lives for the elderly in the future

- discuss the fears of a dying person
- describe the relationship of personal beliefs in facing dying and death
- list ways in which family members cope with and help in times of a relative's death
- describe healthy ways to grieve
- discuss the purposes of funerals, hospice care, and living wills
- describe effective methods of teaching death education

REFLECTIONS

Aging: Consider your own relationships with elderly people—your grandparents and relatives or other elderly around you. Reflect on how you can increase the quality of these relationships.

Death and Dying: As you read through this chapter, consider the ways that you and those around you practice and observe the denial of death and dying—in behavior, in common phrases, on television, and so on.

The Normalcy of Aging

Aging is a normal developmental process, not a pathological phenomenon, as it is often viewed. When we speak of aging, we must avoid the misconception that the process affects only those over sixty-five; each of us is aging every day. We generally consider the changes taking place in the body as "development" until postadolescence and as "aging" after that. Many people view growth as positive and aging as negative—but, in fact, both are part of one process. The process of aging is a continuous experience that begins at birth and ends at death.

Exactly how we age is not clearly understood. Many theories have been advanced, but some aspects of the aging process are still mysteries. In any case, the number of elderly in the United States has risen sharply in the past two decades, and this trend will continue. Because of advances in medical technology, improved health care delivery, reduced infant mortality, and control of diseases, more people are living longer. In this chapter, we examine the ramifications of this fact and consider the ways in which aging is viewed in our society.

The Significance of Aging Education

Aging education is relatively new compared to other health topics. Because the number and proportion of elders are expanding rapidly in the United States, education about aging and the aged is becoming increasingly important. The presentation of correct facts and figures about the elderly and the aging process can counteract many misconceptions (Ferrini and Ferrini 2000, 10). Elders have a tremendous impact on our society through their talents, wisdom, and psychological support for younger age groups.

People face many changes and challenges in life as they age. The problems of the elderly are problems that affect all of us. Major challenges facing the elderly include income, fitness, acute illness, nutrition, housing, sexuality, mandatory retirement, and the changing character of society.

U.S. society places a great deal of emphasis on youth and productivity; the elderly person's role is considered less significant. Also, because of financial reasons (sharing housing costs) and social factors (desiring to live with or near peers and living nearer service-oriented agencies), some elderly people have opted to move into housing and communities for the aged. This further segregates them from the remainder of society and makes them less visible.

Children today are less likely to have significant contact with the older generations than in the past. Some children see older persons daily (such as grandparents), but the interaction is often not as meaningful as in the past (Blieszner and Bedford 1995, 224). This lack of meaningful contact with the elderly, coupled with misleading stories children read and hear, often leads to fears and misconceptions. Students need to be taught about the elderly and aging early in their lives. They need to understand that they themselves will one day be old and that the elderly were once young like themselves.

Intergenerational Contact

Intergenerational contact programs can be one of the most effective ways for secondary teachers to implement an aging education program. Such an experiential approach to intergenerational contact has been implemented in programs throughout the country. Notable examples are the Foster Grandparent Program and the Retired Seniors Volunteer Program. Volunteers and paid aide programs, tutoring projects, free lunches, and guest speaker days have all served to involve the elderly with the schools. Only as students are given the opportunity to understand aging and the aged will many false beliefs be dispelled. The positive attitudes gained from aging education can help students realize their full potential throughout their lives as they themselves age. By studying aging, students will be better able to understand and interact with their parents and grandparents.

There are several things for young adults to consider when planning for later life. For example, the better educated elderly may be better able to cope with the challenges of later life; therefore, younger adults should place an emphasis on continuing their education. A related factor that will help a young adult prepare for later life is the development of hobbies; therefore, one's education does not have to include a program that results in a formal degree. Some courses can be taken to investigate various interests and hobbies. Young adults should become active in organizations and/or movements in which they have concerns or interests—such as environmental issues, women's rights, and charitable organizations. This activity contributes to one's self-concept by providing a purpose in life and can enhance to the quality of life in later years. Finally, young adults should carefully consider financial planning for later years. It is difficult for a young adult to contemplate financial needs that are thirty to forty years away—especially in a society that promulgates instant gratification. Financial concerns usually top the list of problems for elderly people in our society, and this trend is likely to continue; therefore, it is vital for young adults to develop a sound financial plan in order to ensure quality health care, housing, and living standards for themselves in later life.

Population Demographics

According to the National Center for Health Statistics (NCHS), the number of older individuals—those age sixty-five and older—has increased dramatically in the United States between the years 1900 and 2000, from 3.1 million to 35 million, approximately 12.4 percent of the entire U.S. population (NCHS 2003). As the current older population reflects, fewer babies were born during the Great Depression of the 1930s than in subsequent generations. The baby boom generation—those born between 1945 and 1965—for example, will be reaching the age of sixty-five between the years 2010 and 2030, so the older population in the United States is expected to double that of 2000 (NCHS 2003).

The older population itself is getting older. People are expected to live longer, thanks to medical advances and improvements in health-related care reducing the death rates among children, young adults, and the elderly, especially males. A child born in 2000 can expect to live 76.9 years, which is twenty-nine years longer than a child born in 1900 (NCHS 2003).

Women are expected to live longer than men. This sex survival ratio increases with age, primarily because men are more susceptible than women to disease in general at every stage of life and are more prone to health problems related to stress. People who are very nervous will probably not live as long as those who are more relaxed. Some personality types may be more aggressive or prone to taking risks or may pursue a more physically taxing lifestyle.

Race has played a significant role in life expectancy in the past, though this is projected to be less of a factor in the future. As of the year 2000, whites had a longer life expectancy than nonwhites, but the reverse is projected to be true in coming years. (The current difference may be attributable to differences in education, economic levels, living conditions, nutrition, and health care and to the fact that some nonwhites, especially black males, are more prone to hypertension than whites.) Of the increased population of older people expected by the year 2030, the various minority groups (including Hispanics, African Americans, Native Americans, Asians, and Pacific Islanders) are likely to be more represented (NCHS 2003).

The higher the level of education an individual has, the better the chances are that the person will get a better or higher paying job and will be aware of the importance of good diet and proper exercise, and the dangers of tobacco, alcohol, and drug misuse and abuse. College graduates have a greater life expectancy than nongraduates. The educational level of the older population is increasing. Between 1970 and 2000, the percentage of older individuals who had completed high school rose dramatically, though it varies considerably by race (whites, Asians, and Pacific Islanders have the highest graduation rates). By 2000, approximately 16 percent of the older population had at least a bachelor's degree (NCHS 2003).

The Aging Process

Aging is a complex process influenced by physiological, psychological, and sociological factors. Before the specific changes associated with the aging process are discussed, it should be emphasized that the changes occur to different people at different times. Most of theses changes are gradual, and adjustments can often be made to offset them. Many changes can be slowed through proper exercise, nutrition, and other preventive health maintenance.

BIOLOGICAL ASPECTS OF AGING

Gender, genetics (a person's hereditary predisposition toward or resistance to certain diseases and conditions), and general environment (exposure to various hazards or special benefits that affect health and well-being) are all factors that affect how long people live and how healthy they will be over their lifespan.

Many physical changes occur with the passage of time (Pruitt and Stein 1999, 488). These include:

- wrinkling of the skin and thinning of the epidermis
- graying of the hair or baldness
- increase in proportional body fat
- diminishing bone mass
- declining visual capacity
- hearing loss
- reduced sex drive and problems with erections among men
- vaginal dryness or a decline in sexual responsiveness among women

Dementia and Alzheimer's Disease. The majority of people over the age of eighty retain normal brain function, but various biological phenomena involving progressive degeneration of mental functions may occur as people age. **Dementia** is a general term for the progressive loss of cognitive and intellectual functions and is caused by a variety of disorders, the most common of which is structural brain disease. It may affect individuals of any age but is most common in older people. (If the affected person is younger than sixty-five, it is called *presenile dementia;* if the affected individual is older than sixty-five, it is called *senile dementia.*) An estimated 10 to 30 percent of older people who have intellectual impairment are actually suffering from treatable conditions. These include the use and misuse of drugs (sleeping pills, tranquilizers, and some pain medications), nutritional deficiencies (especially vitamins such as B_{12}), depression, reduced blood flow (from bronchitis or other chest infections, stroke, heart attack, atherosclerosis, etc.), hypoglycemia (low blood sugar), and even hypothermia (American Medical Association [AMA] 2002; University of Missouri, Kansas, Institute for Human Development 2003).

The majority of all cases of dementia, however, are due to **Alzheimer's disease,** a progressive and irreversible disease involving the death of nerve cells and deposition of plaques of amyloid (a protein) in the brain. An estimated 11 percent of the general U.S. population under age eighty-five and 47 percent over the age of eighty-five may develop the disease. The cause(s) of Alzheimer's are not yet known, though genetic factors may be involved; research is continuing in an effort to find a treatment. Alzheimer's affects individuals at different rates, and the appearance of symptoms may be so gradual as to be barely noticeable. Memory loss (beginning with recent memories) and difficulty finding the appropriate words during casual conversation may be accompanied by emotional instability, mood swings, and unpredictable behavior. The ability to comprehend and reason becomes impaired, resulting in a decline in personal hygiene, loss of interest in surroundings and interactions with others, and disorientation. Behavior may become less inhibited, even antisocial. The Alzheimer's patient is at increased risk of having accidents, misusing medication, and having nutritional problems; body weight may drop by 20 to 30 percent. As the disease progresses (typically over the course of many years), arms and legs begin to lose their ability to move, and the ability to perform basic skills (such as eating, drinking, walking, maintaining balance, and controlling bowels and bladder) is destroyed. Death usually results from inactivity, increased risk of infection, and pneumonia (NCHS 2003).

A diagnosis of Alzheimer's disease is made only after a thorough examination by a doctor to rule out other treatable causes of dementia. Such an examination should include, among other things, a complete physical examination and medical history, a mental status examination, and clinical imaging tests such as a CT (computed tomography) scan and/or an MRI (magnetic resonance imaging) (NCHS 2003). The diagnosis is still not guaranteed to be accurate, since it can only be confirmed by brain biopsy after death, but the clinical imaging is able to detect brain shrinkage and distortion of nerve tracts (AMA 2002).

PSYCHOLOGICAL AND SOCIOLOGICAL ASPECTS OF AGING

The psychological and sociological changes that accompany the aging process affect some elderly more than others. Each individual will respond to aging in a way that reflects his or her personality, philosophy of life, and the way that he or she is treated by society as a whole. Better treatment of and more positive attitudes toward the elderly would do much to limit many of these detrimental attitudes and behaviors.

Health Highlight

MISCONCEPTIONS ABOUT THE ELDERLY

Younger people are quick to emphasize the problems that occur with aging and the aged. Although people do face special problems and challenges as they grow older, the problems are not so widespread as many younger people believe. For example. it is a myth that most elderly are incapacitated. In fact, most older people are able to work and live independently. Only 5 percent of the elderly are institutionalized, and elderly individuals average less than 15 days a year in bed because of ill health. Here are some other misconceptions about the elderly:

1. After age 65, life goes steadily downhill.
2. Old people are all alike.

3. Old people are lonely and ignored by their families.
4. Old people are senile.
5. Old people have the good life.
6. Most old people are sickly.
7. Old people no longer have any sexuality interest or ability.
8. Most old people end up in nursing homes.

SOURCE: Ferrini and Ferrini 2000

Ageism. Many psychological changes are the result of negative attitudes and behavior toward the elderly, who often are treated as sickly and unproductive by the younger generation regardless of their actual health and abilities. Phrases and images in our language and media reflect these stereotypes. The term for discriminating against someone based on his or her age is **ageism.** This form of prejudice is different from other forms (e.g., sexism, racism) because a person's age changes throughout a lifetime, and older age (and thereby discrimination due to older age) is something that the majority of adults will eventually experience, especially in U.S. society, which stresses the importance of being young, healthy, and economically prosperous. A person may exhibit ageism with respect to others, as well as with respect to himself or herself (Woolf 1998). The focus of government policy on the needs of the frail elderly may also do a disservice to their healthier counterparts by reinforcing a negative image of aging (Hively 2003).

If older people accept these social expectations, their own lifestyles and behaviors will certainly be affected as they age. Conversely, recent advertising has depicted happy gray-haired couples engaged in physical activities and displaying financial independence, which may give an unrealistic account of capacities, activities, and interests of older people and may encourage premature withdrawal from the labor force. There may be economic repercussions to society as a whole, since U.S. society requires a full employment economy to function optimally. As the baby boom generation approaches retirement, these social trends are expected to shift significantly (Hively 2003).

Coping with Changes. In helping individuals cope with changes that do occur, it must be recognized that the elderly face many losses, including peers, jobs, spouse, and physical senses. Problems with making adjustments to these losses overwhelm some elderly people, whereas others are able to face the challenges and find satisfaction. Changes may include:

- loss of the child-rearing function (the empty nest syndrome)
- loss of a spouse
- mandatory retirement (or a change in role if retirement is voluntary)
- problems with transportation
- lack of community involvement
- lack of knowledge of community resources
- inadequate medical services
- financial problems
- a need for leisure activities and ways to use their time
- loneliness
- loss of role identification
- victimization through crime or abuse

Again, it should be noted that many of these sociological aspects of aging are the result of discrimination and inappropriate treatment from younger people. With proper education and attitudinal changes in the general population, many of these detrimental changes could be alleviated among some of the elderly in America. The validity of this premise can be demonstrated by contrasting the role of the elderly in the United States with that of the elderly in some other cultures, such as Japan. In Japan, individuals enjoy higher social status and prestige as they grow older—almost the opposite of what happens in the United States.

Major Challenges Facing the Elderly

INCOME AND EMPLOYMENT

Chief among the challenges facing the American elderly is the lack of financial resources. The primary source of income for older persons in 1999 and 2000, as reported by the Social Security Administration, were Social Security, earnings, income from assets, and public and private pensions. Real median income (after adjusting for inflation) fell from 1999 to 2000 for both men and women (NCHS 2003). Lack of sufficient income is the result of inflation that has eroded the savings many elderly acquired during their working years. Retirement benefits from Social Security are not sufficient to meet all their needs. As of 2003 an elderly person over the age of sixty-five who earns more than $24,000 above his or her Social Security benefits is taxed on the additional income (this does not apply to individuals over the age of seventy).

Poverty level impacts a person's longevity, overall health, and general lifestyle. About 3.4 million older individuals were below the poverty level in 2000, and another 2.2 million were classified as "near poor." (This is not statistically

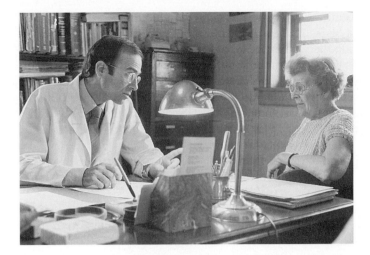

One factor that will determine the quality of life in the elderly is access to medical services.

different from the historic low reached in 1999.) In 2000, higher than average poverty rates for older persons were found among 1) African-American and Hispanic older people than among whites; 2) those who lived in central cities, in rural areas, and in the South compared to other regions; 3) older women more than older men; and 4) older persons living alone or with nonrelatives rather than those living with families. The highest poverty rates were experienced by older Hispanic women who lived alone or with nonrelatives.

In 2000, 4.2 million (12.8 percent) older people were working or actively seeking work; this is 3 percent of the entire U.S. labor force. There was a steady decline in the participation of older men in the labor force between 1900 and 1985, which leveled off and is being maintained at between 16 and 18 percent. The participation of women has fluctuated through the past century but has stabilized between 8 and 10 percent since 1988 (NCHS 2003).

HOUSING AND LIVING ARRANGEMENTS

Housing continues to be a major issue for the elderly. Nearly two-thirds of the elderly in the United States own their own homes. However, even if the house is paid for, the owners are still responsible for taxes and insurance costs, and older homes can have higher maintenance costs. Some elderly have to make a decision between drastic improvements in their current home and moving, but they are sometimes limited financially as to where they can move. Some government housing is available based on current income—the lower the income, the lower the monthly payment. Some elderly share housing to reduce the monthly costs. For many elderly, however, there are few housing options. Some housing alternatives are apartments for the aged that are sponsored by private, public, and nonprofit church-related groups. Also, for older persons requiring assistance, boarding homes and nursing homes that provide both intermediate and skilled care are available.

Over half of older noninstitutionalized individuals (73 percent of older men and 41 percent of older women) lived with their spouses in the year 2000, but this proportion decreases with age. Because men tend to die younger, women are more likely to be living without their spouse or others as they advance in age. About 633,000 grandparents over the age of sixty-five maintained their own households with grandchildren present, and another 510,000 lived with family members in households headed by others and that also included their grandchildren. Only a small percentage of the older population of the United States (4.5 percent, or 1.56 million individuals) lived in nursing homes in 2000. As individuals age, they are increasingly likely to be living in a nursing home (NCHS 2003).

HEALTH

Maintaining good health is a major challenge of growing old. An individual's health affects every aspect of life—relationships to spouse, family, and community; income-producing ability; and leisure pursuits. The health problems that beset the elderly are usually associated with the aging process, in addition to those related to environmental causes and trauma. Chronic ailments, such as heart disease, are the most common affliction of the elderly.

Escalating medical and health-related expenditures are a major concern for the older population. Of economic necessity, the health care of many elderly people is crisis oriented. Because they cannot afford to visit a physician every time they are ill, many do not seek help until they feel it is absolutely necessary—and their more advanced illnesses may be more difficult to treat. At the same time, there are many areas in which the elderly needlessly spend money on health remedies or could spend their money more wisely for greater health benefits. Federal programs such as Medicare and Medicaid have helped in some ways, but even these programs do not pay enough of the health care bills of some elderly because of the ever-increasing costs of health care delivery.

Medicare and Medicaid. The U.S. government provides financial assistance for medical care through two major programs authorized through the Social Security Act and administered by the Centers for Medicare and Medicaid Services (CMS). **Medicare** is the nation's largest health insurance program, providing coverage for nearly forty million individuals who are either age sixty-five and older or are qualifying younger but medically disabled individuals. Generally, older individuals or their spouses must have worked for at least ten years in a Medicare-covered job (i.e., they are entitled to Social Security or railroad retirement benefits) and must be a citizen or permanent resident of the United States in order to receive Medicare benefits. Most of these individuals are covered by Medicare Part A, which helps pay for care in a hospital or skilled nursing facility, home health care, and hospice care, and they will not need to pay additional costs to participate in the program. Additional coverage may be obtained by qualified individuals through a subscription (i.e., at additional cost) to Medicare Part B, which is a supplemental medical insurance to help pay for doctors' fees, outpatient hospital care, and other medical services.

Medicaid is a federal subsidy program for state programs that finance health care for qualified (usually low-income) individuals. Each state makes its own health care regulations, has its own program administration, and determines its

Health Highlight

A THREE-STEP PRESCRIPTION FOR HEALTHY AGING

Diet—The wrong foods are responsible for many of the physical characteristics of premature aging, including a tired, drawn, and doughy complexion; weak muscle tone; wrinkled or leathery-looking facial skin; fatigue; and poor brain power. Eating properly will produce an increase in energy and general well-being.

Supplements—Supplements can enhance a person's health and rebuild and rejuvenate the body and skin from the inside out. The proper use of targeted antioxidants, amino acids, vitamins, and minerals can accomplish everything from sharpening brain power to repairing cells, burning fat to increasing muscle tone, restoring memory to heightening libido.

Exercise—Regular exercise improves cardiovascular conditioning, muscle strength, and flexibility and has a positive effect on the body's cells and organs.

SOURCE: Perricone 2002

own benefits and rates of payment, but these must remain within limits set by federal regulations. A large portion of Medicaid spending is used as reimbursement for nursing facilities.

Nutrition. Some of the health problems faced by the elderly result from improper nutrition. Nutrition is as important for the elderly as it is for other age groups. Because of limited finances, loneliness, various disease states, and a reduction in the senses of smell and taste, many elderly skip meals or do not otherwise eat well. Sometimes emotional problems, such as depression, keep elderly people from eating.

Because an elderly person's basal metabolism is reduced, the person's caloric requirements are also reduced. For this reason, better planning is required to ensure proper nutrition. Less food is required, but the quality must remain high. Programs such as Meals on Wheels, which delivers meals to homebound elderly, and the federal government's Food Stamp Program and Nutrition Program for the Elderly (Title VII of the Older Americans Act of 1965, which is updated every three years) help defray the cost and improve the nutrition of the poor elderly.

Medications. Drug use in older adults may cause greater problems than in younger people because of slower metabolic rates and more illnesses. Older people take more medications than any other segment of the population. Because the older population has the highest rate of chronic or long-term illnesses, this group also tends to take more than one drug at the same time. Prolonged use of multiple drugs increases the risk of dangerous drug interactions (Floyd, Mimms, and Yelding-Howard 1998, 462).

According to the Center for Substance Abuse Prevention, an increasing number of seniors may be abusing drugs, prescription medication (taken for a variety of illnesses that tend to accompany senior citizenship) and alcohol, often for the purpose of dealing with the stresses of older age. Many of them are unaware that their behavior constitutes abuse, or they are ashamed to admit that they have an addiction (Click10.com 2001).

Some normally harmless over-the-counter drugs (OTC) can be dangerous if taken in conjunction with certain prescription medications. Prescription drugs may interact with each other. Many drugs react poorly with alcohol. It is critical to check with a pharmacist before taking any medication and to make sure the pharmacist is aware of *all* medications (OTC, prescription, and even vitamin supplements) so that such interactions can be avoided.

Prescription medications can pose further risks when in the homes of seniors who have young grandchildren. Accidental poisonings can happen when children explore the medicine cabinets and nightstands of their grandparents. The danger of accidental poisoning increases when an elderly person moves in with family members who have young children.

The responsibility for overseeing and safekeeping a senior's medication often falls to a caretaker or family member. This responsibility includes frequent communication with the older person's physician in order to make sure the drugs are being taken appropriately. Using a dispenser or chart to keep medication and dosages organized will help avoid mix-ups and uncertainty about what has been taken. Suicides among the elderly are often due to an overdose of prescription drugs, so a caretaker needs to monitor dosage carefully and discard old medications (preferably down a toilet). The best caregivers will make sure that elderly persons in their charge stay vital and active by encouraging exercise, good eating habits, and social activities (Richard Young Center 2003).

Crimes against the Elderly. Medical quackery also affects the elderly. Arthritis sufferers, mostly older individuals, spend $300 million yearly on quack remedies. Other types of crime against the elderly range from muggings and theft to financial exploitation and physical abuse by members of their own family.

Transportation is a major challenge for some older individuals, many of whom do not drive or have not adjusted to today's complicated traffic patterns. Those who drive with failing eyesight and hearing are more likely to be involved in accidents. The cost of automobile maintenance and gasoline prohibits some older people from operating a car. Nondrivers must seek other means of transportation. Taxis can be expensive, but public transportation, although cheaper, is much less convenient because it requires more walking and takes more time. Often it is not designed with the elderly in mind. For these reasons, many elderly are restricted to their homes and apartments except for going out to get health care, groceries, and other necessities.

Considering Death

Death is a vital part of the life cycle for every creature on earth. Death is included in the natural order of birth, growth, aging, and dying. Death is very democratic—it is a respecter of no person. Death is a certainty—it will come to every person. These seem like elementary statements, but many people in contemporary society believe that life and death are mutually exclusive phenomena.

The contemplation of death can be trying. The various aspects of dying and death are extremely complex and confusing because there is so much about

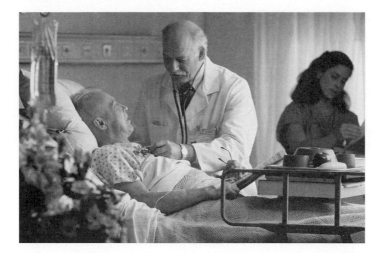

Recognizing that death is a natural end to our lives can have a profound influence on our lives.

death we do not comprehend. Many questions regarding death, such as "If we are born to die, then why do we live?" and "If death is natural, why do so many people regard it as bad?" have still not been answered satisfactorily. None of the numerous attempts to come up with answers to such questions have been able to satisfy everyone. The unknowns have caused much confusion and put an aura of mystery around death, but they have also been the source of many interesting attitudes and philosophies on the subject.

Death is as much a part of human existence, of human growth and development, as birth. Death sets a limit on our time in this world, and life culminates in death. Recognizing that death is a natural end to life can have a profound influence on our lives. Our lifestyles can depend on our attitudes toward death. Much information on death and dying is now available, but many misconceptions and problems concerning issues of death and dying still exist. For example, medical and nursing schools do not do enough to prepare their students to handle end-stage care issues related to dying and death. Therefore, these health professionals may be trained to cure but may avoid the crucial issues surrounding death, thereby complicating the dying process (Dickinson, Leming, and Mermann 2000, 26). Thankfully, with medical education reforms, the number of death education courses is increasing for health care professionals (Ferrini and Ferrini 2000, 487).

Another problem with death and dying concerns students of secondary school age. Parents often protect their children from the trauma of death-related events, thinking they are doing the best thing for the child. However, this treatment tends to propagate fears and misconceptions. For example, children tend to regard death as happening only to the old. This is a result of parents telling them not to worry about death until they are older.

In the remainder of this chapter, we examine these and other death-related issues. We also look at attitudes toward death, the needs of dying people and their families, the grief experience, funerals and related rituals, death education for students, personal beliefs about death, and other issues surrounding death.

Common Attitudes toward Death and Dying

The current attitude of Americans toward death is contradictory. We are both intimidated and fascinated by death. We enjoy living, but we take risks by driving dangerously and taking part in high-adventure sports. We want safety and happiness, but we behave in self-destructive ways, for instance by abusing drugs. We consider the subject of death to be a social taboo but insist on reading and talking more about it now than we did in the past. We say we need nuclear weapons, but at the same time we are concerned about spiritual rebirth.

Our typical response to death is denial. This results from our resistance to imagining death and is predicated on our fears of death. We deny death by not planning for it (for example, by not making out a will) and by participating in high-risk activities as if we were impervious to dying. Students often feel they are impervious to death and will live forever; but death is inevitable, and they need to learn to live with and accept this fact of life. Some of the many reasons students may fear death are given below (University of Buffalo 2002).

- They fear the effects it may have on family, friends, and classmates.
- They fear dying in an undignified manner, such as after being kept alive by a machine.
- They fear what comes after death.
- They fear the premature interruption of life activities.

Many people display an outright hatred of death. They hate death because they think people die too young or because they are afraid of what comes after death. The hate and fear might not result so much from the unknown factor as from the hopelessness regarding what is beyond death.

Open, honest discussions of dying and death are often denied because of the belief that death should be considered a taboo topic for discussion. Taboo means forbidden, profane, or unclean. Death also may be a taboo topic because of the mystery and danger associated with it, an attitude that is influenced by society's emphasis on youth and secularism.

Attitudes toward death are influenced by past experiences with death, by early parental messages, cultural influences, life experiences, religious beliefs, level of education, and maturity. Attitudes are formed largely by childhood experiences and carried into adulthood. Findings from research indicate that negative attitudes toward death tend to be higher among females, blacks, youth, and those who do not characterize themselves as religious (DeSpelder and Strickland 2002, 217–221).

It is interesting that many people today who would rather not discuss death in an open and frank manner actually talk about death in other ways. For example, "You'll be the death of me yet" or "My shoes are killing me" or "That loud noise scared me to death!" In other cases, death is the subject of humor, like the jokes about Saint Peter at the "Pearly Gates." People who talk about death in these ways show both an aversion to death as a topic of conversation and a fascination with death. They may be subconsciously trying to show themselves and others that death really doesn't bother them, even though serious contemplation of the subject makes them extremely uncomfortable.

We also treat death in a very special way. We set aside special places for death—the funeral home, cemeteries, hospices, and hospitals. We set aside special times for remembering deaths—Memorial Day, the Day of the Dead in Mexico, and Good Friday, a day celebrated by Christians for remembering the death of Jesus. The deaths of other celebrated and martyred persons are remembered with special days. We have special symbols for death, such as black armbands worn by athletes when a teammate has died or a flag flown at half-mast in memory of someone who has died.

Several factors have contributed to our very narrow and stereotyped attitudes toward death and dying. Because many people encounter death so infrequently, we fail to accurately contemplate its nature. We blindly believe in modern medicine to the point that we subconsciously feel we may never die. Many never come to realize that death is a fact of life which all people must cope with and reason out for themselves. Most Americans say they want to die quickly or in their sleep. This response reflects reluctance to accept the possibility of a painful or slow death in which one is conscious of what is going on.

Our attitudes toward death and dying are confusing and contradictory. We normally detest the taking of another person's life, as in homicide, yet we train soldiers to do just that in war. In fact, we make heroes of soldiers who tempt death and kill the enemy. In every state in the nation there is serious debate regarding capital punishment. Is it right to kill people because they have committed heinous crimes, such as murder? Is the use of capital punishment a statement that we condone the killing of a criminal and that killing under these circumstances will solve the problem? Another controversial issue involving death is abortion. Such groups as the Right to Life organization say that abortion is murder, akin to genocide. Yet abortion is legal if certain guidelines are followed—for example, if it is performed in the first trimester of pregnancy or if the mother's life is at risk.

Some Americans have very negative attitudes toward death, primarily because they are uncomfortable with their own mortality. Many people associate death only with loss, pain, suffering, frustrated desires, and uncompleted goals. They see death as a separation from people they love, from places or objects they treasure, and from a part of their own self-identity, and they fail to see anything positive in death.

Otherwise mature individuals often find themselves unable to cope with the thought of death. These people generally choose to try to ignore death, to pretend on a subconscious level that they are immortal. This attitude is assumed primarily out of a fear of death. Furthermore, other people's deaths remind us of our own vulnerability, causing us to feel totally helpless, as if nothing we can say or do can change a thing.

Many people try to avoid even mentioning death. When the subject of personal death or the death of someone close comes up, there are often looks of dismay and discomfort until someone changes the subject. When people refer to death, they often use euphemisms that do not imply the finality, totality, and complete separation from life that death is. These euphemisms include "passed away," "departed," "gone to his rest," and "gone to her great reward." Such phrases make it easier to talk about and think about death because they soothe the harshness of its reality. The use of euphemisms is an extension of the denial attitude that many Americans take toward death.

These attitudes can have a profound influence on people's lives. If death is nothing but fear, and if fear prevents people from thinking and acting, they then become less than human. Also, if the fear of death does limit an individual's view of the future, this negative attitude can hinder the person's ability to plan ahead, to anticipate both hazards and opportunities in life.

POSITIVE APPROACHES TO DEATH

Death should not be considered taboo. It should be seen as a natural part of our existence. The more absolute death becomes, the more meaningful life can become. Death is as much a part of human existence and the life cycle as birth. It is not an enemy to be conquered, but an integral part of life that gives meaning to human existence. Death sets a limit on our time in this life, urging us to do something meaningful with that time as long as it is ours to use. Dying is the final chance to grow, to become more truly who you are. Those who truly are reconciled to their own mortal existence are the ones who get the most out of life. Such a positive approach to death frees one to focus on the daily tasks of living life more fully.

A normal and healthy fear of death is considered essential to the preservation of life because this fear leads us to take certain precautions. But we should not allow this fear to affect our emotional health in a negative way. We must find ways to cope effectively with death and dying, and it is not enough to intellectualize. The quality of our life depends on our ability to acknowledge reality and to deal appropriately with death and dying. The first step in overcoming a fear of death is to face it openly and resolve any unrealistic fears by looking into the causes of those fears. Frank and open discussion about death can help a person to diminish fear, anxiety, aggression, and other conflicts associated with death and to develop a positive attitude.

Various media that have been used to help people confront death are religion, art, music, and poetry. For example, those who characterize themselves as religious tend to report less death anxiety than those who do not characterize themselves in this way (DeSpelder and Strickland 2002, 540). Most religions believe that death comes only to the physical self and that one's spirit (or soul) will survive.

Furthermore, people who have shared in the death of someone who understood death's meaning tend to develop a more positive attitude toward dying and death. Those who have a healthy attitude toward death and who consider it truly one phase of existence have profited from this frame of mind. Positive attitudes toward dying can enhance the meaningfulness and richness of life for many, even for the terminally ill.

Personal Beliefs about Death

Personal beliefs are helpful in coping with the reality of death and dying, whether these beliefs are called ethics, thoughts, meditations, or religion. People rely on personal beliefs to find comfort in the face of death. Some use religious beliefs as an escape, as if to gain personal exemption from the reality of death. However, belonging to any particular religious group does not guarantee that death will be faced any more positively. Religious beliefs or philosophical and spiritual systems can be very helpful. They can give one's life a sense of significance. They can also provide a sense of forgiveness—to oneself and to others (Dickinson, Leming, and Mermann 2000, 96).

Needs of a Dying Person

Fear is the most typical psychological response that a dying person experiences. Dying people often fear humiliation, a sense of failure, a loss of self-worth, and anxiety about the future. Other common fears of the dying are the fear of the unknown (that is, not knowing what will happen after death), fear of being disfigured, fear of pain, fear of indignity, and a fear of abandonment by friends and relatives (Marrone 1997, 79–81).

In a sense, dying people have no model to follow. They feel like strangers to the healthy living because no one understands what they are going through. Most dying people want to talk about death and their own illness; unfortunately, sometimes they cannot find anyone willing to discuss these matters.

ADJUSTING TO DYING

Adjusting to dying during the grief process consists of a number of phases, such as shock and numbness, denial, intense grief (which consists of yearning, anger, guilt, and disorganization), and finally reorganization or resolution. This adjustment period occurs differently in each individual and does not necessarily happen in sequential process. Understanding these stages of adjustment to impending death is critical in understanding the needs of the dying person. These phases occur to the person who learns that he or she is going to die as well as to the bereaved person grieving the loss of the deceased.

Shock and numbness are the most immediate reactions to death—the dying person cannot accept the fact that he or she is going to die, and the bereaved cannot consciously believe that the death just occurred. They are typically followed by a period of denial. This is the mind's normal reaction to protect the person from something he or she may not be able to handle emotionally at that time.

Intense grief includes a collection of fears (as discussed earlier in this chapter) on the part of the dying person and a subconscious searching for the deceased by those still living because the thoughts and behavior of the bereaved are

Health Highlight

EMOTIONAL AND PSYCHOLOGICAL RESPONSES

TO LIFE-THREATENING ILLNESS

Elisabeth Kübler-Ross developed an early model of stages associated with emotional and psychological responses to life-threatening illness.

1. **Denial and isolation**—learning of the diagnosis of a terminal condition, the patient reacts with disbelief.

2. **Anger**—the reality of impending death begins to seep into the patient's consciousness, and anger is the reaction.

3. **Bargaining**—the patient is accepting the inevitability of death and begins to bargain (with God and others) for more time.

4. **Depression**—the patient is saddened by the fact that death is approaching and then starts the grief process for the losses death will entail.

5. **Acceptance (or Resolution)**—the patient resolves the issue of death.

SOURCE: DeSpelder and Strickland 2002, 156

focused on the deceased. Hallucinations are not uncommon because of the intense desire for the return of the deceased. Anger is manifested by irritability directed at anyone who comes in contact with the dying person or the bereaved, and it is sometimes even directed at God. The anger may be directed at oneself because of thoughts such as "If I had only done this with my life" or "If I had only done this while he or she was alive." During this intense grief, the dying person and the bereaved often experience despair. Apathy, aimlessness, futility, emptiness, and disorganization are all manifested during this time.

Reintegration is a time of recovery or resolution. This phase occurs when the dying person comes to grips with his or her own mortality and when the bereaved begins to function normally once again. This indicates that the bereaved has resolved the meaning and the purpose of the death and has decided that he or she is going to be healthy and can function even in light of the loss that has occurred. Even when reintegration occurs, there can still be pain during special times, such as anniversaries, birthdays, and holidays (Hales 1999, 606).

It should be noted that each person is as unique in death as in life, and everyone responds differently. Some may progress naturally through these phases, whereas others might reach one of the latter phases of adjustment, then regress. Further, not all dying people will reach the phase of resolution before they die.

The Family of a Dying Person

Impending death affects family members of the dying person in various ways. Sometimes there is a strong prohibition in the family against talk of death because family members feel this may bring about death more quickly. Some family members think that a discussion of death would make the others in the family more uncomfortable, and any discussion may seem to be related to an undue interest in the estate of the dying person. The loss of an important family member, such as the head of a household, can threaten certain social and psychological arrangements. This can lead to enormous stresses and cause tension among all remaining members.

Besides grief, emotional reactions to the death of a family member may range from guilt and anger to fear, anxiety, and money worries. Sometimes the anger is directed toward the person who died: "He died and left me with all these debts" or "She deserted us during a crucial time in our lives." Further, death is a reminder of the survivors' own vulnerability, which evokes fear in itself. If the dying person lives in the home before death, tension and resentment can develop. When family members have to sacrifice their own friends and activities to provide care, feelings of hostility and anger toward the dying person can develop. Then the anger turns to guilt, which has been described as anger turned inward. Some family members tend to feel inadequate when confronted with this overwhelming situation. They tend to want to protect themselves and the dying relative by not speaking to the person. This is wrong because it leads to emotional abandonment, making the situation all the more difficult for the dying person. Compassion, not isolation, should be given.

When circumstances permit, the family can help the most by maintaining an emotional and social environment consistent with the person's past life. This means keeping the person at home or in a hospice rather than in a hospital or nursing home, if possible. The family should include the dying relative as a participant in every discussion, especially those that involve decisions about that person's care and welfare. The family should do all they can to show their love and concern without doing it in ways that make the person feel guilty for being a burden to them. Family members should not allow their inability to face death to hinder the dying person's adjustment. When the person is ready to accept the reality of dying, the family should share that acceptance. An absence of support at this crucial time will mean that the person will die without dignity.

The Grief Experience

Grief is usually described as sorrow, mental distress, emotional agitation, sadness, suffering, and related feelings caused by a death. **Bereavement** refers to a state of experiencing grief. **Mourning** is composed of culturally defined acts that are usually performed when death occurs.

The closer the relationship of the bereaved to the deceased, the stronger the emotional response. Among these emotions and patterns of behavior are sadness, anger, fear, anxiety, guilt, loneliness, tension, loss of appetite, weight loss, loss of interest in things once interesting, a decrease in socialization, and disrupted sleep. These responses are usually greater when the death is unexpected.

Grief and mourning are generally much less formal in the United States than in some other cultures or than they were in early America. Today people generally have greater freedom to determine for themselves what kind of grieving, bereaving, and mourning are appropriate (DeSpelder and Strickland 2002, 225).

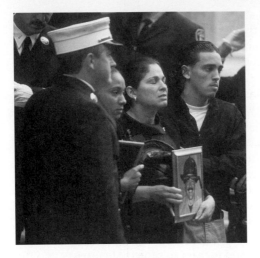

Funerals meet many emotional needs of the survivors.

Studies of mourning show that it is therapeutic for survivors to talk about the deceased and work through their death-related problems in counseling sessions (Hales 1999, 606). Another form of therapy involves going to work, going to school, or participating in organizational activities. Americans seem in need of much more elaboration of death ceremonies than some other cultures. This may explain why many in our society place a strong emphasis on the rituals of funerals and burials.

FUNERALS AND RELATED RITUALS

The funeral is an organized, group-centered response to death. It involves rituals and ceremonies during which the body of the deceased is usually present. The traditional funeral includes speaking to the needs of the mourners. Some religions include a eulogy of the deceased, and some include an open casket that survivors view as part of the ceremony.

An alternative to the traditional funeral is a memorial service. Memorial services are sometimes held in conjunction with a cremation (with the urn present or absent) or when the body is not present for some reason (such as being donated to a medical school immediately on death or the family preferring not to have the body present). This service is held in a church, chapel, home, or whatever place is considered appropriate by the family. The service is not a eulogy but a chance to show thankfulness for having known the person. It also gives an opportunity for the expression of grief and sharing with family members. Generally, individuals who hold a memorial service are using this time to celebrate the life of the deceased while on earth, as opposed to mourning. Memorial services are most common among families who have strong religious convictions and the belief in life after death. Memorial services are becoming more common even among the nonreligious.

A primary purpose of the funeral is to dispose of the body. It also meets many emotional needs, like grief and mourning, of the survivors. The visitation part of the funeral ceremony is important for friends to show their respect for the deceased and support for the survivors. Also, viewing the casket, which is part of some funeral home visits, is important to some for realization (seeing and thus believing that the person is dead) and recall (providing an acceptable image for recalling the deceased). For these reasons, the funeral home visitation can be therapeutic for friends as well as family.

Cemeteries, with markers for each grave, formerly were thought of as very sacred places where relatives and friends could go in quiet and peace to show their respect to the dead. Now, however, many cemeteries are crowded, congested, and impersonal. The relatives and friends of the deceased may also live many miles from the burial site. For these reasons, cemetery visits are less common than they once were. This ritual is not used as often in working out grief and mourning among the survivors.

Issues Surrounding Death

Some topics related to death have become the focal point of controversy in recent years. These issues include the definition of death, organ transplants and donations, the right to die, wills, and suicide.

DEFINITIONS OF DEATH

For thousands of years, the time of death was clearly defined as the time of cessation of life functions. Now, however, with advanced medical technology, life can be sustained beyond when death formerly would have occurred. The problem of defining it is much more complex—for example, not just knowing when a person is dead, but being able to determine the exact moment of death. This is important in the case of potential organ transplants, when every second is critical. Some say that a person is brain dead when the entire brain is dead, even if respiration and circulation could be maintained artificially. Others argue that a person is dead when the outer surface of the cerebrum of the brain has ceased to function (see pages 188–191). (This individual may still breathe spontaneously via control of the brain stem, but thinking and reasoning ability would have ceased.)

Definitions of death center around "brain," "heart," or "physiological" death when various organs cease to function and "clinical" death when there is a total lack of response to any external or internal stimuli, lack of spontaneous respiration, fixed and dilated pupils, lack of brainstem reflexes, and a flat electrocardiogram (i.e., no heartbeat). The significance of the definition of death is not just for the purpose of organ transplants. It also indicates which human lives can be saved, possibly with life-support systems such as heart–lung machines.

Some people wish to donate their organs or entire body for scientific and medical uses. This sometimes involves an urgent decision at the time of the donor's death. Biological, medical, and legal ethics are all involved in this issue. For those who wish to donate an organ, the Uniform Anatomical Gift Act of 1978 sets guidelines underlying the donor laws of each state. Some individuals donate their entire bodies to medical schools for dissection. Other parts of the body that can be donated include eyes for corneal transplants; ear bones to temporal bone banks for use in research into ear diseases; kidneys for kidney transplants; pituitary glands for use in producing growth hormone for those who lack this vital substance; and hearts for heart transplants.

Virtually no religion in our country places restrictions on organ donations to help another patient regain health. Further, the donation of an organ does not interrupt or modify the planned funeral service for the donor in any way. A donor needs to have a signed and witnessed donor card, usually carried at all times. These donor cards are available from many agencies in the community, such as the local kidney dialysis clinic or the Department of Motor Vehicles.

Many organs and body parts can be transplanted successfully. Decisions about who will receive a donated organ can be difficult and painful. An average of sixty-three people will receive a donated organ via transplant on a given day, while another sixteen people will die for lack of a transplanted organ. The question of who receives the organ is usually determined by who will most benefit from the transplant. Candidates who are more likely to die or suffer complications if not given a transplant are given priority over those in less dire circumstances. Among the most often donated organs are the heart, kidneys, pancreas, lungs, liver, intestines, cornea, skin, bone marrow, heart valves and connective tissue (U.S. Department of Health and Human Services 2003; United Network for Organ Sharing 2003). The donor must die in a hospital, since surgery must be performed within hours if the organ(s) is to be used. For example, the heart is suitable for transplantation for only four to five hours. For this reason, surgeries are usually begun simultaneously for the donor and the recipient. The liver must also be transplanted within four to five hours, but the kidneys are suitable for transplantation for thirty-six to forty-eight hours.

It is not always known for sure who will receive the transplant, nor is such information as the donor's name or hometown usually given. General information is provided, though. An example of this would be the information that the kidney of a thirteen-year-old who died in an automobile accident was used. Anyone eighteen years or older and of sound mind may donate by signing a donor card. Anyone under eighteen years may become a donor if either a parent or the legal guardian gives permission. Most body parts from a person who is over fifty-five are not accepted for donation.

Although much of transplant surgery is still classified as experimental, the future is encouraging. Medical knowledge and technology are improving every day. Today two-thirds of the patients receiving liver transplants live beyond the first year. Even when a transplant patient lives only a few months, most families consider the operation worthwhile, because the patient's quality of life was probably vastly improved.

THE RIGHT TO DIE AND EUTHANASIA

Euthanasia, or death with dignity, is not just a medical problem because it also involves legal, ethical, social, personal, and financial considerations. For this reason, the debate over euthanasia involves many professionals and paraprofessionals, as well as the patients and their families. The arguments now have to do with the dignity of the patients, the quality of their lives, their mental state, and sometimes their usefulness to society. For example, the patient who is in a vegetative state is considered dead by some but not by others, and this case presents substantial ethical and logistical problems. Some say that to intervene in any way is to "play God," while others maintain that the rights of the patient are violated if the medical staff does not allow the patient to die. Such procedures as using a life-support machine to sustain life are sometimes seen as heroic acts, but others think this only prolongs the suffering of the patient. Therefore, the line between heroic procedures (or unnecessary care) and giving up (or neglecting the patient) is difficult to draw. This distinction would be simple if we could just ask patients which treatment they wanted, but this is not possible in a majority of such cases.

Today we are being forced to rethink our ideas and choices about life, dying, and death. The issue of euthanasia is an excellent example of this. Currently, there is a change in emphasis in the euthanasia debate. The focus is less on allowing people to die a natural and painless death and more on allowing death to occur by withholding medical treatment. Typically, patients involved in a case of euthanasia are severely deformed or severely diseased infants or the terminally ill. Often the decision to practice euthanasia is more of a decision between letting the person die now or later, rather than a choice between life and death. Some argue that the movement in favor of euthanasia may be rooted in our fear of facing death, and that euthanasia is used to hasten death so that we will not have to cope with the consequences associated with the actual process of dying. A related issue that intensifies the problem is that many times the life, living, dying, or death decision is made by medical staffs or families about someone else's life or death.

Euthanasia has come to imply a contract for the termination of life in order to avoid unnecessary suffering at the end of a fatal illness. Direct (or active) euthanasia is defined as a deliberate action to shorten life. It involves a procedure such as injecting air or a chemical substance into the bloodstream. This is termed *mercy killing* and is still considered murder in our country, although some feel it should be permissible. A related phenomenon is physician-assisted suicide in which the physician supplies the equipment and medicine needed, and the patient performs the act necessary to cause death (Ferrini and Ferrini 2000, 472).

In the early 1990s, Dr. Jack Kevorkian intensified the debate over assisted suicide. He created a suicide machine that delivered an anesthetic and a lethal injection of potassium chloride through an intravenous line. Though he was not convicted for providing such assistance with this machine, Kevorkian was convicted of second degree murder for actively administering lethal drugs to an incurably ill person, even though that person had requested his assistance. Kevorkian's actions provoked discussion of the thin line separating passive euthanasia, which is legal in this country, and active euthanasia. Opponents of

Kevorkian's actions state that he is practicing assisted suicide, which is illegal. Proponents of Kevorkian's actions argue that the patient's right to control his or her medical treatment is sufficient justification for assisted suicide.

In the United States and Canada, a physician is permitted legally to accede to a mentally competent patient's desire to refuse medical treatment, even if the refusal will result in death. These laws do not permit physicians to assist a patient to die—this is considered a form of murder or manslaughter. Today the majority of states have legislation defining suicide assistance as a felony punishable by several years in prison. The Criminal Code of Canada also prohibits suicide assistance. Kevorkian is currently appealing his conviction; in the last several years, those who favor legalizing assisted suicide in the United States and Canada have challenged the constitutionality of these laws. The Supreme Court of the United States allows each state to determine whether or not to prohibit or permit assisted suicide (Beauchamp 1997–2003).

Rapid advances in medical technology have given the medical profession the ability to sustain or prolong life through extraordinary methods, so that those who might have died quickly now have a chance of survival with life-sustaining artificial support mechanisms. An adult in this country is considered to have the right to determine whether this type of medical technology should be employed. The person has the right to expressly prohibit life-saving surgery or other medical treatments. In other words, the right to die with dignity is inherent for every individual, as much as the right to live. Some individuals fear the indignity and humiliation of existing merely as a vegetable, with others making decisions for them and caring for their every need. These people would rather die a "good death" than exist in this manner. The proponents of euthanasia state that saving a life is not always the same as saving people, as some do not wish to go on living or be revived. They argue that further extension of life should not be forced on the person just so life itself is preserved. This places an emphasis on the quality of life rather than just the literal existence of life.

Some families are using Health Care Advance Directives to handle this situation. Such a directive allows a person who is unable to speak for him- or herself to designate a person to make health care decisions (such as the kind of health care desired in such a situation) for him or her.

One example of a Health Care Advance Directive is a living will. In this type of document, a person is allowed to state his or her desires about life-sustaining medical treatments in case it becomes impossible to state those wishes later. Another document, a Health Care Power of Attorney, allows a person to appoint a designated person to make medical treatment decisions for him or her. If you do not wish to name such a person, you may state very specific wishes, such as the desire to donate certain organs.

A Health Care Advance Directive is intended to be used when a person cannot make or communicate decisions because of a temporary or permanent illness or injury. Such a document allows a person to keep control over important health care decisions through a designated agent.

Special care should be taken in choosing an agent for a Health Care Advance Directive because this person will be making significant medical decisions on your behalf. If you do not appoint such a person to speak on your behalf, the health care provider may make the decisions for you or the court will appoint a guardian on your behalf. The advance directive permits the family to know your desires and keeps them from having to make such stressful decisions.

Every state and the District of Columbia has laws that permit advance directives. Though the state laws vary in their wording, the basic principle of serving as a written statement of the patient's values and preferences is present in each law. Most states require two witnesses for advance directives, and some require a notarized signature for those witnesses.

If a person changes his or her mind, an advance directive may be amended or canceled in writing. If an advance directive is amended or canceled, the old or superseded directive should be destroyed. Also, anytime a person writes an advance directive, he or she should ensure that his or her closest relatives are aware of the directive. It is a good idea to give those relatives a copy of the directive, as well as providing a copy to his or her physician (American Association of Retired Persons 1995).

WILLS

The last will and testament is a legal instrument declaring a person's intentions concerning the disposition of property, the guardianship of children, or the administration of the estate after a person's death. A will is a legal document in which a person states how he or she wants property and possessions to be distributed after his or her death. By making such a document, people can ensure how their property will be distributed, the cost and time of settling the estate can be reduced, consequences of estate and inheritance taxes may be avoided, an executor can be named, family quarrels can be avoided, a guardian can be appointed, and a testamentary trust can be created. For most people, ensuring the desired distribution of their property and possessions is sufficient reason for writing a will. Further, a person can enact a living trust that entrusts an estate to another person while the owner of the estate is still alive. A living trust keeps the estate private instead of public, even when the owner of the estate dies. A living trust can avoid probate, attorney fees, and some taxation when the owner of the estate dies.

Perhaps because ours is a society that denies death, most people delay writing a will. It is not surprising that most Americans, even many with sizable estates, do not have a will since writing a will reminds people of their own mortality. For individuals who die without wills, property passes according to state law. In other words, the state will decide which relatives get which part of the estate, even if the deceased person may have wished otherwise.

NEAR-DEATH EXPERIENCES

The near-death experiences that have been reported are remarkably similar to each other, whether they occur in young people or old, whether the result of an accident or illness, and whether the person is actually near death or just thinks he or she is. This has led many to believe that these experiences are not merely dreams, as was thought initially. Some physicians report not only that their patients have similar experiences, but also that the events occur in much the same sequence. Some report being able to watch events transpiring from several feet in the air (including resuscitation attempts on themselves) or feeling a sense of passing into another dimension or foreign region. Some see light, often as if at the end of a tunnel, with their vision clearer and their hearing sharper. Some recall seeing scenes from their earlier life and/or seeing loved ones who have died.

Many people who experience near-death experiences as hospital patients undergoing surgery can recall procedures used on them and remember what each person in the room said. One patient, a nurse in a coma, had total recall of the exact procedures used. These patients also reported an instant replay of their own lives. Some patients have multiple experiences during a prolonged illness—some of these experiences are bad (usually the first ones), while others are very good. The patients themselves interpret whether the experience is good or bad. Sometimes the unpleasant experiences are so frightening that the conscious mind cannot cope with them, and the patient suppresses them into the subconscious (DeSpelder and Strickland 2002, 520–527).

HOSPICES

A hospice is a program, type of care, or facility that cares for the terminally ill and their families. Sometimes hospice care is given in the patient's home and at other times in a separate wing of a hospital. Generally the goal of hospice care is to enhance the quality of a dying person's life during the last days and to allow the person to live as comfortably and inexpensively as possible.

SUICIDE

During the last half of this century, suicide among school-age students has increased dramatically. Suicide is now one of the leading causes of death for U.S. youth (Marrone 1997, 187).

There is more guilt associated with suicide than with any other type of death. Parents or relatives often feel they are somehow to blame. Some feel that a suicide reflects badly on the parents and family, but this is not always the case. Some hold a religious view that suicide is morally wrong or that one who commits suicide cannot enter heaven.

Any suicidal threat, however subtle, must be taken seriously. Most individuals who commit suicide provide significant clues to their contemplated action. These include obvious changes in mood or behavior, excessive use of drugs, changes in any set of habits, preoccupation with personal health, decreased academic performance, and insomnia.

There are four commonly recommended steps for helping someone who seems in danger of suicide. First, one should talk to the person who threatens suicide and determine how deeply troubled the individual really is. Second, one should not challenge the individual to act on the threat. Such a challenge may force the person to act to prove the validity of the threat. Third, someone can help the person postpone the decision and offer other options to consider. Fourth, one should be knowledgeable about resources that can provide aid. The person threatening suicide might have exhausted all personally known avenues of assistance and might need professional help.

Suicide prevention is a community responsibility, and everyone can play an important part in its resolution. However, many people have misconceptions about suicide. For example, they think a person who talks about suicide will not commit suicide; that a person talking about suicide just wants attention; or that a person who is suicidal at one point in his or her life is suicidal forever.

Young People and Death

Many young people in the United States no longer experience many former aspects of the traditional life cycle. Most do not live with grandparents or on farms, so they do not observe aging and death in their immediate environment. Death education is necessary for the proper development of children. Death education should be viewed as a natural topic for inclusion in education because students are not immune to experiencing the death of a loved one, a pet, or a classmate.

Youth in our country continue to commit suicide. In fact, suicide is the third leading cause of death for fifteen- to twenty-four-year-olds and the sixth leading cause of death for five- to fourteen-year-olds. For younger children (five to fourteen), the causes for increasing numbers of suicides are stress, confusion, pressure to succeed, and financial uncertainty. For older youth, causes include divorce, problems in adjusting to a blended family, or making new friends in a new school or community.

Many of these stated reasons are treatable through counseling, especially if the problems are recognized and diagnosed appropriately. However, some parents fail to recognize the warning signs for suicide in their own children. Parents and teachers should be aware of the following signs in adolescents who may try to kill themselves:

- change in eating and sleeping habits
- withdrawal from friends, family, and regular activities
- violent actions, rebellious behavior, or running away repeatedly
- drug and alcohol use
- unusual neglect of personal appearance
- marked personality change
- persistent boredom, difficulty concentrating, or a decline in the quality of schoolwork
- frequent complaints about physical symptoms, often related to emotions, such as stomachaches, headaches, fatigue, etc.
- loss of interest in pleasurable activities
- not tolerating praise or reward
- complaining of being a bad person or feeling "rotten inside"
- giving verbal hints with statements such as: "I won't be a problem for you much longer," "Nothing matters," "It's no use," and "I won't see you again"

- putting his or her affairs in order—for example, giving away favorite possessions, cleaning his or her room, and throwing away important belongings
- becoming suddenly cheerful after a period of depression
- showing signs of psychosis (hallucinations or bizarre thoughts)

If anyone makes a statement indicating a desire to take his or her own life, the statement should be taken seriously, and the person should be referred to a psychiatrist or psychologist. Though most people refrain from talking about death, a person making such a statement should be asked if he or she is depressed or thinking about suicide. This will let the young person know that you care and that you are willing to listen to his or her problems. With support from family and professional treatment, children and teenagers who are suicidal can heal and return to a healthier path of development (Youth Suicide Prevention 2001).

Death is inseparable from the whole of human experience. Education about death can bring insights concerning the true nature of young people and help them discover more about themselves. The study of death and dying leads naturally to choices of an emphatically personal nature. Death education could appropriately be renamed "life and loss education" because only through awareness of our lifelong losses and appreciation of our mortality are we free to be in the present, to live fully (DeSpelder and Strickland 2002, 34).

DEATH EDUCATION

Positive attitudes toward death can help prepare succeeding generations to face death more realistically. We can help young people accept the reality of death by preparing them properly for funerals and by allowing them to mourn, cry, recover from the loss of a pet or a relative, and express grief as part of the healing process. We should talk to them about death in terms they can understand. This discussion can be either from a religious or a factual point of view, depending on the preference of the parents and of the student.

We should explain the cause of death in order to eliminate any fear or guilt the young person might develop as a result of experiencing a death. Do not deceive them by using euphemisms or half-truths. One way to teach young people about death is to allow—but not force—them to attend a funeral or burial service. A recommended method is to take them first to the funeral of a neighbor or distant relative. Because the parents would not be as physically or emotionally involved in such a situation, they could devote time and energy to their children. Make the funeral a learning experience. Prepare the children before the funeral, ask them to watch for certain things during the funeral, and encourage their questions afterward. Education through attendance at a funeral will help young people gain a more complete understanding of death and make it more likely that they will develop a healthy attitude about death.

Finally, young people should be encouraged to talk openly about their fears and feelings. This will help eliminate any misgivings they have and help the parents to respond more appropriately to the emotions expressed. Of course, this assumes that the parents know how to respond and that they will share their own emotions with their children.

Fortunately, people today are more willing than before to discuss death and dying. The many books available on the subject; the courses being taught in schools and universities; the increased number of bereavement societies and hospice groups, and the increasing number of documentaries, specials, and films are evidence of this. The new openness about death is refreshing—a challenge to the previous treatment of death as a taboo topic for conversation, research, and writing. Communication about death can improve the quality of our lives and help us grow as individuals. Even if we fumble through a discussion on death, as a friend or parent, our effort is very helpful.

Death is a universal part of living, even though it is often a taboo topic in our society. Young people are interested in knowing more about the subject of death, but they are generally shielded from such exposure. Many parents are reluctant to talk with their children about death because they wish to protect their children (and themselves) from the pain of loss. Young people are often prohibited from some hospital wards, health care institutions, and other places where people are dying. Such apparent secretiveness may result in fear or curiosity, and as a result of their lack of first-hand knowledge, young people tend to learn about death through the media, which can be confusing and misleading.

Sooner or later, students must confront death to understand the needs of the dying, to have some preparation for the experience, and to deal with their own feelings. Education about death is a legitimate subject for students. It is an important topic worthy of open, informed, and sensitive discussion. Death education can guide students toward greater understanding about death and dying, and, even though it might be painful for them and for the teacher, gaining such understanding can be essential for sound mental health.

In death education, the teacher should come to terms with his or her own feelings about death and not just learn the material. He or she needs to be aware of the students' willingness to express their feelings on this sensitive topic and be ready to let them discuss the subject openly and frankly. Never tell students they need to wait until they are older to talk about death. Many adults use this ploy as an excuse to avoid their own insecurities about death. Teachers need to answer any question at the students' level of understanding. The students' feelings and emotions related to death should also be allowed to be expressed in the classroom, even encouraged. Teachers can use experiences in the classroom, such as the death of a flower, a pet, or a classmate, to teach students about death feelings and rituals.

Summary

- Aging is a normal part of the life cycle, not a pathological condition. We are all aging every day.
- The number of elderly has risen sharply in the past two decades, and this trend is predicted to continue.
- The life expectancy for all Americans is increasing.

- The majority of older Americans still own their own homes, and fewer than 5 percent are institutionalized.

- Both intrinsic and extrinsic factors affect the aging process for each individual.

- Many biological, psychological, and sociological changes occur as a person ages. Some of these changes present unavoidable problems for the elderly, but successful adjustments can be made to other changes.

- Elderly Americans face many challenges in life, but these issues affect all members of society, not just the aged. Among these challenges are income, retirement, housing, health problems, nutrition, crime, and transportation.

- Some of the problems facing the elderly are the result of discrimination and misconceptions.

- Stereotypes about the elderly largely result from lack of knowledge and insufficient contact with the elderly.

- Intergenerational contact programs in schools can be one of the most effective ways to help students understand aging and the elderly, helping dissolve some of the many myths about aging.

- The elderly of the future will generally enjoy a better standard of living.

- Death is the natural end to life, yet many in our society try to deny its existence.

- Death is mysterious because we do not know what is beyond death.

- Many people fear death and refuse to discuss the topic openly and frankly.

- Everyone has personal beliefs about death. Some of these beliefs are helpful in facing death because they help demystify it.

- Facing death is a traumatic experience for both the dying person and survivors.

- The dying person has many emotional needs that often go unmet by relatives and the medical profession. This may leave the dying person feeling lonely and abandoned.

- An individual goes through various stages of adjustment to impending death. If we understand these stages, we can better help the dying person.

- Controversies and issues surround death, including the definition of death, the person's right to die, organ donation and transplants, wills, and suicide.

- Most young people in our society are not exposed to the dying process and lose relatively few individuals with whom they are close.

- Young people go through definite stages in their understanding of death.

- Young people are interested in knowing more about the subject of death. Thus, death education is a legitimate, worthy topic in schools.

DISCUSSION QUESTIONS

1. Discuss the significance of aging education and death education in the school curriculum.

2. Describe the benefits of intergenerational contact.

3. Discuss the current demographics of the elderly in the United States.

4. Predict the lifestyle of the elderly in the United States in the year 2020.

5. Why do most people fear death?

6. How can the family help in the adjustment of a dying person?

7. Differentiate between grief, bereavement, and mourning.

8. Why is there more guilt associated with a death by suicide than with other types of deaths?

CRITICAL THINKING QUESTIONS

1. Rate your personal health in relation to the aging process. In other words, what health skills and behaviors do you possess that will help you age in a healthy way?

2. What are three things that you consider most positive about getting older? What are three concerns you have about aging?

3. It is likely that you will be the primary caregiver for your parent or grandparent. What steps can you take now to prepare for this event?

4. Consider a situation in which you or a close relative have received a diagnosis of a terminal illness. What activities or tasks would you accomplish? What type of circumstances would you desire for your impending death?

5. Contemplate your own attitude toward death—is it negative or positive? What factors in your own life experiences have affected your attitude toward dying and death?

6. Some argue that without proper legislative controls, passive euthanasia may lead to active euthanasia. Propose several controls to prevent this from occurring.

7. Think about the most recent funeral you attended. How would you want your own funeral to be similar or different?

8. How would you design a suicide prevention program specifically for the age of the students you desire to teach?

WEB SITE ACTIVITIES

Go to the Administration on Aging Web site at *www.aoa.dhhs.gov/aoa/stats/ profile,* and determine the five states with the largest elderly population.

Go to the Partnership for Caring Web site at *www.partnershipforcaring.org.* Follow the links to find the Analysis of the Supreme Court Decisions on Physician Assisted Suicide and summarize your interpretation of the analysis.

WEB SITES OF INTEREST

American Association of Retired Persons (AARP): *www.aarp.org*
AARP is a nonprofit, nonpartisan association dedicated to shaping and enriching the experience of aging for all Americans; it is the nation's largest organization of midlife and older persons.

National Institute on Aging (NIA): *www.nia.nih.gov*
The NIA is one of the National Institutes of Health—the principal biomedical research agency of the United States government. It promotes healthy aging by conducting and supporting public education and biomedical, social, and behavioral research.

Administration on Aging (AoA): *www.aoa.gov*
The AoA is emerging as the focal point for the nation's expression of its concern for the needs of its elders and is tasked with the responsibility for assuring that the needs of older Americans are considered in the formulation of policy and cross-cutting initiatives that have an impact on an aging society.

National Council on the Aging (NCOA): *www.ncoa.org*
NCOA is an association of organizations and individuals dedicated to promoting the dignity, self-determination, well-being, and continuing contributions of older persons through leadership and service, education, and advocacy by providing leadership, education and training, publications, research and development, community services, employment programs, coalition building, public policy, and advocacy efforts.

Association for Death Education and Counseling (ADEC): *www.adec.org*
ADEC is a multidisciplinary professional organization that uses theory and quality research to provide information, support, and resources and is dedicated to promoting excellence in death education, bereavement counseling, and care of the dying.

Choice in Dying: *www.choices.org*
Choice in Dying, the inventor of living wills in 1967, is a nonprofit organization that provides advance directives, counsels patients and families, trains professionals, advocates for improved laws, and offers a range of publications and services dealing with communication about complex end-of-life decisions.

Raindrop: A Treatment on Death Education for Children of all Ages:
    www.iul.com/raindrop
A reader on death education, primarily written for children ages six to ten.

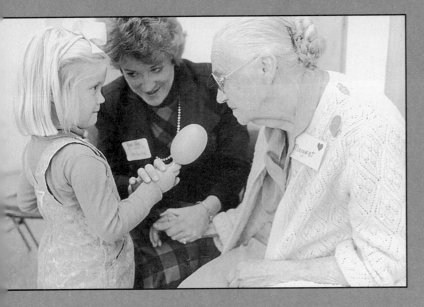

CHAPTER TWENTY-FOUR

Strategies for Teaching about Aging, Dying, and Death

We need to present realistic and accurate information to students about aging, the aged, and death.

VALUED OUTCOMES: AGING

After doing the exercises in this chapter, the students should be able to express and illustrate the following statements:

- Aging is a natural part of the life cycle.
- The body changes as a person ages.
- Exercise and proper diet can slow down the aging process to some degree.
- Most elderly people are healthy and alert.
- Responsibilities change as a person ages.
- People use their retirement years for different activities from those done in preretirement times.
- Elderly people make positive contributions to society.

- Grandparents and grandchildren can share activities.
- Older people face many changes and challenges.
- Medications affect older people differently than they do younger people.
- Nutritional needs change as one ages.
- Everyone needs to continue to exercise throughout one's lifetime.
- The elderly in the United States are often discriminated against.
- Many social agencies provide services for the elderly.

VALUED OUTCOMES: DYING AND DEATH

- Death is a natural end to the life cycle.
- Our society generally avoids the topics of death and dying in discussion and conscious thought.
- Personal beliefs about death and dying can affect mental health and lifestyle.
- There are vastly contrasting views on what happens to us after we die.
- There are many misconceptions about how to treat a dying person.
- Dying people have special needs.
- The family of a dying person has special needs.
- Grief and bereavement naturally follow the death of a close friend or relative.
- Funeral and burial rituals have significant meaning in our society.
- The number of suicide attempts among young people is increasing.
- There are ways to help a friend who is contemplating suicide to reconsider the action.
- Organ donation can be considered an "ultimate gift of life."

REFLECTIONS

Aging: As you teach about aging, have the students reflect upon the positive aspects (e.g., more experience, more confidence, more wisdom) of getting older.

Death and Dying: As you teach about the rituals and customs of death and dying, consider how to use these strategies to help your students internalize their feelings about the customs. Ask them to reflect on how a positive attitude about the concepts of death and dying can enable them to add to the quality of their life and how they can help their friends and family develop positive feelings about these issues.

Introduction: Aging

The percentage of elderly adults in our population is growing extremely fast; therefore, the study of aging is becoming important to everyone. Our culture typically propagates ageism through inaccurate portrayals of elderly people in television, movies, and literature. These stereotypes are shared by young people

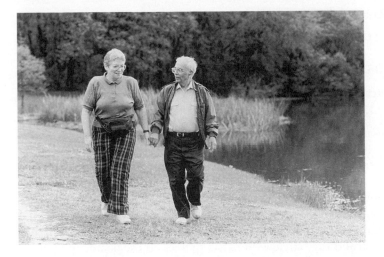

Most elderly people are healthy and alert.

in this country, primarily because of a lack of opportunity to learn about aging and the aged and through a lack of contact with older people. Young people often fear older people and the aging process.

We need to present realistic and accurate information to students about aging and the aged. This will allow students to decide for themselves what aging and the elderly are really like. When students are able to understand and develop healthy attitudes toward aging (including their own aging process), they will be able to live a higher-quality life as they grow older.

Introduction: Dying and Death

The death of a relative, close friend, or even a pet can be traumatic to people of all ages, including children. For this reason, some parents approach the problem by trying to shield their children from experiences related to dying and death. Rather than solving the problem, this avoidance leaves the child unprepared to face a natural part of the life cycle. Many children, though they may not have an accurate concept of death, want to know about the many aspects of life related to dying and death, such as funerals and cemeteries. Death education in the elementary schools can help meet this need. Its objectives are to allow students to clarify their values about death and dying, to provide factual information about the subject, and to encourage students to discuss openly the vital issues concerning the natural end of the life cycle.

Shown to the right of each activity title in this chapter is the suggested grade level(s) for which the activity might be appropriate. However, many of the suggested activities could be modified for use at various grade levels.

Value-Based Activities: Aging

HOW DOES IT FEEL TO BE OLD?   Grades (K–3)

Valued Outcome: The students will understand thoughts we associate with the word *old* and how they affect everyone around them (including themselves).

Description of Strategy: Draw a big circle on the board with the word *kids* in the center. Then draw lines coming from the outside of the circle in toward the word at the center. Ask the class what words they think of when they hear, see, or think the word *kids*. Write the words on the lines of the board. After about three minutes, ask the class how people think of young people their age. Ask how negative and positive attitudes have made them feel. Introduce ageism, a form of discrimination that places people in a limited position because of their age. Draw a second large circle with radiating lines on the board, and put the word *old* instead of *kids* in the center. After three minutes, ask the students how people think of old people and how they think negative and positive attitudes make older people feel.

Materials Needed: board and markers or overhead projector and pen

Processing Question: How do you feel about growing old?

RANK ORDERING   Grades (3–5)

Valued Outcome: The students will be able to decide which qualities associated with aging they most desire.

Description of Strategy: Prepare a list of positive qualities often associated with aging. After discussing these qualities, have students individually rank order each, using the format shown here. Follow with a discussion of why some students feel certain qualities are more desirable than others. Note the importance of individual preferences. Number each of the following from 1 to 5. Use 1 to show the quality or condition about becoming older that appeals to you most, 2 for the second most appealing quality or condition, and so on.

> _____ retirement
>
> _____ wisdom
>
> _____ grandchildren
>
> _____ leisure time
>
> _____ satisfaction

Materials Needed: overhead or handout for each student with list of positive aspects of aging

Processing Question: Why are some qualities associated with aging more desired than others?

AGING TIME LINE   Grades (3–5)

Valued Outcome: The students will be able to state the most important events in their lives.

Description of Strategy: Draw a long timeline on the board. Have different students come to the board and mark on the line the most important dates in their lives, such as date of birth, birthdates of other siblings, date entering school. Stress that many events happen during our lives, but only some are considered most important. Have them notice on the line how much more time they have for birthdays, holidays, and other important events.

Materials Needed: board and markers

Processing Question: Do you think events in the future will be as significant to you as events that have already happened?

AGING VOTING   Grades (K–5)

Valued Outcome: The students will be able to determine for themselves if they agree with aging-related statements.

Description of Strategy: Have students vote by raising their hands if they agree or disagree with the following statements about aging:

- Good health habits may affect the length of your life.
- Having good health habits always means that you are going to live longer than people with bad health habits.
- Bad health habits can shorten the life span.
- It is important to develop good health habits in order to be able to enjoy more years of life.
- Retirement is the worst part about growing old.
- Grandparents are fun to be around.
- Growing old makes a person wiser.
- Growing old is a normal part of life.
- Old people are not very bright.

Materials Needed: list of statements

Processing Question: What factors determine your attitudes about growing old?

SENTENCE COMPLETION   Grades (3–5)

Valued Outcome: The students will be able to complete statements related to aging.

Description of Strategy: Create a handout from the sentences shown below. Instruct students to complete each sentence on the handout by writing down their immediate reaction to the statement. Point out that statements should be honest, even if some are negative. After the exercise, discuss the responses on a volunteer basis. Note varying points of view and discuss possible reasons for these opinions. After the discussion, pass out another copy of the handout for students to fill out and see how their answers may be different.

1. Aging is _____.
2. Growing old is _____.
3. My grandparents are _____.
4. Retirement from full-time work is _____.
5. I think that old people are _____.

Materials Needed: handouts with sentences and pencils for each student

Processing Question: Are your immediate responses the same as they were after you thought about the statement for awhile?

PHYSICAL ACTIVITY IN OLDER AGE   Grades (3–5)

Valued Outcome: The students will be able to describe their feelings when viewing older people exercising.

Description of Strategy: This activity could be done in two different ways. Show a video or DVD (digital video disk) of older people exercising during a fitness class. Have the students write their responses, feelings, and perceptions after seeing older people exercise.

Materials Needed: paper, pens or pencils for each student, video or DVD player and recording of older people exercising

Processing Question: How can exercise in old age improve the quality of life?

VALUE VOTING   Grades (4–5)

Valued Outcome: The students will be able to verbalize their bioethical values regarding death-related issues.

Description of Strategy: Present a series of controversial statements such as those shown below to your class. Explain that each statement represents the way some people feel about death-related issues, then ask students to raise their hands if they basically agree with the stance or to keep their hands down if they disagree. After each show of hands, allow students who wish to comment on the statement to do so. Follow the activity with a general discussion of issues that came up.

- Euthanasia is murder.
- Euthanasia is a peaceful way to die.
- Euthanasia is murder only if the patient is conscious.

Materials Needed: list of statements

Processing Question: Why is euthanasia (or other topic discussed in class) such a controversial issue?

Value-Based Activities: Dying and Death

VALUES STATEMENTS

Grades (K–5)

Valued Outcome: The students will be able to clarify their values regarding death.

Description of Strategy: Have the students complete each of the following statements on a handout with their immediate reaction to the statement. Point out that statements should be honest, even if some are negative. Afterward, discuss how different individuals react and feel about each issue raised in the statements.

    1. When I think about death, I _____.

    2. To me, death means _____.

    3. If I could choose how I will die, I would _____.

    4. My greatest fear about dying is _____.

    5. When I think about relatives who have died, I _____.

Materials Needed: handouts with statements and pencils for all students

Processing Question: What events in your life have determined your attitudes about death?

PERSONAL VIEWS ON SUICIDE

Grades (4–5)

Valued Outcome: The students will be able to clarify their values regarding suicide.

Description of Strategy: Have students answer and discuss these questions:

    1. Do you feel that an individual has the right to make the ultimate decision as to whether he or she should live or die?

    2. What would you do if a friend said to you, "I think I might commit suicide—would you help me?" Would you:
        a. call the police
        b. do nothing
        c. ask why
        d. call a doctor
        e. send your friend away with the statement "Sorry, but I can't help you!"
        f. try to help by talking to him or her

    3. What do you feel might be one possible answer to suicide prevention?

Materials Needed: list of questions

Processing Question: Why do some people feel more positive (or more negative) about suicide as opposed to other types of deaths?

ON LIVING AND DYING

Valued Outcome: The students will be able to decide if death-related ideas are acceptable to them.

Description of Strategy: Have students look over the various statements on a handout created from the list below. Have the students ask themselves, "Would this idea be acceptable or unacceptable to me?"

Rating Scale: Death, Dying, and Living

1 = very acceptable   2 = acceptable   3 = unsure
4 = unacceptable   5 = not acceptable at all

_____ being killed in an auto accident

_____ living forever

_____ dying slowly

_____ dying of cancer

_____ being saved through medical help but unable to walk again

_____ being able to choose when you will die

_____ living to age 110

_____ dying before your spouse

_____ dying after your spouse dies

_____ choosing how you will die

Materials Needed: handouts with statements and pencils for each student

Processing Question: Why should we consider our own deaths?

THE MEDIA AND SEPTEMBER 11, 2001

Valued Outcome: The students will evaluate how their reactions to certain images have changed due to the events of September 11, 2001, in the United States; they will speculate about why these impressions have changed.

Description of Strategy: Have students fold a piece of paper lengthwise down the middle, creating two columns. Students should label the left column Before September 11, 2001 and the right column After September 11, 2001. Explain to the class that they will be viewing a series of images that they may or may not associate with the disastrous events of September 11, but they should record their associations with each of these images from the two perspectives labeled in the headings of the columns. Students can respond in whatever way they wish: jotting down related words, full sentences, or free-writing. Then show the following images, each for two to three minutes at a time to allow students to record their reactions: a jet plane, an American flag, a fireman, and an image of the Manhattan skyline that includes the World Trade Center towers. After students have recorded their reactions to these images, have them share how their impressions of these images may have been altered by the traumatic events of September 11, 2001. Ask the following questions:

- Do you believe that our impressions of these images will be forever altered by the events of that day?

- What circumstances might alter our impressions of these images yet again?

- How does the media contribute to the portrayal of death?
- How do our personal experiences shape the way we interpret these images, both now and in the future?

Materials Needed: photographs of a jet airplane, an American flag, a fireman, and an image of the Manhattan skyline that includes the World Trade Center towers; paper and pencils or pens for each student

Processing Question: How do you feel about the events of September 11, 2001?

Decision Stories: Aging

Follow the procedures outlined in Chapter 4 on pages 80–83 for presenting decision stories.

GOING FOR A VISIT   Grades (K–5)

Fleshika's grandparents live in a retirement village in another state. Her family is going to fly there for a visit next month, but Fleshika doesn't want to go. She visited her grandparents a few years ago, when she was younger. She remembers that there was nothing for her to do at her grandparents' home. There were no other kids around, and her grandparents made such a fuss over her. They were nice, but they treated her like a baby. Fleshika doesn't like that, and she wishes her grandparents would realize that she is growing up.

Focus Question: What should Fleshika do?

Decision Stories: Dying and Death

Follow the procedures outlined in Chapter 4 on pages 80–83 for presenting decision stories.

SALLY'S GRIEF   Grades (3–5)

The mother of Maki's best friend, Sally, died in an automobile accident. Sally had not called Maki yet, but Maki knew that she needed to talk to Sally. She had heard that Sally was not coping with her mother's death well at all. Maki also wanted to see Sally, but she was unsure of what to say or do once she saw Sally.

Focus Question: What could Maki say or do?

A GIFT OF LIFE

Grades (3–5)

Loretta is dying of kidney disease. She knows it and has accepted her coming death. Now her doctors would like to use her heart in a transplant operation. They tell her that her heart could be used to help another person live. Loretta isn't sure about the matter.

Focus Question: What should Loretta do?

Dramatizations: Aging

ROLE-PLAYING LIFE STAGES

Grades (3–5)

Valued Outcome: The students should have a better understanding of the aging process.

Description of Strategy: Assign different roles to students—any role from the family baby, to a teenager, to a grandparent. Students should be encouraged to use costumes and other props to support their role-playing. The role-playing may be performed in mime or otherwise, but it should clearly demonstrate the characteristics of the people they represent. The role-playing exercise in this case would be best performed when showing the response as a member of a family to other members in the family who are aging.

Materials Needed: costumes and props representing various age groups

Processing Questions:

1. What is your response to getting older?
2. What is your favorite stage of life? Why?

GRANDPARENTS AND GRANDCHILDREN

Grades (K–5)

Valued Outcome: The students will be able to discuss relationships with grandparents.

Description of Strategy: Assign several students to role-play a situation involving grandchildren and grandparents. The roles will be grandfather, grandmother, mother, father, sister, and brother. The scene is a visit from the grandparents. The dad will ask the children to remain at home for the day and visit with the grandparents. One child will be instructed to play the role with a lot of enthusiasm, while the other child will resent being made to stay home because of missing the afternoon playing with friends.

Materials Needed: none

Processing Questions:

1. How should a child relate to grandparents—with enthusiasm or resentment?
2. Do you have any meaningful relationships with an older or elderly person?

ELDERLY PUPPET SHOW   Grades (K–2)

Valued Outcome: The students will be able to describe physical attributes of the elderly.

Description of Strategy: Have three students enact the following: A young boy and girl set out on a hike in the morning and come to a bridge. An old troll there is angered by their presence and casts a spell on them to make them "old for a day." They examine themselves and find the following traits, which they discuss with each other: wrinkled skin with age spots, gray hair (boy becomes bald), inability to move quickly, lack of strength, and shortness of breath on their hike.

Materials Needed: five puppets (young boy, young girl, old troll, old man, old woman), puppet bridge

Processing Question: What physical effects occur during the aging process?

NOW I AM OLD   Grades (3–5)

Valued Outcome: The students will be able to differentiate between an active and an inactive retirement lifestyle.

Description of Strategy: Have two volunteers role-play situations in which two elderly retirees are planning the day's activities. One situation could include two retirees who are very active, and another could involve two retirees who are inactive. Follow up the activity by asking the students with which of the characters they most identified.

Materials Needed: none

Processing Question: Can a retiree be healthy if he or she chooses an inactive lifestyle during retirement?

Dramatizations: Dying and Death

SUICIDE   Grades (4–5)

Valued Outcome: The students will be able to discuss ways to help a suicidal friend.

Description of Strategy: Have two students role-play that one friend is calling the other to tell him or her that their best friend just attempted suicide by taking an overdose of pills. Let the students bring the role-play to closure by discussing ways they can help their mutual friend.

Materials Needed: none

Processing Question: How can a person untrained in suicide prevention help a suicidal friend?

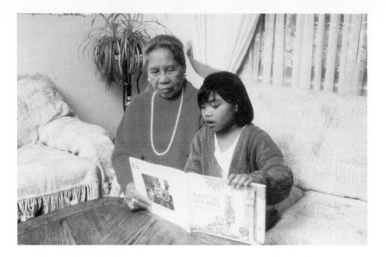

Good relationships with grandparents can enhance a child's life.

TALK CAN HELP   Grades (4–5)

Valued Outcome: The students will be able to describe how to visit a friend who is dying in the hospital.

Description of Strategy: Have one student play the role of a dying patient in a hospital. Have another play the role of a close friend who comes to visit. Role-play the situation for five minutes per pair of students. Ask each student to play the part in the way that seems most comfortable and natural. Have the students switch roles so all will have the opportunity to play the dying patient. Discuss the different approaches used in acting out this situation.

Materials Needed: bed for "dying" patient

Processing Question: What should one say when visiting a dying friend in the hospital?

ONLY ONE WEEK TO LIVE   Grades (4–5)

Valued Outcome: The students will be able to discuss what they would consider most important in their lives if they were facing death.

Description of Strategy: Have volunteers act out their responses when asked what they would do if they had only one week to live. This activity could be spontaneous, or you could allow the volunteers some time to think about the activities and list them.

Materials Needed: none

Processing Question: How does facing death affect our values and desires?

Discussion and Report Techniques: Aging

LIFE COLLAGE   Grades (K–5)

Valued Outcome: The students will create and present a visual representation of their lives from birth to present.

Description of Strategy: Have students bring in items from home that are special to them and that they feel help explain who they are. Encourage them to bring things from their early childhood as well as newer things. Stress that items should be small enough to be glued or taped to poster board. (Students may also bring items to display with their poster if they don't want to tape or glue them.) Distribute magazines, and have students cut out anything that relates to their life up to the present (toys they have or had, baby for sibling). Remind them only to cut out things that already apply to them, not things they hope for in the future. Have students glue or tape items to their poster board. When they have finished, have students explain how the things they chose are significant to their life.

Materials Needed: magazines, personal items, poster board, glue, tape, and scissors for each student

Processing Questions:

1. Why is it important to include items from your early childhood?
2. What part of your collage best represents who you are? Why?

PANEL DISCUSSION   Grades (4–5)

Valued Outcome: The students will be able to discuss the social and emotional problems faced by elderly people.

Description of Strategy: Divide the class into small groups, and have each group research a problem area for elderly Americans. These areas should include health problems, financial problems, problems due to stereotypes and misconceptions, forced retirement, crime, and loneliness. After research is complete, have each group present a panel discussion of their findings. Group members should be prepared to answer questions from the class about the problem area that they have researched.

Materials Needed: research books, such as *World Book* or *Encyclopedia Britannica*

Processing Questions:

1. What health problems do elderly people face?
2. What social problems do elderly people face?
3. What financial problems do elderly people face?

SERVICES FOR THE ELDERLY   Grades (4–5)

Valued Outcome: The students will be able to explain how the Social Security program benefits the elderly.

Description of Strategy: Ask a member of a local Social Security office to come to class and explain the Social Security system provided to elderly people, or have students research the Social Security program and present a lecture on it.

Materials Needed: materials on the Social Security system (if students do research in lieu of a presenter)

Processing Questions:

1. How does the Social Security program benefit elderly people?
2. How does an elderly person become involved in this program?

QUALITY TIME WITH ELDERLY FRIENDS OR RELATIVES   Grades (2–5)

Valued Outcome: The students will be able to relate a positive experience with an elderly person.

Description of Strategy: Have students write a paragraph on the best time they have spent with a grandparent or elderly friend. Have volunteers share the essay with the class.

Materials Needed: paper and pens or pencils for each student

Processing Question: What type of positive experiences can a young person have with an elderly person?

FOUNTAIN OF YOUTH   Grades (4–5)

Valued Outcome: The students will be able to discuss the implications of having a population that never grew old and died.

Description of Strategy: Have students debate whether a fountain of youth would be good or bad for humans.

Materials Needed: none

Processing Questions:

1. What if everyone stayed young and did not die?
2. What implications for overpopulation would there be if no one died?

AGING INTERVIEWS   Grades (3–5)

Valued Outcome: The students will be able to detect stereotypical views of the elderly through interviews with others.

Description of Strategy: Go over the list of misconceptions about the elderly on page 677. Have students interview at least three family members or friends of various ages. Have them make a list of the stereotype-related comments the family members or friends make during the interviews. Have the students share the stereotype-related comments in small groups and then with the class. Some sample questions for the interview are:

1. What is it like to be old?

2. Are you happier now than when you were younger?

3. Have you experienced any discrimination because you are old?

Materials Needed: paper and pens or pencils for each student

Processing Question: How can a stereotype of a group harm that group?

THE ELDERLY IN THE MEDIA   Grades (4–5)

Valued Outcome: The students will be able to compare the media's view of the elderly with their own view.

Description of Strategy: Have students watch television programs, newscasts, and television commercials and look through magazines and newspapers. Have them write comments about whether the media's view of older people is consistent with their own view of the elderly.

Materials Needed: television, magazines, newspapers, paper and pencils

Processing Questions:

1. What are the similarities between the media's view of the elderly and yours?

2. What are the differences between the media's view of the elderly and yours

3. Do you think your view of the elderly has been influenced by the media?

AGE, DYING, AND DEATH   Grade (K–2)

Valued Outcome: The students will be able to identify and list physical characteristics of aging.

Description of Strategy: Introduce the lesson by talking to students about people they know who are older. Let them raise their hands and tell about the person they know. Ask questions such as: "Do the people you just talked about look different from you? Of course, they do because they are older. But how can we tell someone is older just by looking at them?" Let them respond. Give each student a piece of paper and markers or crayons. Have students divide the paper into four sections. In the corner of each square, write 10, 20, 40, and 60.

Example of table:

10	20
40	60

In each square, have the students draw a picture of themselves and how they think they will look at each age.

Point out that aging is not something that happens only to elderly people, but rather something that happens to everyone all the time, beginning at birth. Go over some factors related to aging, including sex, race, personality, genetics, and education. Let students share which attribute of aging they would least want (e.g., wrinkles, gray hair, etc.). Say in closing: "Today we learned that many factors cause us to age in different ways. Whether it is our personality or our genetics or other attributes, we all will age and all end up looking different from the way we do now. However, aging is a normal process, and we can learn a lot from it." Tell students to try and ask a few people older than them to show them a picture of themselves when they were younger and compare how they looked then to how they look now.

Materials Needed: markers or crayons and paper for each student

Processing Questions:

1. What are some factors related to aging?
2. What are some things that will change about our bodies as we age?

THE SCIENCE OF AGING   Grades (4–5)

Valued Outcome: The students learn how scientists study aging by reviewing experiments related to the effect of caloric reduction on aging.

Description of Strategy:
Ask the following questions to stimulate discussion from the class:

- Why do you think people have always been so fascinated with trying to stay young?
- Do you think you can have any control over how you age?
- What factors do you think may have an effect on how long people live? (Remember to consider both emotional as well as physical factors. Factors may include nutrition, economic conditions, environmental conditions, a positive attitude, and genetics.)
- What types of studies do you think scientists would use to determine if there was a relationship between these factors and aging? (Cross-sectional and longitudinal studies of populations of humans and of animals may be used. Cross-sectional studies compare different subgroups within a large group of humans or animals at one point in time, and longitudinal studies compare a group to itself at different points in time.)
- How might nutrition affect aging? How might scientists study the effects of nutrition on aging?

Have students write an answer the following questions:

- What can we learn about the aging process by studying humans directly?

- What can we learn from studying the aging processes of other animals?
- How might that apply to humans?

Materials Needed: pencils or pens and paper for each student

Processing Question: What health behaviors affect how you age?

SOURCE: Science Net Links 2002

CALORIC COMPARISON   Grades (4–5)

Valued Outcome: The students will be able to describe the different nutritional needs and caloric requirements of a person their age and an elderly person.

Description of Strategy: Discuss and show in graphic form the caloric needs of a person your students' age. Then, do the same for an elderly person. Have the students compare the differences and brainstorm why the differences exist.

Materials Needed: charts on caloric needs for elementary students and for elderly persons

Processing Questions:

1. How will your caloric needs differ as you age?
2. How will you need to modify your habits to accommodate this change and still remain healthy?

Discussion and Report Techniques: Dying and Death

HOW IT FELT TO GO TO A FUNERAL   Grades (3–5)

Valued Outcome: The students will demonstrate, through artistic expression, what they think a funeral is.

Description of Strategy: Allow students to tell stories about a funeral they have attended or what they think a funeral involves, using felt boards with felt cutout figures and objects that represent things associated with funerals (such as flowers, religious symbols, cemeteries, coffins, guns, blood, crashed cars, and so on). Offer each child an opportunity to create a story about being at the funeral home, the funeral or memorial service, the cemetery, or the family gathering after the funeral.

Materials Needed: felt board and cutouts

Processing Questions:

1. What do you associate with funeral experiences?
2. Are they positive or negative things? Why?

DETERMINING CAUSES OF DEATH

Valued Outcome: The students will be able to determine the diseases that cause death.

Description of Strategy: Have students identify a list of ten or fifteen diseases that may result in death; write this list on the board or on the overhead projector as the diseases are suggested. Discuss the list briefly to be sure only potentially fatal diseases are included. Have students compare their list to a list of the most common causes of death in the United States in the year 2000. Ask the following types of questions:

- How many diseases in the student-originated list are on the list of actual causes of death?
- What types of diseases are the killers?
- Are they infectious or degenerative diseases?
- Do the diseases tend to strike older or younger people?
- How many of the diseases listed are considered curable?

Now compare the list from the year 2000 with a list of the most common causes of death in the United States in the year 1900, and answer the same questions for causes of death a century ago.

Materials Needed: board and marker or overhead projector and pen, lists of causes of death in the United States for the years 1900 and 2000

Processing Question: How do you think the causes of death will change in the twenty-first century?

MOURNING AND FUNERALS

Valued Outcome: The students will be able to describe ways of dealing with the grief process. They will write about their experiences with funerals.

Description of Strategy: Introduce the topics of death and grieving by asking students about their feelings when something bad happens. Discuss the words *grief* and *mourning*. Ask students to help figure out these words. (**Grief** is sorrow, mental distress, emotional agitation, sadness, suffering, and related feelings caused by death. **Mourning** involves culturally defined acts that are usually performed when death occurs.)

Talk about ways to deal with grief. Students may tell how they deal with grief (reading, talking about it, etc.). Talk about mourning rituals (funerals, memorial services, etc.). Allow students to act out a funeral. Close by saying that grief is acceptable and can be coped with using a variety of techniques. You may wish to repeat coping strategies that the students identified during the discussion.

Materials Needed: none

Processing Question: What is the purpose of a funeral?

DYING: TRUE/FALSE

Grades (K–5)

Valued Outcome: The students will better understand dying.

Description of Strategy: Write on the chalkboard the following facts and have students determine whether they are true or false.

- Mature individuals often find themselves unable to cope with the thought of death.
- Individuals generally choose to ignore death.
- When death is brought up in conversation, it is usually in the form of a joke.

Engage the class in a round robin to discuss the responses.

Materials Needed: board and markers or overhead projector and pen

Processing Question: Why is our society considered a death-denying society?

WHY SHOULD I HAVE A WILL?

Grades (4–5)

Valued Outcome: The students will be able to explain why every adult should have a will.

Description of Strategy: Discuss with the class the reasons for having a will. Describe the format of the will. Have the students prepare wills for themselves, with two classmates acting as witnesses to sign the document. Have students list their important possessions and the people to whom they would like to bequeath these things.

Materials Needed: paper and pencils for each student

Processing Question: Should adults without a lot of possessions have a will?

DYING

Grades (3–5)

Valued Outcome: Students will see that adjusting to dying and understanding the five stages of dying are critical to understanding the needs of a dying person.

Description of Strategy: Create a handout from the list below. Give the following directions to the students: "There are five stages of dying, and they are listed on your handout out of order. Please put the stages in order by placing the number of the stage beside the sentence where it belongs."

_____ **Depression**—the patient is saddened by the fact that death is approaching and then starts the grief process for the losses death will entail.

_____ **Denial and isolation**—learning of the diagnosis of a terminal condition, the patient reacts with disbelief.

_____ **Bargaining**—the patient is accepting the inevitability of death and begins to bargain (with God or others) for more time.

_____ **Anger**—the reality of impending death begins to seep into the patient's consciousness, and anger is the reaction.

_____ **Acceptance or resolution**—the patient resolves the issue of death.

Materials Needed: handouts with descriptions of stages and pencils for each student

Processing Question: Why is it important for each of us to understand the stages of grief?

DYING AND DEATH: INDIVIDUAL RIGHTS
Grades (3–5)

Valued Outcome: The students will establish what they think their rights are as human beings facing death.

Description of Strategy: Divide the class into groups of four or five. Have the students brainstorm what they perceive as their rights as human beings who will be faced with death at some point in their lives. Ask them to list the things that are important to them regarding their feelings about personal issues in their lives and what they would have done to ensure their wishes were done in the event that they knew they were dying. Have the students report on their findings. Assign yourself the role of recorder; on the board, write The Dying Person's Bill of Rights. As the students report their findings, add them to the list of the Bill of Rights. Discuss the importance of coming to terms with one's rights as a human being facing death.

Materials Needed: board and markers or overhead projector and pen

Processing Questions:

1. How do I want to be treated as an individual?
2. Should this treatment change if I may be dying? Why or why not?

ORGAN AND TISSUE DONATION
Grades (4–5)

Valued Outcome: The students will be able to identify organs or tissues that can be transplanted after death and will write out their feelings on transplantation. Also, they will be able to decide what organ or tissue they would or would not want to give away.

Description of Strategy: Introduce the topic of organ and tissue transplants by saying: "We have talked about death and many issues surrounding it. We know death can be very sad. However, today we are going to discuss a way that it can be very positive. Even when people die, they can help others. They can do this by organ donation." Ask the students if they know what organ donation is, and give them time to answer or figure it out. Then explain organ donation—If someone dies, everything in his or her body doesn't immediately stop working. Therefore, doctors can perform surgery to remove certain parts and give them to other people. "The doctor takes one thing from someone and gives it to someone else. We call this transplantation." Explain why we need organ donations for research and dissection in medical schools, and for sick people who can be cured with a new organ. Their body may accept the organ as their own, and they will be able to function normally, at least for a while. Discuss the following organs and tissues and their purposes:

eyes (corneas)	pancreas
kidneys	cartilage
pituitary glands	bone marrow
heart	lungs
liver	bones (including ear bones, or ossicles)
skin	

Talk about the circumstances of an organ or tissue transplant. Tell the students that a potential donor usually must die in a hospital, and the organ removal surgery is performed soon afterward (e.g., a heart must be transplanted within four to five hours of the donor's death). Sometimes living people can donate organs or tissues, such as a kidney (everyone has two), a lobe of their liver (what is left of the liver will regrow), and bone marrow or blood (both of which are replaced by the body). Also, the donor must be eighteen years old or older (anyone under eighteen must have a parent's or guardian's signature). The donor and the recipient do not usually know each other, since the organ or tissue typically goes to someone on a transplant waiting list.

Finally, close by saying: "Today we learned about organ and tissue donation and how it can help people. We learned about organs and tissues that can be donated. We can now see how much medical technology is important." Give students an outline of the body with cutouts of each organ and have them glue onto the body which organs they would donate.

Materials Needed: handout with outline of the body and cutouts of each organ and glue for each student

Processing Questions:

1. How has technology in the medical field helped many people?
2. How can a person die and still help people?

WHY PEOPLE DIE   Grade (5–8)

Valued Outcome: The students will be able to discuss why people die and how they can express themselves in a healthy fashion when a relative dies.

Description of Strategy: Begin by asking students why people die and in what ways people can live longer today. Divide the class into groups and talk about why people get older and what types of people live the longest. Have the students share their responses with their group, and then as a group, have them make a poster with the best answers from their group (or any other answer their group comes up with). Have them include a written description and a picture on the poster to help give a mental image of their answers. Hang up their posters around the room, and then have each group look at the other group posters to see how their poster differed from those of other groups.

Make a class poster and have the students come up with different responses and explain them to the class. Hang the class poster outside the room in the hallway for others to see. Tell students that people who are good to their bodies, who eat right, exercise, and don't drink and smoke are likely to live longer. People who die at an early age often do so because they did not take care of their body. This includes drinking while driving, smoking, eating nonnutritious snacks and fatty foods, and not exercising. Have students share any stories that they may have about people they know who have died, and why they have died. (This has to been done very carefully without upsetting anyone, so let the students know that they don't have to share their story if they don't want to do so.)

Materials Needed: poster board, markers, tape, and pens or pencils for each student

Processing Questions:

1. Why do people die?
2. What makes a person live longer?

MY PET DIED   Grades (K–5)

Valued Outcome: The students will be able to describe the experience of having a pet die.

Description of Strategy: Most students have had pets that died—dogs, cats, hamsters, fish, or other small animals. Ask students who have had the experience of having a pet die to draw a picture or write a short report about the event. The reports should emphasize the things about the pet that the child liked most. Explain that we can remember those qualities and talk about the pleasure or companionship of a past pet, even though the pet will never return to us. Note the comfort that such fond memories can bring.

Materials Needed: paper, pens or pencils, or markers or crayons for each student

Processing Question: Why should we recall qualities of pets who have died?

Experiments and Demonstrations: Aging

LAST YEAR'S CLOTHING   Grades (K–5)

Valued Outcome: The students will be able to discuss how they are aging and the implications of the aging process for them.

Description of Strategy: Have students bring in articles of clothing that they wore a year earlier and try them on. Use this activity as a springboard for a discussion of growth and aging. Note that the process is a continuum and a normal part of the life cycle.

Materials Needed: clothing (brought in by students)

Processing Questions:

1. Why do we grow as we age?
2. Is aging a positive part of the life cycle?

AGING IN PLANTS   Grades (K–5)

Valued Outcome: The students will be able to explain the aging process in a plant.

Description of Strategy: As a year-long or seasonal project, have the students observe the changes that take place in plants. Observation of annuals, such as many flowers, will permit a view of an entire life cycle, from budding stage, through flowering, to withering. Long-term growth can be observed and compared in different trees.

Materials Needed: pots, soil, and plant seeds

Processing Question: How does the life cycle of a plant help us understand aging in ourselves?

AGING IN HUMANS   Grades (K–5)

Valued Outcome: The students will be able to describe how the aging process affects a person's facial features.

Description of Strategy: Bring in photographs of a well-known person taken over a period of many years. Have the students note the aging process in the person's features from year to year.

Materials Needed: photographs of a person taken at several stages of his or her life

Processing Question: How do a person's features change as he or she ages?

LIFE CYCLE OF A FROG   Grades (3–5)

Valued Outcome: The students will observe and record the stages in the life cycle of a frog.

Description of Strategy: Order tadpoles for the classroom, and place them in a shallow, clear container. Explain the different stages of a frog's life (growing back legs, growing front legs, losing tail). When the tadpoles start to go through the first noticeable change, have students observe and record these changes in their journals. They may either write the information or draw a picture. Have students repeat this procedure for each stage in the life cycle until the tadpoles have all lost their tails.

Materials Needed: tadpoles, container, and journals and pencils for each student

Processing Questions:

1. How long did it take for the tadpoles to start growing their back legs?
2. What is the very first stage in a frog's life?

Puzzles and Games: Aging

AGING WORD SEARCH   Grades (4–5)

Valued Outcome: The students will be able to find specific aging-related words in a word search.

Description of Strategy: Provide a handout with the word search from the Teaching in Action box "Aging Word Search." Instruct the students to find the aging-related words in the puzzle.

Materials Needed: handout for each for each student

Processing Question: How many social issues facing the elderly can you find in the word search?

Other Ideas: Aging

ADOPT A GRANDPARENT   Grades (K–5)

Valued Outcome: The students will be able to develop a meaningful, positive relationship with an elderly friend.

Description of Strategy: Have the class choose (possibly with the cooperation of the local senior citizens' group) an elderly person(s) as an adoptive grandparent. The class could invite the elderly person to class for special occasions, such as birthdays, art projects, storytime, and so forth.

Materials Needed: none

Processing Question: How can a positive relationship with an elderly person enhance the quality of a child's life?

ELDERLY HEALTH FAIR   Grades (4–5)

Valued Outcome: The student will be able to discuss the positive aspects of the talents of elderly people.

```
R  L  F  I  N  A  N  C  I  A  L
V  I  N  C  O  M  E  S  B  L  S
I  F  M  E  D  I  C  A  L  M  M
S  E  D  U  C  A  T  I  O  N  E
U  E  C  A  R  C  K  U  V  L
A  X  X  R  A  O  A  E  T  U  L
L  P  E  A  S  I  M  E  O  W  H
P  E  R  S  O  N  A  L  I  T  Y
S  C  A  L  C  I  U  M  A  N  T
T  T  D  M  D  Y  O  E  S  E  T
R  A  G  E  I  S  M  D  O  M  O
E  N  E  D  I  C  A  I  D  Y  U
N  C  T  I  H  I  N  C  A  O  C
G  Y  T  C  A  L  L  A  U  L  H
T  D  S  A  H  U  T  I  P  P  W
H  H  A  R  T  D  I  D  Y  M  O
S  R  A  E  F  A  S  R  A  E  Y
T  N  E  M  E  R  I  T  E  R  F
```

ageism	
calcium	
education	
employment	
fear	
financial	
income	
life expectancy	
Medicaid	
medical	
Medicare	
personality	
race	
retirement	
sex	
smell	
strength	
touch	
visual	

Description of Strategy: Have the students plan a health fair designed for the elderly. Provide health screening services and information about health services in the community. Present arts and crafts made by the elderly. This is a great opportunity for the students to interact with the elderly and acquire an appreciation for the talents of another generation.

Materials Needed: arts and crafts made by elderly people, brochures and pamphlets about health services available in the community for the elderly

Processing Question: How can younger people appreciate the talents of the elderly?

WHAT WAS IT LIKE THEN?   Grades (4–5)

Valued Outcome: The students will be able to explain how society during an elderly person's childhood was different from today's society.

Description of Strategy: Present a living American heritage lesson to your students. Have an older person in the community report on past lifestyles and historic moments for your community. Or, find a veteran of World War II or someone who lived through the Depression and have that person report on his or her experiences.

Materials Needed: none

Processing Question: How was the world different when today's elderly people were young?

Other Ideas: Dying and Death

OBITUARY   Grades (6–8)

Valued Outcome: The students will write their own obituaries as they would appear in the newspaper.

Description of Strategy: Read several obituaries from the newspaper aloud to the class. Have students write their own obituaries modeled after the ones that they heard. Require students to include the date and cause of death and a list of survivors. Any other information provided is the student's choice (such as occupation, achievements, residence, and so on). Have students type and print out their obituaries on the computer. Display the obituaries on the class bulletin board.

Materials Needed: several obituary notices from newspapers, paper and pencils for each student, computer and printer

Processing Question: Why did you choose the lifestyle that you did for yourself?

POETRY   Grades (4–5)

Valued Outcome: The students will be able to compose a poem about dying and death.

Description of Strategy: Some of the greatest works of poetry in literature concern death and dying. Find short poems about death that are appropriate to the level of your class, and read them aloud. Discuss the meaning of each poem. Have the students write poems of their own on aspects of death and dying. Post the completed poems around the room for all to see and appreciate.

Materials Needed: poems about death and dying

Processing Question: Why do so many poems have dying and death as a central message?

WHAT DOES A FUNERAL DIRECTOR DO?   Grades (4–5)

Valued Outcome: The students will be able to discuss the funeral arrangements that need to be made when a family member dies.

Description of Strategy: Invite a funeral director to speak to the class about how funeral arrangements are made. Ask your guest to explain what is done, how costs are determined, and how family members are involved. The funeral director should explain any special considerations that must be taken into account for religious, cultural, or family reasons. Allow time for a question-and-answer session after the presentation.

Materials Needed: none

Processing Questions:

1. What funeral arrangements have to be made when a family member or relative dies?

2. What is the significance of funeral rituals?

Resources

BOOKS

Backer, B. A., N. Hanoi, and N. A. Russell. 1994. *Death and dying: Understanding and care.* 2d ed. Albany, NY: Delmar.

Blieszner, R., and V. H. Bedford, eds. 1995. *Handbook of aging and the family.* Westport, CT: Greenwood Press.

Corless, I. B., B. B. Germino, and M. Pittman, eds. 1994. *Dying, death, and bereavement: Theoretical perspectives and other ways of knowing.* Boston: Jones & Bartlett.

DeSpelder, L. A., and A. L. Strickland. 2002. *The last dance.* 6th ed. Mountain View, CA: Mayfield.

Ebersole, P., and P. Hess. 1994. *Toward healthy aging: Human needs and nursing response.* 4th ed. St. Louis: Mosby.

Ferrini, A. F., and R. L. Ferrini. 2000. *Health in the later years.* 3d ed. Madison, WI: Brown & Benchmark.

Hockey, J., and A. James. 1993. *Growing up and growing old.* London: Sage.

Marrone, R. 1997. *Death, mourning, and caring.* Pacific Grove, CA: Brooks/Cole.

Spirduso, W. W. 1995. *Physical dimensions of aging.* Champaign, IL: Human Kinetics.

Williamson, J. B., and E. S. Shneidman. 1995. *Death: Current perspectives.* 4th ed. Mountain View, CA: Mayfield.

WEB SITES

Batesville Casket Company: *www.batesville.com*

OncoLink: *www.oncolink.upenn.edu/*

Suicide Awareness Voices of Education *www.save.org*

United States Public Health Services *phs.os.dhhs.gov/ophs/default.htm*

Educational and Community-Based Programs

CDC National Center for Chronic Disease Prevention and Health Promotion *www.cdc.gov/nccdphp*

Health Resources and Services Administration *www.hrsa.dhhs.gov*

Healthy Cities Online: *www.healthycities.org*

Office of Minority Health Resource Center, Washington State Department of Health *www.doh.wa.gov*

continued

Death and Dying
Euthanasia Research and Guidance Organization
www.efn.org/~ergo/
GriefNet: *www.rivendell.org/*
Hospice Hands: *www.hospicecares.com*

Surveillance and Data Systems
CDC National Center for Health Statistics
www.cdc.gov/nchs

General Sites
American Medical Association: *www.ama-assn.org*
MedicineNet: *www.medicinenet.com*
Medscape: *www.medscape.com*
Oncolink: *www.oncolink.upenn.edu*
ParentsPlace.com: *www.parentsplace.com*

Links Only
Hardin Meta Directory of Internet Health Sources
www.lib.uiowa.edu/hardin/md

VIDEOS
Teen suicide: A Phil Donahue show
Brings together parents of teen suicide victims, teens who have attempted suicide, and a psychotherapist to seek ways to stem the tide of increasing suicide rates among young people and to help youngsters and adults recognize the signals and warning cries of potential suicides. Available from Films for the Humanities and Sciences, P.O. Box 2053, Princeton, NJ 08543. (28 minutes, Item BVL1250)

The right to die
The medical, ethical, and legal dilemmas of cases are discussed by a physician–attorney and a nurse. Available from Films for the Humanities and Sciences, P.O. Box 2053, Princeton, NJ 08543. (28 minutes, Item BVL1577)

Children die, too
A couple whose three-year-old daughter died suddenly, a teenage girl whose sister died from leukemia, a mother whose six-month-old died from multiple birth defects, and a young woman who has undergone two miscarriages and two stillborns talk about their experiences. Available from Films for the Humanities and Sciences, P.O. Box 2053, Princeton, NJ 08543. (26 minutes, Item BVL2374)

Video focus on health
Discusses several topics related to aging, dying, and death, such as successful aging and medically assisted suicide. Available from Films for the Humanities and Sciences, P.O. Box 2053, Princeton, NJ 08543.

The biology of death
Discusses the various definitions of death and the importance of knowing when a patient is considered dead for the purpose of organ transplantation. Available from Films for the Humanities and Sciences, P.O. Box 2053, Princeton, NJ 08543. (29 minutes, Item BVL3420)

Healthy aging
Healthy aging shows the connection between your daily lifestyle habits and your potential for both a longer life and health span. Available from School House Videos & CDs, 4205 Grove Ridge Drive, Durham, NC 27703. (60 minutes, Item 6066)

Someone I love has Alzheimer's disease
The message of this video is you are not alone. You will meet kids aged 7 through 15. All are caring for and coping with a loved one who has this confusing disorder. Available from School House Videos & CDs, 4205 Grove Ridge Drive, Durham, NC 27703. (17 minutes, Item 7917)

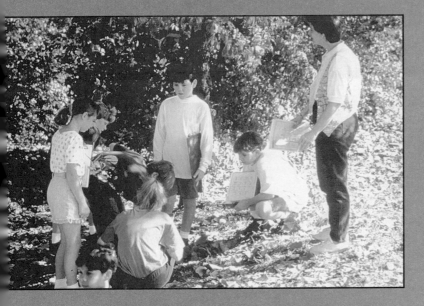

CHAPTER TWENTY-FIVE

Environmental Health

In order to survive, all animals, including human beings, require a certain amount of high-quality air, water, food, and shelter. If people are deprived of any essential environmental factors, or if the environment is polluted with toxic substances, health is adversely affected.

—Edlin, Golanty, and Brown
(1999, 482)

VALUED OUTCOMES

After reading this chapter, you should be able to:

- discuss the responsibility of every human being in caring for the environment
- describe an ecosystem
- describe the impact of pollution on all members of the ecosystem
- relate the connection between overpopulation and environmental pollution
- explain the impact of air pollution on the environment
- detail the conditions that lead to water pollution
- suggest what individuals can do to remedy the different types of environmental pollution

- describe the sources of indoor pollution in a classroom
- discuss the Environmental Protection Agency's Superfund attempt at solid waste cleanup and control
- give examples of legislation designed to control environmental pollution
- describe the Clean Air Act that is enforced by the Environmental Protection Agency

REFLECTIONS

As you read through this chapter, consider the major hazards to the survival of the planet that you face daily; the ways you can protect yourself from these hazards; and the steps you can take personally to reduce these hazards or improve your personal environment and your community's environment.

Living in a Healthy Environment

Maintaining personal health is largely an individual responsibility. Yet, none of us lives in a vacuum. We are all subject to the influences of our environment. Thus, a person may attempt to exercise the most positive personal health behavior and still be subjected to health hazards in the form of contaminated drinking water, polluted air, and urban stress factors, such as noise and overcrowded living conditions. Clearly, our environment has an impact on our health.

Human beings are the dominant species on earth because of our power to control, manipulate, and alter our surroundings. To a large extent, we have learned to use the natural resources of the planet for our own benefit. But in doing so, we have also created a host of environmental problems. For a long time, many of these problems went unrecognized. However, with the growth of technology and industry, the problems became more and more obvious. Even then, many preferred to ignore what was happening to our environment, attributing it to the price of progress. In any case, there seemed to be no way of correcting many of the problems.

Today, more and more people are becoming aware of the negative impact human activity has had on the environment. Many of the negative changes that have occurred did not have to happen. Certainly, most do not have to keep getting worse. We can no longer plead ignorance about how many of our activities affect the world in which we live. We also are increasingly recognizing our responsibility toward protecting the environment and preserving our natural resources for future generations.

Ecology is the study of interactions in the environment. From this study, three basic natural laws have been determined:

1. Every system within nature is connected to every other system.

2. Matter is never destroyed but is recycled in one way or another.

3. Natural resources are finite, and nature's capacity to absorb the by-products of human technology is limited.

The implications of these three laws, separately and together, have great bearing on the health of all people and the state of the environment. At first, it may seem that these principles are beyond the control of the individual, but this is not so. Each of us has a responsibility both to understand the laws of ecology and to realize that as individuals what we do affects the operation of these laws. This is the single most important concept in the teaching of environmental health education.

Students must be taught that humans are part of the overall ecosystem of our planet, and as intelligent members of that ecosystem they have both rights and responsibilities concerning the environment. This is a vital concept that must be stressed.

Ecosystems and Ecology

Each living thing, whether plant or animal, is part of an immediate ecosystem, or habitat, in which the living and nonliving components interact and interrelate. For example, all the organisms in a particular field or pond form an ecosystem. By interacting in a balanced fashion with all other parts of the ecosystem, a given species can generally continue to thrive while perpetuating its population. This interrelationship and interdependence with other animals and plants in the environment produces a web of common sharing of most natural resources, including air, water, territorial space, sunlight, and soil minerals. Nonliving natural resources are usually referred to as the *physical,* or *abiotic, environment* of the given ecosystem, while living organisms are referred to as the *biotic environment* of the ecosystem.

Each environmental component of an ecosystem influences the other. When the physical environment is altered significantly, the biotic environment will be correspondingly altered, and vice versa. As a result, ecosystems are governed by and operate through an interwoven natural organization of cycles between groups within the system. These cycles ensure that balance and stabilization of the community are sustained. Yet, balance and stability are dynamic processes, always changing in response to the alterations in these cycles as they themselves are changed by the varying interactions between the residents of the neighborhood and their use of natural resources. Thus, since ecosystems are inherently unstable, an input of energy is required in order to maintain equilibrium, or homeostasis. This input of energy produces a closed and self-sustaining cycle wherein chains of interconnections arise. For example, life is nurtured from decomposition within the system, one species feeds off another, and so forth. All resources, by nature's rules, are recycled and continually reused in one form or another because energy is always constant. In addition, ecosystems are in continuous interaction with one another and are joined by the actions of the various physical and biotic environments to form a total worldwide ecosystem called the *ecosphere,* or *biosphere.*

The human species, unlike any other species, can extensively manipulate both the physical and biotic environments of ecosystems, indirectly affecting

Health Highlight

GLOBAL WARMING AND OZONE LAYER DEPLETION

As inhabitants of the Earth, we are protected by the ozone layer, which protects us from the sun's radiation. Unfortunately, several of our daily activities (as discussed in this chapter) have damaged this ozone layer. This damage has resulted in less protection for us from the ultraviolet lights, and eventually will lead to higher skin cancer and cataract rates.

Global warming, or rising global temperatures, is expected to affect our world in several ways: sea levels will be raised, there will be increased precipitation, and local climate conditions will be changed. Global warming will cause an overall trend toward more intense rainstorms and drier soils in some areas of the country. The changing climate conditions could change the way forests appear, lessen the amount of crops yielded by farmland, and deplete our water supplies. Further, deserts may grow into current rangelands. Global warming should be expected throughout much of the United States and North America, although sulfates may limit the effects of global warming somewhat.

Fortunately, the United States, in cooperation with over 140 other countries, is phasing out the production of ozone-depleting substances in an effort to safeguard the ozone layer.

SOURCE: Environmental Protection Agency 2003a

the ecosphere as a whole. Although many of these alterations are not inherently damaging, the cumulative impact on the ecosphere has taken its toll, and the natural recycling mechanisms have sometimes been overwhelmed. Ecologists have pleaded for all of us to develop a greater understanding of the scientific principles that govern ecosystems so that an increased awareness about our impact on the ecosphere will result. Then more of our decisions regarding the ways in which we choose to interact with the environment will be based on knowledge and logic rather than on ignorance or greed. Ecologists have also warned of the grave danger facing our entire planet from depletion or pollution of its rich natural resources, which are finite and must be preserved for future generations.

Human Impact and Health

Human activity can have detrimental effects on the environment. For example, a growing number of diseases in children are linked to the unsafe environments in which they live, play, learn, and grow. Children, since they are still growing and their immune system and detoxification mechanisms are not fully developed, are especially vulnerable to chemical, physical, and biological hazards in air, water, and soil. In both industrialized and developing countries, their development, health, and well-being are threatened by unsafe food and chemicals in household products and consumer goods and by the overuse of antibiotics and antibacterial products (which increase the number of antibiotic- and antibacterial-strains of bacteria when used improperly). Air pollution causes

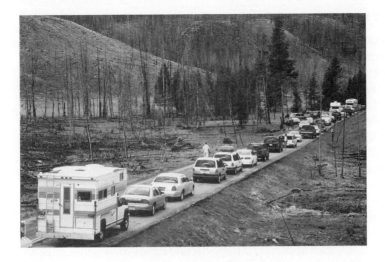

Environmental problems arise from overpopulation.

adverse health effects, such as asthma, leukemia, and respiratory cancer. In the United States each year, about 900,000 people get sick from unsafe drinking water (Pruitt and Stein 1999, 531, 537).

The physical, social, and intellectual development of children from conception to the end of adolescence requires an environment that is both protected and protective of their health.

OVERPOPULATION

Many environmental health problems arise not so much from misuse of technology, but from the sheer number of people who exist. There are simply not enough natural resources to support an unlimited human population. For example, a rapidly growing population often exceeds the food resources, and an unresolved question is whether the world can provide enough food to feed its people (Edlin, Golanty, and Brown 1999, 495). Joblessness, environmental devastation, and uncontrolled urban growth are also concerns. In the last decade or two, many countries have attempted to deal with the problem of overpopulation by means of governmental incentives to limit births. However, ethical and moral controversies surround the issue, which is understandably a very delicate and highly personal one to most individuals.

Regardless of the ethical or moral considerations, however, overpopulation is a serious environmental problem that must be addressed—not only by governmental and private agencies, but by the schools as well. Information about family planning and parenthood should be provided to junior high and high school students after a foundation about families and population has been provided at the elementary school level. Children need to understand that our planet will soon be unable to house the growing human population if reproduction continues at the present rate. Although the solutions are not easy and decisions must ultimately be made by each individual, a world perspective should be provided.

POPULATION CONTROL

World population is expanding exponentially. In 1800, about one billon people lived on earth. The world's population grew to two billion in 1930; to three billion in 1960; to four billion in 1975; to five billion in 1987; and to six billion in 1997. With the increase in the number of people comes an increase in the demand for resources (Hales 1999, 644).

The problems resulting from overpopulation are well recognized in such countries as China and India, where governmental incentives have been established to limit childbearing. Before condoms and diaphragms became available in the nineteenth century, birth control methods were generally unsafe and were not widely used. However, with the introduction to the general public of the birth control pill and the intrauterine device (IUD) in the 1960s, as well as improved female sterilization and male vasectomy techniques introduced in the 1970s, birth control has become more accepted throughout the world. New contraceptive methods, such as hormone implants and male birth control pills, are being introduced.

Dissemination of information about contraceptive methods (and protection against sexually transmitted infections) has been increased to include preteens, teenagers, young adults, and older adults alike. Although some individuals and groups believe instruction about birth control is ill advised in a school setting, many school systems nevertheless have incorporated such instruction into the curriculum. The establishment of various kinds of family planning services throughout the United States and in many other nations has also aided in increasing contraceptive education.

In the United States, population growth has stabilized. The average age for marriage has increased, and many young couples delay parenthood in order to advance educationally or professionally. In developing nations, where population control is more of a problem, efforts must be made to provide the same kind of education and services that are offered in more technologically advanced nations. It must be recognized, however, that decisions about pregnancy are deeply personal, cultural, religious, and social in nature and should be based on free choice.

Pollution of the Ecosphere

Human activity is a major cause of environmental pollution, but humans often experience the results of contamination much less quickly than other members of the ecosphere. As a result, although pollution of the environment has been occurring for centuries, only relatively recently has an awareness developed that polluting constitutes self-destructive behavior. The most crucial areas of concern include problems caused by overpopulation (which in turn contribute heavily to other pollution problems, see page 735), air pollution, water pollution, hazardous chemical pollution, solid waste pollution, radiation pollution, and noise pollution.

AIR POLLUTION

Human beings—all six billion of us—need air more desperately than any other resource for survival. People can endure drought, famine, and drastic temperature changes, but oxygen deprivation will result in death after only a few minutes. Yet, most of us think very little about the air we breathe, what it is composed of, or how, as a finite supply, it is replenished and kept clean. Almost no oxygen was present in the atmosphere at the earth's creation, but an abundance of carbon dioxide was available for sustaining plant life. Green plants, over an evolutionary period, were responsible for producing oxygen as a waste product of photosynthesis so that today the atmosphere is composed of approximately 80 percent nitrogen and 20 percent oxygen. Humans have contributed a variety of harmful gases and other substances to the atmosphere, resulting in air pollution (and thereby some of the water and soil pollution) and an increasing environmental health problem affecting the ecosphere as a whole—including the plants that provide our oxygen. Exposure to sufficiently high concentrations of air pollutants can cause a variety of health problems ranging from sneezing and coughing to labored breathing and death. Those most sensitive to air pollution are usually older adults and people who have chronic respiratory or cardiovascular conditions.

Major Air Pollutants. The chief air pollutants include carbon monoxide and nitrogen oxides, sulfur oxides, hydrocarbons, and particulate matter. Other toxic air pollutants that are products of technology include arsenic, mercury, polyvinyl chlorides, and pesticides, all of which can cause cancer and death.

Carbon Monoxide and Nitrogen Oxides. **Carbon monoxide,** which is by far the most plentiful air pollutant, is a colorless, odorless poisonous gas produced by the incomplete burning of carbon in fossil fuels. The chief source of carbon monoxide pollution is internal combustion engines, most of which are gas-powered motor vehicles. Because hemoglobin has a greater affinity for carbon monoxide than for oxygen, carbon monoxide replaces oxygen in the blood. An environment in which heavy traffic is present provides significant levels of carbon monoxide, and diminished physical and mental functioning can result from long-term exposure. Adverse effects include affected breathing, heart failure, and impaired perception and thinking (Pruitt and Stein 1999).

Nitrogen oxides, which account for about 6 percent of air pollutants, are chemically very similar to carbon monoxide, and poisonous nitrogen oxides (such as nitrogen dioxide and nitric acid) produce comparable physiological disturbances in the circulatory system. Nitrogen oxides form the brownish component of photochemical smog and combine with water vapor in the air to form nitric acid, which is capable of corroding metal and destroying vegetation.

Automobiles and other internal combustion engines produce most man-made carbon monoxide and nitrogen oxides. Most experts agree that shifting away from automobiles as the primary source of transportation is the only way to reduce air pollution significantly. Many cities have encouraged this shift by setting high parking fees, imposing bans on city driving, and establishing high road-use tolls. Local governments have also been implementing plans for electric buses and bicycle lanes to encourage low-impact transportation (Natural Resources Defense Council 2003). Some automobile companies have introduced hybrid electric vehicles that use less gas *and* produce very low emissions to the market (HybridCars.com 2003).

Sulfur Oxides. After carbon monoxide, sulfur oxides are the most abundant air pollutant and are a product of combustion of sulfur-containing coal and fuel oil. Sulfur dioxide, a poison that irritates the eyes, nose, and throat and damages the lungs, is highly injurious to human health, to property, and to vegetation (Edlin, Golanty, and Brown 1999, 483–484). In the atmosphere, sulfur dioxide is converted to sulfuric acid, which is the major source of acid deposition.

Hydrocarbons. Although no specific ailments or irritations can be directly attributed to the release of hydrocarbons—compounds composed of hydrogen and carbon—these substances constitute an important component of smog. They account for 10 to 15 percent of all air pollution emissions.

Particulate Matter. Particulate matter is any nongaseous pollutant found in the air, whether liquid or solid. These pollutants include such substances as ash, soot, asbestos, and lead. It is estimated that particulate matter comprises approximately 8 percent of air emissions. Prolonged exposure to these pollutants can cause deterioration of the respiratory tract surfaces, particularly the cilia.

> **Lead**—Sources of airborne lead are primarily smelters and automobile exhausts. (Unleaded gasoline has somewhat eased the problem of automobile exhaust pollution.) Health hazards from high concentrations of lead include irritability, anemia, convulsions, severe intestinal cramps, loss of consciousness, and kidney and brain damage. Lead enters the body primarily through the respiratory tract and sometimes through the stomach walls. Signs of lead poisoning are behavioral problems, anemia, decreased mental functioning, vomiting, and cramps.
>
> **Asbestos**—In the past, asbestos was widely used in construction and manufacturing; most exposures occur in occupational settings. Asbestos can cause serious respiratory problems, such as emphysema, and has been implicated in lung cancer.

Damage Resulting from Air Pollution. Air pollution causes serious damage in terms of human well-being, property, and plant and animal life. Air pollution negatively affects such human respiratory illnesses as coughs, colds, asthma, pneumonia, and bronchitis, as well as cancer and even heart disease. Animals and plant life can also be severely harmed by air pollution that interferes with normal physiological functions. Buildings become darkened and discolored and public works of art and monuments are damaged by contaminants. Unfortunately, today's advanced technology produces pollutants faster than the scientific community is able to study their results. These by-products may pose serious health problems that are currently unknown.

Chemicals. When pesticides are sprayed by crop dusters, only one-fourth lands on the crop, less than 1 percent may hit the target insects, and the rest drifts miles away. The insecticides kill birds, frogs, and predatory insects. Falcons and eagles have become extinct in some local areas as a result of pesticide spraying. Herbicides sprayed on forest lands have caused miscarriages, cancer, and birth defects, and they often wipe out local wildlife as well as pets and livestock.

Vegetation may change color or fail to pollinate. Animals grazing on affected land can be contaminated.

Acid Rain. The primary cause of acid rain is the burning of fossil fuels in electricity-generating plants. The sulfur in fuel is converted to sulfur oxides, and sulfur oxides and nitrogen oxides combine with rain, snow, dew, or mist to form sulfuric and nitric acids. Of the two, sulfuric acid is responsible for the most damage. Most sulfur pollution in the United States originates east of the Mississippi River and much of the pollution that originates in the United States is deposited in Canada. Throughout the eastern parts of Canada and the United States, acid rain changes soil acidity levels and causes lakes and streams to become more acidic. As the water becomes more acidic, life begins to disappear from the water as the lives or reproductive capacities of amphibians and fish are destroyed and the chemical balance of the ecosystem shifts. Mercury levels, for example, tend to rise in acidic waters and thereby also in the organisms living there or that eat food from those sources. Warnings have been issued to fishermen not to eat fish caught in the Great Lakes of the United States because of the mercury contamination (Nebel and Wright 1993, 364).

The impact on other aspects of human lives varies widely. Acid rain has accelerated the erosion of limestone buildings and monuments. It corrodes outdoor equipment and mobilizes other toxic elements (such as aluminum and lead) that may then contaminate soil and groundwater supplies. Springtime snowmelt can cause a surge of acid contamination. Forests and other foliage may be damaged by the acid, and even croplands have been affected.

Temperature Inversions. When a warm air mass moves over cooler air near the ground, a temperature inversion results. The cooler air cannot be dissipated. Temperature inversions decrease visibility and allow a buildup of pollutants, making the air unsafe for breathing. The pollutants are trapped and subjected to the action of sunlight and then produce other pollutants (known as secondary pollutants), such as ozone. The temperature inversion eventually disperses, but illness and even death have resulted from this condition.

Air Pollution Control. The Environmental Protection Agency (EPA) was established in 1970 by Congress to become the federal environmental enforcement agency. Under the provision of the Clean Air Act of 1970, the EPA set national ambient air quality standards for "criteria" pollutants, the most common air pollutants. The criteria pollutants are ozone, suspended particulate matter, carbon monoxide, sulfur dioxide, lead, and nitrogen oxides (see Major Air Pollutants on page 737). According to the EPA, at least 74 million people have lived in areas that still exceeded at least one air quality standard, and as many as 140 million people may have lived in areas that had ozone levels or smog (a combination of smoke and fog) in excess of national standards during that year.

Some progress has been made in controlling air pollution through mandating the reduction of pollutants in auto exhaust. This was accomplished by switching to lead-free gasoline and introducing catalytic converters in automobiles. As a result, automobile emissions of carbon monoxide and hydrocarbons have dropped 96 percent and nitric oxide emissions have fallen 88 percent. Emissions from industrial sources are also heavily regulated and have been reduced as new technologies and procedures were implemented.

The EPA also lists "hazardous" air pollutants and establishes safety standards for their emission. For example, asbestos now has been banned in new construction, and materials containing asbestos have been removed from schools and other public buildings (Floyd, Mimms, and Yelding-Howard 1998, 497–498). Other examples of hazardous pollutants are beryllium, mercury, vinyl chloride, arsenic, benzene, radionucleotides, and coke oven emissions.

WATER POLLUTION

Like air, water is essential to life. The demand for clean water has increased with the growth in population, in irrigation demands, and in manufacturing. These areas of growth, plus the conversion of land that formerly held water, have caused a significant and dangerous reduction in water tables in many areas of the country.

Most people in the United States have clean water to drink, but there are significant pockets of the country where the water supply is contaminated. About 80 percent of U.S. drinking water has chlorine added to it to prevent outbreaks of waterborne illnesses that were once endemic. In areas where drinking water is polluted, health diseases such as cholera, typhoid, and dysentery abound due to infectious agents and toxins in the water (Pruitt and Stein 1999, 536–537).

Despite water's importance, we dump everything from animal fertilizer and detergents to industrial wastes and sewage into our precious water supply. In addition, when pollutants are channeled into nonflowing bodies of water, such as lakes, eutrophication (accelerated growth of algae) occurs. As algae growth skyrockets on a diet of inorganic pollutants, especially nitrogen and phosphorus, a blanket of slime covers the water. Eventual death of the algae results in bacterial decomposition that consumes the oxygen present. This oxygen deficit kills fish and other lake inhabitants, many of which are valuable as food resources, and, as recently suggested, disrupts freshwater animals' endocrine systems (Morgan 2003). Eventually, the body of water becomes contaminated beyond use. Even flowing bodies of water, such as streams and rivers, that undergo natural purification can be badly polluted if sufficient quantities of wastes are dumped into them.

Major Water Pollutants. There are numerous sources of water pollution. The main ones are industrial wastes, human sewage, and thermal pollution.

Industrial Wastes. Chemical byproducts from the manufacture of paper, steel, oil, pesticides, and the like account for more than half of the water pollution in this country. Despite water pollution laws, an abundance of diverse industrial wastes continues to be deposited in lakes, streams, and rivers throughout the country. Many, like lead and mercury, are known to be toxic to humans. Of great concern regarding the danger of any industrial waste product is the length of time it takes to be broken down by the environment and the concentration that is tolerable by given organisms, particularly humans.

Human Sewage. Although contamination of water from human waste is much less serious than it once was, it nevertheless can occur in varying degrees if a community's sewage treatment system is antiquated or not inspected regularly. It is recommended that sewage treatment consist of two stages: primary

Health Highlight

SELECTED GOALS FROM HEALTHY PEOPLE 2010—

ENVIRONMENTAL HEALTH

Harmful air pollutants—*Outdoor (ozone and particulate matter):* reduce the proportion of persons exposed to air that does not meet the EPA's health-based standards for harmful air pollutants. *Indoor:* reduce indoor allergen levels

Safe drinking water—increase the proportion of persons served by community water systems who receive a supply of drinking water that meets the regulations of the Safe Drinking Water Act

Waterborne diseases—reduce waterborne disease outbreaks arising from water intended for drinking among persons served by community water systems

Lead poisoning—eliminate elevated blood lead levels in children

Radon—increase the proportion of persons who live in homes tested for radon concentrations

Disaster planning—ensure that state health departments establish training, plans, and protocols and conduct annual multi-institutional exercises to prepare for response to natural and technological disasters

Lead paint—increase the proportion of people living in pre-1950s housing that has been tested for the presence of lead-based paint

Global burden of disease—reduce the global burden of disease due to poor water quality, sanitation, and personal and domestic hygiene

SOURCE: Partners in Information Access for Public Health Professionals 2003

and secondary. The primary stage rids the water, which has been allowed to settle in a holding tank, of large objects through a filtration process of passing the liquid over a series of screens. During the secondary stage of treatment, smaller particles of organic material and microbes are removed through additional filtration techniques, dispersement over beds of stone, and chemical purification. The final step usually involves the addition of chlorine to disinfect the water of any remaining bacteria so it is safe for recycling. There has been rising concern over the presence of antibiotics, prescription medications, and radioactive waste (from medical treatments) in human sewage.

Thermal Pollution. Numerous industries, including those involved in generating nuclear power, use water as a coolant for their equipment. Water absorbs heat from the equipment and is channeled back to its source, where it produces a rise in temperature of the source water itself. Although this process seems harmless enough, the warmer the water is, the less oxygen it will absorb, and the less oxygen absorbed, the less quickly the lake or river decomposes its organic material. Since power-generating plants in particular heat large volumes of water, the parent waterway is certainly at risk. In addition, much of the aquatic life is drastically affected by extreme temperature variation from the norm.

Damage Resulting from Water Pollution. Polluted water can be responsible for transmitting many pathogens. For example, the infectious agents that cause typhoid fever, dysentery, and cholera are just a few of the microorganisms that can be transmitted through polluted water. Viruses from human wastes carried in contaminated water can cause hepatitis. Bacteria found in polluted water can cause intestinal disorders. Parasitic worms and protozoa found in water may cause such health problems as giardiasis, also known as traveler's diarrhea. Other materials found in polluted water, such as asbestos fibers, can cause cancer.

Polluted water can be particularly harmful to fish, birds, and animals. For example, herbicides, phosphates, fertilizers, sewage, and industrial wastes kill numerous fish and birds, and some may act as estrogen mimics that disrupt reproductive hormones and even development of reproductive organs. These products also promote the growth of algae, which changes the ecological balance and produces odors and foul-tasting drinking water. Aquatic organisms may be affected by rising water temperature, which retards their reproduction, destroys their food supplies, or kills them.

The oil slicks of recent years have been widely publicized. The devastation to birds and fish has been apparent. The oil coats the gills of fish, thus killing them. Feathers of birds are coated so that the birds cannot fly, and preening their feathers leads to ingestion of the oil. Oil-covered beaches are also expensive to clean, and the public loses recreational areas. Floating debris may entangle wildlife or even be mistaken as food and swallowed.

Water Quality Control. Although federal controls regarding water pollution have not been as extensive as those for air pollution, the enactment of the Federal Water Pollution Control Act in 1973 was conceived as a means of developing a national system that would require any institution, industry, or company that discharges substances into waterways to meet EPA standards.

The Clean Water Act, enacted in 1972, was implemented to protect and restore the nation's waters. Its main purpose is to eliminate discharge of pollutants into our waters and to keep our waters at levels that are fishable and swimmable (EPA 2003c). In 1996 Congress renewed the Safe Drinking Water Act of 1974. Under the new act, consumers must be notified whenever contaminants are found in drinking water and not merely when the water does not meet federal standards for contamination and safety (Edlin, Golanty, and Brown 1999, 490). The EPA also provides Internet access to information on water standard violations (National Center for Health Statistics 2000, 123).

HAZARDOUS CHEMICAL POLLUTION

The hazardous chemicals that pollute our environment are numerous and varied. They include not only the toxins deposited in our air and waterways, but also the pesticides sprayed on crops, the chemicals transported along our railways and highways for use in industry, and those contained in commonly used household products.

Major Hazardous Chemicals.

Pesticides. With the 1962 publication of Rachel Carson's *Silent Spring,* people began to become more conscious of the hazards of pesticides, toxic chemicals used to kill insects, and other pests that destroy crops. In past decades, the harm caused by the widespread use of chlorinated hydrocarbons such as DDT (dichlorodiphenyltrichloroethane), dieldrin, and chlordane as pesticides was not fully recognized. These chemicals have been restricted or banned by the EPA (for example, DDT use was banned more than twenty years ago) because they may cause cancer, birth defects, neurological disorders, and damage to wildlife and the environment. They are persistent, sometimes remaining in the environment for as long as fifteen years before degrading (Hales 1999, 658).

Chlorinated hydrocarbons decompose very slowly and remain toxic to a wide variety of animal life for long periods. Organophosphate pesticides such as diazinon, parathion, and malathion exhibit similar properties and are even more poisonous than the chlorinated hydrocarbons.

Although worldwide food production needs to be increased to meet the demands of a growing population, extensive use of pesticides can cause great harm to environmental health in the process. Questions still need to be answered concerning the implication of long-term exposure to moderate or even minimal levels of pesticides. There is evidence that these chemicals can damage the human reproductive and nervous systems, for example. The use of pesticides must be limited and controlled in order to protect all inhabitants of our ecosphere.

Industrial Chemicals. One of the newer and most dangerous environmental threats is the transportation of industrial chemicals from state to state and from country to country. Although transportation itself is not inherently harmful, leakage or spills of chemical substances most certainly is. In fact, hardly a week goes by without news of such an accident that causes disability or death. For example, accidents involving the transportation of oil and other petroleum products have resulted in several major oil spills that have damaged some of our nation's most beautiful beaches and killed or endangered countless birds and marine life.

In response to this increasingly dangerous threat, many state governments and the federal government have formed special subcommittees to study the problem of transportation of industrial chemicals. Particularly with regard to the movement of radioactive material for industrial and burial purposes, many states have indicated an unwillingness to continue to allow such toxins to cross their borders. More controls and safeguards need to be implemented in transporting hazardous chemicals of any kind, whether by trucks, ships, or trains.

Household Products. Before the recent ban on spray cans containing propellant fluorocarbons and detergents containing phosphates, numerous household products served as contaminators of the environment by releasing these agents into the air and water, respectively. Fluorocarbons destroy the protective ozone layer of the atmosphere that shields us from damaging ultraviolet rays of the sun, while phosphates serve as nutrients for bacteria, protozoa, and algae, promoting eutrophication of lakes, streams, and rivers. These examples serve as an excellent illustration of the dangers involved in releasing seemingly harmless compounds into our surroundings from heavily used household products like cleansers, polishes, waxes, and sprays of all kinds without first studying their environmental impact.

Hazardous Chemical Control. Several federal laws have been passed that have focused on the dangers of pesticides. For example, the Federal Insecticide,

Fungicide, and Rodenticide Act was passed in 1948 originally (and the last amendment was in 1988) to regulate the use of pesticides. Also, the Food, Drug and Cosmetic Act regulates the tolerances for pesticide residues in foods. As a result, more environmentally sustainable approaches to crop spraying have evolved. Alternative means of pest control are being implemented in the United States and elsewhere, the best known of which is integrated pest management, a combination of controls including chemical and biological methods. The global use of pesticides still poses a danger to environmental health.

In 1976, the U.S. government created the Resource Conservation and Recovery Act (RCRA) to enforce proper management of hazardous wastes. This law has helped to regulate the production, handling, and cleanup of hazardous materials and to reduce illegal disposal of such wastes (Office of Environmental Policy & Guidance 2003).

SOLID WASTE POLLUTION

Until recently, the public virtually ignored the problems related to the disposal of solid wastes. The majority of these solid wastes are buried in landfills, many of which have been identified as hazardous waste sites and unacceptable health risks. Solid waste is made up of everything from paper packaging and durable goods to plastic containers, food, grass and other yard wastes, and motor oil. Hazardous wastes consist of materials that are flammable, corrosive, toxic, or chemically reactive (Donatelle 2002, 575–576).

Today, we use more and more convenience products that are easily disposed of and replaced. Everything from disposable diapers, dishes, and food containers to plastic wraps, sanitary products, and paper napkins are available. The price of this convenience has been the growing problem of solid waste disposal. The unsightly junkyards, dumps, and scattered litter are more than just eyesores. They are a public health hazard as well.

Many solid waste materials are not biodegradable; they remain in the environment for long periods of time because they do not decay or cannot be burned easily. The piles of refuse serve as breeding grounds for microorganisms, rats, insects, and other disease carriers. In addition, agricultural waste products from orchards, feedlots, and farms add significantly to the total solid waste that must be disposed of each year. How then do we rid ourselves of all our refuse?

Solid Waste Control. In 1980, the United States created the Superfund, a $1.6 billion trust fund designated to clean up abandoned hazardous waste sites. Under this law, the EPA can clean up a dump site and then recover the costs, through lawsuits, from those responsible. In 1986, realizing the problem was greater than originally thought, the U.S. federal government added another $8.5 billion to the Superfund. Progress has been slow. The government has identified 1,219 sites as hazardous and an additional 32,000 as potentially hazardous. As many as forty million Americans live within four miles of the nation's worst hazardous waste sites. As a result, they are susceptible to birth defects, nervous system disorders, cancer, cardiovascular problems, respiratory irritation, and skin irritation (Floyd, Mimms, and Yelding-Howard 1998, 504–505).

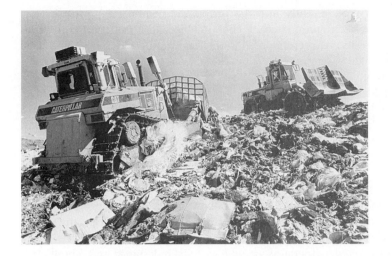

The benefits of a well-functioning landfill can be numerous.

The United States, like many other nations, is still struggling with the problem. Until citizens recognize that many solid waste disposal programs are ineffective or unacceptable, the situation is unlikely to change. Individual efforts toward decreasing the daily use of disposal products that are not easily biodegradable as well as efforts aimed at recycling can assist greatly, but more public awareness and action are needed to draw attention to the problem of solid waste disposal. Current methods of solid waste disposal primarily include dumps, landfills, incineration, and recycling.

Dumps. Most solid waste in this country is deposited in open, minimally managed dumps. Some burning of garbage does take place in order to condense the material. Besides being unsightly, open dumping grounds can pose a serious threat to a community's health if the insect or rodent population gets out of control. The widespread use of dumps results from the short-term cheapness of this method of solid waste disposal.

Landfills. Unlike the procedures of open disposal in a dump, those in a landfill require the solid waste to be covered by dirt each day after it has been compacted. Once covered with dirt, the landfill is bulldozed to smooth out and compress the area. A properly operated landfill requires predetermined designing and engineering of the site as well as continued daily maintenance from a crew of workers within a city sanitation department. However, the benefits of a well-functioning landfill can be numerous. Because refuse is covered daily, risk of a contaminated water supply or of disease due to the breeding of flies, mosquitoes, rats, and the like is diminished considerably. Because burning is not necessary, the technique does not contribute to air pollution. In addition, after the location has been completely filled in, it can serve some other valuable purpose, such as a site for housing, recreation, or industry. (Burial of some types of hazardous wastes in a landfill will preclude its use for some types of construction.)

There are problems, nevertheless, associated with the use of landfills. Land itself is becoming more scarce and more expensive, not all types of terrain are suitable to serve as landfills, and the surrounding water table must be low enough to not be contaminated by chemicals leeching from the landfill. In addition, residents are often opposed to the establishment of a landfill nearby for fear that it will lower property values.

Incineration. Like dumping, incineration is a very old method of waste disposal that adds to environmental pollution because of the release of particulate matter into the atmosphere during burning. Of particular danger is the release of hydrogen chloride from burning plastic materials, which are mainly composed of polyvinyl chloride. On contact with moisture in the air, hydrogen chloride forms hydrochloric acid, an especially corrosive agent that causes respiratory irritation.

However, the energy and heat produced as by-products of incineration can be used in homes and industry. Incineration of solid wastes has been employed successfully for this purpose in many locations throughout Europe and is now being used in the United States. To accomplish this throughout the entire United States, many incinerators would have to be redesigned and rebuilt. As it stands, incineration is already one of the more costly waste-disposal methods. Nevertheless, incineration as a generator of energy deserves more investigation.

Recycling. Many products can be recycled, or reused in another mode. For example, paper, glass, and metal products can all be recycled. This method of solid waste control was widespread before World War I and regained some popularity during the environmentally conscious era of the late 1960s and early 1970s. Many communities provide recycling centers to which residents can bring recyclable materials. Some communities merely ask residents to place recyclable materials out for collection in front of their homes. These projects have significantly decreased the amount of unrecycled solid waste.

Many schools around the country also participate in recycling programs. For example, Madison County in Illinois has implemented the Madison County Solid Waste Recycling Program, which emphasizes recycling, reduction, and reusing. With regard to recycling, it is suggested that you recycle every item that you can, and be sure to use curbside programs and recycling stations, when available. We can reduce the amount of material needed to be thrown away by buying items with less packaging; buying in bulk when possible; avoiding single-use packaging; and packing waste-free lunches, such as not using paper bags, foil, and/or plastic wraps. Finally, try to use materials that can be reused. For example, use lunch containers instead of paper bags, ceramic drinking cups instead of foam, and cloth rags instead of paper towels (Madison County Recycles 2003).

RELATED ENVIRONMENTAL RISKS

Radiation Exposure. Individuals are exposed to radiation daily, both from natural sources such as sunlight and from man-made sources. The man-made sources of radiation are of most concern. Radioactive materials release energy in the form of a stream of particles generally referred to as *radiation*. Alpha and beta radioactive particles do not easily penetrate the human body, but gamma radiation does. Gamma rays are much like X rays. If an individual is exposed to a

Health Highlight

WHAT YOU CAN DO TO PROTECT OUR PLANET

1. Plant a tree. This helps absorb carbon dioxide and produce cooling.

2. Look for simply packaged items. Look for items packed in recycled materials or something recyclable.

3. Bring your own bag. Avoid using plastic or paper bags for items you could carry in a cloth carryall.

4. Hit the switch. Turn off electrical appliances when you are not in the room.

5. Avoid disposables. Use a mug instead of a paper or Styrofoam cup, a sponge instead of a paper towel, a cloth napkin instead of a paper one.

6. Be water wise. Turn off water while you shave or brush your teeth. Install water-efficient faucets and showerheads.

7. Cancel junk mail. It consumes 100 million trees a year. To get off mailing lists, write: Mail Preference Service, Direct Marketing Association, 11 East 42nd St., P.O. Box 3861, New York, NY 10163-3861.

8. Spare the seas. If you live near the coast or are picnicking or hiking near the ocean, don't use plastic bags or plastic 6-pack holders (which can get caught around the necks of sea birds).

9. Don't buy products made of endangered substances. Examples include coral, ivory, tortoise shell, or wood from endangered forests.

10. Be politically active. Monitor environmental legislation. Write letters to legislators, campaign for environmental candidates, or start projects at school or in your community.

SOURCE: Hales 1999, 650

sufficiently high dosage of gamma radiation, several adverse effects occur, ranging from nausea, hair loss, and diarrhea to cell mutation, anemia, and death.

In the United States, individuals come into contact with radiation mainly through medical testing and X rays. Although X rays are generally considered safe, many instances of unnecessary exposure have been reported. Intervals of several months should elapse between exposures to X rays. Pregnant women, particularly during the first trimester, should avoid being x-rayed if at all possible because radiation can cause cell damage and mutation to the developing fetus.

Exposure to low-level radiation for a prolonged period is also of great concern for individuals whose work surroundings or home environment may be near a radioactive source. The health effects of radiation exposure depend on many factors, including the duration, type, dose of exposure, and individual sensitivity. Lesser exposure can affect egg and sperm production and embryonic development, and cause irreversible changes to the eyes and skin. Heavy exposure can produce radiation sickness or immediate death (Hahn and Payne 1997, 436). As a result, opponents to the use of nuclear power as an energy source are becoming more vocal. They fear both the dangers of mishandling the disposal of nuclear wastes and the potential for a nuclear accident like those that occurred at Three Mile Island in Pennsylvania in March 1979 and at the Chernobyl plant in the Soviet Union in April 1986. On the other hand, supporters of nuclear power believe that, through the implementation of the Nuclear Regulatory

Table 25.1	*Typical Noise Levels*
Source of Noise	**Decibels**
Whispering	30
Air conditioner at twenty feet	60
Busy traffic	70
Truck noise	90
Airplane overhead	100
Chainsaw	100
Rock band concert in front of speakers	120
Shotgun blast	140
Rocket pad during launch	180

Commission's guidelines, nuclear power can be a safe, viable, and much needed energy source for the future.

Radiation Exposure Control. Guidelines exist that indicate allowable ranges of radiation exposure from medical testing, X rays, and consumer products emitting small amounts of radiation, such as television sets. However, the long-term effects on health of even low or "safe" levels of radiation are still poorly understood. Any radiation at all may in fact be deleterious to health. Certainly as individuals we must become more educated and aware of both the benefits and the dangers of using radiation and nuclear power.

Noise Pollution. With more and more of the U.S. population living in metropolitan areas, the problem of noise as a pollutant is also growing. Noise pollution is a problem for almost every urban dweller and a particular cause of concern among people living near airports; employees working in manufacturing or industry; and commuters who must endure hours of noise each week traveling in cars, trains, buses, and subways. Also, listening to loud music, especially through earphones, is a noise pollutant that is a potential cause of hearing loss.

Noise levels are calculated in decibels (dB), a measurement for which 1 dB represents the minimum level of hearing for humans. A sound that is 10 times as loud would be 10 dB, another 100 times as loud would be 20 dB, one 1,000 times as loud would be 30 dB, and so forth. Sounds exceeding 80 to 85 decibels can cause hearing damage (see Table 25.1). The damage is initially reversible; however, with continued exposure, the changes become permanent (Hahn and Payne 1997, 438–439).

Many detrimental effects apart from hearing impairment can occur due to noise because of its stressful nature. Headaches, difficulty sleeping, increase in anxiety, and elevated blood pressure are just a few. As a result, increased efforts must be made toward minimizing noise pollution.

Noise Pollution Control. No uniform standards regarding acceptable noise levels for school, home, or work environments have been formulated. Therefore, each individual must exercise personal judgment in deciding how much noise exposure is not only tolerable but safe. Employees in industry are, of course, issued protective ear devices, but the general public is not guaranteed the same protection on noisy highways or in neighborhoods near loud noise sources. Greater awareness of the harmful physical and psychological effects of noise may lead to public action and legislation in the years ahead.

Wildlife is also affected by noise pollution. Studies have shown that in response to common human activities that cause large amounts of noise, animals have injured themselves, lost energy due to decreases in food intake, avoided and abandoned their habitat, and suffered reproductive losses. Noise stresses these animals to the point of endangering their population (Noise Pollution Clearinghouse 2003).

Indoor Air Pollution. When people think of pollution, they do not consider their most familiar environment, the indoors, as a factor. Most people do not know that indoor air pollution can also have significant health effects. The EPA has stated that indoor levels of pollutants may be two to five times, and occasionally more than 100 times, higher than outdoor levels. These levels of indoor air pollutants may be of particular concern because most people spend about 90 percent of their time indoors.

In the home, there are many sources of pollution that can have significant effects on health. Tobacco smoke, pet dander, mold, and dust mites are all environmental asthma triggers. Some problems arise from asbestos-containing insulation; household cleaners; gas stoves that emit carbon monoxide; containers of oil, gas, and kerosene; fumes from new carpeting, etc. Any kind of unsanitary conditions such as excess dirt, old food, and trash can lead to vermin and insects within the home as well.

Indoor pollution sources that release gases or particles into the air are the primary cause of indoor air quality problems in homes. Inadequate ventilation can increase indoor pollutant levels by not bringing in enough outdoor air to dilute emissions from indoor sources and by not carrying indoor air pollutants out of the home. Radon, a gas that cannot be smelled or tasted, has become a problem in many homes. Breathing air containing radon can led to lung cancer. High temperature and humidity levels can also increase concentrations of some pollutants. Indoor pollutants are also a concern within schools and classrooms. Chalk dust from boards and erasers, old air conditioning, old insulation, mildew, and public bathrooms can all contribute to classroom pollution (EPA 2003b).

Preservation of the Ecosphere

Conservation and protection of our natural resources must stem from both individual and public action. Both are needed to stabilize and eventually reverse the harmful cycle of contamination that currently plagues the ecosphere. Legislation and implementation of healthier environmental practices have been instituted. The enactment of additional measures could serve to improve the quality of living for us and for future generations.

Summary

- Individuals should act responsibly and diligently with regard to their environment to ensure high-level wellness.

- The environment in which one lives must be free of dangerous levels of pollutants and therefore conducive to quality living—not just mere survival.

- In order to maintain the natural resources on which all living things depend, it is essential that we understand how we interact with and influence our ecosystem, our immediate habitat.

- Many man-made changes have caused havoc in ecological chains or webs within ecosystems.

- Because ecosystems, like the residents within them, are interdependent and thus form one worldwide ecosphere, the harmful impact of human growth and technology is felt throughout the entire planet.

- Population growth is causing our species to stretch the capacity of land, water, and food supplies to accommodate us.

- Particularly in the highly industrial nations, human lifestyles have resulted in an abundance of pollution problems that cannot be dealt with by the buffering capacities of natural cycles within the ecosphere.

- With our automobiles, we release dangerous pollutants into the air.

- Industry adds still other toxins, and runoff from agriculture and industrial dumping contaminates our water.

- Incidents involving the accidental leakage or spillage of highly lethal substances during transport occur fairly frequently.

- These environmental health problems, coupled with problems of solid-waste disposal, radiation exposure, noise pollution, and indoor air pollution, have resulted in unprecedented ecological crises.

- Through continued research, education, and responsible action on the part of both governments and individuals, preservation of the ecosphere is possible.

- It is our job as educators to provide instructional and consciousness-raising experiences to the children we teach so that their children and grandchildren will enjoy continued health and well-being in a sound environment.

DISCUSSION QUESTIONS

1. Define and differentiate between the terms *environment* and *ecology*.

2. What is the ecosphere, and how do human beings interact with elements of the ecosphere?

3. What impact does overpopulation have on the state of the environment, and what problems directly or indirectly stem from overpopulation?

4. What are the major sources of air pollution? Describe the harmful effects of specific air pollutants on human health.

5. What are the objectives that the U.S. government has set for regulation of contaminants by the year 2010?

6. What individual steps can be taken to more effectively manage and control air pollution?

7. What threats to environmental health does the transportation of hazardous substances pose?

8. What is indoor air pollution? How does it affect environmental health?

9. How can each individual help to preserve the ecosphere? Give specific suggestions.

CRITICAL THINKING QUESTIONS

1. After reading this chapter and considering the "Reflections" at the beginning of this chapter, what have you decided are the major environmental hazards that you face personally? What are some steps you have decided to take to protect yourself from these hazards?

2. Are there any environmental hazards to which your behavior may contribute? Consider the Health Highlight box on page 747, "What You Can Do to Protect Our Planet." What are some steps you can incorporate in your lifestyle?

3. The steps to control overpopulation in our world are considered controversial by some. Consider the pros and cons of these steps and your values and beliefs regarding each step.

4. This chapter has challenged you to become proactive in reducing the threat of environmental health problems. Research a piece of environmental health legislation currently being considered by your county or state. Draft a letter to your local or state legislator regarding your stand on this legislation.

WEB SITE ACTIVITY

Go to the EPA Web site at *www.epa.gov*. Follow the links provided there to find information about the effects of acid rain.

WEB SITES OF INTEREST

American Environmental Health Foundation (AEHF): *www.aehf.com*
The AEHF is a nonprofit organization founded to provide research and education on chemical sensitivity.

The Envirolink: *www.envirolink.org/start_web.html*
EnviroLink is a nonprofit organization that unites hundreds of organizations and volunteers around the world in more than 150 countries.

Environmental Protection Agency (EPA): *www.epa.gov*
The mission of the EPA is to protect human health and to safeguard the natural environment—air, water, and land—upon which life depends.

National Resources Defense Council (NRDC): *www.nrdc.org*
NRDC uses law, science, and the support of its membership to protect the planet's wildlife and wild places and to ensure a safe and healthy environment for all living things.

The Sierra Club: *www.sierraclub.org*
The Sierra Club promotes exploration, enjoyment, and protection of the earth's ecosystems and resources through responsible use and by lawful means.

Science News: *www.sciencenews.org*
Provides a weekly overview of research articles published in scientific journals.

Scientific American: *www.scian.com*
Provides in-depth review articles of topics of current interest in the scientific arena.

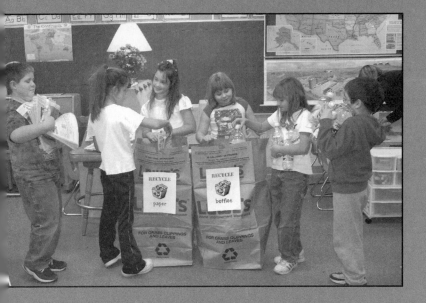

Strategies for Teaching Environmental Health

Environmental protection contributes to making our communities and ecosystems diverse, sustainable, and economically productive.

—U.S. Environmental Protection Agency Mission Statement (2000)

VALUED OUTCOMES

After doing the activities in this chapter, the student should be able to explain and illustrate the following statements:

- High levels of personal wellness can only be sustained if the environment is conducive to well-being.

- All the animals, plants, and natural resources in any particular habitat form a self-sustaining ecosystem.

- All parts of an ecosystem are interdependent.

- Each ecosystem is linked to all other ecosystems to form a global network called an ecosphere. Thus, change in one ecosystem has the potential to affect any other ecosystem and the ecosphere as a whole.

- Because human beings have the ability to alter and manipulate the environment, human activities have the greatest impact on ecosystems.

- Human activities have caused extensive harm to the environment, which has affected environmental health.

- The major sources of pollution are air impurities, water contaminants, hazardous chemicals, solid waste, radiation, and noise.

- Overpopulation has resulted in environmental problems.

- Conservation of natural resources, preservation of ecosystems, and protection of the environment from pollution are essential for preserving the ecosphere.

- Preservation of the ecosphere must stem both from individual and public action.

REFLECTIONS

As you review this chapter, think in terms of where and how the classroom teacher can foster a concern for environmental issues. Where should the emphasis begin and what types of strategies would you use at the lower elementary, upper elementary, and middle school levels?

Fostering Environmental Appreciation

All living species have had to adapt to its environment or face extinction. This adaptation has resulted in an amazing variety of life-forms on the planet. Thick-skinned cacti have adapted to the harsh environment of our deserts. Luminescent fish live successfully in the perpetual darkness of the ocean depths. Polar bears carry on their life cycles in the frozen landscape above the Arctic Circle.

Human beings have also had to adapt to the physical environment; but, unlike any other form of life on the planet, human beings can also extensively adapt the environment to suit their needs. We build cities, dam rivers, mine the earth, and farm the land. To a large extent, we can manipulate and control our environment. This unique ability has sometimes resulted in the misconception that we are the masters of our environment. This has led to abuse of natural resources and consequent pollution, waste, and lowering of environmental quality.

In the last few decades, we have become more aware that human beings are not free to alter the environment—we pay a price. We have recognized that we are part of a worldwide ecosystem, interacting and interrelating with every other part. This increased environmental awareness has not come too soon. We now know all too well that nature's resources are finite and must be conserved and used wisely. We have begun to see that change to any part of the environment can have a wide-ranging impact on many other parts. Failure to understand the consequences could mean disaster not only for ourselves but also for the entire planet.

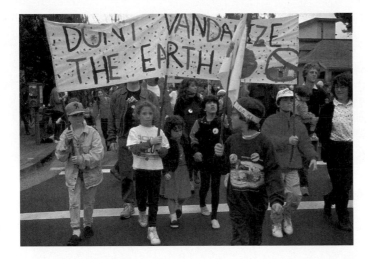

We are the stewards of our land and water.

Students need to learn about the importance of healthy environment. They must recognize that it is up to each of us to maintain the environment. Doing so will more easily foster high-level wellness. Instruction about environmental health should build a sense of appreciation for all life and natural resources and encourage personal practices that will help to ensure the continued preservation of the ecosphere. The activities suggested in this chapter will help you attain this goal for your students.

Shown to the right of each activity title is the suggested grade level(s) for which the activity might be appropriate. However, many of the suggested activities could be modified for use at various grade levels.

Value-Based Activities

MAJOR ENVIRONMENTAL PROBLEMS   Grades (4–6)

Valued Outcome: The students will identify the biggest problem they believe is affecting our environment.

Description of Strategy: Have students research the problems affecting our environment such as overpopulation, pesticides, land pollution, air pollution, water pollution, and noise pollution. Then have a class discussion about each environmental area and the issues associated with each area. After the discussion have the students prepare posters showing the effects of the environmental problems in question. The processing questions are good guidelines for the questions to be answered on the posters. Pictures, graphs, and illustrations should be part of the poster.

Materials Needed: poster board and markers for each student

Health Highlight

THINGS KIDS CAN DO TO PROTECT THE ENVIRONMENT

Our natural resources are important, and there are many things we can do to protect and preserve them. Some things kids can do include the following:

■ purchase recycled products

■ ask family members to reuse shopping bags

■ recycle metals, including all aluminum

■ recycle newspapers

■ use as few paper products as possible

■ recycle cardboard

■ recycle plastics

■ recycle tin cans

■ recycle glass containers

Processing Questions:

1. Why do you believe this is the biggest problem?

2. How is this problem affecting the environment?

3. How does this problem affect you and your family?

4. What can your family do to help relieve this problem?

ECOLOGICAL FOOD CHAIN   Grades (2–6)

Valued Outcome: The students will be able to describe an ecological food chain.

Description of Strategy: The following are the major parts of an ecological food chain: predators, scavengers, consumers, and producers. Have the students make a poster illustrating an ecological food chain. The students may add links to make a more elaborate food chain: water, birds, fish, humans.

Materials Needed: paper, markers, and pictures

Processing Questions:

1. What happens when pesticides affect one link in the ecological model?

2. What is an example of an endangered animal that has been affected by pesticides or pollution?

3. What are some ways you can help eliminate environmental pollution?

LET'S RANK OUR   Grades (6–8)
ENVIRONMENTAL PROBLEMS

Valued Outcome: The students will be able to identify the most hazardous environmental problems.

Description of Strategy: Have the students rank the environmental problems listed in the Teaching in Action box "Environmental Problems," from most

Air Pollution

_____ carbon monoxide and nitrogen

_____ sulfur oxides

_____ lead

Water Pollution

_____ animal fertilizers

_____ human sewage

_____ industrial wastes

Solid Waste Pollution

_____ dump

_____ landfills

_____ recycling

Hazardous Chemical Pollution

_____ pesticides

_____ industrial chemicals

_____ household products

hazardous to least hazardous, with 1 being the most and 3 being the least hazardous. Once the class is finished, write the problems on the board and rank them as a group. Have an open class discussion about the answers.

Materials Needed: list of environmental hazards for each student

Processing Questions:

1. Why are some hazards more dangerous than others?
2. What are some ways we can prevent pollution of our environment?

Decision Stories

Follow the procedure discussed in Chapter 4 (pages 80–83) for presenting decision stories such as the following.

THE FISHING TRIP   Grades (K–3)

Ramon is going fishing with his grandfather and is very excited. They have fixed a picnic lunch because they plan to stay all day. Ramon and his grandfather drive to the river. As they walk along the riverside, Ramon notices some dead fish floating in the water. "Grandfather, what killed those fish?" Ramon asks. "They were killed because people put garbage into the river," Grandfather replies. Then they sit down and start to fish. Ramon and his grandfather catch several fish apiece.

Focus Questions:

1. Should they take the fish home and cook them? Why or why not?
2. What can Ramon and his grandfather do to make the river cleaner?

A BIRD'S NEST   Grades (K–3)

Jim and Richard are good friends who live next door to one another. They are now old enough to walk home from school, and today is their first time to do so. On the way home they cut through a small park. Richard discovers a bird's nest with three eggs in it. He wants to take it home. Jim has been taught that it is important not to disturb the natural surroundings, but Richard is such a good friend.

Focus Question: What should Jim do?

IS RECYCLING WORTH THE WORK?   Grades (3–8)

Kathy has heard about a recycling center in her town. People can bring bottles and aluminum cans there. The material is crushed and then sold to industry to be used again. Kathy tells her mother about the recycling center and asks if the family can bring in their bottles and cans. "It sounds like a good idea," Kathy's mother says, "but it's too much work. We would have to clean and sort all our old bottles and cans. Anyway, the recycling center has enough bottles and cans without us."

Focus Question: Should Kathy try to convince her mother that recycling is worth the effort? If so, how could she do this?

BAD AIR   Grades (4–6)

Esther's mother always comes home from work coughing and wheezing. "What's wrong, Mom?" Esther asks. "It's all that dirty air I have to breathe riding the bus to and from work," her mother replies. "Maybe you could find a job closer to home," Esther says. "It's not that easy to find jobs these days," her mother says. "I guess I'll just have to put up with the bad air on the bus."

Focus Questions:

1. Is there anything Esther can do to help her mother?
2. Who can Esther contact to find out about lowering air pollution?

Dramatizations

ROLE-PLAYING ENVIRONMENTAL HAZARDS   Grades (4–6)

Valued Outcome: The students will be able to discuss environmental hazards.

Description of Strategy: Divide the students into groups of four to five. Have the groups pick an environmental hazard, then have one group at a time come up and act out the problem. Examples of hazards that might be used include water pollution and air pollution—pretend to be using hair spray, littering, and so on. The group that can guess what environmental hazard is taking place receives a point. If no one can guess the environmental hazard, then that group receives a point. Have the students draw index cards that have the hazards listed on them. Have several cards for each type of hazard. Instruct the students that they may *not* portray the same aspect of that hazard as has already been performed. List hazards on the board. Have students brainstorm to come up with hazards that weren't covered. Keep playing until everyone has had several turns. At the end of the lesson, have the students brainstorm all the hazards and write them down on the board.

Materials Needed: board and marker or overhead projector and pen

Processing Question: Where can environmental hazards be found?

WATER POLLUTION: OIL SPILLS   Grades (K–3)

Valued Outcome: The students will be able to describe how oil spills hurt the environment.

Description of Strategy: Have five to ten students pretend that they are living plants, fish, animals, and other living things in a body of water. Have three or four other students act as if they are the sun shining on the water and helping the plants and other living things to live. Then have five to ten students come marching in and pretend they are an oil spill in the water. Have each "organism" explain the effect the oil spill will have on its species.

Materials Needed: none

Processing Questions:

1. What exactly happens during an oil spill?
2. What other environmentally dangerous events can oil spills cause?

POPULATIONS AND RESOURCE USE   Grades (3–4)

Valued Outcome: Students will be able to discuss how to conserve resources.

Description of Strategy: Have three of the students act as if they are horses in the wild. Provide several bottles around the room for water and little snacks such as cereal for food. Tell the horses they must eat and drink to survive. The snacks represent the grass they must have, and the water represents a stream of water. Add three more horses, then three more, and keep going until everyone is a horse. Have them "go to sleep," and tell them that when they wake up there will only be a small amount of water and food left. Ask them to explain to you what they will do. Have several of the horses die. Then ask a variety of questions about what actually happened. Relate the story to human beings and our resources. Explain what happens to other animals and the whole ecological system when resources become limited for a species.

Materials Needed: water bottles, bags of cereal

Processing Questions:

1. What was the problem?
2. What would happen once there was no more food or water?

PLANTS AND ANIMALS NEED PROTECTION, TOO

Grades (K–3)

Valued Outcome: The students will role-play a community of plants and animals in environmental danger.

Description of Strategy: Divide students into groups and use a story such as "Smokey the Bear," "Bambi," or any other suitable example for the specific grade level to inspire students to role-play a community of plants and animals that is in danger from an environmental threat. Tell students not only to voice their concerns as the animals and plants, but also to try to decide whether they as plants and animals can do anything to either prevent or diminish the environmental threat.

Materials Needed: none

Processing Question: How do environmental health dangers affect animals?

HOME HUNTING

Grades (2–6)

Valued Outcome: The students will role-play selling a house and identify several examples of a safe neighborhood.

Description of Strategy: Divide the class into small groups. Each group is responsible for describing a home that is for sale. One or two people in the group act as the sellers, while one or two people act as the buyers. The buyers come to look at the house and ask questions, many of which focus on environmental concerns, such as: What is the average monthly heating bill and cooling bill? How many miles from downtown is the neighborhood? How far away are the schools and shopping centers? Where is the nearest industrial site? Is there much noise in the neighborhood? Give only minimal guidance, such as a few examples of environmentally related questions. Allow each group five minutes for the presentation, and keep track of the commonly asked questions by listing them on the board. Then summarize by emphasizing the importance of living in a safe environment.

Materials Needed: board and markers or overhead projector and pen

Processing Question: What environmental concerns are involved with owning and maintaining a house?

FUTURE LIFESTYLES

Grades (4–8)

Valued Outcome: The students will be able to portray what life will be like in the future.

Description of Strategy: Divide students into small groups; assign each group a different social role—for example, factory workers, business professionals, and small-scale farmers. Ask each group to portray what they think life will be like for their members in fifty years, paying particular attention to possible environmental changes and their influences on the surroundings.

Materials Needed: none

Processing Question: What environmental changes likely will affect people's lives fifty years from now?

CITY CRISIS   Grades (6–8)

Valued Outcome: The students will enact a hypothetical dilemma concerning an environmental issue.

Description of Strategy: Provide the class with a hypothetical dilemma involving a voting question about a proposed city ordinance concerning an environmental issue. Give enough detailed information so that the viewpoints of various special interest groups can be developed. Then divide the class into three groups. Assign two groups the task of presenting a scenario and possible solution to the problem at a town meeting; the purpose is to have each group come up with its own solution to the same problem. Let students within each group volunteer to role-play identical characters, such as meeting moderator, mayor, union representatives, and conservation spokespeople. Allow both groups a few days to prepare a fifteen-minute dramatization. Dramatizations are presented as the third group acts as observers. Following the presentations, the third group then objectively critiques the ideas by highlighting strong points of each presentation and suggesting additional alternatives.

Materials Needed: description of hypothetical city and its problems (may be in handout form) for each student

Processing Questions:

1. What environmental concerns are being debated, discussed, and voted on by your city politicians?
2. How will their discussions affect you and your family?

DISASTER PREPARATION PRACTICE   Grades (4–6)

Valued Outcome: The students will identify an environmental disaster and its effects on communities.

Description of Strategy: Divide students into groups of five, and assign each group to research an environmental disaster that could affect communities, such as an air pollution crisis, train derailment of hazardous chemicals, or a highly toxic pollutant entering municipal water systems. Ask each group to dramatize a preparation plan that demonstrates the actions that should be taken or contributions that could be made by various community organizations in dealing with the environmental danger, should it ever occur.

Materials Needed: none

Processing Questions:

1. What are examples of environmental danger plans?
2. Does your community have a plan for a radiation disaster or other danger?

ALIEN IMPRESSIONS   Grades (4–6)

Valued Outcome: The students will be able to discuss how aliens from another planet would react to our environmental conditions.

Description of Strategy: Divide the class into groups of about five students. Tell each group that they are aliens from outer space who have suddenly landed in the heart of the city. Ask the groups to act out their reactions to our earthly surroundings, placing special emphasis on impressions about noise levels, traffic, air pollution, crowding, and use of natural resources.

Materials Needed: none

Processing Question: How would our environmental conditions appear to someone not familiar with our planet?

Discussion and Report Techniques

NATURE WATCH   Grades (4–6)

Valued Outcome: The students will observe behaviors in the environment with regard to plants and animals.

Description of Strategy: Divide students into groups of three, and place each group in a spot on or near the school premises in as natural an environment as possible. Have each group silently observe and record on paper the happenings in the environment for ten to fifteen minutes, particularly those associated with plants and animals. Then have each group discuss their observations. Later, ask the members of the class as a whole to focus on their feelings and attitudes about nature, based on this observation experience.

Materials Needed: pens or pencils and paper for each student

Processing Questions:

1. What aspects of nature did you observe?
2. How did you feel about the environment you observed?

ACTIVITIES AND THEIR   Grades (1–3)
ENVIRONMENTAL EFFECTS

Valued Outcome: The students will list ten activities and describe how these activities affect the environment.

Description of Strategy: Ask each student to list ten hobbies or activities he or she enjoys doing. After listing the activities, students should examine each activity in terms of its effects, if any, on the environment. As a result of this exercise, students will observe the relationship between their behavior and the environment in which they live.

Materials Needed: pens or pencils and paper for each student

Processing Question: What effects, if any, do your hobbies have on the environment? Are the effects positive or negative?

ME AND MY SURROUNDINGS   Grades (4–6)

Valued Outcome: Students will recognize their perceptions of the environment.

Description of Strategy: Ask each student to keep a daily log for a week about his or her perceptions of environmental influences by writing a short paragraph that describes an event or events of each day in terms of environmental awareness. Students should emphasize not only facts, but also feelings about these influences. For example, "Heavy rain against my window last night sounded nice. The noisy and crowded school bus made me feel irritable." At the end of the week, divide the class into seven discussion groups, each one representing one day of the week. Have groups compare their logs for that day and summarize major perceptions about surroundings. One group member should then present a five-minute report to the class outlining summary findings for the group.

Materials Needed: pens or pencils and paper for each student

Processing Questions:

1. What environmental influences did you observe?
2. What influences need to be changed in order to protect the environment?

CAN I RECYCLE?

Valued Outcome: The students will become acquainted with a variety of ways to recycle resources on a daily basis.

Description of Strategy: Using the Internet, students will find at least ten different ways to recycle at home and at school. Assign each method to a different group to learn about and describe to the class. Students will discuss how to make each recycling method a part of their daily life.

Materials Needed: computer with Internet access, pens or pencils and paper for each student

Processing Questions:

1. What are some things we can do every day to reduce environmental waste?
2. Why should we consider recycling every day?

SPREAD THE WORD   Grades (6–8)

Valued Outcome: The students will write and produce their own infomercials about recycling and easy ways to recycle every day.

Description of Strategy: Using the information they have gathered from researching recycling methods on the Internet, students will divide into groups (one for each recycling method) and write their own infomercials about how easy recycling can be, demonstrating their assigned method. The infomercials can be videotaped and played for the class, in other classes, and for special presentations for parents.

Materials Needed: computer with Internet access, pens or pencils and paper for each student, video camera, VCR, television

Processing Questions:

1. Why do we need to let others know the importance of recycling?
2. What is the best way to get that message across to other people?

RECYCLING AND YOU   Grades (6–8)

Valued Outcome: The students will design pamphlets that stress the importance of recycling.

Description of Strategy: Divide students into groups of four or five. Using information they have gathered from the Internet and other sources, have each group design a pamphlet about the importance of recycling. They can include illustrations and suggestions for recycling. When completed, groups present their pamphlets to the class. Additional pamphlets can be made and distributed throughout the school.

Materials Needed: computer with Internet access; research references; colored pens, markers, pencils, tape or glue, and paper for each group

Processing Questions:

1. Why do you think people should recycle?
2. What is the most important aspect of recycling?
3. What can you say that would make others want to recycle?

FOR THE LOVE OF THE EARTH   Grades (3–6)

Valued Outcome: The students will list different things that make up their natural environment and select the ones they think are most important.

Description of Strategy: Conduct a class discussion about the environment: what it is and how it affects our lives. As a group, have students name and list on the board different aspects of our environment (water, air, land, sunshine, petroleum, weather, etc.). After making a comprehensive list, divide students into groups of three. Have each group name the part of their environment they consider the most important and list three reasons why. Then, have them draw a picture showing this vital resource with the reasons why it is important listed below. Each group will present their completed assignment to the class.

Materials Needed: board and markers or overhead projector and pen; large sheets of butcher paper, markers, crayons, and pencils or pens for each group

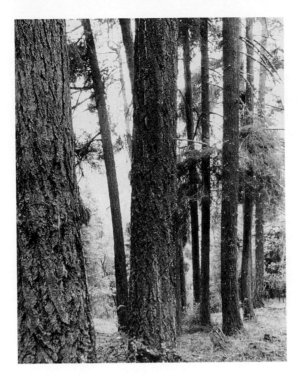

Trees can have a positive influence upon our environment.

Processing Questions:

1. What would our world be like if we did not have the resources we have today?

2. Which resources could we live without? Which ones do we need in order to live?

3. Which resources are most important to you?

ENVIRONMENTAL STORIES   Grades (4–8)

Valued Outcome: The students will create a story about the environment.

Description of Strategy: Select a colorful, eye-catching, and appropriate picture depicting an aspect of the environment. Have each student write a story about the picture. Allow about twenty minutes, and encourage both creativity and the exploration of thoughts. Have volunteers read their stories to the class.

Materials Needed: picture of the environment, pens or pencils and paper for each student

Processing Questions:

1. What did you notice about the environment from the picture?

2. Was the environment in the picture a pleasant scene?

ENVIRONMENTAL NEWSWATCH AND COMMENTARY

Grades (5–8)

Valued Outcome: The students will choose various environmental articles and identify the purpose of the articles.

Description of Strategy: Divide students into small groups; provide each student with three sheets of colored construction paper. Have them to paste an article on an environmental topic onto each sheet. Use of newsletters, supplementary magazines, and books that are written for the students' grade level should be encouraged. Underneath each article, have the students write a caption that describes the purpose of the article. Have each group then compile their articles into a booklet. Similar articles should be grouped within the booklets.

Materials Needed: three sheets of construction paper and pencils or pens for each student, markers, newspapers, magazines, glue

Processing Questions:

1. What were your environmental articles about?
2. Did the stories portray any lessons about conservation?

LET'S BE CREATIVE

Grades (5–8)

Valued Outcome: The students will be able to present solutions for various environmental hazards.

Description of Strategy: Have the students draw a cartoon series, write a story, or make up a poem about an environmental problem, then have volunteers share what they did with the class. Discuss what was said, problems, and solutions for the environmental hazard. After completing the activity, have students hang their work around the room. Let them observe each other's displays.

Materials Needed: paper, markers, pens or pencils for each student

Processing Questions:

1. What environmental hazards did you identify?
2. What solutions did you present for each hazard?

RECYCLING CENTERS

Grades (3–6)

Valued Outcome: Students will be able to discuss their community's recycling plan.

Description of Strategy: Have the students tell you where they can go to recycle in their community and what they can recycle. Then have a guest speaker come in from one of the recycling centers to talk with the students. Ask the speaker to explain the activities conducted at the center, what he or she does, and what the students should do to help their community's recycling efforts.

Materials Needed: none

Processing Question: What is the purpose of a recycling plant or center?

WHAT DO YOU THINK?   Grades (4–6)

Valued Outcome: The students will be able to discuss alternatives to activities that are environmental hazards.

Description of Strategy: Divide the students into groups of four to six. Assign each group an environmental hazard. Have the group list all of the pros and cons related to the presence of that environmental hazard, and ask them to think of what hazards it can cause and of different alternatives that might be used. Have them think of a solution for any problem that may be associated with the hazard. Depending on what the environmental factor is, suggest some possibilities for them to think about. Then have each group discuss what their item is and their conclusions from it. Have the whole class discuss the problem, and ask the group different questions concerning the item.

Materials Needed: paper and pencils or pens for each group; list of environmental hazards and a few pros, cons, and solutions for each

Processing Questions:

1. What are some environmentally dangerous activities you participate in daily?
2. Are there alternatives to these activities that would be less dangerous to our environment?

BANNER   Grades (K–5)

Valued Outcome: The students will be able to describe the positive and negative environmental aspects of their surroundings.

Description of Strategy: Place a long blank banner on one side of the room and another long banner on the other side of the room. Write Positive on one and Negative on the other. Have the students draw and write positive and negative environmental factors on the correct banners, then have the students volunteer to show what they drew or wrote to the class and discuss each item.

Materials Needed: two long banners, markers or crayons for each student

Processing Questions:

1. What environmental factors in your surroundings should be considered?
2. What are the positive and negative aspects of each of those factors?

ECOSYSTEM EXPLANATION   Grades (5–8)

Valued Outcome: The students will be able to explain an ecosystem.

Description of Strategy: Using the dairy cow as an example of the relationships that exist in an ecosystem, explain with pictures, posters, and diagrams how cows eating grass produce milk we drink. Then ask each student to think of another animal that is part of a food chain, and have the students describe the workings of that food chain.

Materials Needed: pictures, posters, and diagrams of a dairy cow's role in a food chain

Processing Questions:

1. What is an ecosystem?
2. How does an ecosystem affect your environment?

POPULATION PROBLEMS   Grades (4–8)

Valued Outcome: The students will be able to discuss overpopulation as an environmental hazard.

Description of Strategy: To stimulate discussion about the concerns of overpopulation for very young students, have them recite the nursery rhyme, "There was an old woman who lived in a shoe./She had so many children she knew not what to do." Have students tell you what this rhyme means to them. Older students can be asked to make a graph of the world's population increases since the beginning of recorded years (see population statistics on page 736). Note especially the curve for the last twenty years. Then provide further information about the problem of overpopulation, and have students discuss suggestions to curb overpopulation.

Materials Needed: pens or pencils and graph paper for each student

Processing Questions:

1. Does your community have an overpopulation problem?
2. What measures can be taken to reduce the overpopulation problem?

HUNGER HURTS   Grades (4–8)

Valued Outcome: The students will be able to discuss world hunger.

Description of Strategy: As a class, have students research information about the impact of hunger on children throughout the world. Ask the librarian to suggest a few sources that each class member can read. Also have students determine the three leading causes of death among infants and children in the United States compared to those of several other countries you select. Be sure to include both European and developing countries. Allow students to discuss their ideas concerning the reason for these differences. You may need to remind students that food, medicine, and access to quality health care are all resources.

Materials Needed: library books

Processing Questions:

1. What is the incidence of hunger in Europe and other countries?
2. Is hunger a problem in our country? In your community?

GENERAL POLLUTION PROBLEMS   Grades (5–8)

Valued Outcome: The students will be able to describe the impact of major environmental problems.

Description of Strategy: Divide the class into several small groups, and assign each group a different major pollution problem. After researching the general aspects of the problem, each group should give a short oral panel presentation. Within the groups, each member is then assigned a specific aspect of the given pollution problem, such as oil spills, effects of sulfides in the air, or the banning of pesticides such as DDT. Have the students prepare individual written reports.

Materials Needed: pens or pencils and paper for each student; references

Processing Question: What are the major environmental problems that directly affect you? That indirectly affect you?

ENERGY SAVINGS   Grades (4–6)

Valued Outcome: The students will be able to explain how to conserve energy.

Description of Strategy: Have a general class discussion concerning ways to save energy in the United States. Discuss how rising costs of fuel have made Americans more energy conscious in recent years. Individual students may wish to volunteer how their families are doing more to save energy. For older students, ask them to formulate a rationale for why they think their suggestions will save energy.

Materials Needed: none

Processing Questions:

1. What are the types of energy used in your homes?
2. What are ways you and your family can save energy?

SOLID WASTE   Grades (4–6)

Valued Outcome: The students will be able to identify the terms associated with handling and disposing of solid waste.

Description of Strategy: Ask the students to identify the terms associated with solid waste. Put the terms on an overhead; discuss each of the terms and provide examples or illustrations of each. After reviewing the terms, pass out a worksheet containing the terms and their definitions (see the Teaching in Action box "Solid Waste Worksheet" on page 770.). Have students match the words with the definitions.

Materials Needed: worksheet and pens or pencils for each student

Processing Questions:

1. What three important ideas came out of discussing the solid waste terms?
2. What are ways we can reuse, reduce, or recycle solid waste in our daily lives?
3. Why are biodegradable products important to our environment?

Directions: Place the correct letter in the blank to the left.

_____ 1. biodegradable

_____ 2. compost

_____ 3. conservation

_____ 4. decompose

_____ 5. ecosystem

_____ 6. garbage

_____ 7. incinerator

_____ 8. landfill

_____ 9. leachate

_____ 10. microorganisms

_____ 11. recycle

_____ 12. reduce

_____ 13. reuse

_____ 14. solid waste

_____ 15. wasteland

b. a material that can be broken down by microorganisms into simpler forms

d. a mixture of degraded organic materials such as grass, leaves, and garden and kitchen wastes; the mixture is usually used as fertilizer

f. the preservation and wise use of natural resources to minimize loss and waste

h. to rot or break down into the simplest form possible

j. a unit of the environment that consists of living and nonliving things that interact with each other

l. solid waste or trash; things that we throw away

n. a furnace used for burning waste

o. a place where solid waste or trash is dumped and covered with dirt

m. a solution of water that streams through a dump or landfill and picks up pollutants and other soluble molecules along the way

k. minute living organisms that can be seen only through a microscope

i. to make materials such as plastic, glass, and paper into new products

g. to decrease the amount of trash or waste produced by buying only what is needed and contained in packages that are not excessively wrapped

e. to extend the life of an item by repairing it or creating a new use for it

c. the things that we throw away such as trash, yard and kitchen waste, and old machinery

a. ravaged land that is unable to support life

Answers: 1. b   2. d   3. f   4. h   5. j   6. l   7. n   8. o   9. m   10. k   11. i   12. g   13. e   14. c   15. a

SOURCE: Adapted from the Manchester College Elementary Education Program 2000. Used with permission.

Experiments and Demonstrations

DEADLY PRECIPITATION   Grades (6–8)

Valued Outcome: The students will be able to define acid rain and its potential effects on the environment.

Description of Strategy: Before the class date, assign students to work in groups of five to collect samples of rainwater either at school or at home. Have them also collect and label samples from the school's drinking water, a nearby lake or stream, and other local water sources. (Masking tape labels should include the date and where the sample was collected.) On the activity day, define the term *acid rain* and write the definition on the board. Give each group its own containers for each water source. Have students test the water in each container for acidity by dipping litmus paper into it. Record the results on the label on each container. A pH less then 7.0 is acidic; a pH higher than 7.0 is alkaline (or basic). Water is considered "clean" at 5.4. A pH less than 5.0 is a pollution concern. Have students graph the results for their group and present the data to the class.

Materials Needed: multiple small containers for water samples; water samples; litmus paper, masking tape, graph paper, pencils or pens for each group

Processing Questions:

1. Could acid rain be an environmental hazard in our area?
2. How much of a problem do you think acid rain is in your community?

RESOURCE REDUCTION   Grades (4–6)

Valued Outcome: The students will identify common products and compare the usage of different products.

Description of Strategy: Divide the class into small groups, and assign each group a common environmental product or resource, such as paper, plastic, water, electricity, or natural gas. For a few days, ask each group member to keep a daily list of his or her specific uses of the resource or products they use that may impact that resource (such as plastic milk jugs contain milk to drink, paper towels used to mop up a spill). Have students compare lists. On butcher paper, prepare a master list outlining the most typically used products, most common uses, amount students think has been used by the total group, and ways to reduce the use. Lists might look something like this:

Product	Frequency	Amount	Ways to Reduce
Paper napkins			
Facial tissues			
Toilet paper			
Notebook paper			

Materials Needed: daily log for each student, butcher paper and markers

Processing Questions:

1. Did you observe any patterns in your use of the various products?
2. Do you think you can conserve products in order to help the environment?

RECYCLABLE CONTAINERS   Grades (1–5)

Valued Outcome: The students will be able to explain the positive aspects of recycling.

Description of Strategy: Have the students bring a box or paper bag to class to make into a recycle container. Have the students draw, color, or write whatever they want on their containers. Place the containers around the school and in different classes. At the end of the week, collect the recyclable cans and paper. Discuss with the class how they feel about the project and the results from it.

Materials Needed: box or bag, markers, crayons or other writing and drawing tools for each student

Processing Questions:

1. What is the purpose of recycling?
2. How does recycling help our environment?

SIGNS   Grades (4–6)

Valued Outcome: The students will be able to produce some helpful environmental hints.

Description of Strategy: Have the students make a variety of signs to display around the school—such as, "Turn off the water when you're finished," "Throw away your trash," "Recycle your cans." Ask the students how they might monitor any changes in behavior that might occur in response to their signs, and have them implement their plan. After a week, discuss the results and note any changes in behavior. If there are no changes, ask why. Think of another alternative, and try it. If it works, congratulate them on a job well done.

Materials Needed: paper, markers, pens or pencils for each student

Processing Question: What can we do to help advance the cause of environmental conservation?

WATER CONSERVATION   Grades (K–3)

Valued Outcome: The students will be able to describe ways to conserve resources in order to help the environment.

Description of Strategy: Bring two toothbrushes and a tube of toothpaste to class. Have two students volunteer to brush their teeth. Put one bucket under the faucet to catch the water run by each student. One student will leave the water running while brushing his or her teeth, and the other student will turn the water off. Ask students to compare the quantity of water used by each student and to notice how much water was wasted. Have them explain what would happen to our water supply if everyone did this. Have them also describe other ways we waste water and how we can prevent this from happening.

Materials Needed: two toothbrushes, toothpaste, two buckets

Processing Question: What are some habits that you can change in your daily life that will conserve water resources and help the environment?

WATER POLLUTION   Grades (4–8)

Valued Outcome: The students will be able to describe the negative effects of used engine oil on the environment.

Description of Strategy: Add some engine oil to a small jar half filled with water. Show the students what happens to the water. Then use a bigger container (again half filled with water) and place the same amount of oil in it. Show the students the results. Have them describe what they observed. Explain to them that it doesn't matter how much oil is spilled because it spreads. Ask the students how many of their parents change the oil in their own cars. Ask what they do with the used oil once they are through. Tell them that the average car uses four quarts of oil. Have them guess how much water would be polluted with four quarts of oil (thirty to forty square feet). Have them tell you how their parents can recycle the engine oil.

Materials Needed: one small jar, bucket or other similar-sized container, bottle of engine oil

Processing Question: What are some ways you and your family can recycle oil in order to protect the environment?

WASTE PRODUCTION   Grades (4–8)

Valued Outcome: The students will be able to discuss the impact of solid waste (such as household trash) on the environment.

Description of Strategy: Have the students observe in their homes how many bags of trash they fill a day. Have them do this for three days. Every day before class starts, tally up the bags of trash used the day before. After three days, have the students place a recycling container by the trash and ask all family members to put recyclable items in it. Calculate the number of bags of trash for the next three days and keep a class tally as before. Have the students explain what has happened and what they have observed. This will show how much they waste. Tell students how many people were living in the United States at the last population census and point out how much people in our country waste. Discuss what will happen if we keep doing this. Discuss what might happen if we start recycling, or what happens to the recycled products if there is already a recycling program.

Materials Needed: tally sheets, pencils

Processing Questions:

1. What is the impact of solid waste products on our environment?

2. What are some ways you and your family can dispose of or recycle some solid wastes to help protect the environment?

SEASONAL ADJUSTMENTS   Grades (3–6)

Valued Outcome: The students will be able to explain the environmental influences of trees and plants.

Description of Strategy: Divide students into small groups, and ask each group to select a favorite tree or shrub in the school yard to observe once a month for the school year. Have groups record their observations in relation to environmental influences on the changes of the tree or shrub.

Materials Needed: journal to record monthly data, and pencils or pens for each group

Processing Questions:

1. What changes take place in trees from season to season?

2. What effects can planting trees have on our environment?

TERRARIUMS AND AQUARIUMS   Grades (3–6)
AS ECOSYSTEMS

Valued Outcome: The students will be able to describe the interrelationships involved in ecosystems.

Description of Strategy: As a class project—either in small groups or the entire class—help students make a terrarium or an aquarium. Refer to science textbooks as resources to help you do this. Use the terrarium or aquarium to demonstrate the interrelationships between inhabitants of each ecosystem.

Materials Needed: terrarium(s) or aquarium(s), science textbooks

Processing Question: How do inhabitants in a terrarium or aquarium depend on each other for their existence?

WATER IMPURITIES   Grades (5–8)

Valued Outcome: The students will be able to discuss the environmental implications of impurities in drinking water.

Description of Strategy: Have each student bring in a small glass jar of water from a tap at home. Even though the water may all come from the same municipal supply, there will be differences in the samples because of rust or chemical residues in the water pipes in each home. Examine the water samples using a light microscope.

Materials Needed: glass jars, tap water from each student's home

Processing Questions:

1. What are the implications of impurities in drinking water?

2. How can we ensure that we have safe water to drink?

CROWDING PROBLEMS   Grades (2–6)

Valued Outcome: The students will be able to discuss the effects of overcrowding (overpopulation) on the environment.

Description of Strategy: Divide students into groups, and give each group two milk cartons with the tops cut off and a few holes punched in the bottom for drainage. Ask students to fill each carton about two-thirds full with potting soil, and in one carton plant two or three bean seeds one inch apart just under the surface of the soil. In the other carton, students should plant fifteen seeds about one-half inch apart. Have them water the seeds every four days and record their observations. As an extension of this activity, crowd students into a confined space for a few minutes, and then ask them to describe how it felt.

Materials Needed: two milk cartons for each group, potting soil, bean seeds, water, journals and pencils or pencils for each student to record observations

Processing Question: What are the problems of overcrowding as it relates to the use of natural resources?

NOISE LEVELS   Grades (4–8)

Valued Outcome: The students will be able to discuss unwanted noise as an environmental hazard.

Description of Strategy: Use a decibel meter to check noise levels in various locations throughout the school. Record the location, time of day, and meter reading. Noise levels will vary during different times of day. Which locations are noisiest? Are there any sources of particularly loud sounds, such as school bus engines?

Materials Needed: decibel meter, journals, and pencils to record data

Processing Questions:

1. How can some sounds become environmental hazards?

2. What are some ways to diminish noise pollution in the school environment?

Puzzles and Games

HEALTH HAZARD   Grades (3–8)

Valued Outcome: The students will be able to name and suggest solutions to environmental hazards.

Description of Strategy: Ask the students various questions about their environmental health. Examples: How many of you like to drink soda? How many of you recycle your cans when you're done? Why? Why not? How many of you have an electric can opener in your house? Do you think you're wasting electricity by using it instead of a manual one? What are some other hazardous behaviors we have that can threaten our environmental health? (Answers might include not conserving water or electricity; polluting the air, water, environment; not recycling other items; and so on.)

Have a student put on a jersey to represent one of the health hazards in our environment. The student will be "it." He or she will try to tag the other students. Once the students are tagged, they must sit down because they are now health hazards. After two minutes, have all the students who have not been tagged come to you. Ask them to tell you something that we can do to correct the problem. For instance, if the health hazard was "waste," the students may suggest that we recycle. The game starts again with another student as a different health hazard. At the end of the lesson, have three or four health hazards be "it" simultaneously to illustrate that the more health hazards we have, the greater the chance of having a highly unhealthy environment.

Materials Needed: jerseys or bandannas

Processing Question: What are some specific ways that each of us can correct some environmental hazards?

TREASURE HUNT   Grades (2–8)

Valued Outcome: The students will be able to describe the recycling process and how recycling helps protect the environment.

Description of Strategy: Divide the students into groups of five to eight. On several tables have a variety of items (recyclable, nonrecyclable, hazards, and helpful things for our environment) such as notebook paper, a coin, a leaf, plastic wrap, clean water, rubber stopper, cleansers, oil bottle, and so on. Ask the students various questions about environmental health. Some questions might relate to the items on the table, and some questions may not. Students must write down the answers. An example of a question that might be asked is "Who can show me a recyclable item?" The group with the student who raises a hand first and can give the right answer will get a point. Another example: "Name three types of pollution" (water, air, noise, radiation, chemical, thermal). The game continues until all the questions are answered. The group that answers the most questions correctly is considered the winner.

Materials Needed: a variety of objects that are recyclable, nonrecyclable, harmful, or helpful to the environment; pencils and paper; list of environmental health questions

Processing Questions:

1. What is the purpose of recycling?
2. How does recycling help protect the environment?
3. How can recycling help your health?

BRAINSTORM   Grades (4–6)

Valued Outcome: The students will be able to discuss the meaning of several environmental terms.

Description of Strategy: Divide the class into groups of four to six. Write a word on the board, such as *recycle*. Have groups brainstorm everything that comes to their minds when they hear the word *recycle*. Then have each group work as a team and make a list of terms related to the environment—for example, glass, paper, plastic, newspapers, water. After one minute, start with group 1 and have them tell one item on their list. Group 2 will then go, naming a different item. Write all the words on the board for the class.

After each group has been asked, go around the room again. The group that has the most responses gets a point. Then the game starts again with another word. Specific questions can also be asked. For example, what are the effects of water pollution? Answers might include destroys or injures animals, depletes food supplies, harms reproduction, produces odors, makes foul tasting drinking water, causes diseases, and pollutes beaches.

Materials Needed: paper and pens or pencils for each student; board and markers or overhead projector and pen

Processing Question: What are the effects of various types of pollution on the environment?

AIR POLLUTION WORD SEARCH   Grades (4–6)

Valued Outcome: The students will be able to identify words associated with air pollution.

Description of Strategy: After reviewing terms and conditions associated with air pollution, provide the students with the word search in the Teaching in Action box on page 778 and have them find the words. After identifying each word, have them write the definition of the word.

Materials Needed: copy of word search and pencils or pens for each student

Processing Questions:

1. When you found the words, were you able to define them?
2. Of the words on the list, which causes the most air pollution?

SOURCE: Ohio Department of Natural Resources 1990

Find each of the words listed below and circle them. The words may read in any direction—up, down, across, or diagonally. The words may even intersect.

```
I  X  I  H  A  V  L  C  F  H  N  F  X  B  O  J  D  D  V  L       air
K  U  S  Y  T  U  R  F  B  O  G  P  L  G  K  U  A  Q  K  C       breathe
Q  C  O  P  K  K  H  A  I  M  I  P  R  S  B  P  H  F  W  Y       bus
T  F  G  O  P  C  I  T  C  E  L  Z  F  S  I  C  K  Q  D  I       car
H  T  Q  X  W  Y  Y  N  G  Q  K  X  M  L  T  R  P  I  U  N       clouds
J  X  V  H  V  Q  R  N  M  V  W  L  U  A  Q  K  O  H  S  T       dust
U  I  S  O  N  Q  P  Q  R  Y  X  S  H  S  M  O  G  S  T  O       eyes
Z  M  F  R  E  S  H  M  C  O  P  O  L  L  U  T  I  O  N  X       fresh
M  X  B  W  R  V  G  D  O  Y  P  R  G  S  J  Z  N  J  I  Y       lungs
Q  X  Z  J  I  E  B  U  S  H  M  P  L  L  V  F  J  T  W  G       nose
E  J  Q  U  S  T  N  E  O  A  E  B  C  U  W  X  P  R  B  E       oxygen
Z  F  Y  T  V  W  E  U  S  C  M  I  V  N  K  G  D  U  H  N       pollution
H  F  G  Q  M  B  I  A  T  L  S  M  J  G  L  T  T  C  X  Y       sick
T  F  R  T  W  O  C  I  G  O  I  A  B  S  U  Q  I  K  C  P       smog
L  V  S  N  B  C  L  Y  U  U  E  R  V  T  B  S  I  R  A  X       truck
W  O  X  Y  C  K  E  R  C  D  E  Z  E  N  J  S  E  K  R  X
H  S  O  X  Z  I  E  Y  E  S  P  M  Z  F  D  Z  Q  R  Z  I
P  N  C  L  G  W  D  N  T  X  N  S  N  D  L  E  Z  D  X  J
B  O  L  R  B  I  Z  A  F  L  A  F  U  M  F  N  O  S  E  Q
M  W  M  A  B  R  E  A  T  H  E  J  S  W  M  C  A  I  R  F
```

Other Strategies for Learning

POSTER CONTEST

Grades (3–8)

Valued Outcome: The students will be able to create a poster with an environmental message.

Description of Strategy: Ask each student to make a poster entitled Energy. Give minimal details about what might be included. Let the students use their creativity. Number each poster anonymously and hang each around the room. Have another class view the posters and select the five best, which are then hung in the hallway or school library.

Materials Needed: poster board, markers, crayons for each student

Processing Question: What are some environmental messages we can portray through posters?

ILLUSTRATING ENVIRONMENTAL ASPECTS   Grades (4–6)

Valued Outcome: The students will illustrate ideas concerning various environmental resources.

Description of Strategy: Create a handout from the list below and give one to each student. Then ask the class to draw or illustrate their ideas about the items on the list. Have students share their pictures with each other to compare ideas.

- most important environmental resource
- most abundant environmental resource
- most depleted environmental resource
- most dangerous environmental threat to the world
- most environmentally helpful family measure practiced
- least environmentally helpful family measure practiced
- most environmentally helpful personal measure practiced
- least environmentally helpful personal measure practiced

Materials Needed: pencils or pens, paper, handout for each student

Processing Questions:

1. What did you learn from this activity that will help protect our environment?
2. What can you personally do to protect the environment?

SURVIVAL LISTS   Grades (4–6)

Valued Outcome: The students will be able to compile a list of supplies needed in the time of an environmental disaster.

Description of Strategy: Divide students into small groups. Ask each group to prepare two lists. One list should include necessary supplies for a family of four to survive on the earth for the next year in the event of a disaster. The other list should include the twenty most important items to take on a trip to outer space. Let groups compare lists and discuss ideas. If enough agreement can be reached, make a class master list.

Materials Needed: paper and pens or pencils for each student

Processing Questions:

1. What are some environmental disasters that might necessitate the prior accumulation of supplies?
2. What supplies would be the most important to gather prior to such a disaster?

Resources

WEB SITES

EE—Link: *www.eelink.net*

The Enviro Link
envirolink.org/start_web.html

Environmental Protection Agency
www.epa.gov

The Use Less Stuff Report page
www.use_less_stuff.com

VIDEOS

Can buildings make you sick? (Grades 6–8)
Discusses "bad" air in buildings, homes, schools, and hospitals. Available from Library Video Company at *www.libraryvideo.com* (55 minutes, Item N5761).

The greenhouse effect (Grades 5–8)
Computer animation and live-action video combine to develop a fundamental understanding of the greenhouse effect. Available from Library Video Company at *www.libraryvideo.com*. (16 minutes, Item N4203)

Green means (Grades 6–8)
Series of 32 short programs concerning environmental issues. Available from *www.envmedia.com*. (180 minutes, two videocassettes, Item GM203)

Wormania (Grades 2–5)
Demonstrates the usefulness and work that worms play in our lives. Produced by Flowerfield Enterprises; available through *www.wormania.com*. (26 minutes, ISBN: 0-942256-09-023)

References

Chapter One: The Need for Health Education

Brown, G. I. 1990. *Human teaching for human learning: An introduction to confluent education.* New York: Gestalt Journal Press.

Centers for Disease Control and Prevention (CDC). 1993. *Comprehensive school health education programs: Initiatives, policies, and issues in setting standards.* Atlanta: CDC.

——. 1998. 1997 Youth risk behavior surveillance system (YRBSS). *Morbidity and mortality weekly report* 47 (No. SS03; 001).

——. 2002a, August 30. Healthy youth: An investment in our nation's future. *www.cdc.gov/nccdphp/aag/aag _dash.htm* (15 November 2002).

——. 2002b. *Comprehensive health education curriculum. www.cdc.gov/nccdphp/dash/about/comprehensive_ed.htm* (15 November 2002).

Chapman, L. E. 1987. Developing a useful perspective on spiritual health: Love, peace and fulfillment. *American journal of health promotion* 2(22): 12–17.

Children's Defense Fund. 1999. *The health of American children yearbook.* Washington, DC: The Fund.

Dunn, H. L. 1991. *High-level wellness.* Arlington, VA: Beatty.

Federal Interagency Forum on Child and Family Statistics. 2002. *America's children: Key national indicators of well-being 2000.* Washington, DC: Federal Interagency Forum on Child and Family Statistics.

Green, L. W., and M. W. Kreuter. 1999. *Health promotion planning: An educational and ecological approach.* 3d ed. Mountain View, CA: Mayfield.

Hacker, K. 1996. Integrating a school-based health center into managed care in Massachusetts. *Journal of school health* 66(9): 317–322.

Hoyman, H. S. 1975. Rethinking an ecologic-system model of man's health, disease, aging, death. *Journal of school health* 45: 9.

Joint Committee on Health Education Standards. 1995. *The national health education standards: Achieving health literacy.* Atlanta: American Cancer Society.

Joint Committee on Health Education Terminology. 1991. Report of the 1990 joint committee on health education terminology. *Journal of health education* 22: 97–108.

Making the Grade. 1995. *Medicaid managed care and school-based health center: Proceedings of a meeting with policy makers and providers.* Washington, DC: Robert Wood Johnson Foundation.

Marx, E., S. Wooley, and D. Northrop, eds. 1998. *Health is academic—a guide to coordinated school health programs.* New York: Teachers College Press.

National Education Goals Panel. 2002, March. Goals. *www.negp.gov/page3.htm* (23 January 2003).

National Center for Injury Prevention and Control. 2002. *Ten leading causes of death, United States 1998.* Atlanta: CDC.

National School Boards Association, American Association of School Administrators, American Cancer Society, and National School Health Education Coalition. 1995. *Be a leader in academic achievement.* Alexandria, VA: National School Boards Association, American Association of School Administrators, American Cancer Society, and National School Health Education Coalition.

Office of Disease Prevention and Health Promotion. 2002, May. *Healthy people 2010: National health promotion and disease prevention objectives.* U.S. Department of Health and Human Services. *www.cdc.gov/nchs/about/otheract/ hpdata2010/2010fa28.htm.*

Seffrin, J. R. 1994. America's interest in comprehensive school health education. *Journal of school health* 64(10): 397–399.

U.S. General Accounting Office. 1994. *Report to the chairman, committee on government operations, U.S. House of Representatives: Health care reform school-based health centers can promote access to care.* Washington, DC: U.S. General Accounting Office.

World Health Organization. WHO definition of health. *www.who.int/about/definition/en* (October 2002).

Chapter Two: The Role of the Teacher in Coordinated School Health Programs

Indiana Professional Standards Board. 2002. Teachers of health education and physical education. *www.in.gov/psb/ standards/HealthPhysEdContStds.html* (15 January 2003).

Marx, E., and D. Northrop. 1995. *Educating for health: A guide to implementing a comprehensive approach to school health education.* Newton, MA: Education Development Center.

National Task Force on the Preparation and Practice of Health Educators. 1988. *A framework for the development of competency-based curricula for entry-level health educators.* New York: National Task Force on the Preparation and Practice of Health Educators.

Rose, L. C., and A. M. Gallup. 2002. The 34th annual Phi Delta Kappa/Gallup Poll of the public's attitudes toward the public school. *Phi Delta Kappan* 84(1):41–46, 51–56.

Sciacca, J., et al. 1999. *Journal of health education* 30(1): 42–46.

Smith, M., et al. 1999. *Journal of health education* 30(3): 157–165.

Chapter Three: Planning for Health Instruction

Association for the Advancement of Health Education (AAHE). 1995. *National health education standards— achieving health literacy.* Reston, VA: AAHE.

Bloom, B. S. 1956. *Taxonomy of educational objectives, handbook I: Cognitive domain.* New York: McKay.

Joint Committee on National Health Standards. 1995. *Achieving health literacy: An investment in the future.* Atlanta: American Cancer Society.

National Diffusion Network. 1995. *Education programs that work—The catalogue of the National Diffusion Network,* 21st ed. Longmont, CO: Sopris West.

Popham, W. J. 1995. *Classroom assessment—What teachers need to know.* Boston: Allyn & Bacon.

Chapter Four: Strategies for Implementing Health Instruction

Barth, R. P. 1996. *Reducing the risk—Building skills to prevent pregnancy, STD and HIV.* Santa Cruz, CA: ETR Associates.

Carr, R. 1992. *Peer helper handbook to accompany just for me.* Bloomington, IN: AIT.

Concept to classroom: Tapping into multiple intelligence— Implementation. 2002, June 15. *www.thirteen.orgedonline/ concept2class/month1/index.html* (15 June 2002).

Curtis, J., and R. Papenfuss. 1980. *Health instruction: A task approach.* Minneapolis: Burgess.

Educational Materials Center. 2003. *Michigan model for comprehensive school health education curriculum.* Mt. Pleasant, MI: Central Michigan University.

Evertson, C. M., E. T. Emmer, B. S. Clements, and M. E. Worsham. 1997. *Classroom management for elementary teachers.* Boston: Allyn & Bacon.

Foder, G. T., and G. T. Dalis. 1989. *Health instruction: Theory and application.* 4th ed. Philadelphia: Lea & Febiger.

Gardner, H. 1993. *Frames of mind: The theory of multiple intelligence.* New York: Basic Books.

Gold, R. S. 1991. *Microcomputer applications in health education.* Dubuque, IA: Brown.

Greenberg, J. S. 1989. *Health education—Learner-centered instructional strategies.* Dubuque, IA: Brown.

Hamrick, M., D. Anspaugh, and D. Smith. 1980. Decision making and the behavioral gap. *Journal of school health* 50: 455–458.

Hochbaum, G. M., S. M. Rosenstock, and S. S. Kegeles. 1960. *Determinants of health behavior.* Washington, DC: White House Conference on Children and Youth, 1960.

Jung, C. G. 1976. *Psychological types.* Princeton, NJ: Princeton University Press.

Komoski, P. K., and E. Plotnik. 1995. Seven steps to responsible software selection. *www.ericfacility.net/ericdigests/ ed382157.html* (20 June 2002).

McCarthy, B. M. 1987. *The 4-mat system.* Barrington, IL: Excell.

McKenzie, W. 1999. It's not how smart you are—It's how you are smart!. *http://surfaquarium.com/mi.html* (1 December 2002).

National School Boards Association, American Association of School Administrators, American Cancer Society, and National School Health Education Coalition. 1995. *Be a leader in academic achievement.* Alexandria, VA: National School Boards Association, American Association of School Administrators, American Cancer Society, and National School Health Education Coalition.

Price, G. E., and R. Dunn. 1997. *Learning style inventory (LSI): An inventory for the identification of how individuals in grades 3 through 12 prefer to learn.* Lawrence, KS: Price Systems.

Rivard, J. D. 1997. *Allyn & Bacon quick guide to the Internet for educators.* Boston: Allyn & Bacon.

Smith, D., M. Hamrick, and D. Anspaugh. 1981. Decision story strategy: Practical approach for teaching decision making. *Journal of school health* 51(10): 637–643.

Stone, D., L. O'Reilley, and J. Brown. 1980. *Elementary school health education.* Dubuque, IA: Brown.

Timmreck, T. 1978. Creative health education through puppetry. *Health education* 9(1): 40–41.

Wagner, B., S. Gregory, M. Daniel, and J. Sapers. 1997. Where computers do work. *U.S. News & World Report* 121(22): 82–93.

Chapter Five: Measurement and Evaluation of Health Education

Baumgartner, T. A., and A. S. Jackson. 1999. *Measurement for evaluation in physical education and exercise science.* Boston: WCB McGraw-Hill.

Council of Chief State School Officers, The. Health education assessment project. *www.ccsso.org/scass/p_heap* (November 2002).

Hamilton County Department of Education (Tennessee). 2002. *www.hcde.org/standards* (November 2002).

King, A. 1990. Enhancing poor interaction and learning in the classroom through reciprocal questioning. *American educational research journal* 27: 664–687.

Linn, R., and N. Gronlund. 1999. *Measurement and assessment in teaching.* 8th ed. Bellevue, WA: Merril Press.

Marx, E., and S. F. Wooley. 1998. *Health is academic: A guide to coordinated school health programs.* New York: Teachers College Press, Columbia University.

Marzano, R., and J. Kendall. 1996. *A comprehensive guide to designing standards-based districts, schools, and classrooms.* Aurora, CO: McREL.

McCown, R., M. Driscoll, and P. G. Roop. 1996. *Educational psychology—A learning-centered approach to classroom practice.* 2d ed. Boston: Allyn & Bacon.

Morrow, J. R., A. W. Jackson, J. G. Disch, and D. P. Mood. 1995. *Measurement and evaluation in human performance.* Champaign, IL: Human Kinetics.

National Council on Measurement in Education. 2002, October. *www.ncme.org.*

Read, D. A. 1997. *Health education—A cognitive-behavioral approach.* Boston: Jones & Bartlett.

San Diego State University, College of Education. 2002. *http://webquest.sdsu.edu/* (November 2002).

Shor, I. 1992. *Empowering education: Critical teaching for social change.* Chicago: University of Chicago Press.

Simons-Morton, B. G., W. H. Greene, and N. H. Gottlieb. 1995. *Introduction to health education and health promotion.* 2d ed. Prospect Heights, IL: Waveland Press.

Tennessee Department of Education. 2002, October. *www.state.tn.us/education/ci/cicomphealth/cich35.htm* (January 2003).

Tennessee.gov. Tennessee's K–8 healthful living curriculum standards. *www.state.tn.us/education/ci/cistandards2001/ health/cihlthk2stand.htm* (April 2003).

Woolfolk, A. E. 1995. *Educational psychology.* 6th ed. Boston: Allyn & Bacon.

Chapter Six: Mental Health and Stress Reduction

American Academy of Child and Adolescent Psychiatry. 1999a, December 15. Children's major psychiatric disorders. *www.aacap.org/publications/factsfam.*

———. 1999b, December 20. Children's major psychiatric disorders. *www.aacap.org/publications/factsfam/ divorce.htm.*

———. 1999c. Panic disorder in children and adolescents. *www.aacap.org/publications/factsfam.*

———. 1999d, December 20. Panic disorder in children and adolescents. *www.aacap.org/publications/factsfam/ panic.htm.*

———. 2002. Children's major psychiatric disorders. *www.aacap.org/publications/factsfam/suicide.htm.*

American Psychiatric Association (APA). 1987. *Diagnostic and statistical manual of mental disorders.* 3d ed., rev. Washington, DC: APA.

———. 1999, December 20. Depression. *www.psych.org.*

Bean, R. 1992. *The four conditions of self-esteem in the classroom: A handbook for teachers and parents.* Santa Cruz, CA: ETR Associates.

Chandler, C., and C. Kolander. 1988. Stop the negative, accentuate the positive. *Journal of school health* 58(7): 295–297.

———. 1989. Depression. *Mayo Clinic health letter—Medical essay.*

Deming, W. E. 1994. The new economics for industry, government, education. Cambridge, MA: W. Edward Deming Institute.

DeSpelder, L., and A. Strickland. 1987. *The last dance.* 2nd ed. Mountain View, CA: Mayfield.

Fredlund, B. S. 1984. Children and death from the school setting viewpoint. In *Death and dying in the classroom: Reading for reference.* J. L. Thomas, ed. Phoenix, AZ: Oryx Press.

Garcia, R. L. 1991. *Teaching in a pluralistic society: Concepts, models, strategies.* 2d ed. New York: HarperCollins.

Goodwin, L., W. Goodwin, and J. Cantrill. 1988. The mental health needs of elementary school children. *Journal of school health* 58(7): 282–287.

Greenberg, J., and G. Dintiman. 1992. *Exploring health— Expanding the boundaries of wellness.* Englewood Cliffs, NJ: Prentice Hall.

Grollman, E. A. 1988. *Suicide.* Boston: Beacon Press.

Hales, D. 1992. *An invitation to health.* Redwood City, CA: Benjamin Cummings.

Hamrick, M., D. Anspaugh, and G. Ezell. 1986. *Health.* Columbus, OH: Merrill.

Jones, J. 1985. Promoting mental health of children and youth through the schools. Paper presented at the American School Health Association Convention, October, Little Rock, AK.

Katz, L. G. 2002. How can we strengthen children's self-esteem? *http://npin.org* (15 February 2003).

Kuersten, J. 1999. Healthy young minds: Rx for children's emotional and mental health. *Our children magazine.* Taken from *www.pta.org/parentinvolvement/ helpchild/hc_ aa_health_minds.asp* (5 December 2002).

Magg, J. W., and S. R. Forness. 1991, September. Depression in children and adolescents: Assessment and treatment. *Focus on exceptional children* 24:14–19.

Martin, C., and S. Martin. 2002. Self-esteem: What is it? *www.cyberquotations.com/articles/self-esteem.htm* (1 December 2002).

Maslow, A. 1983. *The farther reaches of human nature.* New York: Penguin Books.

Nelson, R. E., and B. Crawford. 1991. Suicide among elementary school–age children. *Elementary school guidance and counseling* 25: 123–128.

Olsen, L., K. Redican, and C. Baffi. 1986. *Health today.* 2d ed. New York: Macmillan.

Page, R. M., and T. S. Page. 2000. *Fostering emotional well-being in the classroom.* Boston: Jones & Bartlett.

Patros, P. G., and T. K. Shamoo. 1989. *Depression and suicide in children and adolescents: Prevention, intervention, and postvention.* Boston: Allyn & Bacon.

Payne, W.A., and Hahn, D.B. 2002. *Understanding your health.* 7th ed. Boston: McGraw-Hill.

Psychological Trauma Center. 2002, June 26. Terrorism. What does one say to children? *http://ptcweb.org/terror.html.*

Ricci, I. 1982. *Mom's house, Dad's house.* New York: Macmillan.

Rinholm. J. 1999, December 15. Classroom behavior strategies—Self-esteem building. *www.ottawa.net/~rinholm/self-esteem.htm.*

Selye, H. 1975. *Stress without distress.* New York: New American Library.

Stepfamily Foundation. 2003. Ten steps for steps. *www.stepfamily.org* (15 February 2003).

Stroher, D. B. 1986. Latchkey children: The fastest-growing special interest group in the schools. *Journal of school health* 56(1): 16.

U.S. Department of Health and Human Services. 2002. *Child health USA 93.* Washington, DC: U.S. Government Printing Office.

Wallerstein, J., and J. Kelly. 1981. *Surviving the break-up.* New York: Basic Books.

Chapter Eight: Body Systems

Betts, J., and J. Shkolnik. 1999. *Educational evaluation and policy analysis* 21(2): 193–213.

Jancke, L. et al. 2000. *Cognitive brain research* 10(1–2): 177–183.

Mueller, C. M., and C. S. Dweck. 1998. *Journal of personality and social psychology* 75(1): 32–52.

Nunley, K. F. Hot topics in current research. *www.brains.org/hottopics.htm#learning* (February 2003).

Chapter Nine: Personal Health

American Academy of Dermatology. 1997. Nail health. *www.aad.org/pamphlets/nailhealth.html* (November 2002).

Centers for Disease Control and Prevention. 2000. Summary of physical activity and health: A report of the Surgeon General. *www.cdc.gov/nccdphp/sgr/summ.htm* (November 2002).

Cosmetics, Toiletries and Fragrance Association. 2000, September. *www.fda.gov/ohrms/dockets/dailys/00/Sep00/090600/c000573.pdf* (November 2002).

Graham, G. S., A. Holt-Hale, and M. Parker. 1998. *Children moving.* 4th ed. Mountain View, CA: Mayfield.

Metlife Consumer Education Center (reviewed by the American Heart Association and the National Heart, Lung and Blood Institute). 2000. "Life Advice® about fitness and exercise." *www.hoptechno.com/book11.htm* (November 2002).

MedicineNet, Inc. 1998. *www.medicinenet.com/script/main/art.asp?li=mni&articlekey=7745* (November 2002).

Neuropsychiatric Institute, University of California, Los Angeles. *www.npi.ucla.edu/sleepresearch/encarta* (November 2002).

Ohio Department of Health, Vision Conservation Programs for Children. 2001. *www.odh.state.oh.us/odhprograms/HVSCR/Vision01.pdf* (November 2002).

President's Council on Physical Fitness and Sports, U. S. Department of Health and Human Services, Office of Public Health and Science, Washington, DC. *www.fitness.gov* (November 2002).

U.S. Department of Health and Human Services. 2002. *Healthy people 2010 objectives.* Washington, DC: Office of Public Health and Science.

Chapter Ten: Strategies for Teaching Body Systems and Personal Health

A to Z Teacher Stuff, LLC. 2002a, November. Glitter germs. *www.atozteacherstuff.com/lessons/GlitterGerms.shtml.*

———. 2002b, November. Stay away tooth decay. *www.atozteacherstuff.com/lessons/ToothDecay.shtml.*

American Heart Association (AHA). 1996. *Heart power, kindergarten through second grade level.* Dallas: AHA.

Bajah, S., and IICBA Organization. 2002, March 23. Home page. *www.unescoiicba.org/electronic_library/science/science_pages/science_lessons/caring_for_your_body.htm.*

Bentley, M. 1995. The body systems being. *Journal of health education* 26(4): 245–247. Reston, VA: American Association for Health Education.

Berenstain, S., and J. Berenstain. 1981a. *The Berenstain bears go to the doctor.* New York: Random House.

———. 1981b. *The Berenstain bears visit the dentist.* New York: Random House.

BioRAP. 2000, August. Here's looking at you . . . Healthy skin. *www.biorap.org/br5contents.html* (October 2002).

Bourgeois, P. 1996. *Franklin and the tooth fairy.* New York: Scholastic.

Calvert County Public Schools (Prince Frederick, MD). 2002, November. *www.calvertnet.k12.md.us.*

Dauer, V., and R. Pangrazi. 1998. *Dynamic physical education for elementary school children.* 13th ed. New York: Macmillan.

Ezell, G. 1992. *Healthy living.* Grand Rapids, MI: Christian Schools International.

Health Strategies, Inc. 2002a, February 2. Home page. *www.healthteacher.com/lessonguides/personal/k-1/pch5elk1/index.asp.*

———. 2002b, February 9. Home page. *www.healthteacher.com.*

———. 2002c, March 2. *www.healthteacher.com/lessonguides/personal/2-3/pch5el23/index.asp.*

Johnson, K. 1997. *Celebrate the months—February.* Cypress, CA: Creative Teaching Press.

MEDtropolis. 2002, November. Virtual body. *www.medtropolis.com/Vbody.asp.*

Mace-Matluck, B. J., and N. G. Hernandez. 1993. Five senses in *Integrating mathematics, science, and language (Paso Partners): An instructional volume I (Grades K–1).* Austin, TX: Southwest Education Development Laboratory. Retrieved 6 December 2002 from *www.sedl.rg/scimath/pasopartners/senses.*

Merritt, K. 2002, October. Dental health. Information Institute of Syracuse, ERIC Clearinghouse on Information & Technology, Syracuse University, Syracuse, NY. *http://askeric.org/cgi-bin/printlessons./cgi/Virtual/Lessons/Health/Body_Systems_and_Senses/BSS0008.html.*

Netter, F. H. 1989. *Atlas of human anatomy.* Dover, NJ: Ciba-Geigy.

Pluckrose, H. 1998. *Touching and feeling.* Austin, TX: Steck-Vaughn.

Santiago, T. 2002, April 7. Education world. *www.education-world.com/a_tsl/archives/00=2/lesson0002.shtml.*

Sevaly, K. 1997. *February idea book.* Riverside, CA: Teacher's Friend.

Smoak, D. W. 2002, October. Brushing and flossing to a healthy smile. Information Institute of Syracuse, ERIC Clearinghouse on Information & Technology, Syracuse University, Syracuse, NY. *http://askeric.org/cgi-bin/print-lessons./cgi/Virtual/Lessons/Health/Body_Systems_and_Senses/BSS0015.html.*

South Carolina State University. 2002, May 10. Body systems. *http://askeric.org* (17 January 2002).

University of Richmond. 2000, August. *www.richmond.edu/~ed344/98/health/touch.html* (October 2002).

Chapter Eleven: Sexuality Education

Administration for Children & Families. 2002. National clearinghouse on child abuse and neglect information. *www.calib.com/nccanch/pubs/factsheets/canstats.cfm* (22 April 2003). Washington, DC: U.S. Department of Health and Human Services.

Allen, L. S., and R. A. Gorski. 1989. Sexual orientation and the size of the anterior human brain. *Proceedings of the National Academy of Sciences USA* (15):7199–7202.

American Academy of Child and Adolescent Psychiatry. 2002. Gay and lesbian adolescents. *www.aacap.org/publications/factfam/63.htm* (10 June 2002).

Byer, C. O., and L. W. Shainberg. 1994. *Dimensions of human sexuality.* Madison, WI: Brown and Benchmark.

Childhelp USA. 2000. Child abuse. *www.childhelpusa.org/abuse.htm* (8 June, 2002).

Denney, N. W., and D. Quadagno. 1992. *Human sexuality.* 2d ed. St. Louis: Mosby-Yearbook.

Eshleman, J. 1996. *The family: An introduction.* 8th ed. Boston: Allyn & Bacon.

Fromm, E. 1989. *The art of loving.* New York: Harper & Row.

Gevinger-Woititz, J. 1993. *The intimacy struggle.* Dearfield Beach, FL: Health Communications.

Haas, K., and A. Haas. 1993. *Understanding sexuality.* St. Louis: Mosby.

Henry J. Kaiser Foundation, The. 2002. *Talking with kids about tough issues: A national survey of parents and kids.* New York: The Henry J. Kaiser Foundation.

Kilander, F. H. 1968. *Sex education in the schools.* Toronto: Macmillan.

Monahan, T. 1970. Are interracial marriages really less stable? *Social forces* 48: 461–473.

Nelson, K. L. 1996. The conflict over sexuality education: Interviews with both sides of the debate. *Sexuality Information and Education Council of the United States (SIECUS) Report,* 24(6): 12–16. New York: SIECUS.

Office of the Attorney General. 1985. *Child abuse prevention handbook.* Sacramento, CA: Office of the Attorney General.

Ogletree, R. J., J. V. Fetro, J. C. Drolet, and B. A. Rienzo. 1994. *Sexuality education curricula—The consumer's guide.* Santa Cruz, CA: ETR Associates.

Prevent Child Abuse America. 2002. Fact sheet: Sexual abuse of children. *www.preventchildabuse.org* (1 June 2002).

Scales, P. 1984. *The front line of sexuality education.* Santa Cruz, CA: Network Publications.

Sexuality Information and Education Council of the United States (SIECUS). 1996. *Guidelines for comprehensive sexuality education: Grades K–12.* New York: SIECUS.

———. 2002a. *Guidelines for comprehensive sexuality education: Grades K–12.* New York: SIECUS.

———. 2002b. State mandates: Sex education and HIV/AIDS/STD education. *www.siecus.org/school/sex_ed/Mandate* (16 December 2002.)

Single Parent Central. Did you know? *www.singleparent central.com/factstat2.htm* (16 December 2002).

Spalt, S. W. 1996. Coping with controversy: The professional epidemic of the nineties. *Journal of school health* 66(9): 339–340.

Strong, B., C. DeVault, and B. Sayad. 1999. *Human sexuality: Diversity in contemporary America.* Mountain View, CA: Mayfield.

U.S. Bureau of the Census. 2002. *Statistical abstract of the United States.* Washington, DC: U.S. Government Printing Office.

Chapter Twelve: Strategies for Teaching Sexuality Education

Heesacker, M. 1994. *Portraits of adjustment.* Boston: Allyn & Bacon.

Tambrands, Inc. 1989. *From fact to fiction—The menstrual cycle.* Lake Success, NY: Tambrands.

Chapter Thirteen: Substance Use and Abuse

Abadinsky, H. 2001. *Drugs: An introduction.* 4th ed. Belmont, CA: Wadsworth.

Barry, J. D. 2002. Barbiturate abuse. *eMedicine consumer journal* 3 (3) (March 2002). *www.emedicine.com/ consumerjournal.htm* (23 April 2003).

Carroll, C. 2000. *Drugs in modern society.* 5th ed. Boston: McGraw-Hill.

Centers for Disease Control and Prevention. 1999. *www.cdc. gov/nccdphp/dash/yrbs.*

———. 2001. Surgeon General's report. *www.cdc.gov/tobacco/ sgrpage.htm* (22 April 2003).

Davis, M. M., and A. Jain. 2001. Paediatrics. *British medical journal* 322 (7300): 1469.

Donatelle, R. 2002. *Access to health.* 7th ed. San Francisco: Benjamin Cummings.

Hahn, D., and W. Payne. 1998. *Focus on health.* St. Louis: Mosby.

Hanson, F., P. Venturelli, and A. Fleckenstein. 2001. *Drugs and society.* 7th ed. Boston: Jones & Bartlett.

Levinthal, C. F. 1999. *Drugs, behavior, and modern society.* 2d ed. Boston: Allyn & Bacon.

National Clearinghouse for Alcohol and Drug Information (NCADI). 1998. *www.health.org/pubs/nhsda/98hhs/ findings/4cocaine.htm.*

National Household Survey on Drug Abuse. 2002. Volume 1: Summary of national findings. *www. samhsa.gov/oas/ nhsda/2k1nhsda/vol1/toc.htm* (22 April 2003).

National Reye's Syndrome Foundation. 2002. What is the role of aspirin? *www.reyessyndrome.org/aspirin.htm.*

Neergaard, L. 2002, 19 June. Abuse-resistant OxyContin hits snag in lab. *Chattanooga Times Free Press.*

Pinger, R., et al. 1998. *Drugs: Issues for today.* 3d ed. Boston: WCB McGraw-Hill.

Ray, O., and C. Ksir. 2002. *Drugs, society, and human behavior.* 9th ed. Boston: WCB McGraw-Hill.

U.S. Drug Enforcement Administration (DEA). 2002. Depressants. *www.usdoj.gov:80/dea/pubs/abuse/abuse_ 07.htm* (23 April 2003).

Chapter Fourteen: Strategies for Teaching about Substance Use and Abuse

American Lung Association. 2002. T.A.T.U. (Teens against tobacco use). *www.lungusa.org/smokefreeclass/ index.html.*

———. 2003, January. State of the air—2002. *www.lungusa. org/tobacco/teenager_factsheet99.html.*

Foster, C. W. 2002, January 2. To smoke or not to smoke. *http://lessonplanspage.com/PESmoking78.htm.*

Furtado, D. B. 1994, May. Substance abuse influences. *http://askeric.org/Virtual/Lessons/Health/Substance_Abuse_ Prevention/SBA0003.html.*

Geiger, B., and D. Reynolds. 2000, May 18. Drugs abstinence skills. *www.pecentral.org/lessonideas/ViewLesson. asp?ID=929.*

Gerne, P., and T. Gerne. 1991. *Substance abuse prevention activities for secondary students.* Englewood Cliffs, NJ: Prentice Hall.

Hawley, C. 1997, August 13. Most people don't use drugs. *http://education.indiana.edu/cas/tt/v3i3/normative. html.*

Health Teacher. 2001. To air is human. *www.healthteacher. com/lessonguides/alcohol/4–5/aod1eh45/index.asp.*

National Clearinghouse for Alcohol and Drug Information. 2002, October. Drugs of abuse. *www.health.org/govpubs/ rpo926/#Top.*

Nemours Foundation, The. 1995–2003a. Kids and alcohol. *www.kidshealth.org/teen/drug_alcohol/index.html* (October 2002).

———. 1995–2003b. Kids and alcohol, why shouldn't I drink? *www.kidshealth.org/kid/stay_healthy/body/ alcohol.html* (October 2002).

———. 1995–2003c. Smoking stinks. *www.kidshealth.org/kid/ watch/house/smoking.html* (October 2002).

———. 1995–2003d. What you need to know about drugs. *www.kidshealth.org/kid/grow/house/drugs_alcohol/know_ drugs.html* (October 2002).

PE Central. 2000a. Marshmallows. *www.pecentral.org/ lessonideas/ViewLesson.asp?ID=888.*

———. 2000b. Public service announcements. *www.pecen- tral. org/lessonideas/ViewLesson.asp?ID=909.*

———. 2000c. Smoking aerobics. *www.pecentral.org/ lessonideas/ViewLesson.asp?ID=930.*

U.S. Department of Education. 2001. The gateway to educa- tional material. *www.thegateway.org.*

Utah Lesson Plans. 1996, November. Prevention dimensions: 100+ things to do instead of drugs. *www.uen.org/Lessonplan/preview.cgi?LPid=25.*

Wolfanger, S. 2001, August 24. Impaired. *www.pecentral.org/LessonIdeas/ViewLesson.asp?ID=931.*

Wright, B. 2000a. Do you wish you never had started smoking? *www.pecentral.org/lessonideas/ViewLesson. asp?ID=926.*

———. 2000b. Tendon damage from steroids. *www.pecentral.org/lessonideas/ViewLesson.asp?ID=927.*

Chapter Fifteen: Infectious and Noninfectious Conditions

American Cancer Society. 2002. *Cancer facts and figures.* New York: American Cancer Society.

American Diabetes Association. 2002. Fact sheet. *www.diabetes.org* (5 July 2002).

Anderson, K. N., L. E. Anderson, and W. D. Glanze, eds. 1998. *Mosby's medical, nursing, & allied health dictionary.* 5th ed. Boston: Mosby.

Brooks, G. F., J. S. Butel, and S. A. Morse. 2001. *Jawetz, Melnick, & Adelberg's medical microbiology.* 22d ed. New York: McGraw-Hill.

Centers for Disease Control and Prevention (CDC). 1997. HIV/AIDS surveillance report in *Morbidity and Mortality Weekly Report* 9(2):1. *www.cdc.gov/hiv/pubs/MMWR.htm* (23 April 2003).

———. 1999. America Responds to AIDS. *AIDS prevention guide—Deciding what to say to younger children.* Atlanta: CDC.

———. 2000. HIV/AIDS prevention: CDC update. *www.cdc. gov/nchstp/hiv_aids/pubs/facts/hiv2.htm* (5 July 2002).

———. 2002. Viral hepatitis: A fact sheet. *www.cdc/diseases/hepatitis/a/index.htm* (14 June 2002).

———. 2003. HIV/AIDS update—A glance at the HIV epidemic. *www.cdc.gov/nchstp/od/news/at-a-glance.pdf* (16 January 2003).

Cray, D., and A. Park. 1996. The exorcists. *Time,* Special Issue 148(14): 64–68.

Crocker, A. C., A. T. Lavin, J. S. Polfrey, S. M. Porter, D. M. Shaw, and K. S. Weill. 1994. Support for children with HIV infection in school: Best practices guidelines. *Journal of school health* 64(1): 33–34.

Donatelle, R. J., L. G. Davis, and C. F. Hoover. 1991. *Access to health.* Englewood Cliffs, NJ: Prentice Hall.

Elster, A. B., and N. J. Kuznets. 1994. *AMA guidelines for adolescent prevention services (GAPS).* Baltimore: Williams & Wilkins.

Guyton, A. C., and J. E. Hall. 1997. *Human physiology and mechanisms of disease.* 2d ed. Philadelphia: W. B. Saunders.

Lichtenstein, P., N. V. Holm, P. K. Verasalo, A. Iliadou, J. Kaprio, M. Koskenvuo, Z. Pokkala, A. Skytthe, and

K. Hemmink. 2000. Environmental and heritable factors in the causation of cancer—Analysis of cohorts of twins from Sweden, Denmark, and Finland. *New England journal of medicine* 343(2):78–85.

Mange, E. J., and A. P. Mange. 1990. *Basic human genetics.* Sunderland, MA: Sinauer Associates.

National Immunization Program. Recommended childhood immunization schedule. *www.cdc.gov/nip* (17 June 2002).

Palella, F. L., K. L. Delaney, A. C. Moorman, M. O. Loveless, J. Fuhrer, G. A. Satten, D. J. Aschman, and S. D. Holmberg. 1998. Declining morbidity and mortality among patients with advanced human immunodeficiency virus infection. *New England journal of medicine* 338(13):853.

Peterman, T. A. 1986. Sexual transmission of human immunodeficiency virus infection in the United States. *Journal of the American Medical Association* 256: 2222–2226.

Scott, R., and A. D. Kessler. 1988. *A child with sickle cell anemia in your class.* Washington, DC: Center for Sickle Cell Disease, Howard University College of Medicine.

Spence, A. P., and E. B. Mason. 1992. *Human anatomy and physiology.* 4th ed. New York: West Publishing Company.

Task Force on Blood Pressure Control in Children. 1987. Report of the second task force on blood pressure control in children. *Pediatrics* 79(1):1–25.

Tate, P., R. R. Seeley, and T. D. Stephens. 1994. *Understanding the human body.* St. Louis: Mosby.

Thibodeau, G. A., and K. T. Patton. 1993. *Anatomy and physiology.* St. Louis: Mosby.

———. 1995. *The human body in health and disease.* St. Louis: Mosby.

Chapter Sixteen: Strategies for Teaching about Infectious and Noninfectious Conditions

White, D. M., and L. Rudisill. 1987. Analyzing cigarette smoke. *Health education* (August–September): 50–51.

Chapter Seventeen: Nutrition

Blanco-Molina, A., G. Castro, D. Martin-Escalante, D. Bravo, J. Lopez-Miranda, P. Castro, F. Lopez-Segura, J. Fruchart, J. M. Ordovas, and F. Perez-Jimenez. 1999, January 16. Effects of different dietary cholesterol concentrations on lipoprotein plasma concentrations and on cholesterol efflux from fu5ah cells. Agricultural Research Service. *www.nal.usda.gov/ttic/tektran/data/000009/82/0000098210.html* (February 2003).

Cantuti-Castelvet, I., B. H. Shukitt, and J. A. Joseph. 2000, May 31. Neurobehavioral aspects of antioxidants in aging. Agricultural Research Service. *www.nal.usda.gov/ttic/tektran/data/000010/51/0000105128.html* (February 2003).

Corbin, C. B., R. Lindsey, G. J. Welk, and W. R. Corbin. 2002. *Concepts of fitness and wellness: A comprehensive lifestyle approach.* 4th ed. Boston: McGraw-Hill.

Donatelle, R., and L. Davis. 1998. *Access to health.* 5th ed. Boston: Allyn & Bacon.

Floyd, P., S. Mimms, and C. Yelding-Howard. 1988. *Personal health: Perspectives and lifestyles.* 2d ed. Englewood, CO: Morton.

Garza, C., et al. 2000. U.S. Department of Agriculture. Dietary guidelines for Americans. U.S. Department of Health and Human Services. *www.health.gov/dietary guidelines/dga2000/document/summary/default.htm* (February 2003).

Glickman, D. 2002, January 31. Healthy eating helps you make the grade! U.S. Department of Agriculture. *www.fns. usda.gov/ccnd/Breakfast/AboutBFast/nutrition-learning.html* (February 2003).

Hales, D. 1999. *An invitation to health.* 8th ed. Pacific Grove, CA: Brooks/Cole.

irishwizards Council. Food and water: Water content of vegetables, fruits, nuts and seeds. U.S. Food and Drug Administration. *www.irishwizards.com/resources/water_food.html* (February 2003).

Mayfield, E. 1999, January. A consumer's guide to fats. *www.cfsan.fda.gov/~fdfats.html* (February 2003).

National Dairy Council. 2003a. Children's nutrition and physical activity are not making the grade. *www.national dairycouncil.org/lv104/nutrilib/digest/dairydigest_736b. html.*

———. 2003b. Creating a healthy school environment. *www.nationaldairycouncil.org/lv104/nutrilib/digest/ dairydigest_736.html.*

React. 1999. Water and food. *www.react.ie/Health/Nutrition/ Waterfood.htm* (February 2003).

Saari, J. T. Grand Forks Human Nutrition Research Center. 2002, April 12. Vitamins and minerals, free radicals and aging. *www.gfhnrc.ars.usda.gov/News/nws0005a.htm* (February 2003).

Satcher, D. Department of Health and Human Services. 1998, February 13. Progress review: Nutrition. *www. healthypeople.gov/data/progrvw/nutrition/default.htm* (February 2003).

U.S. Department of Agriculture (USDA). 1996, April 18. What and where our children eat. *www.barc.usda.gov/bhnrc/ foodsurvey/Kidspr.html* (February 2003).

———. 1998. Glickman challenges experts to turn the tide of childhood obesity. *www.usda.gov:80/news/releases/1998/ 10/0444* (25 April 2003).

———. 1999, May. USDA dietary guidelines for Americans. *www.warp.hal.usda.gov:80/fnic/consumer/intra.htm.*

———. 2002a, August. School lunch program fact sheets: National school lunch program. *www.usda.gov/CND/ Lunch/AboutLunch/faqs.htm* (February 2003).

———. 2002b, October. Evaluation of the school breakfast pilot project: Findings from the first year of implementation. *www.fns.usda.gov/oane/MENU/Published/CNP/FILES/ BreakfastPilotYr1.pdf.*

———. 2003. Why breakfast? *www.fns.usda.gov/cnd/ Breakfast/Downloadable/Time4SchoolBfast.pdf* (February 2003).

U.S. Department of Health and Human Services: Office of Disease Prevention and Health Promotion. Healthy people 2010. *www.healthypeople.gov* (3 April 2003).

U.S. Food and Drug Administration (FDA). 1995, September. Alternatives to high-sodium foods. *www.cfsan.fda.gov/ ~dms/sodchrt.html* (February 2003).

———. 2002, April 1. Health claims: Fiber-containing grain products, fruits, and vegetables and cancer. *www.cfsan. fda.gov/~lrd/cf101-76.html* (25 April 2003).

Chapter Eighteen: Strategies for Teaching Nutrition

American Dairy Association. 2002. Cheese guide. *www.ilovecheese.com/cheese_guide.asp* (October 2002).

Corbin, B., R. Lindsey, G. J. Welk, and W. R. Corbin. 2002. *Concepts of fitness and wellness: A comprehensive lifestyle approach.* 4th ed. Boston: McGraw-Hill.

Dietz, W. H., and L. Stern (Eds). 1999. *American Academy of Pediatrics guide to your child's nutrition: 1–5.* New York: Villard Books.

Emazing, Inc. 1999. Nutritious snacks for kids. *http:// archives.emazing.com/archives/domestic/1999-08-17.*

Gassiott, L. 1999, April 29. Fun with food: The food pyramid. *http://askeric.org/cgi-bin/printlessons.cgi/Virtual/Lessons/ Interdisciplinary/INT0100.html.*

Geiger, B. F., and S. Willis. 1998, May. Using an egg hunt to teach about nutrition. *www.askeric.org/cgi-bin/ printlessons.cgi/Virtual/Lessons/Health/Nutrition/NUT0014. html.*

Health Strategies, Inc. 2002. *Nutrition. www.healthteacher. com/lessonguides/nutrition.asp.*

National Dairy Council. 2003. Nutrition explorations: The fun and easy way to teach and learn nutrition. *www.nutritionexplorations.org.*

Roger, K. 1994. Food labels in the classroom. *http://askeric. org/cgi-bin/printlessons.cgi/Virtual/Lessons/Health/ Consumer_Health/COH0001.html.*

Sanden, K. 1997. Pyramid relay. *http://ericr.syr.edu/Virtual/ Lessons/Health/Nutrition/NUT0010.html.*

Teacher Store. 1999. A to Z Teacher Stuff Network. *www.lessonplanz.com.*

Timpanelli, P. A. 1999. Good and healthy snacks. *http:// askeric.org/cgi-bin/printlessons.cgi/Virtual/Lessons/Health/ Nutrition/NUT0018.html.*

U.S. Department of Education. Let's be healthy. *www.ed.gov/pubs/parents/LearnPtnrs/healthy/html* (October 2002).

———. The gateway to education materials. *www.thegateway. org* (March 2003).

Utah Education Network. 1996. Breakfast. *www.uen.org/ Lessonplan/preview.cgi?Lpid=960.*

———. 1997a. Feeling good. *www.uen.org/Lessonplan/preveiw. cgi?Lpid=973.*

———. 1997b. What's nutrition? *www.uen.org/Lessonplan/ preview.cgi?Lpid=972.*

Chapter Nineteen: Injuries: Accident and Violence Prevention

Miller, D., S. Telljohann, and C. Symons. 1996. *Health education.* Madison, WI: Brown & Benchmark.

National Center for Chronic Disease Prevention and Health Promotion. 2002, September 3. Fact sheet: Accident and unintentional injury prevention. *www.cdc.gov/nccdphp/ dash/shpps/factsheets/fs00_injury.htm.*

National Center for Education Statistics. 2001, October. Indicators of school crime and safety. *http://ncesed.gov/ pubs2002/crime2001.*

———. 2002a, November. Indicators of school crime and safety. *www.nces.ed.gov/pubs2003/schoolcrime/1.asp.*

———. 2002b, November. Indicators of school crime and safety, 2002. *http://nces.ed.gov/pubs2003/schoolcrime/ 10.asp?nav=3.*

National Center for Health Statistics. 2001, October. Healthy people 2000 final review. *www.cdc.gov/nchs/data/hp2000/ hp2k01-acc.pdf.*

National Center for Injury Prevention and Control. 1999, July 2. Childhood injury fact sheets. *www.cdc.gov/ncipc/ factsheets/childh.htm.*

———. 2002, October 18. Facts about violence among youth and violence in schools. *www.cdc.gov/ncipc/factsheets/ schoolvi.htm.*

National Institute for Occupational Safety and Health. 2002, May. Asbestos. *www.cdc.gov/niosh/topics/asbestos/.*

Product Safety, Health Canada. 1999, September 24. Safety tips—Winter sports. *www.hc-sc.gc.ca/ehp/ehd/catalogue/ psb_pubs/ winter.htm.*

Satcher, D. 2001, January 17. Youth violence: A report of the Surgeon General. *www.surgeongeneral.gov/library/ youthviolence/chapter2/sec1.html#epidemic.*

Sondik, E. J. 1999, August 5. Healthy people 2000 progress review on unintentional injuries. *www.cdc.gov/nchs/ about/otheract/hp2000/injury/ injurycharts.htm.*

Sturt, Gary. Gary Sturt's Web site. *www.garysturt.free-online. co.uk/* (28 February 2003).

Chapter Twenty: Strategies for Teaching about Injuries: Accident and Violence Prevention

Chaiet, D., and F. Russell. 1998. *The safe zone: A guide to personal safety.* New York: Morrow Junior Books.

Governale, F. 2002, July 25. Number bingo. *http://askeric. org/cgi-bin/printlessons.cig/Virtual/Lessons/Foreign– Language/French/FRN0202.html.*

iVillage, Inc. 2000, March 19. Asthma and allergies QA. *www.ivillagehealth.com/conditions/respiratory/articles/ 0,11299_165874,174569,00.html* (October 2002).

Media Awareness Network. 2003. Perceptions of youth crime. *www.media-awareness.ca/english/resources/ educational/lessons/secondary/crime/youth_and_crime.cfm.*

National Highway Traffic Safety Administration. 2003. Bus safety. *www.nhtsa.dot.gov/kids/bussafety/index.html.*

P. E. Central. 2000a. *www.pe.central.vt.edu/lessonideas/ health/firstaidkits.html.*

———. 2000b. School violence. *www.pe.central.vt.edu/ lessonideas/health/schoolviolence.htm.*

———. 2000c. Rescue 911. *www.pe.central.vt.edu/lessonideas/ classroom/rescue911.html.*

Tennessee Department of Safety. 2003. Tennessee driver license handbook and study guide. *www.state.tn.us/ safety/cntents.html.*

University of Northern Iowa. 2003. National program for playground safety. *www.uni.edu/playground/home.html.*

University of Oklahoma Police Department. 2003. Bike safety. *www.ou.edu/oupd/bikesafe.htm.*

U. S. Environmental Protection Agency. 2002. Pesticides. *www.epa.gov/pesticides/* (17 March 2003).

WGBH Play and Learn with Arthur Vol. 1. 2003. Sidewalk safety. *http://pbskids.org/arthur/grownups/activities/play_ learn1/sidewalk_safety.html.*

yoursafety.ca. 2003. Mommy, what does this do? *www.yoursafety.ca/kids_safe.html.*

Chapter Twenty-One: Consumer Health

Anspaugh, D. J., M. Hamrick, and F. D. Rosato. 2002. *Concepts and applications of wellness.* 5th ed. Boston: McGraw-Hill.

Barrett, S., W. Jarvis, M. Kroger, and W. London. 2002. *Consumer health.* 7th ed. New York: McGraw-Hill.

Cornacchia, H., and S. Barrett. 1993. *Consumer health: A guide to intelligent decisions.* 5th ed. St. Louis: Mosby-Yearbook.

Corry, J. 1983. *Consumer health: Factors, skills, and decisions.* Belmont, CA: Wadsworth.

Corry, J., and N. Galli. 1985. The role of the school in consumer health education. *Journal of school health* 55:4.

Devita, E. 1995. The decline of the doctor–patient relationship. *American health* 13(7): 63–65, 105.

Greenberg, J. S., and G. B. Dintiman. 1992. *Exploring health—Expanding the boundaries of wellness.* Englewood Cliffs, NJ: Prentice Hall.

Health with Web MD. 2000, July. *www.webmd.com.*

Nordenberg, T. 2000. FDA takes action to enforce the law. *FDA consumer* 34(3): 7–8.

Payne, W. A., and D. B. Hahn. 2002. *Understanding your health.* 7th ed. Boston: McGraw-Hill.

Propecia. 1998. Propecia and Rograine: Extra strength for alopecia. *The medical letter* 40 (February 27): 25–27.

Chapter Twenty-Three: Aging, Dying, and Death

American Association of Retired Persons. 1995, January. Shape your healthcare future with healthcare advance directives. *www.ama-assn.org/public/booklets/livgwill.htm.*

American Medical Association. 2002. *Family medical guide.* Westwood, MA: Dorling Kindersley, CD-ROM.

Beauchamp, T. L. Microsoft Encarta Encyclopedia. 1997–2003. Assisted suicide. *http://encarta.msn.com/encnet/refpages/RefArticle.aspx?refid=761589503.*

Blieszner, R., and V. H. Bedford, eds. 1995. *Handbook of aging and the family.* Westport, CT: Greenwood Press.

Click10.com. 2001. Prescription drug abuse among elderly is up. *www.click10.com/mia/health/kristisgoodhealth/stories/kristisgoodhealth-100206520011003-131029.html.*

DeSpelder, L. A., and A. L. Strickland. 2002. *The last dance.* 6th ed. Boston: McGraw-Hill.

Dickinson, G., M. Leming, and A. Mermann, eds. 2000. *Dying, death, and bereavement.* 5th ed. Guilford, CT: Dushkin/McGraw-Hill.

Ferrini, A., and R. Ferrini. 2000. *Health in the later years.* 3d ed. Boston: McGraw-Hill.

Floyd, P., S. Mimms, and C. Yelding-Howard. 1998. *Personal health: Perspectives and lifestyles.* 2d ed. Englewood, CO: Morton.

Hales, D. 1999. *An invitation to health.* 8th ed. Pacific Grove, CA: Brooks/Cole.

Hively, J., Vital Aging Network. 2003. Combating ageism. *www.van.umn.edu/advocate/3a_ageism.asp.*

Marrone, R. 1997. *Death, mourning, and caring.* Pacific Grove, CA: Brooks/Cole.

National Center for Health Statistics. Health of the elderly. *www.cdc.gov/nchs/fastats/elderly.htm* (8 April 2003).

Perricone, N. 2002, August 14. Healthy aging: The Perricone prescription. Public Broadcasting Station. *www.pbs.org/whatson/dbs/description.html?nola_root=HAGI&date=2002-08-01.*

Pruitt, B., and J. Stein. 1999. *Health styles: Decisions for living well.* 2d ed. Boston: Allyn & Bacon.

Richard Young Center. 2003. Welcome to the Richard Young Center. *www.richardyoungcenter.org.*

United Network for Organ Sharing. 2003. Resources and policies. *www.unos.org/policiesandbylaws/policies/docs/policy_70.doc* (20 March 2003).

U.S. Department of Health and Human Services. 2003. Organ donation. *www.organdonor.gov.*

University of Buffalo—Student Affairs. 2002, August 29. The grieving process. *http://ub-counseling.buffalo.edu/process.shtml.*

University of Missouri, Kansas, Institute for Human Development. 2003. Alzheimer's disease. *www.ihd.umkc.edu/ITC/aging1.htm.*

Woolf, L. M. 1998. Ageism. *www.webster.edu/~woolflm/ageism.html.*

Youth Suicide Prevention. 2001. Youth. *www.yspep.org/youth.html.*

Chapter Twenty-Four: Strategies for Teaching about Aging, Dying, and Death

Science NetLinks. 2002, January. Aging2: How scientists study aging. *www.sciencelinks.com/lessons.cfm?Grade=6-8&BenchmarkID=6&DocID=200* (28 March 2003).

Chapter Twenty-Five: Environmental Health

Donatelle, R. 2002. *Access to health.* 7th ed. Boston: Allyn & Bacon.

Edlin, G., E. Golanty, and K. Brown. 1999. *Health and wellness.* 6th ed. Boston: Jones & Bartlett.

Environmental Protection Agency (EPA). Global warming—Impacts. 2003a. http://yosemite.epa.gov/oar/globalwarming.nsf/content/impacts.html (5 May 2003).

———. 2003b. Indoor air quality. *www.epa.gov/iaq* (27 March 2003).

———. 2003c. Wetlands, oceans, & watersheds. *www.epa.gov/owow* (27 March 2003).

Floyd, P., S. Mimms, and C. Yelding-Howard. 1998. *Personal health: Perspectives and lifestyles.* 2d ed. Englewood, Colorado: Morton.

Hahn, D., and W. Payne. 1997. *Focus on health.* 3d ed. St. Louis: Mosby-Yearbook.

Hales, D. 1999. *An invitation to health.* 8th ed. Pacific Grove, CA: Brooks/Cole.

HybridCars.com. What's new at hybridcars.com? *www.hybridcars.com* (27 March 2003).

Madison County Recycles. Madison county recycling. *www.madisoncountyrecycles.com* (27 March 2003).

Morgan, K. 2003. Sexual hang-up. *Science news* 163(9): 132.

National Center for Health Statistics. 2000. *Healthy people 2000 review, 1998–99.* Washington, D.C.: National Center for Health Statistics.

Natural Resources Defense Council. Clean air and energy: Transportation. *www.nrdc.org/air/transportation/brief.asp* (27 March 2003).

Nebel, B., and R. Wright. 1993. *Environmental science.* 4th ed. Englewood Cliffs, NJ: Prentice Hall.

Noise Pollution Clearinghouse. NPC online library. *www.nonoise.org/library.htm* (27 March 2003).

Office of Environmental Policy & Guidance. Federal Environmental Laws. *www.tis.eh.doe.gov/oepa* (27 March 2003).

Partners in Information Access for Public Health Professionals. Healthy people 2010—Environmental health. *http://nnlm.gov/partners/hp/eh.html* (27 March 2003).

Pruitt, B., and J. Stein. 1999. *Health styles: Decisions for living well.* 2d ed. Boston: Allyn & Bacon.

Chapter Twenty-Six: Strategies for Teaching Enviromental Health

Manchester College Elementary Education Program. Robinson, R. 2000, September 5. Solid waste management. *www.manchester.edu/Adademic/Programs.*

Ohio Department of Natural Resources. 1990, June 1. *www.Ohiodnr.com/education.*

A coordinated approach to addressing students' health can become one of the means to meet a shared outcome: productive and capable students. Similiarly, a primary objective of health care reform is cost savings; health education and prevention play central roles in accomplishing that goal.*

Epilogue

It is the intention of the authors that this textbook portray the necessity for providing a sound cognitive base for health education complemented by opportunities for weighing and formulating a value system. This process enables students to begin to make more intelligent decisions pertaining to their health. The message is that all teaching efforts are aimed at the development of a value system resulting in a positive and healthy lifestyle. Ultimately, the decisions about lifestyle rest with each individual. Although the ability of children to fully control their health patterns may be limited, the seeds of critical thinking, wise decision making, and positive health choices must be planted and nourished. It is the teacher's professional, societal, and personal responsibility to facilitate the understanding of a wellness lifestyle that will result in the highest possible quality of life for every student.

We believe that health education should be viewed as a planned series of experiences that promote disease prevention behaviors and reinforce positive health experiences in each student. The ultimate goal of health education is the development of individuals who take charge of their lives and promote their own well-being, as well as that of their family and their community. To accomplish this goal, our nation must strive for the development of a comprehensive health education program. This necessitates effort beginning in kindergarten and continuing through grade 12. Each step in the educational ladder should be predicated on what has previously occurred in the learning situation. Health is the most fundamental of the basics. Health education must be allotted time in the same manner as mathematics, reading, and science.

The content areas of health education are many and varied. Health is not just physical education, although this is an important component. Truly healthy individuals are more able to accept themselves and others, are more physically fit, and are more capable of making informed decisions concerning the many components of living a more healthy wellness type of lifestyle. Without the best possible health, people become less productive, less satisfied in their personal lives, and less capable of contributing to other people's lives and the society of which they are a part.

As health educators, we should seek to enhance the life of each person we touch. It is our desire to help people feel better about themselves, to enhance their personal esteem, to help them select positive health habits, and to become better critical thinkers. There is no one blueprint to accomplish these goals. Each state, many school systems, and individual teachers have plans and strategies that can serve as springboards to better provide responsible health education.

Each year new crises evolve requiring health educators' efforts. The issues are constantly changing. New needs and new knowledge are continually evolving. According to the U.S. Surgeon General, childhood obesity should be a primary concern among parents and educators. Nationwide crime statistics indicate that American children are increasingly at danger for violence while at school, en route to and from school, and at school-related events. Also, with the recent terrorist events occurring on American soil, school administrators and teachers need to address the possibility of terrorist threats at school.

*Marx, E., and S. F. Wooley, eds. with D. Northrop. 1998. Health is academic: A guide to coordinated school health programs. New York: Teachers College Press.

New challenges in the areas of HIV education, nutrition education, substance abuse education, sexuality education, and environmental education are ongoing. The one constant in all of this is the classroom teacher. His or her professional dedication and love for the student must remain, if health education is to be successful.

Other than parents, no one person has a greater impact on a child than a teacher. What children learn about themselves, others, and their society begins with the classroom teacher.

We hope this book helps point out the necessity for health education and provides part of the blueprint for becoming successful in the teaching of health education. After all, each teacher deals with our most precious of resources—our children.

If our values are straight and we value human health above all else, then health education becomes one of the master areas in all of American education, along with language. It deals, or should deal, with all those phenomena indigenous to being human, that develop or retard, create or kill. Nothing is more important. Time must be found for it.

—Delbert Oberteuffer, April 24, 1982

First-Aid Skills

INFANT AND CHILD LIFESAVING STEPS

Check

- Check the scene for safety.
- Check the victim for consciousness, breathing, pulse, and bleeding.

Call

- Dial 911 or local emergency number (should be posted by phone).

Care

- Care for conditions you find.

GETTING PERMISSION TO GIVE CARE

- Tell victim who you are.
- Tell victim how much training you have and how you plan to help.
- Do NOT give care to a conscious victim who refuses it.
- For an infant or child obtain permission from a supervising adult.
- Permission is implied if an adult is not present or if a victim is unconscious.

DISEASE TRANSMISSION

Universal Precautions: Treat all human blood as if known to be infectious for human immunodeficiency virus (HIV) and hepatitis B virus (HBV). Follow these guidelines to help reduce disease transmission when providing first aid:

- Avoid contact with body fluids when possible.
- Place barriers, such as disposable gloves or a clean dry cloth, between the victim's body fluids and yourself.
- Wear protective clothing, such as disposable gloves, to cover any cuts, scrapes, and skin conditions you may have.
- Wash your hands with soap and water immediately after giving care. Do not eat, drink, or touch your mouth, nose, or eyes when giving first aid. Do not touch objects that may be soiled with blood.
- Be prepared by having a first-aid kit handy.

FIRST PRIORITY WHEN ADMINISTERING FIRST AID IS TO CHECK BREATHING

After checking the scene and checking for consciousness, check breathing for three to five seconds.

Open the airway by using the head tilt–chin lift method. If the victim is not breathing, give two full breaths. Next, you should check breathing and pulse for at least five to ten seconds.

- Check pulse for adult and child (one to eight years): carotid pulse at the side of the neck.
- Check pulse for infant (birth to one year): brachial pulse on the inside of the upper arm.

During the pulse check, if the victim has pulse but is not breathing, perform rescue breathing.

- Adult—one breath every five seconds
- Child and Infant—one breath every three seconds

Check pulse after each minute. If the victim has no breathing and no pulse, begin cardiopulmonary resuscitation (CPR).

- Adult—fifteen compressions and two breaths (counting one and two and three and . . .).

- Child—five compressions and one breath (counting one-two-three-four-five).
- Infant—five compressions and one breath (counting one-two-three-four-five) at a slightly faster rate than for a child.
- Use two hands for an adult.
- Use one hand for a child.
- Use two fingers for an infant.

BLEEDING

Most external bleeding you will encounter will be minor. Minor bleeding, such as a scraped knee, usually stops by itself within ten minutes, when blood clots. Sometimes, however, the damaged blood vessel is too large and clotting does not occur. If you think a wound may need stitches, it probably does.

First Aid for MINOR Bleeding

- Wash the wound thoroughly with soap and water.
- Place a sterile dressing over the wound.
- Apply direct pressure to control bleeding.
- Put an antibiotic ointment on the wound.
- Apply a new dressing and bandage.

First Aid for SEVERE Bleeding

- Do not attempt to cleanse the wound.
- Apply direct pressure with sterile gauze or a clean cloth.
- Elevate the injured area above the heart if there are no broken bones.
- Apply a pressure bandage to hold the gauze or cloth in place.
- If bleeding continues, apply pressure at the pressure point.

  BRACHIAL—inside portion of upper arm (use flat part of fingers).

  FEMORAL—base of upper leg and trunk (use the base of your hand).

- Seek medical help.

NOSEBLEED (MOST NOSEBLEEDS ARE NOT SERIOUS)

First Aid to Control Nosebleed

- Keep victim in a sitting position.
- Tilt victim's head slightly forward.
- Apply steady pressure to both nostrils for five minutes.
- If bleeding persists, have victim gently blow nose and repeat pressure for five minutes.
- Gauze or tissue may be placed in the nostrils to apply pressure.
- Gauze may be placed under the upper lip to apply pressure.
- Ice may be applied to the nose to slow blood flow.

HEAD AND SPINE INJURIES

Head injuries are often minor. However, you should consider the possibility of a serious head and/or spine injury in several situations.

These include:

- A fall from a height greater than the victim's height.
- Any diving mishap.
- A person found unconscious for unknown reasons.
- Any injury involving severe blunt force to the head or trunk.
- A motor vehicle crash where seatbelts are not being worn.
- Any person thrown from a motor vehicle.
- Any injury in which a victim's helmet is broken.
- Any incident involving a lightning strike.

Physical signals of head and spine injuries may include:

- Changes in the level of consciousness.
- Severe pressure in the head, neck, or back.
- Tingling or loss of sensation in the extremities.
- Partial or complete loss of movement of any body part.

- Unusual bumps or depressions on the head or spine.
- Blood or other fluids in the ears or nose.
- Impaired breathing or vision as a result of injury.
- Persistent headache.
- Loss of balance.
- Bruising of the head, especially around the eyes and behind the ears.

These signals alone do not always suggest a serious head or spine injury, but they may when combined with the cause of the injury. Regardless of the situation, always call emergency medical system (EMS) personnel when you suspect a serious head or spine injury.

Caring for a Head or Spine Injury

Immobilize the injured part and control bleeding. To minimize movement of the head and neck, use in-line stabilization. With this technique, you place your hands on both sides of the victim's head, position it gently, if necessary, in line with the body, and support it in that position until EMS personnel arrive.

If there is pain or resistance when attempting to gently position the head, do not try to align but support in its present position.

MUSCULOSKELETAL INJURIES

Regardless of whether the injury is a closed fracture, dislocation, sprain, or strain, apply ice or a cold pack. Apply the RICE principles: Rest, Ice, Compression, Elevation.

- The only way to determine if a simple fracture has occurred is by X ray.
- Immobilize the affected area.
- A splint must include the joints above and below the fracture.

BURNS

Expect that burns caused by flames or hot grease will require medical attention, especially if the victim is under five or over sixty-five years of age.

Four basic core steps for treatment of burns:

- Cool the burned area with cool water—not ice water.
- Cover the burned area with a dry, clean covering.
- Prevent infection by not touching the burned area except with clean covering.
- Do not try to clean or apply any kind of ointment on a severe burn.
- Minimize shock (lie victim down and elevate burned area).

BEE STINGS

First Aid for Bee Stings

- Locate and remove the stinger (scrape the stinger away with fingernail, credit card, and so on).
- Wash the sting site thoroughly.
- Apply an ice pack over the sting site to slow absorption of the venom.
- Relieve pain and itching by using one of the following: calamine lotion, paste made of meat tenderizer and water, paste made of baking soda and water; full-strength household ammonia may be helpful.

ALLERGIC REACTION

Signs include difficulty breathing, facial swelling, fever, chills, or dizziness. Call 911. A dose of epinephrine is the only effective treatment.

Using an Epinephrine Auto-Injector

- Place the tip of injector against victim's thigh.
- Push firmly against thigh.
- Hold injector in place for ten seconds.
- If signs return, inject every fifteen minutes if needed.

POISONING

If you suspect someone has swallowed a poison try to find out:

- what type of poison it was
- how much was taken
- when it was taken

If the victim is conscious, call your regional poison control center (PCC). The number should be posted by the phone. If the victim is unconscious, call 911 or local emergency number and check for breathing and pulse.

- Syrup of ipecac and activated charcoal (with instructions) should be available in your first-aid kit.

SEIZURES

Objectives when caring for seizures are to protect the victim from injury and manage the airway.

- Move away nearby objects, such as furniture, that may cause injury.
- Protect the person's head by placing something soft underneath it.
- Place victim on one side so that fluid can drain from the mouth.
- When the seizure is over, check for other injuries.
- Be reassuring and comforting; stay with the victim until he or she is fully conscious.
- Do not restrain the person or place anything between the victim's teeth.
- EMS personnel should be called if the victim is an infant or child.

SOURCE: Reproduced with permission. *Basic Life Support Heartsaver Guide,* 1997–1999. Copyright American Heart Association.

DIABETES

For a diabetic emergency, give the victim some form of sugar and call for help.

Warning signs and symptoms of type I (Juvenile Diabetes):

- increased urination
- increased hunger and thirst
- unexpected weight loss
- irritability
- weakness and fatigue

CLEAN UP BLOOD AND OTHER BODY FLUIDS

- Use materials from bio-hazardous clean-up kit.
- Flood area with disinfectant (¼ cup household bleach per gallon of water).
- Let disinfectant sit for approximately twenty minutes.
- Wash hands thoroughly with soap and water.

IF IN DOUBT AS TO WHAT SHOULD BE DONE FOR AN INJURY, OR THE SERIOUSNESS OF AN INJURY, DO NOT HESITATE TO ACTIVATE EMS FOR HELP. CALL 911 OR LOCAL EMERGENCY NUMBER.

CONTROLLING BLEEDING

Check-Call-Care

If, when you check, the person is bleeding . . .

1. **APPLY DIRECT PRESSURE (see illustration 1):**
   - Place sterile dressing or clean cloth over wound.
   - Press firmly against wound with your gloved hand.

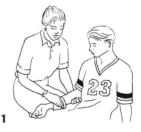

1

2. ELEVATE THE BODY PART (see illustration 2):

■ Raise wound above level of heart.

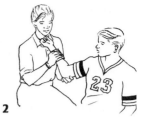

2

3. APPLY A PRESSURE BANDAGE (see illustration 3):

■ Using a roller bandage, cover dressing completely, using overlapping turns.

■ Secure bandage.

■ If blood soaks through bandage, place additional dressings and bandages over wound.

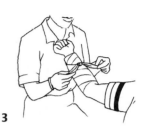

3

If bleeding stops . . .

■ Determine if further care is needed.

If bleeding does not stop . . .

■ Send someone to call EMS personnel.

Then . . .

4. USE A PRESSURE POINT (see illustration 4a):

■ Maintain direct pressure and elevation.

■ Locate brachial artery.

■ Press brachial artery against underlying bone.

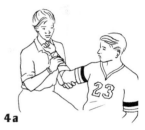

4 a

If bleeding is from leg, press with the heel of your hand where leg bends at hip (see illustration 4b).

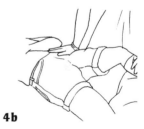

4 b

5. CONTINUE TO TAKE STEPS TO MINIMIZE SHOCK:

■ Maintain direct pressure, elevation, and pressure point.

■ Position person on back.

■ Monitor breathing and pulse.

■ Keep person from getting chilled or overheated.

■ Apply additional dressings and/or bandages as necessary.

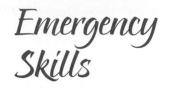

Emergency Skills

Adult One–Rescuer CPR

THE STEPS OF CPR FOR AN ADULT ARE AS FOLLOWS:

1. CHECK RESPONSE: **Check whether the victim is responsive** by gently shaking the victim and shouting, "Are you OK?"

   - If the victim is *unresponsive,* **phone 911 or send someone to phone 911 (or other emergency response number)** and get an automated external defribillator (AED) if available. The call to 911 activates the emergency medical system (EMS) and ensures that professional help is on the way. The American Heart Association (AHA) recommends that in out-of-hospital settings AEDs be stored next to the telephone to ensure rapid access to both 911 and the AED.

   - **If you are alone** and find an unresponsive victim, leave the victim to phone 911 and get an AED if available.

   - When you or someone else has phoned 911, kneel at the victim's side near his or her head to start cardiopulmonary resuscitation (CPR). Carefully turn the victim onto his or her back if needed. If you suspect the victim is injured, turn the head, neck, and body as one unit.

2. AIRWAY: **Open the airway**

   - *Head tilt–chin lift:* Tilt the head back by lifting the chin gently with one hand while pushing down on the forehead with the other hand.

   - *Jaw thrust:* If the victim has a possible injury to the head or neck, use the *jaw thrust* to open the airway. Lift on the angles of the jaw. This moves the jaw and tongue forward and opens the airway without bending the neck.

3. BREATHING: **Hold the airway open and look, listen, and feel to determine if the victim is breathing normally. If the victim is not breathing normally, provide rescue breaths.**

   To check for normal breathing, *look, listen,* **and** *feel for breathing:*

   a. Place your ear next to the victim's mouth and nose and listen for sounds of normal breathing, turning your head to look at the chest.

   b. Look for the chest to rise. Listen and feel for air movement on your cheek.

   If the victim is not breathing normally, give rescue breaths. To give rescue breaths:

   a. Place your mouth around the victim's mouth and pinch the nose closed.

   b. Continue to tilt the head and lift the chin (or perform the jaw thrust).

   c. Give two slow breaths (approximately two seconds each).

   d. Be sure the victim's chest rises each time you give a rescue breath. If the chest does not rise when you give a rescue breath, reopen the airway (using head tilt–chin lift) and try to give the rescue breaths again.

   e. If a barrier device is available for CPR in the workplace, use the barrier device to provide rescue breathing.

Table B.1   *Adult 1–Rescuer CPR Performance Guidelines*

1. Establish that the victim is unresponsive. Phone 911 (or other emergency response number).

2. Open airway (head tilt–chin lift or, if trauma is suspected, jaw thrust). Check for normal breathing (look, listen, and feel).*

3. If normal breathing is absent, give 2 slow breaths (2 seconds per breath), ensure adequate chest rise, and allow for exhalation between breaths.

4. Check for signs of circulation (normal breathing, coughing, or movement in response to the 2 rescue breaths). If signs of circulation are present but there is no normal breathing, provide rescue breathing (1 breath every 5 seconds, about 10 to 12 breaths per minute).

5. If no signs of circulation are present, begin cycles of 15 chest compressions (about 100 compressions per minute) followed by 2 slow breaths.*

6. After 4 cycles of compressions and breaths (15:2, about 1 minute), recheck for signs of circulation.* If no signs of circulation are present, continue 15:2 cycles, beginning with chest compressions. IF signs of circulation return but breathing does not, continue rescue breathing (1 breath every 5 seconds, or about 10 to 12 breaths per minute).

*If the victim is breathing or resumes normal breathing and no trauma is suspected, place in the recovery position.

---

4. **CIRCULATION:** After you deliver two rescue breaths, look for signs of circulation:

   a. Look for any response to the two rescue breaths. The victim may start breathing normally, coughing, or moving.

   b. Do not take more than ten seconds to check for signs of circulation.

   c. If you are not confident that signs of circulation are present, start chest compressions.

   Note: If the victim has signs of circulation, chest compressions are *not* required. If the victim is not breathing normally but signs of circulation *are* present, the victim is in **respiratory arrest** and you must continue to give rescue breaths (one breath every five seconds).

   d. To provide chest compressions, place the heel of one hand on the center of the breastbone right between the nipples. This positions the hand on the lower half of the breastbone.

   e. Place the heel of the second hand on top of the first hand.

   f. Position your body directly over your hands. Your shoulders should be above your hands, your elbows should be straight (not bent), and you should look down on your hands.

   g. Provide 15 compressions at a rate of about 100 per minute. (**Note:** The rate of compressions is slightly less than two compressions per second. You will actually deliver fewer than 100 compressions per minute because you will stop compressions to provide rescue breaths.)

   - Push the breastbone in (compress) 1½ to 2 inches with each compression.

   - Allow the chest to relax (return to its normal shape) between compressions, but leave your hands on the chest between compressions (do not lift your hands off the chest).

5. **"PUMP AND BLOW"**: Provide cycles of fifteen chest compressions and two rescue breaths.

   a. Continue CPR with fifteen chest compressions (pump) and two slow breaths (blow).

   b. After approximately one minute of CPR (about four cycles of fifteen compressions and two breaths), check for signs of circulation. Check for signs of circulation every few minutes. If signs of circulation return, stop chest compressions and continue to provide rescue breathing as needed (one breath every five seconds).

6. **RECOVERY POSITION**: If the victim develops signs of circulation, chest compressions are no longer necessary. If the victim resumes normal breathing, it is no longer necessary to provide rescue breathing. Place the victim in a position that will hold the airway open and continue to monitor the victim's breathing. If there are no signs of trauma, turn the victim onto his or her side in the recovery position. If trauma has occurred, leave the victim on his or her back and hold the airway open using a jaw thrust as needed.

Adult Foreign-Body Airway Obstruction

FIRST AID FOR SEVERE OR COMPLETE AIRWAY OBSTRUCTION

Use the **Heimlich maneuver** (abdominal thrusts) to relieve severe or complete obstruction of the airway caused by a foreign object. Victims with severe or complete airway obstruction will not be able to cough forcefully or speak.

The Heimlich maneuver quickly forces air from the victim's lungs. This expels the blocking object like a cork from a bottle. Repeat abdominal thrusts until the object is expelled or the victim becomes unresponsive.

If the choking victim is *responsive* and *standing*, perform the Heimlich maneuver:

1. Make a fist with one hand.

2. Place the thumb side of the fist on the victim's abdomen, slightly above the navel and well below the breastbone.

3. Grasp the fist with the other hand and provide quick upward thrusts into the victim's abdomen.

Table B.2   *Adult Foreign-Body Airway Obstruction in Responsive Victim (and Responsive Victim Who Becomes Unresponsive) Performance Guidelines*

RESPONSIVE VICTIM

1. Ask "Are you choking?" If yes, ask "Can you speak?" If no, tell the victim you are going to help.

2. Give abdominal thrusts (chest thrusts for victim who is pregnant or obese). Avoid pressing on the bottom of the breastbone (xiphoid).

3. Repeat thrusts until foreign body is expelled (obstruction relieved) or victim becomes unresponsive.

VICTIM BECOMES UNRESPONSIVE

4. Phone 911 or other emergency response number (or send someone to do it). Return to the victim.

5. Attempt CPR. (Each time you open the airway, look for a foreign object in the mouth; if you see it, remove it.)

4. Repeat the thrusts and continue until the object is expelled or the victim becomes unresponsive.

If severe or complete foreign-body airway obstruction is not relieved, the victim will stop breathing. Then the brain and heart will lack oxygen-rich blood. The victim will become unresponsive. When the victim becomes unresponsive and you are alone, *activate the EMS system by phoning 911 or other emergency response number (and get an AED if available)*. Then attempt CPR. If someone else is present, send that person to phone 911 while you begin CPR.

There are two reasons why CPR may be effective for the person who becomes unresponsive from choking. First, when a victim becomes unresponsive, the muscles of the upper airway relax, and a *complete* airway obstruction may become an *incomplete* obstruction. If this happens, you may be able to deliver rescue breaths successfully past an incomplete obstruction. Second, evidence indicates that chest compressions may help relieve choking.

The steps you use to provide CPR for the victim who has become unresponsive after choking are the same as those described earlier in this chapter with one addition. When you open the airway to check for breathing and every time you open the airway to provide rescue breaths, open the mouth widely and look for a foreign body. If you see an object in the throat, remove it. Do not, however, spend a lot of time looking, and do not perform blind finger sweeps. If you do not see an object, continue the steps of CPR.

Infant and Child One–Rescuer CPR

This section presents the basic approach to CPR for an infant or child. The term *infant* refers to a child less than one year old; *child* refers to a child who is one to eight years. For a child older than eight years, use the steps of CPR for adults.

1. **CHECK RESPONSE: Check whether the victim is responsive** by shouting, "Are you OK?" and gently tapping the victim.

- **If the victim is unresponsive, shout for help and begin CPR.** If anyone responds to your shout, tell the responder to phone 911 (or other emergency response number). This activates the EMS system and ensures that professional help is on the way.

- **If you are alone** and find an unresponsive infant or child, **begin CPR** and provide approximately one minute of CPR and then call 911.

- Kneel at the victim's side near his or her head. The victim should be on his or her back on a firm surface, such as a table or the floor. If necessary, carefully turn the victim onto his or her back. Support the head and neck as you turn the victim. If you suspect the victim is injured, turn the head and neck and body as a unit.

2. **AIRWAY: Open the airway.**

- *Head tilt–chin lift:* Tilt the head back by lifting the chin gently with one hand while pushing down on the forehead with the other hand. When lifting the chin, place your fingers on the bony part of the chin and avoid compressing on the soft tissues of the neck or under the chin. Lifting the chin moves the tongue away from the back of the throat and prevents obstruction of the airway by the tongue. It creates an open airway.

- *Jaw thrust:* If trauma to the head or neck is suspected, do not tilt the head or neck. Instead use the jaw-thrust technique to open the airway. Lift on the angles of the jaw. This moves the jaw and tongue forward and opens the airway without bending the neck.

3. **BREATHING:** Hold the airway open and look, listen, and feel to determine if the victim is breathing normally. If the victim is not breathing normally, you will provide rescue breaths.

To check for normal breathing, *look, listen, and feel* for the victim's breathing.

Table B.3   *Child 1–Rescuer CPR Performance Guidelines*

1. Establish unresponsiveness. If a bystander is available, send that person to phone 911 (or other emergency response number).

2. Open the airway (head tilt–chin lift or, if trauma is suspected, jaw thrust). Check for normal breathing (look, listen, and feel).*

3. Give 2 slow breaths (1 to 1½ seconds per breath), ensure adequate chest rise, and allow for exhalation between breaths.

4. Check for signs of circulation (normal breathing, coughing, or movement in response to 2 breaths). If signs of circulation are present but normal breathing is absent, provide rescue breathing (1 breath every 3 seconds, about 20 breaths per minute).*

5. If no signs of circulation are present, provide cycles of 5 chest compressions, typically with the one-hand technique (rate of about 100 compressions per minute), followed by 1 slow breath.

6. After about 1 minute of rescue support, check for signs of circulation.* If the rescuer is alone, phone 911 (or other emergency response number). If no signs of circulation are present, continue cycles of chest compressions and ventilations (5:1 ratio). If signs of circulation are present but normal breathing is absent, continue rescue breathing (1 breath every 3 seconds, about 20 breaths per minute).

*If the victim is breathing or resumes normal breathing and no trauma is suspected, place in the recovery position.

---

a. Place your ear next to the victim's mouth and nose, turning your head to look at the chest.

b. **Look** for the chest to rise. **Listen** and **feel** for air movement on your cheek.

If the victim is not breathing normally, give rescue breaths.

To perform rescue breathing in an infant, do the following:

a. Cover the infant's mouth and nose with your mouth. If your mouth is too small to cover the infant's nose and mouth, cover the infant's nose with your mouth and deliver the rescue breaths through the infant's nose. You may need to hold the infant's mouth closed to prevent air from escaping through the mouth.

b. Continue to tilt the head and lift the chin or perform jaw thrust.

c. Give two slow breaths (1 to 1½ seconds for each breath).

d. Be sure the infant's chest rises each time you give a rescue breath. The chest will rise if you are delivering enough air into the infant's lungs. Deliver just enough air to cause the infant's chest to rise. If the chest does not rise, reopen the airway and reattempt ventilation.

e. If a barrier device suitable for infants is available for CPR in the workplace, use the barrier device to provide rescue breathing.

To perform rescue breathing in a child, do the following:

a. Cover the child's mouth with your mouth while pinching the child's nose closed.

b. Continue to hold the airway open by using a head tilt–chin lift or a jaw thrust.

c. Give two slow breaths (1 to 1½ seconds for each breath).

d. Be sure the child's chest rises each time you give a rescue breath. The chest will rise if you are delivering enough air into the

Table B.4   Infant 1–Rescuer CPR Performance Guidelines

1. Establish unresponsiveness. If a bystander is available, send that person to phone 911 (or other emergency response number).

2. Open the airway (head tilt–chin lift or, if trauma is suspected, jaw thrust). Check for normal breathing (look, listen, and feel).*

3. Give 2 slow breaths (1 to 1½ seconds per breath), ensure adequate chest rise, and allow for exhalation between breaths.

4. Check for signs of circulation (normal breathing, coughing, or movement in response to 2 breaths). If signs of circulation are present but normal breathing is absent, provide rescue breathing (1 breath every 3 seconds, about 20 breaths per minute).*

5. If no signs of circulation are present, begin cycles of 5 chest compressions with the 2-finger technique (rate of about 100 compressions per minute), followed by 1 slow breath.

6. After about 1 minute of rescue support, check for signs of circulation.* If the rescuer is alone, phone 911 (or other emergency response number). If no signs of circulation are present, continue 5:1 cycles of chest compressions and ventilations. If signs of circulation are present but normal breathing is absent, continue rescue breathing (1 breath every 3 seconds, about 20 breaths per minute).

*If the victim is breathing or resumes normal breathing and no trauma is suspected, place in the recovery position.

child's lungs. If the chest does not rise, reopen the airway and reattempt ventilation.

e. If a barrier device is available for CPR in the workplace, use the barrier device.

4. CIRCULATION

a. **Assess or check for signs of circulation in response to the two rescue breaths.** The victim has no signs of circulation if there is no response (no normal breathing, coughing, or movement) to the two breaths.

b. Do not take more than ten seconds to check for signs of circulation.

c. **If you are not sure there are signs of circulation, begin chest compressions.**

d. Note: If the victim has signs of circulation, chest compressions are *not* required. If the victim is not breathing normally but signs of circulation *are* present, the victim is in respiratory arrest. Continue rescue breathing (**one** breath every **three** seconds).

To provide chest compressions for an infant:

a. Imagine a line drawn between the infant's nipples.

b. Place two or three fingers of one hand on the infant's breastbone (sternum) about one finger's width below the imaginary line. Maintain head tilt with your other hand.

c. Do not press over the very bottom of the breastbone (the xiphoid).

d. To provide compressions, press the infant's chest downward about *one-third to one-half the depth* of the chest. Provide compressions at a rate of at least 100 compressions per minute.

e. Release your pressure completely to allow the chest to expand after each compression, but do not move your fingers off the infant's chest.

f. Give **one** breath after every **five** compressions.

To provide chest compressions for a child:

a. Find the middle of the breastbone. Place the heel of one hand on the lower half of the breastbone but not over the very bottom of the sternum (the xiphoid).

b. Maintain head tilt with your other hand (this will keep the airway open and facilitate the delivery of rescue breaths when needed).

c. Do not press over the very bottom of the sternum (the xiphoid).

d. To provide compressions, press the child's chest downward about *one third to one-half the depth* of the chest. Provide compressions at a rate of approximately 100 compressions per minute.

e. Release your pressure completely to allow the chest to expand after each compression, but do not remove your hand from the child's chest.

f. Give **one** breath after every **five** compressions.

5. **"PUMP AND BLOW": Provide cycles of five chest compressions and one rescue breath.**

a. Continue CPR with five chest compressions ("pump") and one slow breath ("blow").

b. After providing CPR for approximately one minute (about twenty rescue breaths or twenty cycles of five compressions and one breath; these will actually take a little longer than one minute), check for signs of circulation (normal breathing, coughing, or movement).

c. If no signs of circulation are present and no one has phoned for help, leave the victim and **phone 911**. If the child is small and un-injured, you may carry him or her to the telephone to activate the EMS system. After you answer all of the dispatcher's questions, resume CPR.

Infant and Child Airway Obstruction (Choking)

FIRST AID FOR SEVERE OR COMPLETE CHOKING

This section describes the **actions you perform to dislodge a foreign object** that is causing severe or complete obstruction of the airway in a responsive infant or child. Perform these actions when the responsive infant or child has signs of *severe or complete* airway obstruction and you suspect the obstruction is caused by a foreign object (for example, if a child playing with a small toy suddenly starts to cough forcefully and then cannot talk or make other sounds). **Do not follow these steps** if the cause of obstruction is illness (for example, if the infant or child has been ill with asthma or has a croupy or hoarse cough).

Relief of Complete Foreign-Body Airway Obstruction in a Responsive Infant

1. Position the infant face down and head down while you support the infant's jaw and head with your hand. Often you will need to sit or kneel, resting the arm holding the infant's torso on your lap or thigh.

2. Deliver up to **five** back blows with the heel of your free hand. If the object is expelled and the infant begins to breathe after fewer than five back blows, discontinue the back blows.

3. If the obstruction is not expelled after five back blows, turn the infant onto his or her back while supporting the head and deliver up to **five** chest thrusts using two to three fingers positioned over the breastbone (sternum) in the same position used for chest compression during CPR. Deliver each thrust with the intention of dislodging the object by deliberately compressing the chest. Stop chest compressions if the object is dislodged.

4. Alternate performing **five** back blows and **five** chest compressions until the object is dislodged or the infant becomes unresponsive.

Table B.5   *Infant Foreign-Body Airway Obstruction in Responsive Victim (and Responsive Victim Who Becomes Unresponsive) Performance Guidelines*

RESPONSIVE VICTIM

1. Check for serious breathing difficulty, ineffective cough, and weak or absent cry. If severe or complete airway obstruction is present, proceed.

2. Support the infant on rescuer's knee or lap and give 5 back blows with heel of hand followed by 5 chest thrusts (using 2-finger technique).

3. Repeat step 2 until the object is expelled (obstruction relieved) or the victim becomes unresponsive.

VICTIM BECOMES UNRESPONSIVE

4. If a second rescuer is available, send that rescuer to phone 911 (or other emergency response number).

5. Attempt CPR. (Each time you open the airway, look for a foreign object in the mouth. If the object is seen, remove it, but *do not perform blind finger sweeps.*)

6. If the infant is unresponsive after about 1 minute of CPR and the rescuer is alone, phone 911 (or other emergency response number), then continue CPR.*

*If the victim is breathing or resumes normal breathing and no trauma is suspected, place in the recovery position.

Table B.6   *Child Foreign-Body Airway Obstruction in Responsive Victim (and Responsive Victim Who Becomes Unresponsive) Performance Guidelines*

RESPONSIVE VICTIM

1. Ask "Are you choking?" If the child indicates yes, ask "Can you speak?" If child shakes head "no" or cannot make any sound, tell the child you are going to help. Give abdominal thrusts.

2. Stand or kneel behind the child and wrap your arms around child. Give abdominal thrusts, avoiding compression on the bottom of the breastbone (xiphoid).

3. Repeat step 2 until the object is expelled (obstruction relieved) or the victim becomes unresponsive.

VICTIM BECOMES UNRESPONSIVE

4. If a second rescuer is available, send that rescuer to phone 911 (or other emergency response number).

5. Attempt CPR (each time you open the airway, open it widely and look for a foreign object in the mouth. If you see an object, remove it, but *do not perform blind finger sweeps*).

6. If the victim is not responsive after about 1 minute of CPR and the rescuer is alone, phone 911 (or other emergency response number). Continue CPR.*

*If the victim is breathing or resumes normal breathing and no trauma is suspected, place in the recovery position.

Relief of Complete Foreign-Body Airway Obstruction in a Responsive Child

In children the **Heimlich maneuver** (abdominal thrusts) is used to relieve complete obstruction of the airway caused by a foreign object. The Heimlich maneuver quickly forces air from the victim's lungs, similar to a cough. The rapid air movement expels the blocking object like a cork from a bottle.

1. Tell the child you are going to help him or her. Stand behind the child and wrap your arms around the child so that your fists are in front of the child.

2. Make a fist with one hand.

3. Place the thumb side of the fist on the child's abdomen slightly above the navel and below the breastbone.

4. Grasp the fist with the other hand and provide quick upward thrusts into the child's abdomen.

5. Give sets of five abdominal thrusts and watch to see if the object is expelled.

6. Repeat sets of abdominal thrusts until the object is expelled or the child becomes unresponsive.

If complete airway obstruction is *not* relieved, the infant or child will become unresponsive and may turn blue. The infant or child may also stop breathing. When this happens, the brain and heart do not have enough oxygen-rich blood to function well. When the child becomes unresponsive, shout for help and begin CPR. Open the airway widely and look for the object. If you see it, remove it. If the child is not breathing, give two rescue breaths. If the child has no signs of circulation after you deliver two rescue breaths, begin chest compressions. The chest compressions may dislodge the object. If these interventions are not effective after about one minute, **phone 911** unless another rescuer has already done so.

Photo Credits

p. 1: David Young-Wolff/PhotoEdit; p. 23: Bonnie Kamin/PhotoEdit; p. 30: Stephen McBrady/ PhotoEdit; p. 35: James Pickerell; p. 39: Frank Siteman/PhotoEdit; p. 63: Rob Crandall/The Image Works; p. 97: Mary Kate Denny/PhotoEdit; p. 122: Bonnie Kamin/PhotoEdit; p. 126: Anne Vega/Merril Education; p. 143: Porter Gifford/Stock Boston; p. 153: Will Faller; p. 186: Will Hart/PhotoEdit; p. 207: Petit Format, P. Bruce/Photo Researchers; p. 213: Robert Finken/Inde Stock Imagery; p. 227: Will Faller; p. 255: Will Faller; p. 280: Janice Fullman/ Inde Stock Imagery; p. 282: Will Faller; p. 296: Jeff Persons/Stock Boston; p. 297: Laura Dwight; p. 315: Michael Newman/PhotoEdit; p. 325: Michael Newman/PhotoEdit; p. 345: Efrem Lukatsky/AP Wideworld Photos; p. 376: Syracuse Newspapers/ Gary Walts/The Image Works; p. 417: Lon C. Diehl/ PhotoEdit; p. 422: Pictor; p. 427: Dimitra Lavrakas/ Inde Stock Imagery; p. 438: Richard Gross/CORBIS; p. 458: Charles Gupton/CORBIS; p. 473: Laura Dwight; p. 481: Bob Daemmrich/Stock Boston; p. 510: Joe Raedle/Getty Images; p. 518: Myrleen Ferguson Cate/PhotoEdit; p. 540: Doug Martin/Stock Boston; p. 545: Will Faller; p. 562: Kathy McLaughlin/ The Image Works; p. 569: James Pickerell; p. 570: Mike Mazzaschi/Stock Boston; p. 581: Bob Daemmrich/The Image Works; p. 585: W. Marc Bernsau/The Image Works; p. 591: Michelle Gabel/Syracuse Newspapers/ The Image Works; p. 608: Lewin Studio, Inc., Elyse/ Getty Images; p. 617: David Young-Wolff/PhotoEdit; p. 620: Felicia Martinez/PhotoEdit; p. 632: Nathaniel Antman/The Image Works; p. 640: Bob Daemmrich/ The Image Works; p. 650: Ryan McVay/Getty Images; p. 671: Michael Newman/PhotoEdit; p. 679: Bob Daemmrich/The Image Works; p. 683: Bruce Ayres/Getty Images; p. 690: Les Stone/The Image Works; p. 705: Marianne Gontarz/Inde Stock Imagery; p. 735: Klein/Hubert/Peter Arnold, Inc.; p. 745: Norman Rowan/Stock Boston; p. 753: Dennis MacDonald/PhotoEdit; p. 755: Lisa Law/The Image Works; p. 765: Frank Siteman/Inde Stock Imagery.

Index

Page references followed by *fig* indicates a figure; those followed by *t* indicates a table.